EPIDEMIOLOGY
Concepts and Methods

William A. Oleckno
Northern Illinois University

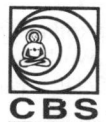

CBS

CBS Publishers & Distributors Pvt. Ltd.

New Delhi • Bengaluru • Chennai • Kochi • Kolkata • Mumbai
Hyderabad • Uttarakhand • Nagpur • Patna • Pune • Jharkhand

Epidemiology: Concepts and Methods

Waveland ISBN: 978-1-57766-522-9

Copyright © 2008, by Waveland Press, Inc.

The worldwide edition of this book is published by Waveland Press, Inc., 4180, IL, Route 83, Suite 101, Long Grove, Illinois 60047, United States of America

This edition has been published in India with the permission of Waveland Press, Inc. for sale in India, Bangladesh, Myanmar, Pakistan, Sri Lanka, Maldives, Bhutan and Nepal.

CBS Reprint: 2015
Reprint: 2019

CBS ISBN: 978-81-239-2565-3

Published by **Satish Kumar Jain** and produced by **Varun Jain** for
CBS Publishers & Distributors Pvt. Ltd.,
4819/XI Prahlad Street, 24 Ansari Road, Daryaganj, New Delhi - 110002
delhi@cbspd.com, cbspubs@airtelmail.in • www.cbspd.com
Ph.: 23289259, 23266861, 23266867 • Fax: 011-23243014

Corporate Office: 204 FIE, Industrial Area, Patparganj, Delhi - 110 092
Ph: 49344934 • Fax: 011-49344935
E-mail: publishing@cbspd.com • publicity@cbspd.com

Branches:
• *Bengaluru:* 2975, 17th Cross, K.R. Road, Bansankari 2nd Stage,
  Bengaluru - 70 • Ph: +91-80-26771678/79 • Fax: +91-80-26771680
  E-mail: cbsbng@gmail.com, bangalore@cbspd.com
• *Chennai:* No. 7, Subbaraya Street, Shenoy Nagar, Chennai - 600030
  Ph: +91-44-26681266, 26680620 • Fax: +91-44-42032115
  E-mail: chennai@cbspd.com
• *Kochi:* Ashana House, 39/1904, A.M. Thomas Road, Valanjambalam,
  Ernakulum, Kochi • Ph: +91-484-4059061-65
  Fax: +91-484-4059065 • E-mail: cochin@cbspd.com
• *Kolkata:* 6-B, Ground Floor, Rameshwar Shaw Road, Kolkata - 700014
  Ph: +91-33-22891126/7/8 • E-mail: kolkata@cbspd.com
• *Mumbai:* 83-C, Dr. E. Moses Road, Worli, Mumbai - 400018
  Ph: +91-9833017933, 022-24902340/41 • E-mail: mumbai@cbspd.com

Representatives:

• Hyderabad: 0-9885175004	• Nagpur: 0-9021734563
• Patna: 0-9334159340	• Pune: 0-9623451994
• Jharkhand: 0-9811541605	• Uttarakhand: 0-9716462459

Printed at Neekunj Print Process, Haryana, India

In Memory of
Barbara and Adolph

Contents

11 Cohort Studies   315

12 Experimental and Quasi-Experimental Studies   371

13 Screening for Disease and Other Conditions   447

Preface

Epidemiology: Concepts and Methods is a comprehensive textbook of epidemiology suitable for graduate or upper division undergraduate students taking their first, and often their only, course in epidemiology. It is appropriate for use in schools or programs of public health as well as those in other health-related disciplines, including medicine, nursing, and allied health. In addition, it should be a valuable resource for practicing health professionals who often need to refresh themselves on fundamental ideas and procedures in epidemiology. In fact, it is the author's dream that this book would be considered valuable enough to be on the bookshelf of every practicing public health professional.

The text covers major concepts, principles, methods, and applications of both conventional and modern epidemiology using frequent examples to illustrate important ideas. Key terms appear in boldface type to aid students in quickly becoming conversant in the language of epidemiology. Alternate terminology is included where appropriate so as to be as thorough as practicable. Unlike many texts with similar objectives, *Epidemiology: Concepts and Methods* introduces several important design and analytical issues that are only rarely approached in fundamental epidemiology textbooks. Topics like identifying additive and multiplicative effects in epidemiologic studies, deciding whether to use a fixed or random effects model in a meta-analysis, and accounting for the effect of clustering in group randomized trials are all discussed in this text in addition to various other topics sometimes considered "too advanced" for a such a text. The wide range of concepts covered can be quickly ascertained by scanning the glossary at the end of the book. This voluminous glossary contains definitions of over 700 terms that are discussed in one or more of the fourteen chapters that comprise the text. Concepts such as competing risks, maturation, residual confounding, futility, and the prevalence effect are discussed in addition to concise descriptions of sophisticated analytical methods and their variations. Of course, the more customary aspects of conventional and modern epidemiology are treated in much greater depth. The writing style has been adapted to make all topics as clear and understandable as possible.

For convenience, *Epidemiology: Concepts and Methods* can be conceived as being organized into five major parts:

- Part One (chapters 1–4): *Basic Foundations of Epidemiology.* This part introduces epidemiology, describes its historical roots and modern adaptations, reviews basic concepts related to health and disease, and summarizes the major study designs used in epidemiology. These chapters are relatively succinct and provide a basis for the rest of the text.

- Part Two (chapters 5–6): *Statistical Measures in Epidemiology.* This part describes biostatistical measures of occurrence and association commonly used in epidemiology as well as methods of rate adjustment and the appropriate use and interpretation of confidence intervals and statistical significance testing. These chapters also provide a foundation for the statistical measures discussed in subsequent chapters.

- Part Three (chapters 7–8): *Assessing Epidemiologic Studies.* This part describes spurious, noncausal, and causal associations and how to recognize them in addition to various types of causes and guidelines for assessing causation in epidemiologic studies. Also described are the major sources of bias, confounding, and random error in epidemiologic studies that can affect the accuracy of study findings along with specific examples and explanations.

- Part Four (chapters 9–12): *Study Designs in Epidemiology.* This part describes the fundamental design, analysis, and interpretation of ecological, cross-sectional, case-control, and cohort studies as well as that of randomized controlled trials, group randomized trials, and quasi-experimental studies. Meta-analysis is also discussed as are special problems and issues in the conduct and analysis of particular types of epidemiologic studies.

- Part Five (chapters 13–14): *Applications of Epidemiology.* This part describes applications related to screening for disease and other conditions, the investigation of disease outbreaks and disease clusters, and the practice of public health surveillance. Pertinent concepts, methods, and examples are provided including a discussion of syndromic surveillance.

Together these five parts, along with the appendixes and the glossary, provide a comprehensive presentation of the fundamentals of conventional and modern epidemiology that should provide a solid basis for continued study in epidemiology or other health-related fields.

NOTE

My other epidemiology textbook, *Essential Epidemiology: Principles and Applications,* is also available from Waveland Press.* It is a broad introduction to epidemiology aimed primarily at undergraduate students in the health sciences, including public and community health. Those seeking a somewhat more scaled down version of epidemiology may find this textbook of interest. It has received excellent reviews for its clarity and reader-friendly format as well as its outstanding coverage of basic epidemiology.

*Oleckno, W. A. (2002). *Essential Epidemiology: Principles and Applications.* Long Grove, IL: Waveland Press, Inc.

ACKNOWLEDGEMENTS

I am humbly aware that my work is largely possible because of the many contributions of others dedicated to the field of epidemiology. As I reviewed numerous articles and books in preparing the present edition of *Epidemiology: Concepts and Methods*, I became aware of the degree to which my ideas have been shaped by others in the field. I often felt during the writing of this text that I had come to know many of those whose publications I reviewed. Notables in the field like Kenneth J. Rothman, Moyses Szklo, F. Javier Nieto, Neil E. Pearce, and others, many of whom I have never met, have helped me think about aspects of epidemiology in ways that might never have occurred to me had I not become familiar with their works. I am very grateful to have had this opportunity. I also thank the staff at Waveland Press, Inc. for their continuing interest in the project and their care in preparing this textbook. I found the staff very competent and eager to be of assistance and support whenever needed. I extend my personal gratitude to Tom Curtin, who oversaw the project. Tom and the staff did an excellent job.

Finally, I thank my wife, Karen, who has now seen me through the writing of two textbooks in the past several years. Without her patience and understanding during the long hours spent on this project, I doubt that it could have been completed. My motivation for writing this text has been my love of epidemiology, but any talents required for the effort have been a gift from my Creator.

About the Author

William A. Oleckno holds the title of Distinguished Teaching Professor Emeritus from Northern Illinois University in DeKalb where he has been a professor for over two and a half decades and coordinator of the undergraduate and graduate programs in public health. His areas of expertise are in public health epidemiology and environmental health. He obtained his B.S. degree from Indiana University School of Medicine, his M.P.H. from the University of Pittsburgh, and his doctoral degree from Indiana University at Bloomington. He has also taken course work at the University of Michigan. Dr. Oleckno is the recipient of several coveted awards in the areas of teaching, research, and service, including the A. Harry Bliss Editor's Award from the *Journal of Environmental Health*, the Sullivan Award for Excellence in Research, and Northern Illinois University's Presidential Teaching Award. He has been an active member in a number of professional associations at the state, national, and international levels and is a fellow of the Royal Society for the Promotion of Health. He has also worked as a national public health consultant. Dr. Oleckno has authored or co-authored over 50 scientific publications related to his areas of expertise and has made regular scholarly presentations at national and international professional meetings. He has been a reviewer for several journals, including *Preventive Medicine, Public Health Nursing, Psychological Reports*, and the *Journal of Environmental Health*. Formerly, he served as assistant professor and coordinator of the Environmental Health Sciences Program at Indiana University School of Medicine in Indianapolis. He has taught introductory epidemiology courses at the undergraduate and graduate levels for over 25 years.

CHAPTER ONE

The Scope and Significance of Epidemiology

*This chapter provides a succinct overview of the importance,
practical uses, and dimensions of epidemiology as it relates to
public health and medicine.*

Learning Objectives

- Explain the importance of epidemiology.
- Describe at least five common applications of epidemiology.
- Define and give examples of risk factors, risk markers, and the disease iceberg concept.
- Explain the meaning and give an example of a disease outbreak.
- Discuss the meaning and scope of epidemiology.
- Define temporal pattern of disease and compare and contrast short-term fluctuations, cyclic patterns, and secular trends.
- Distinguish among descriptive, analytic, and experimental epidemiology.
- Distinguish between efficacy and effectiveness.

INTRODUCTION

Epidemiology is a dynamic field concerned with the occurrence of disease or other health-related events in human populations. Its scope covers the description of disease patterns, the search for causes of disease, and practical applications related to disease surveillance, prevention, and control. Epidemiology is one of the fundamental disciplines relevant to public health and provides a basis for understanding public health problems, including their distribution, natural history, antecedents, and management. Epidemiology is also important to the practice of medicine since increased knowledge of disease and its causes aids physicians and other health professionals with patient diagnosis, treatment, and

1

prognosis. Before defining epidemiology in greater detail, we will first take a closer look at its importance and applications to public health and medicine.

IMPORTANCE OF EPIDEMIOLOGY TO PUBLIC HEALTH

Epidemiology provides a *basis for describing and explaining disease occurrence in a population*. A typical epidemiologic question might be, "How many new cases of acquired immune deficiency syndrome (AIDS) were reported in a given population in a given year?" If 300 new cases were reported, this tells us something about the occurrence of AIDS in this population. We need a reference point, however, to make sense of this number. We might, for example, want to compare the number of reported cases in the population to numbers in previous years to get an idea of whether AIDS is increasing or decreasing in this population. It would be better, however, to compare risk or rate measures of AIDS since the population may have changed from one year to the next. These measures allow us to make comparisons that account for differences in the sizes of the groups being compared. The importance of using risk or rate measures to make comparisons is discussed in chapter 5.

Describing public health problems from an epidemiologic perspective helps us to understand their potential significance and impact. Through comparisons of epidemiologic measures such as incidence, prevalence, and mortality we can identify potentially high-risk groups and perhaps begin to explain the reasons behind the differences. For example, the estimated rate of new cases of AIDS among adults and adolescents in the United States is almost three times higher in males than females.[1] In seeking an explanation for this difference, one might want to examine differences in behaviors between the sexes as well as biological differences.

Epidemiology is also important to public health because it provides a *basis for developing, prioritizing, and evaluating public health programs*. Public health programs should be developed based on need, and the epidemiologic approach is helpful in needs assessment. As a prelude to developing new programs in public health, one might ask such questions as, "What health problems are present in the community?" "Which problems have the greatest public health impact?" and "Are adequate resources available to implement needed programs?" These questions, and related ones, can be answered epidemiologically. Public health surveillance (chapter 14), a tool of epidemiology, and epidemiologic surveys (appendix B) can be used to assess the frequency and scope of specific public health problems. Measures of morbidity, mortality, years of potential life lost, as well as other epidemiologic measures of occurrence (chapter 5), can be used to characterize the potential impact or significance of public health problems in a population. Epidemiology can also be used to evaluate the success of public health programs. Significant reduction in the rate of risk-taking behaviors, disease incidence, or mortality may be useful measures of a program's long-term success. Other applications of epidemiology are discussed in the following section.

SOME APPLICATIONS OF EPIDEMIOLOGY

Identifying Risk Factors for Disease

A major objective of epidemiology is identifying *risk factors* for disease. This is a step toward understanding disease causation. A **risk factor** may be defined as a behavior, environmental exposure, or inherent human characteristic that increases the probability of the occurrence of a given disease.[2] Therefore it plays a causative role (chapter 7) in disease occurrence. For example, hypertension is a well known risk factor for stroke, and excess sun exposure is an established risk factor for skin cancer. Control of a risk factor should result in a reduction in the risk of the disease. Thus, controlling hypertension should reduce one's risk of stroke. A related concept is **risk marker** (or **risk indicator**), which refers to a factor that is statistically *associated* with an increased risk of a given disease but which is not considered a causal factor for that disease. Elevated C-reactive protein, for example, is a factor statistically associated with coronary heart disease, but it is not considered a cause of the disease. Risk markers are therefore noncausal factors that are presumably associated with other causes of the disease. Eliminating a risk marker will not necessarily result in a lowered risk of the disease because of its noncausal role. Chapter 7 discusses the differences between causal and noncausal factors in greater detail.

Perhaps the most well known risk factor today is cigarette smoking, which the U.S. Surgeon General has determined to be a cause of lung cancer, heart disease, certain chronic lung diseases, and other conditions. Furthermore, epidemiologists have demonstrated convincingly that a reduction in cigarette smoking in a population results in a reduction in the frequency of these diseases. Interestingly, the term *risk factor* was popularized after its repeated use in research papers based on the Framingham Heart Study, one of the most well-known and enduring studies in epidemiologic history.[2]

The Framingham Heart Study, which began in 1948, is a longitudinal study (see chapter 4), which was originally designed to identify risk factors associated with cardiovascular disease (CVD). The study began with a representative sample of approximately 5,200 adult men and women between 30 and 62 years of age residing in Framingham, Massachusetts, a town of about 28,000. The subjects were tracked throughout the years by monitoring hospital admissions and other sources and examining subjects biennially for the presence of CVD. The Framingham Heart Study has contributed significantly to our understanding of the risk factors that predispose individuals to CVD, including hypertension, diabetes, cigarette smoking, and blood cholesterol levels.[3-5] Some significant milestones in the history of the Framingham Heart Study appear in exhibit 1-1.

Evaluating the Efficacy of Various Treatments

Are aromatase inhibitors efficacious in preventing recurrences of breast cancer in postmenopausal women? Should individuals at risk of heart disease

Exhibit 1-1
Some Significant Milestones in the Framingham Heart Study

1948   Start of the Framingham Heart Study
1960   Cigarette smoking found to increase the risk of heart disease
1961   High cholesterol level, high blood pressure, and electrocardiogram abnormalities found to increase the risk of heart disease
1967   Physical activity found to reduce the risk of heart disease
Obesity found to increase the risk of heart disease
1970   High blood pressure found to increase the risk of stroke
1971   Framingham Offspring Study begins
1976   Menopause found to increase the risk of heart disease
1977   Effects of triglycerides and LDL and HDL cholesterol described
1978   Psychosocial factors found to affect heart disease
1988   High levels of HDL cholesterol found to reduce the risk of death due to heart disease
1990   Homocysteine found as a possible risk factor for heart disease
1994   Enlarged left ventricle shown to increase the risk of stroke
Lipoprotein (a) and apolipoprotein E found as possible risk factors for heart disease
Risk factors for atrial fibrillation described
1996   Progression from hypertension to heart failure described

Reference: National Institutes of Health, National Heart, Lung, and Blood Institute (2002). Framingham Heart Study: 50 Years of Research Success. Available: http://www.nhlbi.nih.gov/about/framingham/index.html (Access date: June 28, 2005).

take an aspirin a day to prevent a first heart attack? Is chemotherapy with Taxotere (docetaxel) efficacious in treating advanced lung cancer? Each of these questions can be answered epidemiologically by a randomized controlled trial (see chapter 4), which has become the *gold standard* for determining the *efficacy** of various preventive and therapeutic procedures. The well known Hypertension Detection and Follow-Up Program, for example, evaluated two approaches to treatment using a randomized controlled trial involving 10,940 subjects with hypertension. Subjects were randomly assigned to either stepped care or referred care. Those assigned to stepped care received progressive increases in their prescribed blood pressure medications or additional antihypertensive medicines so as to achieve desired blood pressure levels. Those in the referred care group were advised to see their usual health

*Gold standard** refers to something that is "widely recognized as the best available."[6(p72)] **Efficacy** refers to the benefits of a treatment, procedure, or program among those who use it compared to those who do not. The term is most often used in reference to randomized controlled trials. A related term is **effectiveness**, which refers to the benefits among those to whom a treatment, procedure, or program is offered whether or not they use it.[2, 7] These terms are used again in chapter 12 where experimental studies are discussed. Efficacy and effectiveness are elaborated upon in exhibit 12-1.

care providers for treatment. The study found that the five-year mortality was 17 percent lower for those receiving stepped care compared to those receiving referred care.[8] The implication was for more aggressive treatment of hypertension, a philosophy which has since become standard practice in treating patients with mild to severe hypertension.

Investigating Disease Outbreaks

When routine vaccination for adenovirus types 4 and 7 was suspended at Fort Jackson, South Carolina, due to a vaccine shortage, an outbreak of adenovirus type 4-associated acute respiratory disease arose. The victims of the outbreak were soldiers at the fort completing their basic training. In all, 1,018 men and women trainees were hospitalized from May through December with fever and other acute respiratory symptoms consistent with the disease. The majority of these patients tested positive for adenovirus type 4. Fortunately, in this case, reinstitution of the vaccine was effective in preventing further spread of the disease, and the outbreak quickly subsided.[9]

Disease outbreaks, like that at Fort Jackson, are circumstances where there is a clear increase in the number of cases of a disease compared to what is normally expected for the particular time and place. Disease outbreaks and epidemics (chapter 14) are investigated to identify their causes so as to minimize their immediate impact and, most importantly, to prevent similar situations from occurring in the future. These investigations are a challenging dimension of epidemiology, and one that is important to the maintenance of public health.[10] The investigation of disease outbreaks is discussed in detail in chapter 14.

Other Uses of Epidemiology

In addition to the applications already discussed, there are several other areas where epidemiology is useful. As implied in the section on the importance of epidemiology, the epidemiologic approach can be very helpful in the health planning process, particularly in needs assessment, objective setting, and program evaluation. Epidemiology is also useful in health policy formulation since it can answer vital questions about the benefits or harm resulting from specific interventions.[11]

Epidemiology also increases our understanding of the natural history or life cycle of specific disorders (see chapter 3). Moreover, it can help us estimate an individual's risk of a particular disease based on epidemiologic findings from populations with characteristics similar to the individual. This is the basis for health risk appraisals for diseases like cancer and heart disease, which are based on individual risk factors, such as age, sex, personal behaviors, and medical history. Epidemiology also aids us in completing the clinical picture of a disease by filling in the gaps for health care providers. Physicians, for example, ordinarily have a distorted view of the severity and frequency of disease in the communities they serve due to the fact that not everyone who is ill seeks treatment. This illustrates the **disease iceberg con-**

cept.[12] For example, when a primary care physician sees influenza patients in her office during the "flu season," she often overestimates the severity of the disease since she tends to see only the sicker patients (those requiring medical treatment). Furthermore, if she were to rely on the number of patients seeking medical assistance to quantify the extent of influenza in the community, she would inevitably underestimate its true frequency since many patients rely on self-treatment at home. The disease iceberg concept is so named because of the fact that four-fifths of an iceberg is submerged and out of view. Health care providers typically see only the tip of the iceberg when it comes diseases in a community. Some common applications of epidemiology are summarized in table 1-1.

Table 1-1   Common Applications of Epidemiology

- Describing and Explaining Disease Occurrence in a Community
- Assisting in Developing, Prioritizing, and Evaluating Public Health Programs
- Identifying Risk Factors and Causes of Diseases
- Evaluating the Efficacy or Effectiveness of Various Treatment Options
- Investigating Disease Outbreaks or Epidemics
- Assisting in Health Planning and Health Policy Formulation
- Understanding the Natural History of Diseases
- Estimating Individual Risks of Diseases
- Completing the Clinical Picture of Diseases

DEFINITION OF EPIDEMIOLOGY

By now, you should have a fairly good idea of what epidemiology is and why it is important to the practice of public health and medicine. It would be helpful, however, to have a good, concise definition of this important discipline. For those who are interested in the origin of terms, epidemiology is derived from the Greek words "epi" (on or upon), "demos" (people), and "logos" (word or statement). Literally, it translates as "a statement of what is upon the people."[13] A more practical definition is presented below. This definition can be thought of as the 3-D definition of epidemiology, where each of the "D" words in the definition has special significance.

> *Epidemiology is the study of the distribution, determinants, and deterrents of morbidity and mortality in human populations.* *

---

*It is important to note that in addition to morbidity and mortality, which comprise the major focus of epidemiology, the discipline also deals with a variety of other health-related issues such as cholesterol levels, drug abuse, violence, wellness, and health care practices.

The term *distribution*, the first "D" word in the definition, refers to how **morbidity** (illness, disease, injury, etc.)* and **mortality** (death) are distributed in a given population or community. Specifically, we are interested in describing the frequency and patterns of morbidity or mortality in terms of *person, place,* or *time* variables. Person variables relate to *who* is affected; place variables relate to *where* they are affected; and time variables relate to *when* they are affected. Table 1-2 lists some of the more common person variables that may be used to describe the distribution of morbidity or mortality. As an example, we might describe the distribution of lung cancer in the United States by age group, sex, race, smoking status, and occupation. This description would yield a fairly good picture of who is afflicted with lung cancer in the United States and would suggest what groups appear to be at greatest risk for this disease.

Table 1-2   Commonly Used Person Variables

• Age	• Religion
• Sex	• Marital status
• Race/ethnicity	• Health status
• Socioeconomic status	• Immunization status
• Occupation	• Life style or behavioral practices (e.g., substance use)
• Education	• Environmental exposures (e.g., asbestos exposure)

Place variables include specific geographic areas (e.g., census tracts, neighborhoods, cities, counties, states, regions, countries) and general locations (urban or rural areas, schools or other institutions, indoors or outdoors, at home or at work, along the lake or inland, etc.). Time variables may include the time of onset of a given disease (hour of the day, day of the week, month of the year, etc.) or the time of diagnosis, especially for those health-related conditions where it is virtually impossible to know the actual time of onset (e.g., dementia, arthritis, prostate cancer). Infectious diseases are usually classified by when the first symptoms of disease appear. Chronic diseases tend to be classified by the date of diagnosis. Classifying morbidity or mortality by time can also reveal **temporal patterns of disease**, which refer to changes in disease frequency over time. Common temporal patterns of morbidity and mortality are illustrated in figure 1-1. They include:

- Short-term fluctuations
- Cyclic patterns
- Secular trends

*Morbidity is defined as any departure from physiological or psychological well-being and may include both objective and subjective states.[2] The term is commonly used to describe diseases, injuries, and other nonfatal conditions. It should be thought of in broad terms.

Figure 1-1   Temporal Patterns of Disease

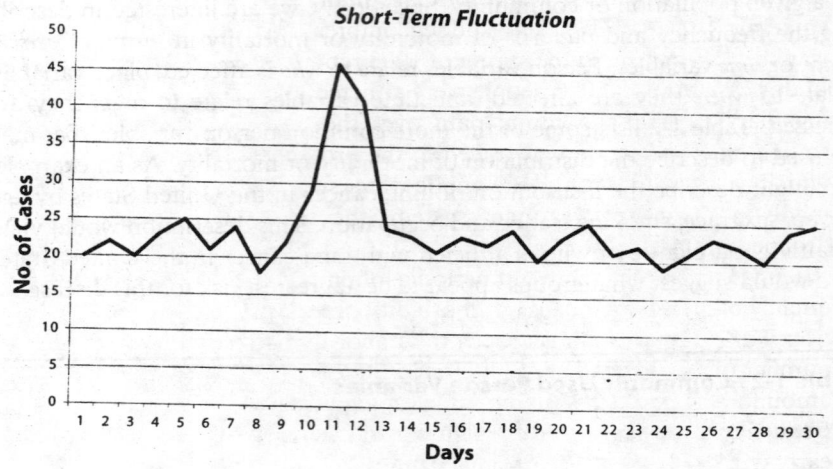

Short-Term Fluctuation

No. of Cases

Days

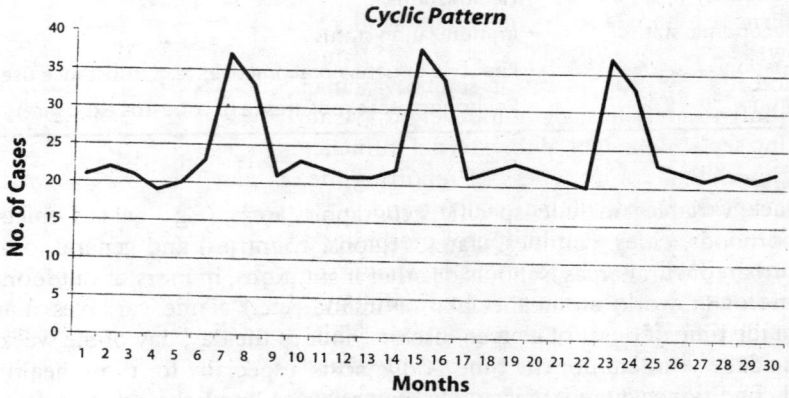

Cyclic Pattern

No. of Cases

Months

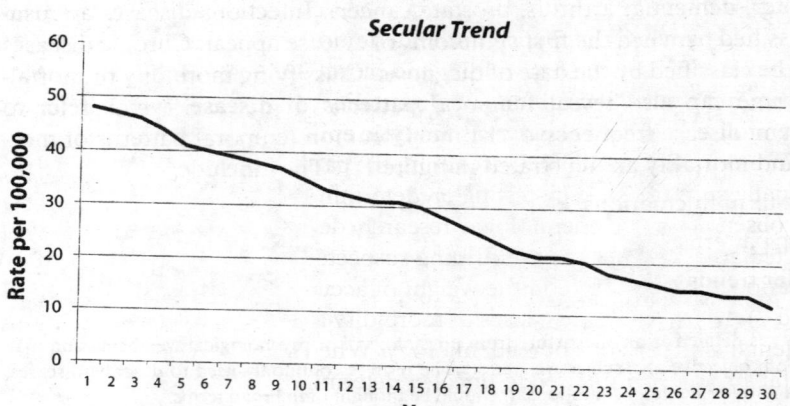

Secular Trend

Rate per 100,000

Years

Generally, **short-term fluctuations** represent relatively brief, unexpected increases in the frequency of a particular disease in a particular population. Short-term fluctuations are commonly manifested in disease outbreaks or epidemics (chapter 14). The sudden outbreak of cryptosporidiosis in Milwaukee, Wisconsin, in the spring of 1993 represents a short-term fluctuation. In this case over 400,000 people were afflicted with a parasitic infection causing diarrhea and abdominal pain over the course of several weeks. The source of the infection was traced to the protozoan *Cryptosporidium parvum*, which was spread through the public water supply. Once improvements were made in the water treatment system, the incidence of cryptosporidiosis dropped dramatically.

Cyclic patterns represent periodic, often predictable, increases in the frequency of a particular cause of morbidity or mortality in a particular population. For example, each year over the Labor Day weekend we expect that the number of traffic deaths in the United States will increase by an anticipated amount. Also, influenza in the midwest tends to show a seasonal variation in frequency each year with the number of cases peaking in the late fall and early winter months.

Secular trends represent long-term changes in morbidity or mortality patterns in a population. The U.S. mortality rate for septicemia, for example, showed a steady increase between 1951 and 1988. During the same time period, the mortality rate for cerebrovascular disease declined significantly and only recently has begun to level off.[14] Caution must be exercised in associating secular changes with external influences. Sometimes changes in diagnostic criteria, completeness of reporting, demographics, and other factors may explain part or all of a secular trend.

Describing the distribution of morbidity and mortality by person, place, or time variables is a major focus of what is sometimes called **descriptive epidemiology**. This dimension of epidemiology is concerned with variations in morbidity and mortality in populations. This information is not only useful in health care planning but can provide clues to the potential causes of disease. The characteristics of descriptive epidemiologic studies are discussed in chapter 4.

While the term *distribution* in the definition of epidemiology refers to the who, where, and when of morbidity and mortality, the second "D" term, *determinants*, refers to why morbidity and mortality occur. The goal of this aspect of epidemiology, generally known as **analytic epidemiology**, is to identify causes of morbidity and mortality. Uncovering the causes of morbidity and mortality is usually accomplished by testing predetermined hypotheses using one of several observational epidemiologic research designs. Initial steps are usually directed at identifying and confirming suspected risk factors. Judgments about causation are then based on the weight of accumulated evidence (see chapters 4 and 7). Discovering the causes of morbidity and mortality is one of the most challenging dimensions of epidemiology. When experimental or quasi-experimental approaches are used to uncover determinants of morbidity and mortality, this aspect of epidemiology is more precisely referred to as **experimental epidemiology**. The main difference is that analytic epidemiology employs observational studies of determinants, while experimental epidemiology uses experimental or quasi-experimental methods. Typically, experimental studies in epidemiology are designed to determine the efficacy or effectiveness of planned interventions (i.e., how well an intervention reduces a particular outcome). Table 1-3 summarizes the important differences among these three dimensions of epidemiology. Chapters 4 and 9-12 discuss various descriptive, analytic, and experimental studies in epidemiology.

The third "D" word in the 3-D definition of epidemiology refers to *deterrents*. From a practical point of view, the ultimate goal of epidemiology is to prevent or reduce morbidity and premature mortality in human populations. In a sense, describing the distribution and identifying the determinants of morbidity and mortality are a prelude to seeking deterrents. Morbidity and premature mortality in a population can sometimes be prevented or reduced without fully understanding their distribution or determinants, as history has shown (see chapter 2). Knowledge of these aspects, however, usually leads to more effective strategies for prevention and control.

Finally, epidemiology is concerned with *human populations*. As a branch of public health, epidemiology is a human science, and epidemiologists seek to understand and explain health-related events in defined groups of people or communities (e.g., the population of a state or region, African Americans, women between 45 and 54 years of age). **Clinical epidemiology**, an offshoot of classical epidemiology, is patient oriented; it seeks to use epidemiology to aid decision making about clinical cases of disease, such as their diagnosis, treatment, and prognosis.[7] Clinical epidemiology can be defined as "the application of epidemiologic principles and methods to problems encountered in clinical medicine."[7(p2)] Unlike classical epidemiology, which is a branch of public health, it is most appropriate to view clinical epidemiology as a branch of medicine. Aspects of clinical epidemiology are discussed in subsequent chapters along with more customary aspects of epidemiology related to public health. Chapter 2 delineates other common specializations

---

Table 1-3   Descriptive, Analytic, and Experimental Epidemiology

Descriptive Epidemiology:
frequency and distribution of morbidity or mortality in a population by person, place, or time variables. Useful in planning health programs and services, identifying potential health-related issues or trends, and suggesting hypotheses for further study.

Analytic Epidemiology: A facet of epidemiology concerned with uncovering the causes of morbidity and mortality using observational methods. Useful in identifying risk factors for disease and explaining disease patterns in a population.

Experimental Epidemiology: A facet of epidemiology concerned with determining the efficacy or effectiveness of various interventions using experimental or quasi-experimental methods. Useful in evaluating treatments, procedures, programs, or services.

in epidemiology. To sum up, epidemiology is a field of study concerned with the patterns, causes, and control of morbidity and mortality in human populations. It is an integral part of public health with applications in medicine and other disciplines as well.

SUMMARY

- Epidemiology is the study of the distribution, determinants, and deterrents of morbidity and mortality in human populations. It seeks to describe, explain, and prevent or reduce public health problems that plague our society. It also provides a basis for developing, prioritizing, and evaluating public health programs.

- Some of the specific applications of epidemiology include identifying risk factors and causes of diseases, evaluating the efficacy or effectiveness of various treatment options, investigating disease outbreaks, explaining the natural history of diseases, estimating an individual's risk of a specific health problem, and completing the clinical picture of disease for health care providers.

- Depending on its purpose, epidemiology may be classified as descriptive, analytic, or experimental epidemiology. Descriptive epidemiology describes morbidity and mortality by person, place, or time variables. Analytic and experimental epidemiology seek to identify the causes of morbidity and mortality.

- Epidemiology is a branch of public health that also has applications in medicine and other disciplines as well. Clinical epidemiology, in particular, is a branch of clinical medicine.

New Terms

- analytic epidemiology
- clinical epidemiology
- cyclic pattern
- descriptive epidemiology
- disease iceberg concept
- effectiveness
- efficacy
- epidemiology
- experimental epidemiology
- gold standard
- morbidity
- mortality
- risk factor
- risk indicator
- risk marker
- secular trend
- short-term fluctuation
- temporal patterns of disease

Study Questions and Exercises

1. Human immunodeficiency virus (HIV) infection is a significant public health issue in the United States and abroad. Untreated, an estimated 90%

or more of those infected with HIV will develop acquired immune deficiency syndrome or AIDS. Research has identified a number of risk factors for HIV infection. Identify and discuss four distinct risk factors and rank them in relative order of importance in the spread of HIV infection in the United States.

2. Planning public health programs at the community level typically involves six major steps: (a) assessment of needs, (b) determination of priorities, (c) development of goals and objectives, (d) design of activities to achieve objectives, (e) implementation of the program, and (f) evaluation of processes and outcomes. Describe how epidemiology can contribute to each of these steps. In which steps is epidemiology likely to make the greatest contributions and in which the least?

3. Because of the disease iceberg concept physicians often have a distorted view of the true nature of a disease in the communities they serve. Since those who seek treatment from physicians often differ from those who do not, a physician's view of the severity or distribution of a disease in the community may not be characteristic of the disease as a whole. Identify three diseases or conditions that are likely to exhibit the disease iceberg concept and indicate why. Also, name three diseases or conditions that are unlikely to demonstrate the disease iceberg concept and again indicate why.

4. Epidemiology has been referred to as the cornerstone or foundation of public health. Other than its role in health planning, how is epidemiology fundamental to the practice of public health?

References

1. Centers for Disease Control and Prevention, National Center for HIV, STD, and TB Prevention, Divisions of HIV/AIDS Prevention (2005). *Cases of HIV Infection and AIDS in the United States, 2003*. Available: http://www.cdc.gov/hiv/stats/2003SurveillanceReport/Table5.htm (Access date: June 14, 2005).
2. Last, J. M., ed. (2001). *A Dictionary of Epidemiology*, 4th ed. New York: Oxford University Press.
3. National Institutes of Health, National Heart, Lung, and Blood Institute (2002). Framingham Heart Study: 50 Years of Research Success. Available: http://www.nhlbi.nih.gov/about/framingham/index.html (Access date: June 28, 2005).
4. Brink, S. (1998). Unlocking the Heart's Secrets. *U.S. News & World Report* (On-Line). Available: http://www2.usnews.com.usnews/issue/980907/7fram.htm (Access date: January 5, 1999).
5. Hennekens, C. H., and Buring, J. E. (1987). *Epidemiology in Medicine*. Boston: Little, Brown and Company.
6. Day, S. (1999). *Dictionary for Clinical Trials*. Chichester: John Wiley & Sons, Ltd.
7. Fletcher, R. H., Fletcher, S. W., and Wagner, E. H. (1988). *Clinical Epidemiology: The Essentials*, 2nd ed. Baltimore: Williams and Wilkins.
8. Meinert, C. L. (1986). *Clinical Trials: Design, Conduct, and Analysis*. New York: Oxford University Press.
9. McNeill, K. M., Hendrix, R. M., Lindner, J. L., Benton, F. R., Monteith, S. C., Tuchscherer, M. A., Gray, G. C., and Gaydos, J. C. (1999). Large, Persistent Epidemic of Adenovirus Type 4-Associated Acute Respiratory Disease in U.S. Army Trainees. *Emerging Infectious Diseases* 5 (6): 798–801.

10. Reingold, A. L. (1998). Outbreak Investigations—A Perspective. *Emerging Infectious Diseases* 4 (1): 21–27.
11. Ibrahim, M. A. (1985). *Epidemiology and Health Policy.* Rockville, MD: Aspen.
12. Duncan, D. F. (1988). *Epidemiology: Basis for Disease Prevention and Health Promotion.* New York: Macmillan.
13. Markellis, V. C. (1986). Epidemiology: Cornerstone for Health Education. *Health Education* 16:14–17.
14. Hoyert, D. L., Kochanek, K. D., and Murphy, S. L. (1999). Deaths: Final Data for 1997. *National Vital Statistics Reports* 47 (19). Hyattsville, MD: National Center for Health Statistics.

CHAPTER TWO

The Evolutionary Roots of Epidemiology

This chapter summarizes the early origins of epidemiology and some of the significant men and women who contributed to its development. Modern specializations in epidemiology are also described.

Learning Objectives

- Describe the cause, source, nature, and historical impact of plague as it relates to public health.
- Discuss some of the major achievements of individuals who contributed to the early development of epidemiology.
- Differentiate among the meaning of endemic, epidemic, and pandemic and give some examples of each.
- Recognize the significance of Bills of Mortality and spot (or dot) maps.
- Identify the major specializations in epidemiology.
- Define multifactorial etiology; antecedent, immediate, and underlying cause of death; notifiable or reportable disease; vital event, record, and statistics; and vital statistics registration system.

INTRODUCTION

Between 1347 and 1351 over 30 percent of the population of Western Europe (some 25 million people) died of a highly contagious disease known as the Black Death, or **plague** as it is properly known.[1, 2] In 1348 alone, Venice lost 100,000 people, and at least 1,200 died daily in Vienna. Worldwide the number of deaths was over 60 million.[3] The desolation caused by plague (see table 2-1) can hardly be overestimated. According to John J. Hanlon and George E. Pickett, the authors of a classic public health text, "Probably nothing ever came so close to exterminating the human species."[3(p15)] So many dead bod-

Table 2-1   Some Basic Facts about Plague

Clinical Forms	Bubonic, Septicemic, and Pneumonic
Causative Agent	*Yersinia pestis*, a bacterium
Major Source	Bite of the infected rat flea, *Xenopsylla cheopsis*
Description	Bubonic plague, which has an incubation period of 2–6 days, generally produces fever, chills, malaise, myalgia, nausea, sore throat, headache, and one or more painful, swollen lymph nodes, known as bubos, near the bite area. Bubonic plague may also be contracted by direct contact with infected tissues or body fluids. Untreated, bubonic plague has a case fatality of 50–60%.
	Septicemic plague results from direct invasion of the circulatory system without node involvement or by secondary spread of bubonic plague. The prognosis is very poor.
	Pneumonic plague, like septicemic plague, can be primary or secondary. In secondary pneumonic plague either of the bubonic or septicemic forms can lead to lung involvement causing pneumonic plague. Primary pneumonic plague is spread person-to-person by infected respiratory droplets. It has an incubation period of 1–3 days. Pneumonic plague is characterized by a severe pneumonia with high fever, chills, cough, and bloody sputum. Untreated, the case fatality is near 100%.
Preventive and Control Measures	While relatively rare today (only about 1000–2000 cases per year worldwide), plague has been the cause of millions of deaths in the Middle Ages. It is a disease with epidemic potential that needs to be taken very seriously when detected. Proper sanitation for rodent control is an important preventive measure. Use of appropriate insecticides and repellants may be recommended in areas where flea bites are possible. Isolation of active cases, antibiotic treatment (e.g., streptomycin), disinfection and proper disposal of discharges and contaminated clothing, and quarantine of contacts may be used as appropriate control measures.

References: Chin, J., ed. (2000). *Control of Communicable Diseases Manual*, 17th ed. Washington, DC: American Public Health Association; Centers for Disease Control and Prevention (1995). Plague Information: Health-care Worker Information. Available: http://www.cdc.gov/ncidod/diseases/plague/hlthcarw.htm (Access date: March 12, 2000).

ies had to be disposed that in some locations they were stacked in layers by the thousands and buried in large pits or discarded in the river.

    This was not the first occurrence of plague as a **pandemic**, which is an epidemic (chapter 14) on a grand scale, causing illness or death over extensive areas that cross international borders and generally afflicting large numbers of people.[4] Plague is estimated to have killed tens of millions of people in Europe and Asia between AD 500 and 650 and another 280,000 in Europe from 1098 to 1101. Altogether, epidemics and pandemics of plague may have accounted for as many as 138 million lives worldwide from AD 500 to 1923.[1] When we consider these and other historical pandemics of diseases, such as leprosy and syphilis,[3, 5] it is not difficult to see why these events were connected with the origins of epidemiology.[6] The great thinkers of the time sought to explain the devastation caused by plague and other diseases, while the more practical souls fought to control the carnage using whatever methods seemed to work. These early efforts to understand and control disease in human populations marked the beginnings of epidemiology.

Before we discuss some of the early contributors to the evolution of epidemiology as a public health discipline it is worth mentioning a more recent pandemic whose devastation was truly global in scope. This was the Great Influenza Pandemic of 1918 caused by the so-called "Spanish" influenza. This massive pandemic may have caused more deaths than the plague during its 1347–1351 rampage across Europe and other parts of the world. Recent research suggests that the death toll from the Spanish flu may have been as high as 50 to 100 million people with most deaths occurring in the fall of 1918.[7] Worldwide, from 1918 to 1919, perhaps as many as 500 million to a billion people were infected. In Geneva, Switzerland, over 50 percent of the population was stricken with the disease, and hospitals were so overextended that other facilities were converted into emergency care sites.[8] In the United States almost 700,000 people were killed by the Spanish flu.[9] By fall 1918, the following rhyme was being repeated in the streets of San Diego:

I had a little bird, / Its name was Enza. /
I opened the window, / And in-flu-enza.[10]

While the original source of the pandemic is still being debated, some believe it began among British soldiers stationed at an army camp in Northern France. It was here that localized outbreaks of a "new" disease produced a high mortality rate among the soldiers in early 1917, and the outbreaks were similar to those occurring in 1918. It was also here where conditions were favorable for the emergence and transmission of influenza—overcrowding; presence of live animals, including pigs and geese; and contamination by toxic gases. In addition, it was near the time when millions of soldiers were returning home from World War I.[11] John M. Barry, however, is convinced that the pandemic had its origin in the United States, specifically in Haskell County, Kansas, based on his review of the early work of other researchers and deductive reasoning.[7] Other theories still persist, and we may never know the true origin.

Subsequent pandemics of influenza, though not as devastating as that of 1918, took place in 1957 (Asian influenza) and 1968 (Hong Kong influenza).[12] Today, public health authorities worry about the possible onset of a new pandemic of a deadly strain of influenza that could begin at any time. According to the U.S. Department of Health and Human Services:

A flu pandemic occurs when a new influenza virus emerges for which people have little or no immunity, and for which there is no vaccine. The disease spreads easily person-to-person, causes serious illness, and can sweep across the country and around the world in very short time.[13]

Pandemics remain a serious concern for epidemiologists. Diseases like HIV/AIDS, malaria, cholera, and SARS (severe acute respiratory syndrome) have been considered pandemic in various places in the world, and many emerging diseases threaten to or have already erupted on an international scale (see table 2-2 and figure 2-1). In the past, as well as the present, epidemics and pandemics have been motivating forces in the search for the causes and control of diseases. They have had an impact on the early origins of epidemiology as well as its continuing development.

Table 2-2   Examples of Emerging Diseases*

Campylobacteriosis	Meningitis
Chagas disease	Moneypox
Cholera	Methicillin resistant *Staphylococcus aureus*
Cryptococcosis	Nipah virus infection
Cryptosporidiosis	Norovirus infection
Cyclosporiasis	Pertussis
Dengue fever	Plague
Diphtheria	Polio
Ebola hemorrhagic fever	Pontiac fever
Escherichia coli infection	Rabies
Group B streptococcal infection	Rift Valley fever
Hantavirus pulmonary syndrome	Rotavirus infection
Hepatitis C	Salmonellosis
Hendra virus infection	Severe acute respiratory syndrome
Histoplasmosis	Shigellosis
HIV/AIDS	Smallpox
Influenza	Trypanosomiasis
Lassa fever	Tuberculosis
Legionellosis	Tularemia
Leptospirosis	Valley fever
Listeriosis	Vancomycin-intermediate/resistant
Lyme disease	*Staphylococcus aureus*
Malaria	Variant Creutzfeldt-Jakob disease
Marburg hemorrhagic fever	West Nile virus infection
Measles	Yellow fever

*Emerging diseases are those that have been increasing in recent decades or are threatening to increase (see chapter 14).
Reference: Centers for Disease Control and Prevention, National Center for Infectious Diseases (2005). Infectious Disease Information: Emerging Infectious Diseases. Available: http://www.cdc.gov/ncidod/diseases/eid/disease_sites.htm (Access date: June 16, 2005)

Figure 2-1   Examples of Emerging Diseases Around the World

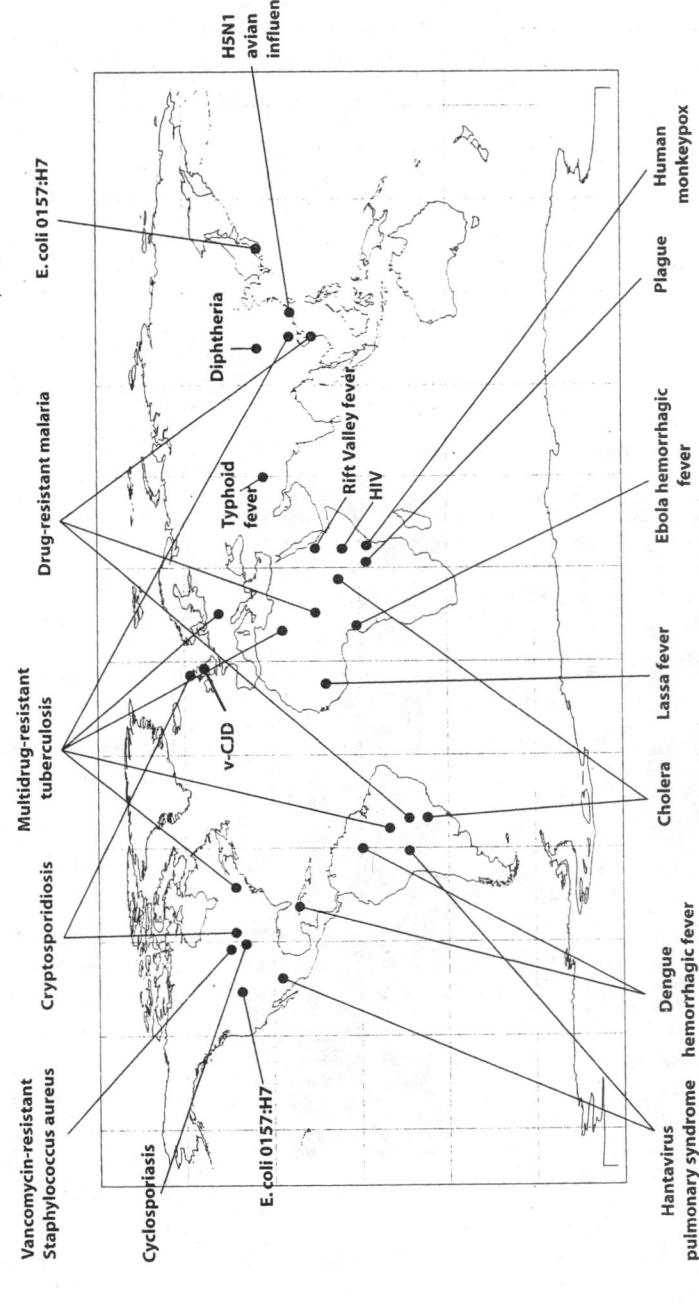

Source: Fauci, A.S. (1998). New and Emerging Diseases: The Importance of Biomedical Research. *Emerging Infections Diseases 4* (3).
Available: http://www.cdc.gov/ncidod/eid/vol4no3/fauci.htm (Access date: June 16, 2005).

EARLY PIONEERS OF EPIDEMIOLOGY

The first "epidemiologists" were those who sought to explain the causes of morbidity and mortality in human populations in a systematic manner. Epidemiology as a discipline evolved slowly as theories of disease causation and methods of disease control were developed, refined, and tested. While many contributed significantly to the early evolution of epidemiology (see table 2-3), the achievements of a few men and women stand out as milestones in the shaping of this dynamic field.

Hippocrates

Hippocrates (see figure 2-2), a Greek physician who lived about 460–377 BC, is often credited as being the *first true epidemiologist*. He is also frequently referred to as the "Father of Medicine." Although not always correct in his beliefs about disease causation, Hippocrates has an honored place in the history of epidemiology because he was one of the first to base his conclusions on observations.[6] Some of his important contributions to epidemiology are summarized below.

Figure 2-2   Bust of Hippocrates

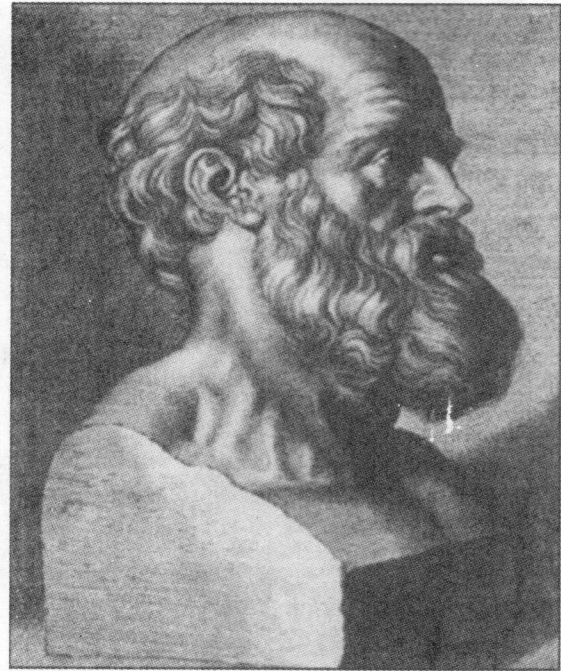

Source: Courtesy U.S. National Library of Medicine.

- He was the first individual who attempted to use rational versus supernatural means to explain disease occurrence.

- He recognized that disease not only affects individuals but populations as well.

- He wrote three books that dealt with epidemiologic concepts— *Epidemic I*, *Epidemic III*, and *Air, Water, and Places*.

- He differentiated between **endemic**, which refers to the constant presence or usual frequency of a specific disease in a given population,[4] and *epidemic* disease, which represents a clear increase in the number of cases of disease

Table 2-3   Selected Historical Contributions of Men and Women to Epidemiology

Individual	Life Span	Selected Contributions
Hippocrates	460–377 BC	The first formally to offer rational versus supernatural explanations for disease occurrence in terms of environmental and other factors
Girolamo Fracastoro	1478–1553	Believed to be the first formally to articulate a theory of disease transmission by contagion
John Graunt	1620–1674	Used the Bills of Mortality to describe disease occurrence in a systematic manner
Thomas Sydenham	1624–1689	Insisted that observation should guide the study of the natural history of disease rather than merely theoretical explanations
James Lind	1716–1794	Used the experimental approach to determine that dietary factors were influential in treating and preventing scurvy
Edward Jenner	1749–1823	Invented a vaccine against smallpox based on careful observation
William Farr	1807–1883	Used vital statistics and other statistical approaches to describe epidemiologic problems
John Snow	1813–1858	Demonstrated that cholera could be transmitted through contaminated water
Ignaz Semmelweis	1818–1865	Used epidemiologic methods to identify the source of childbed (puerperal) fever and introduced hand washing with chlorinated lime to reduce its incidence
Peter Ludwig Panum	1820–1885	Demonstrated that acquired immunity results from infection with measles
Florence Nightingale	1820–1910	Used mortality statistics to justify improved hygienic standards at military hospitals
Louis Pasteur	1822–1895	Demonstrated that microorganisms cause disease and that vaccination could be employed as a sound approach to disease control
Robert Koch	1843–1910	Developed strict criteria for establishing bacterial causes of disease. Together with Pasteur, Koch is credited with firmly establishing the Germ Theory of Disease
Anna Wessels Williams	1863–1954	Isolated a strain of the diphtheria organism that was used to prepare an effective antitoxin against diphtheria
Joseph Goldberger	1874–1929	Used observational and experimental approaches to demonstrate that pellagra was caused by a protein-deficient diet

References: Fox, J. P., Hall, C. E., and Elveback, L. R. (1970). *Epidemiology: Man and Disease*. New York: Macmillan Co.; Lilienfeld, D. E., and Stolley, P. D. (1994). *Foundations of Epidemiology*, 3rd ed. New York: Oxford University Press; Timmreck, T. C. (1998). *An Introduction to Epidemiology*, 2nd ed. Boston: Jones and Bartlett Publishers; Shearer, B. F., and Shearer, B. S., eds. (1996). *Notable Women in the Life Sciences: A Biographical Dictionary*. Westport, CT: Greenwood Press.

compared to what is normally expected for a particular time and place (see chapter 14).

- He recognized associations between environmental and other factors (e.g., water conditions, housing, diet, climate) and certain diseases.[6]

John Graunt

John Graunt (1620–1674) was a London tradesman who is well known for his publication in 1662 of the book, *Natural and Political Observations…Made Upon the Bills of Mortality* (see figure 2-3). This landmark volume can be considered the forerunner of modern **vital statistics**,[3] which are introduced in exhibit 2-1. **Bills of Mortality** was the phrase used for the weekly and annual recording of births and deaths, which started in England as early as 1538.[4] Graunt, who was a founding member of the Royal Society of London, is credited with quantifying disease patterns in London and associating births and deaths with age, sex, and other factors. He was one of the first to demonstrate statistically, for example, that there was a higher frequency of births and deaths among males than among females and that the infant mortality rate in London was unusually high in 1632.

Figure 2-3   Graunt's Bills of Mortality

Natural and Political

OBSERVATIONS

Mentioned in a following INDEX,

and made upon the

Bills of Mortality.

By *JOHN GRAUNT,*

Citizen of

L O N D O N

With reference to the *Government. Religion. Trade. Growth, Ayre, Difeafes,* and the feveral Changes of the faid CITY.

––– *Non, me ut miretur Turba. laboro.*
Contentus paucis Lectoribus –––

LONDON,
Printed by *Tho: Roycroft,* for *John Martin. James Alleftry.* and *Tho: Dicas,* at the Sign of the *Bell* in *St. Paul's* Church-yard. M D C L X I I.

Source: Graunt, J. (1662). *Natural and Political Observations Mentioned in a Following Index and Made Upon the Bills of Mortality.* London: Martin, Allestry, and Dicas. Image accessible at Friendly, M. (2007). *Milestones in the History of Thematic Cartography, Statistical Graphics, and Data Visualization.* Available: http://www.math.yorku.ca/SCS/Gallery/milestone/milestone.pdf (Access date: February 23, 2007).

The impact of Graunt's work with the Bills of Mortality was clearly ahead of its time. In fact, it was almost 200 years later that Graunt's early attempts to describe disease occurrence statistically came to fruition in the work of William Farr, another early pioneer of epidemiology.[6]

Exhibit 2-1
A Primer on Vital Statistics in the U.S.

Vital statistics refer to information derived from **vital events**, which are registered life events, such as births, deaths, marriages, divorces, and certain diseases. In the United States, vital events must be reported by law. Typically, registration forms or certificates are completed and signed by authorized personnel. For example, birth and death certificates are normally completed and signed by the attending physician. **Vital records**, which are the completed registration forms or certificates of birth, death, marriage, etc., are generally filed with a local vital statistics registrar, who maintains the records in the county or parish where they occurred. Copies of the vital records are then forwarded to the state registrar for vital statistics, who forwards copies to the National Center for Health Statistics (NCHS) located in the Centers for Disease Control and Prevention within the U.S. Department of Health and Human Services. This system constitutes the **vital statistics registration system** of the United States. Vital statistics may be combined with census data to develop a variety of statistics that can be used to describe trends, make comparisons, and test hypotheses about the causes of morbidity and mortality. While the NCHS recommends standardized forms for the collection of vital statistics, states may adopt their own forms as long as the required information is collected.

Examples of Vital Records
Birth Certificates: Birth certificates contain demographic information about the child and parents, data relating to birth weight, complications of pregnancy and labor, previous births and terminations, visible birth defects, etc. A copy of the U.S. Standard Certificate of Live Birth may be obtained at the following URL:

http://www.cdc.gov/nchs/data/dvs/BIRTH1.pdf (current as of March 1, 2007)

Death Certificates: Death certificates contain demographic and other information about the decedent along with the causes of death. A copy of the U.S. Standard Certificate of Death may be obtained at the following URL:

http://www.cdc.gov/nchs/data/dvs/DEATH11-03final-acc.pdf
(current as of March 1, 2007)

The causes of death recorded on death certificates include:

• **Immediate Cause of Death:** This is the disease or condition that led directly to death. It specifically excludes *modes* of dying, such as respiratory or heart failure. *Example:* pneumonia

• **Antecedent Causes of Death:** These are the diseases or conditions, if any, that gave rise to the immediate cause of death. They represent the chain of events that preceded the death. *Example:* congestive heart failure

• **Underlying Cause of Death:** This is the cause or injury that *initiated* the chain of events that ultimately produced death. It is the antecedent cause that began the chain of events, and it is the *official cause of death* used in mortality statistics in the U.S. Internationally, the World Health Organization uses a similar definition. *Example:* aortic valve disease

• *Other Significant Conditions:* These are important conditions that contributed to death but are not related to the other immediate, antecedent, or underlying causes of death. *Example:* coronary heart disease, diabetes

(continued)

Instructions for completing the cause-of-death portion of the certificate are available at the following URL:

http://www.cdc.gov/nchs/data/dvs/blue_form.pdf (current as of March 1, 2007)

Reports of Notifiable Diseases: **Notifiable diseases** (also known as **reportable diseases**) are diseases or conditions that must be reported to the appropriate health authority whenever they are diagnosed. Reporting is usually by physicians, laboratories, or hospital personnel. The specific reporting methods and the specific diseases or conditions that must be reported vary from state to state in the U.S. In general, notifiable diseases are those that require prompt public health action because of their severity, communicability, or because they may represent a failure of preventive measures already in place (e.g., immunizations, food safety inspections). There are over 60 nationally notifiable infectious diseases in the United States. Examples include AIDS, botulism, cryptosporidiosis, diphtheria, hepatitis C (acute and chronic), HIV infection, Lyme disease, measles, rabies, smallpox, and syphilis.

William Farr

William Farr (1807–1883), described as the founder of modern epidemiology,[14] extended the work of Graunt by using vital statistics in a comprehensive and systematic manner to describe epidemiologic problems. Working as a medical statistician for the General Register Office for England and Wales from 1839 to 1879, Farr contributed to epidemiology in manifold ways. Some of his accomplishments include:

- Demonstrating the need for population studies to describe disease distribution and explain disease causation
- Promoting the concept of **multifactorial etiology** (i.e., the idea that some diseases, especially chronic diseases, have many causes, often interrelated)
- Recognizing the interrelationship between incidence (new cases of disease) and prevalence (existing cases of disease)
- Classifying diseases in a systematic fashion that eventually led to the International Classification of Diseases*
- Applying his understanding of the distribution and determinants of disease to prevention and control efforts
- Developing standardized statistical measures, such as the infant mortality rate, the standardized mortality rate, life tables, and mathematical models of epidemic curves[14]

Farr is also known for his work with other early pioneers of epidemiology, including John Snow and Florence Nightingale (see table 2-3), and for having had a role in the first modern census conducted in Great Britain in the year 1841.[14, 15]

*The International Classification of Diseases (ICD) is an international system for categorizing health outcomes. The tenth and most recent version, for example, is known as the *International Statistical Classification of Diseases and Related Health Problems,* but is commonly referred to as *ICD-10* for short. It has 21 chapters and uses alphanumeric coding to classify virtually all known diseases.[4]

John Snow

Perhaps the most well known of the early pioneers of epidemiology is Dr. John Snow (1813–1858), a British anesthesiologist who administered chloroform to Queen Victoria during the birth of two of her children[6] and a collaborator with William Farr.[14, 15] Snow (figure 2-4) was a founding member of the London Epidemiological Society, whose initial purpose was to determine the causes of cholera,[16] an acute enteric disease that was epidemic in London at the time and had been pandemic throughout most of the world during the 19th century.[17] Today, Snow's work is looked upon as an eminent example of *analytic epidemiology*[18] (see chapter 1).

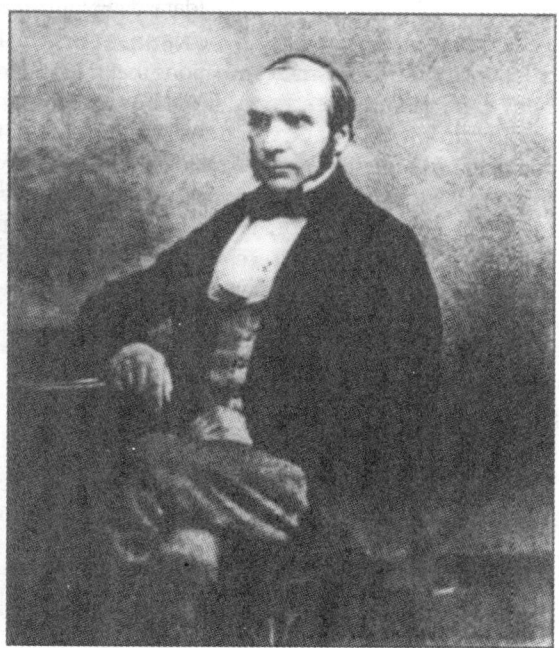

Figure 2-4   John Snow

Source: Courtesy of U.S. National Library of Medicine.

During an investigation of a cholera outbreak in London in 1849, Snow observed that deaths from cholera were highest in districts served by two water companies (the Lambeth Company and the Southwark and Vauxhall Company), both of which obtained their water supplies from sewage-contaminated areas of the Thames River. In 1852, the Lambeth Company relocated its source to a relatively uncontaminated area of the Thames. A subsequent cholera outbreak in 1853 provided Snow with an opportunity to compare cholera death rates in the districts served by each water company. Snow found that the death rate from cholera was over five times higher in districts served exclusively by the Southwark and Vauxhall Company when compared to those served only by the Lambeth Company.[19] There thus appeared to be an association between sewage-contaminated drinking water and cholera deaths. To test this hypothesis, Snow focused on those districts served by *both* water companies. In these districts, the death rate from cholera was intermediate between those served only by the Lambeth Company or only by the Southwark and Vauxhall Company. Fortunately for Snow, in the districts served by both water companies, there was no discernible pattern in terms of which households obtained their water from which source. For all intents and purposes, the households in these districts used one of the two water companies on a completely random basis. Through painstaking and careful data collection, Snow was able to verify that households receiving drinking water from the Southwark and Vauxhall Company had substantially higher death rates from cholera than those served by the Lambeth Company, thus lending support to his original hypothesis that sewage-contaminated water was associated with cholera deaths.[19] Snow's meticulous work demonstrates a *natural experiment* (an unplanned situation in nature that mimics a planned experiment; see chapter 4). Through his work he was able to show that cholera was associated with the ingestion of contaminated drinking water. The impact of Snow's findings was significant. Following publication of his report, legislation was passed requiring that all water companies in London provide filtered water by 1857.[16] Not all, however, were convinced of the link between drinking water and cholera at the time.[20]

In another investigation, Snow examined patterns of an 1854 cholera outbreak in the Golden Square area of London. In this inquiry, known as "The Case of the Broad Street Pump," Snow carefully noted the location of all cholera deaths in the area by place of residence and place of work. He then noted the sites of the water well pumps in the area based on his hypothesis that cholera was transmitted through water. The distribution of deaths and the location of the well pumps were marked on what is commonly known today as a **spot map** (synonym, **dot map**).* Snow noticed that the cases clustered around the pump on Broad Street (see figure 2-5). After carefully eliminating other potential explanations and investigating the actual water sources of those who succumbed to cholera, Snow concluded that contaminated water at the Broad Street pump was the source of the epidemic.[19] As a final gesture, he had the pump handle removed, thereby curtailing the epidemic, which was almost over anyway.

Though John Snow was able to show conclusively that cholera could be transmitted through contaminated water by 1854, it took another 27 years for the etiologic agent, *Vibrio cholerae*, to be identified.[5] In his own work entitled *On the Mode of Communication of Cholera*, Snow discussed common modes of person-to-person transmission and added that cholera could also be spread by "the mixture of the cholera evacuations with water used for drinking and culinary purposes, either by permeating the ground, and getting into wells, or by running along channels and sewers into the rivers from which entire towns are sometimes supplied with water."[21(p45)] What is so amazing is that the *germ theory of disease* (that microorganisms are responsible for infectious diseases) had not been developed at the time of Snow's work. He was clearly ahead of

---

*A spot or dot map is a map showing the geographical location of each case of a disease or other attribute. It is frequently used in investigating localized disease outbreaks to discover place factors where cases cluster. Case clustering may suggest possible causes of the outbreak. Inferences from spot maps can be misleading, however, if the population at risk for the disease is not evenly distributed over the area.[4]

Figure 2-5   A Modern Depiction of Snow's Spot Map

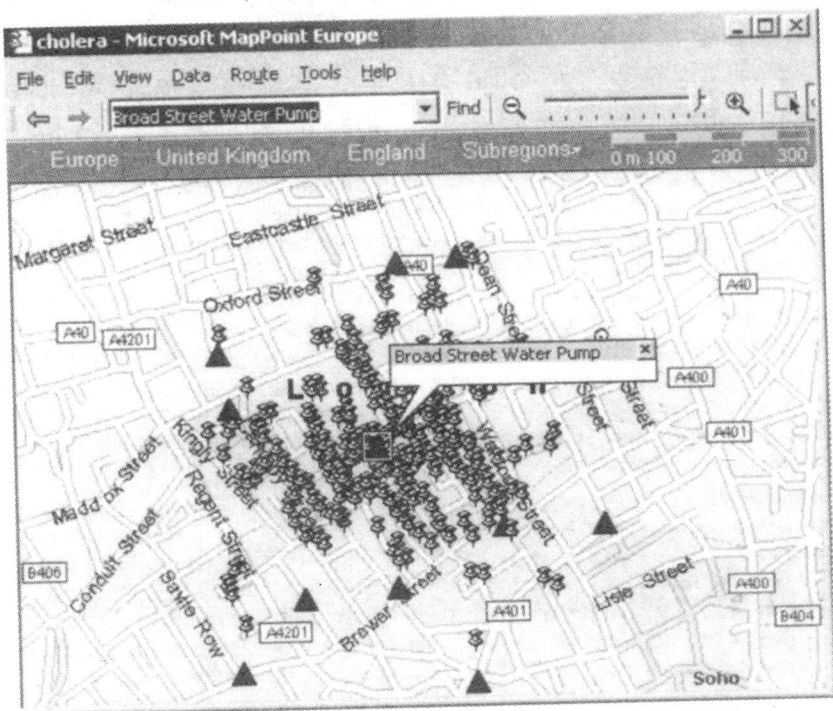

Source: Courtesy Mapping-Tools.com: Tools for Microsoft MapPoint. Copyright 2004–2007, Winwaed Software Technology LLC.

his time. An informative Web site devoted to Dr. John Snow is maintained by the Department of Epidemiology at the University of California at Los Angeles (UCLA). Its Web address is: http://www.ph.ucla.edu/epi/snow.html. For those in or visiting London, the John Snow tavern on Broadwick Street, formerly Broad Street, bears a plaque noting the original site of the Broad Street pump.[22] Trivia lovers may be interested in knowing that John Snow was a vegetarian and a teetotaller.[20] He died at the age of 45.

Joseph Goldberger

Among the many other individuals who contributed to the early development of epidemiology (see table 2-3 and exhibit 2-2) is Joseph Goldberger (1874–1929), an American physician who used experimentation to confirm his observations. In the early part of the 20th century Goldberger studied pellagra, a condition that most believed to be an infectious disease at the time. Goldberger observed that pellagra was associated with rural areas and poverty and that it was prevalent in mental institutions but oddly absent among

Exhibit 2-2
Lady Montagu and Smallpox: From Poet to Epidemiologist?

Background

Lady Mary Wortley Montagu (1689–1782), a daughter of the Earl of Kingston in England, was never trained in medicine, nursing, or epidemiology, but she made a notable contribution to disease prevention during the early 18th century. Lady Montagu has been described as a "brilliant" writer of her time. She was both an essayist and a poet and wrote frequent letters to friends. In 1715 she contracted smallpox at the age of 26. The disease left numerous facial scars, which she covered with a form of make-up. A year later she and her husband, Sir Wortley Montagu, moved to Turkey where Sir Montagu had been appointed Ambassador from England. Here she observed a crude form of inoculation for smallpox known as *engrafting* (see below). After observing the process and being convinced it was safe, she had her son Edward engrafted. Later, when she returned to England she had her infant daughter engrafted. Her daughter was the first person in England to receive the treatment. Through her efforts smallpox inoculation was provided to the children of many prominent English families well before Edward Jenner (table 2-3) introduced a method of vaccination for smallpox in the latter 18th century.

Engrafting

The following description is based on the contents of a letter from Lady Montagu to her friend Sarah Chiswell in April, 1717. Engrafting, a crude inoculation procedure and precursor to vaccination, starts "with a nutshell full of the matter of the best sort of small-pox." The person performing the engrafting, usually an old woman, inserts a large needle into "veins you please to have opened." She "puts into the vein as much venom as can lie upon the head of her needle, and after binds up the little wound with a hollow bit of shell. . . ." On about the eighth day the "fever begins to seize" the engrafted children, who usually recover in about two to three days and by the end of eight days are apparently well except for the scars left by the needle.

References: Story of Lady Montagu and Her Contributions to Smallpox Inoculation (no date). Available: http://www.stanford.edu/~dbmuniz/Montagu.htm (Access date: February 9, 2007); Lady Mary Wortley Montagu, *Letters of the Right Honourable Lady M--y W--y M--e: Written During her Travels in Europe, Asia and Africa. . . .*, vol. 1 (Aix: Anthony Henricy, 1796), pp. 167–169; letter 36, to Mrs. S. C. from Adrianople, n.d. Available: http://www.fordham.edu/halsall/mod/montagu-smallpox.html (Access date: February 23, 2007).

the nurses and attendants. This led him to hypothesize that the disease was caused by a nutritional deficiency. He was able to demonstrate both observationally and experimentally in selected populations that pellagra was caused by a protein-deficient diet. Today, we know that pellagra is due specifically to a deficiency of nicotinic acid, a form of the B vitamin niacin, found in protein-rich foods such as red meat.[5, 23] Dr. Goldberger, it turns out, was not far off the mark.

THE MODERN ERA

In our time, new pioneers are expanding the borders of epidemiology into new areas of clinical practice, health care decision making, environmental risk assessment, and numerous other areas. The increasing diversity of the field can be seen in the many specializations that have developed in addition to *clinical epidemiology* (chapter 1). Some of these are described below.

- **Social epidemiology** focuses on the study of social determinants of health, disease, or death in human populations. Social epidemiologists examine the roles of societal characteristics such as socioeconomic status, social inequality, poverty, gender, race/ethnicity, and other social and cultural factors on health-related outcomes. The use of social theories and advanced statistical approaches, such as multilevel analysis (chapter 9), are common in this specialization. A contemporary concern of some social epidemiologists is health disparities, which refer to differences in health status or access to health care by certain social groups (e.g., racial/ethnic minorities). Social epidemiologic studies may be descriptive, analytic, or experimental.

- **Behavioral epidemiology** involves the study of the role of behavioral factors in health, disease, or death in human populations. Typical factors examined include substance use, activity levels, dietary choices, and sexual practices. A proposed framework for classifying the various phases of study in behavioral epidemiology includes: (a) establishing links between behaviors and health outcomes, (b) developing measures of the behaviors, (c) identifying influences on the behaviors, (d) evaluating interventions designed to modify the behaviors, and (e) translating research into practice.[24]

- **Psychosocial epidemiology** can be conceived as a synthesis of social and behavioral epidemiology in that its focus is on the study of psychological, behavioral, and social determinants of health, disease, or death in human populations. Some use the term synonymously with social epidemiology, since social epidemiology is largely rooted in the social sciences, including psychology and sociology.

- **Environmental epidemiology** has been defined as "the epidemiologic study of the health consequences of exposures that are involuntary and that occur in the general environment."[25(p3)] These exposures include physical, chemical, and biological agents that may be found in air, water, soil, or food. Examples include radiation, carbon monoxide, and the hepatitis A virus. The effects of urban air pollution on the development of respiratory and cardiovascular disease is an example of a topic of current interest in environmental epidemiology. The effects of social-psychological factors relating to the environment, such as the stress or outrage that may be caused by living near a hazardous waste site, is also a concern of some environmental epidemiologists.

- **Occupational epidemiology** can be defined as "the study of the effects of workplace exposures on the frequency and distribution of diseases and injuries in the population."[26(p3)] It is concerned with the effects of physical, chemical, and biological agents in the occupational environment on workers' health and well-being. Studies of the effects of occupational noise on injury rates among exposed workers would be in the domain of occupational epidemiology. This specialization can be conceived as a branch of environmental epidemiology.

- **Genetic epidemiology** has been defined as "The science that deals with the etiology, distribution, and control of disease in groups of relatives, and with inherited causes of disease in populations."[4(p76)] It is concerned with the genetic components of health and disease in human populations and has been recently advanced by the human genome project. The focus of genetic epidemiology is on complex diseases like coronary heart disease that have multifactorial etiologies. Thus, a goal of genetic epidemiology is to discover interactions between genetic and non-genetic factors in the development of various health-related outcomes and the specific roles that the genetic factors play.[27] For example, while it is believed that the increased frequency of obesity and diabetes 2 is primarily due to non-genetic factors, genetic predisposition may play a role in the regulation of food intake and energy expenditure that may be more amenable to treatment than lifestyle changes in attempting to reduce these problems.[28]

- **Molecular epidemiology**, which is broader in scope than genetic epidemiology, uses molecular and biochemical measures (i.e., *biomarkers*; see chapter 9) to study the contribution of potential genetic and environmental risk factors to the distribution, etiology, and prevention of disease in families and across populations.[29] Its scope includes "descriptive and analytical studies to evaluate genetic/environmental factors involved in disease etiology; the development of prevention strategies for the control of bacterial, parasitic, and viral disorders through molecular diagnostics; and the prevention of non-communicable diseases and genetic disorders by assessing risks and identifying exposed and susceptible individuals through molecular screening."[29, 30] For example, molecular epidemiology has been used in applications with the goal of improving assessments of potential risk factors and in defining inherited susceptibility to cancers through DNA fingerprinting.[31] In this context, DNA fingerprinting refers to identifying susceptible persons through identification of unique DNA sequences. Molecular epidemiology is also used to subtype infectious agents, which can be beneficial in epidemic investigations and related applications.

- **Neuroepidemiology** is the application of epidemiologic methods to the study of neurological disorders, such as multiple sclerosis, epilepsy, and Parkinson's disease. Two areas of investigation in neuroepidemiology that have received increased attention in recent years concern damage of the gray matter of the brain, which is characteristic of Alzheimer's disease in the elderly, and damage of the white matter, which is characteristic of periventricular leukomalacia in newborns. It is hypothesized that the damage may share common factors.[32]

- **Pharmacoepidemiology** is the application of epidemiologic methods to the study the drug effects and drug utilization patterns. The U.S. Food and Drug Administration, Center for Drug Evaluation and Research, for example, has a division that monitors drug safety. This unit, the Division of Pharmacovigilance and Epidemiology, uses epidemiologic methods to evaluate and assess the risks posed by drugs in the postmarketing environment.[33]

It is important to realize that each of these specializations, as well as others in epidemiology, all depend on having a firm grasp of the basic principles, concepts, and methods of epidemiology as presented in this text. For the most part, these specializations represent a union of epidemiology and one or more other disciplines. For example, social epidemiology represents a merger of epidemiology and the social sciences, and pharmacoepidemiology is a blending of epidemiology and clinical pharmacology.

SUMMARY

- Historical pandemics of devastating diseases like plague (the Black Death), leprosy, and syphilis were connected with the origins of epidemiology.
- As a discipline, epidemiology evolved slowly as theories of disease causation and methods of disease control were developed, refined, and tested. Later pandemics like the Great Influenza Pandemic of 1918 and the rise of emerging diseases and new threats of epidemics and pandemics continue to shape the practice of epidemiology.
- Among the many noteworthy early pioneers of epidemiology we can cite Hippocrates, who provided the first rational explanations for disease occurrence; John Graunt, who systematically evaluated the Bills of Mortality; William Farr, who brought the statistical analysis of epidemiologic problems to a new level; John Snow, who used epidemiologic methods to uncover the source and mode of transmission of cholera; and Joseph Goldberger, who used observation and experimentation to demonstrate the cause of pellagra.
- In the modern era, new pioneers have expanded the borders of epidemiology into new areas of clinical practice, health care decision making, environmental risk assessment, and other areas. Some of the modern specializations in epidemiology include social epidemiology, behavioral epidemiology, psychosocial epidemiology, environmental epidemiology, occupational epidemiology, genetic epidemiology, molecular epidemiology, neuroepidemiology, and pharmacoepidemiology. These specializations represent the importance and expanding influence of epidemiology.

New Terms

- antecedent cause of death
- behavioral epidemiology
- Bills of Mortality
- dot map
- endemic
- environmental epidemiology
- genetic epidemiology
- immediate cause of death
- molecular epidemiology
- multifactorial etiology
- neuroepidemiology
- notifiable disease
- occupational epidemiology

- pandemic
- pharmacoepidemiology
- plague
- psychosocial epidemiology
- reportable disease
- social epidemiology
- spot map
- underlying cause of death
- vital event
- vital record
- vital statistics
- vital statistics registration system

Study Questions and Exercises

1. Match the historical contributions in Column B with the individuals in Column A.

   Column A

   _____ William Farr

   _____ Joseph Goldberger

   _____ John Graunt

   _____ Peter Ludwig Panum

   _____ Edward Jenner

   _____ Hippocrates

   _____ James Lind

   _____ Florence Nightingale

   _____ Louis Pasteur

   _____ John Snow

   _____ Girolamo Fracastoro

   Column B

   A. Probably first to express formally a theory of contagion

   B. The first to explain disease occurrence on a rational basis

   C. Used mortality data to get improvements at military hospitals

   D. Evaluated the Bills of Mortality

   E. Demonstrated cholera could be transmitted through water

   F. Demonstrated that immunity results from measles infection

   G. Promoted the concept of multifactorial etiology

   H. Showed that diet could prevent scurvy

   I. Invented a vaccine against smallpox

   J. Helped establish the Germ Theory of Disease

   K. Showed pellagra was caused by a protein-deficient diet

2. An 85-year-old woman with type 2 diabetes, osteoporosis, and coronary heart disease tripped on a rug, fell, and fractured her right hip. She was admitted to the hospital within six hours by her daughter-in-law but died two days later at the hospital. Just four hours prior to her death she had extreme difficulty breathing and her skin became bluish in color. The attending physician said this was the result of a massive pulmonary embolism, a condition resulting from a large blood clot in the pulmonary artery. Using the definitions in exhibit 2-1, hypothesize as to the immediate, antecedent, and underlying causes of death.

3. Describe three diseases anywhere in the world that are currently endemic, epidemic, and pandemic, respectively. Explain why these diseases are classified as they are.

4. Suggest a research topic that might be considered within the purview of social epidemiology. Also suggest ones that might be in the purview of environmental epidemiology and molecular epidemiology, respectively.

References

1. Major Plagues and Epidemics (no date). *Compton's Encyclopedia Online*. Available: http://www.optonline.com/Tables/90000f5_T.html (Access date: January 6, 2000).
2. Janis, E. (1996). Bubonic Plague. Available: http://ponderosa-pine.uoregon.edu/students/Janis/menu.html (Access date: January 6, 2000).
3. Hanlon, J. J., and Pickett, G. E. (1979). *Public Health Administration and Practice*. St. Louis: C. V. Mosby Company.
4. Last, J. M., ed. (2001). *A Dictionary of Epidemiology*, 4th ed. New York: Oxford University Press.
5. Goerke, L. S., and Stebbins, E. L. (1968). *Mustard's Introduction to Public Health*, 5th ed. London: Macmillan Company.
6. Fox, J. P., Hall, C. E., and Elveback, L. R. (1970). *Epidemiology: Man and Disease*. New York: Macmillan Company.
7. Barry, J. M. (2004). The Site of Origin of the 1918 Influenza Pandemic and Its Public Health Implications. *Journal of Translational Medicine* 2 (1): 3. Available: http://www.translational-medicine.com/content/2/1/3 (Access date: June 27, 2005).
8. Ammon C. E. (2002). Spanish Flu Epidemic in 1918 in Geneva, Switzerland. *Eurosurveillance Monthly* 7 (12): 190–192. Available: http://www.eurosurveillance.org/em/v07n12/0712-226.asp (Access date: June 27, 2005).
9. Reid, A. H., and Taubenberger, J. K. (2003). The Origin of the 1918 Pandemic Influenza Virus: A Continuing Enigma. *Journal of General Virology* 84 (Pt. 9): 2285–2292.
10. San Diego Historical Society (no date). Stranger Than Fiction: Vignettes of San Diego History (a chapter from *Stranger Than Fiction: Vignettes of San Diego History* by Richard W. Crawford, 1995). Available: http://www.sandiegohistory.org/stranger/flu.htm (Access date: June 25, 2005).
11. Oxford, J. S., Lambkin, R., Sefton, A., Daniels, R., Elliot, A., Brown, R., and Gill, D. (2005). A Hypothesis: The Conjunction of Soldiers, Gas, Pigs, Ducks, Geese and Horses in Northern France During the Great War Provided the Conditions for the Emergence of the "Spanish" Influenza Pandemic of 1918–1919. *Vaccine* 23 (7): 940–945.
12. Kilbourne, E. D. (2006). Influenza Pandemics of the 20th Century. *Emerging Infectious Diseases* 12 (1): 9–14.
13. U.S. Department of Health and Human Services (2006). Pandemicflu.gov/Avianflu.gov: General Information. Available: http://www.pandemicflu.gov/general/index.html#history (Access date: February 9, 2007).

14. Susser, M., and Adelstein, A. (1987). The Work of William Farr. In *Epidemiology, Health, & Society: Selected Papers* (by M. Susser). New York: Oxford University Press, pp. 49–57.
15. Stolley, P. D., and Lasky, T. (1995). *Investigating Disease Patterns: The Science of Epidemiology.* New York: Scientific American Library.
16. Lilienfeld, D. E., and Stolley, P. D. (1994). *Foundations of Epidemiology*, 3rd ed. New York: Oxford University Press.
17. Chin, J., ed. (2000). *Control of Communicable Diseases Manual*, 17th ed. Washington, DC: American Public Health Association.
18. Susser, M. (1987). Epidemiologists in Society. In *Epidemiology, Health, & Society: Selected Papers* (by M. Susser). New York: Oxford University Press, p. 11.
19. Centers for Disease Control and Prevention (1992). *Principles of Epidemiology: An Introduction to Applied Epidemiology and Biostatistics*, 2nd ed. Atlanta: The Centers.
20. The John Snow Society (2004). John Snow Facts. Available: http://www.johnsnowsociety.org/johnsnow/facts.html (Access date: February 16, 2007).
21. Snow, J. ([no date] 1988). On the Mode of Communication of Cholera. In *The Challenge of Epidemiology: Issues and Selected Readings,* C. Buck, A. Llopis, E. Najera, and M. Terris, eds. Washington, DC: Pan American Health Organization, pp. 42–45.
22. Ashton, J. (1994). John Snow, The Broad Street Pump and After. In *The Epidemiological Imagination: A Reader,* J. Ashton, ed. Buckingham: Open University Press.
23. Goldberger, J. ([1914] 1988). Considerations on Pellagra. In *The Challenge of Epidemiology: Issues and Selected Readings,* C. Buck, A. Llopis, E. Najera, and M. Terris, eds. Washington, DC: Pan American Health Organization, pp. 99–102.
24. Sallis, J. F., Owen, N., and Fotheringham, M. J. (2000). Behavioral Epidemiology: A Systematic Framework to Classify Phases of Research on Health Promotion and Disease Prevention. *Annals of Behavioral Medicine* 22 (4): 294–298.
25. Steenland, K., and Savitz, D. A. (1997). Introduction. In *Topics in Environmental Epidemiology,* K. Steenland, D. A. Savitz, eds. New York: Oxford University Press, p. 3.
26. Checkoway, H., Pearce, N., and Crawford-Brown, D. J. (1989). *Research Methods in Occupational Epidemiology.* New York: Oxford University Press.
27. Kaprio, J. (2000). Science, Medicine, and the Future: Genetic Epidemiology. *British Medical Journal* 320: 1257–1259.
28. Permutt, M. A., Wasson, J., and Cox, N. (2005). Genetic Epidemiology of Diabetes. *The Journal of Clinical Investigation* 115 (6): 1431–1439.
29. Graduate School of Public Health, University of Pittsburgh (no date). Molecular Epidemiology Training Program. Available: http://www.pitt.edu/~kkr/task.html (Access date: February 2, 2007).
30. Dorman, J. S. (2000). Molecular Epidemiology: The Impact of Molecular Biology in Epidemiology Research. *Revista Médica de Chile* 128 (11). Available: http://www.scielo.cl/scielo.php?script=sci_arttext&pid=S0034-98872000001100012&lng=en&nrm=i&tlng=en (Access date: February 2, 2007).
31. MacDonald, M. A. (2004). From Miasma to Fractals: The Epidemiology Revolution and Public Health Nursing. *Public Health Nursing* 21 (4): 380–391.
32. Cowan, L. D., Leviton, A., and Dammann, O. (2000). New Research Directions in Neuroepidemiology. *Epidemiologic Reviews* 22 (1): 18–23.
33. Department of Health and Human Services, Food and Drug Administration, Center for Drug Evaluation and Research (1998). *The CDER Handbook.* Available: http://www.fda.gov/cder/handbook/ (Access date: February 3, 2007).

CHAPTER THREE

Selected Disease Concepts in Epidemiology

This chapter summarizes basic concepts of disease, its natural history, levels of prevention, and concepts of disease immunity. Common vaccines administered to children and adults in the United States are also presented.

Learning Objectives

- Define and give examples of communicable and noncommunicable diseases.
- Apply the chain of infection to a common communicable disease and give examples of each of the six components involved in transmission of that disease.
- Apply the ecological model to a given disease.
- Differentiate between models of disease and holistic models of health.
- Use the concepts of natural history of disease and its stages and the three levels of prevention to describe the development, progression, and control of a selected disease.
- Give examples of primary, secondary, and tertiary prevention.
- Describe the differences among active, passive, and herd immunity.
- Give examples of at least three different vaccines commonly administered to children and adults, respectively, in the United States.
- Define disease, health, incubation period, induction period, latency or latent period, subclinical disease, carrier, antibody, and antigen.

INTRODUCTION

Disease, which refers to physiological or psychological dysfunction,[1] is an important concept in epidemiology since much of the field deals with communicable and noncommunicable disease distribution, etiology, prevention, and control. **Communicable diseases**, also known as **infectious diseases**,[2] are those that can be transmitted directly or indirectly to a susceptible person through contact, inhalation, or ingestion. Figure 3-1 illustrates the basic **chain of infection** normally involved in communicable disease transmission, and table 3-1 presents applicable definitions and examples of the components comprising the chain. Vital to communicable disease transmission is the infectious agent, which may be a bacterium, virus, or other type of pathogen, including a prion (an infectious protein) that is implicated, for example, in Creutzfeldt-Jakob disease.[1] **Noncommunicable diseases** are those that cannot be transmitted to others, either directly or indirectly. These are also known as **noninfectious diseases** and include such diverse conditions as diabetes, skin cancer, stroke, and muscular dystrophy. Historically, communicable diseases have often been considered acute diseases, and noncommunicable diseases have often been referred to as chronic diseases. In more recent years this line has become blurred. For example, HIV/AIDS and hepatitis C are chronic infectious diseases, and some types of cervical cancer have been found to have an infectious etiology (i.e., the human papillomavirus).

Epidemiology also deals with other health-related issues that are not technically diseases. For example, epidemiologists may be concerned with the distribution, antecedents, and control of various risk-taking behaviors such as cigarette smoking, sedentary lifestyle, or body piercing; social problems such as child abuse, domestic violence, and alienation; and attributes such as wellness and joy. Epidemiology may also be applied to health care and policy issues as well as other areas. Nevertheless, partly because of the historical concerns of epidemiology (discussed in chapter 2) and partly because of the toll disease still takes on the quality and longevity of human life, diseases remain an important focus of epidemiology and need to be studied and understood.

Figure 3-1   Chain of Infection

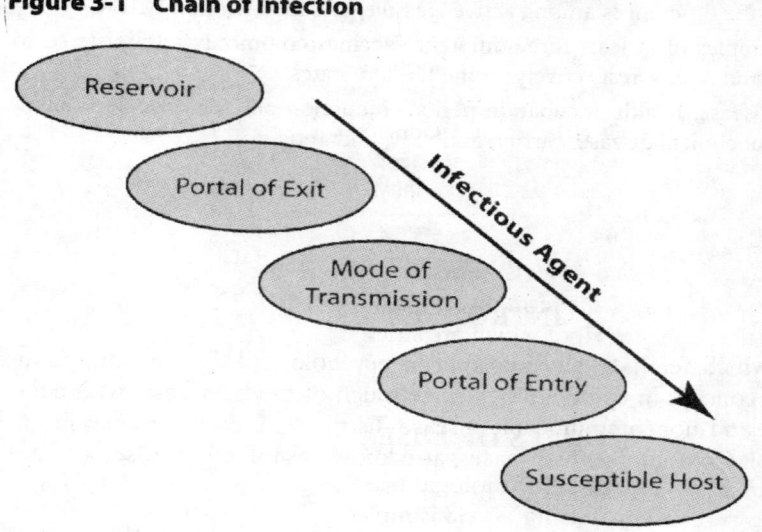

Table 3-1   Components in the Chain of Infection

Infectious Agent	A human pathogen or microorganism capable of causing a communicable disease, such as *Yersinia pestis*, the bacterium responsible for plague.
Reservoir	The normal habitat of the infectious agent (i.e., where the agent lives and grows). Common reservoirs include humans, animals, and the environment (e.g., soil, water). Human reservoirs include actively infected persons as well as carriers.
Portal of Exit	The point at which the infectious agent leaves the reservoir. In human and animal reservoirs portals of exit include the respiratory system, skin or mucous membranes, blood, saliva, gastrointestinal tract, etc.
Mode of Transmission	In general, there are three major modes of transmission from human hosts: (1) *direct transmission*, which includes contact from touching, kissing, sexual intercourse, etc. or through droplet spread during coughing, sneezing, talking, etc.; (2) *indirect transmission*, which includes transmission through *vehicles* (inanimate intermediaries, such as contaminated food, water, or surfaces) or *vectors* (animate intermediaries, such as mosquitoes, flies, ticks, or rodents); and (3) *airborne transmission*, which is transmission through microbial aerosols, including fungal spores (e.g., histoplasmosis, hantavirus pulmonary syndrome) or droplet nuclei (i.e., the dried residue of exhaled droplets) as implicated in the spread of tuberculosis and influenza.
Portal of Entry	The point at which the infectious agent enters the susceptible host. For human hosts portals of entry include the respiratory system, skin or mucous membranes, blood, gastrointestinal tract, etc.
Susceptible Host	The susceptible host may be human or animal. Factors affecting susceptibility in humans include lowered resistance, presence of open cuts or wounds, poor health status, lack of immunity, etc.

Some of the concepts and models of disease may also apply to other health-related problems. In fact, the term disease is often used broadly to encompass a variety of disorders not all of which are strictly diseases. This chapter briefly summarizes some of the more common concepts related to disease and health.

COMMON MODELS OF DISEASE AND HEALTH

The **ecological model,** or epidemiologic triangle, represents an attempt to explain disease causation using a very simple paradigm. According to this model, disease is caused by an imbalance among *host, agent,* and *environmental factors* (see figure 3-2). *Host factors* represent intrinsic characteristics that influence a host's (individual's) susceptibility to disease. These include immune status, general health status, genetic makeup, lifestyle practices, age, sex, and socioeconomic status. *Agents* consist of biological, chemical, and physical hazards that can induce disease or injury. Biological agents include pathogenic microorganisms such as bacteria, viruses, and parasites. Chemical agents are generally toxic substances such as lead, mercury, and carbon monoxide. Physical agents include such things as extreme temperatures, excessive noise, and ionizing radiation. *Environmental factors* are extrinsic characteristics that can affect exposure to the agent, effectiveness or virulence of the agent, or susceptibility of the host. Examples are weather conditions, adequacy of living conditions, general levels of sanitation, population density, and access to health care. According to the ecological model, disease results when the agent, host, and environment are no longer in balance. This can occur when environment (the fulcrum in figure 3-2) shifts or when either the agent or the host are no longer aligned due to changes in agent effectiveness or host susceptibility.

Figure 3-2   Ecological Model of Disease

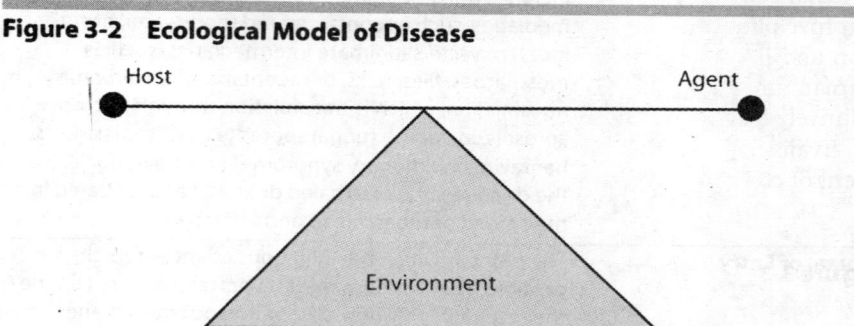

Adapted from Centers for Disease Control and Prevention (1992). *Principles of Epidemiology: An Introduction to Applied Epidemiology and Biostatistics,* 2nd ed. Atlanta: The Centers, p. 36.

Although the ecological model was originally conceived to explain the causes of communicable diseases, it has also been applied to noncommunicable diseases and other health-related problems, but with less success. One of the problems is that it can be difficult to differentiate some agents from environmental factors.[3] Noise, for example, could be classified as an agent because it induces hearing loss or as an environmental factor because it distracts attention, thereby increasing host susceptibility to injuries. In addition, G. E. Alan Dever argues that since the agent is traditionally considered essential for a communicable disease to occur, the ecological model represents a *single cause/single effect model* that is not applicable to noncommunicable diseases.[4] Indeed, he believes that a single cause/single effect model is not valid for most of the serious health problems facing contemporary society. When we consider chronic health problems and conditions, *multiple cause/multiple effect models* appear to make more sense. According to these models, multiple factors like cigarette smoking, excessive alcohol consumption, stress, and poor diet can lead to multiple effects like heart disease, stroke, hypertension, and cancer. The topic of disease causation, including the *causal pie model*, is discussed further in chapter 7.

Holistic models of health go beyond the ecological model by looking at the factors that influence *health* versus disease. **Health** can be conceived as a state of well-being and positive functioning and not just the absence of disease.[5] Holistic models of health can serve as a basis for public health planning and policy making.[4] An example of an early holistic model is the *health field concept* developed by Marc Lalonde, former Canadian Minister of National Health and Welfare (see figure 3-3). Lalonde envisioned environment (e.g., food and water quality), lifestyle (e.g., drug and alcohol use), human biology (e.g., genetics and aging), and health care organization (e.g., accessibility, quality, and quantity of services) to be the key factors determining health.[6] The health field concept says that health exists when its four components are in balance. It is reasonable to conclude from this model that efforts to improve public health must include programs aimed at environmental protection and lifestyle management, as well as those directed toward optimizing human functioning and treating disease. Other models have gone beyond the relatively basic health field concept. One example is a model developed by R. G. Evans and G. L. Stoddart.[7] This model includes prosperity as a key element of community health (see figure 3-4 on the next page).

Figure 3-3   Health Field Concept

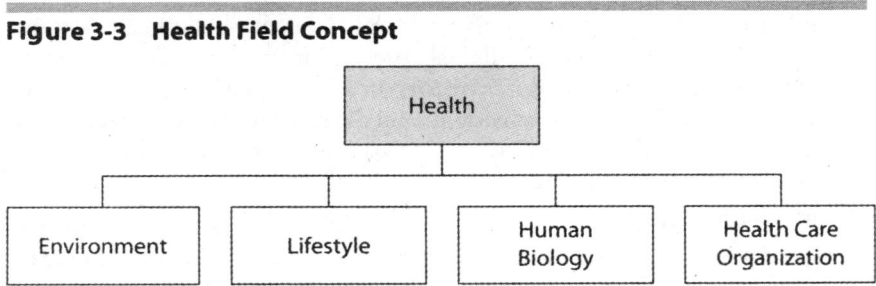

Source: Lalonde, M. (1975). *A New Perspective on the Health of Canadians: A Working Document.* Ottawa: Information Canada.

Figure 3-4   Health Model of Evans and Stoddart

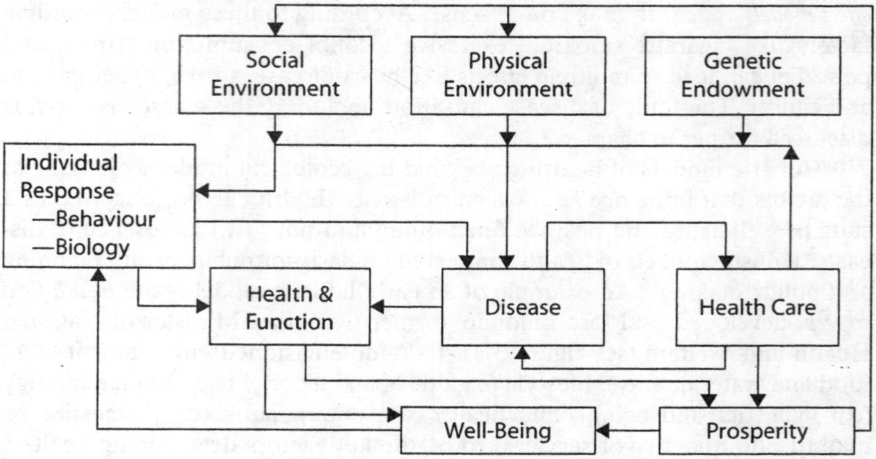

Reprinted with permission from R. G. Evans, Morris L. Barer, and Theodore R. Marmor, eds. *Why Are Some People Healthy and Others Not? The Determinants of Health of Populations.* (New York: Aldine de Gruyter). Copyright ©1994 Walter de Gruyter Inc., New York.

NATURAL HISTORY OF DISEASE

Every disease in a host follows a potentially predictable life cycle from onset to final outcome, which is known as its natural history. Understanding the **natural history of disease** is important to clinicians in establishing appropriate treatment and accurate prognosis, and it is vital to public health professionals in developing effective disease prevention and control strategies. Although the life cycle or natural history of a particular disease will vary somewhat from individual to individual, and different diseases will each have their own distinct natural histories, it is possible to identify four common stages that most diseases manifest:

- Stage of susceptibility
- Stage of presymptomatic disease
- Stage of clinical disease
- Stage of diminished capacity

The **stage of susceptibility** precedes the onset of disease. The disease has not yet developed, but the host is susceptible due to the presence of risk factors for the disease. Individuals with high cholesterol, hypertension, a sedentary lifestyle, and diabetes, for example, have an increased risk of developing coronary heart disease. Likewise, lack of sleep, excessive stress, and poor eating habits may predispose one to the common cold. Epidemiologists are continually seeking to identify and confirm risk factors for the major health problems that affect our societies. Ongoing research to determine specific risk factors for prostate cancer is just one example.[8]

In the **stage of presymptomatic disease** the disease process has begun, but no overt signs or symptoms are evident. For communicable diseases, this stage includes the **incubation period**, which is the time between the invasion of an infectious agent and the development of the first signs or symptoms of the disease. For example, influenza has a typical incubation period of one to three days, and hepatitis A has an average incubation period of 28-30 days.[9] For noncommunicable diseases, the stage of presymptomatic disease includes the **latency period** (also called the **latent period**), which can be defined as the period from disease initiation to disease detection.[1] Cancer, for example, can be conceived as passing through different phases during the latency period. Following *initiation* by a carcinogen, cancer is *promoted* by the same or other agents whereupon it *progresses* as cancerous cells divide and multiply. The latency period ends when cancer is manifested by overt signs or symptoms, or by definition, when it is clinically detected and diagnosed. The initiation process in noncommunicable diseases such as lung cancer may be termed the **induction period**. This is the period from the initial exposure to causative factors to disease initiation. The disease, however, is not apparent at this point. In this conceptualization, the induction period precedes the latency period. Together, they represent the entire phase from the disease-free state to the state of clinical disease. Applied to the paradigm of the natural history of disease, the induction period for noncommunicable diseases represents an interval starting somewhere in the stage of susceptibility and ending in the stage of presymptomatic disease. The latency period corresponds to a subsequent interval starting in the stage of presymptomatic disease and ending in the stage of clinical disease. Of course, these intervals cannot be quantified precisely because of the uncertainty as to when disease initiation actually begins.

In addition to the incubation and latency periods, the stage of presymptomatic disease includes cases of **subclinical disease**, that is, disease that is fully developed but which produces no overt signs or symptoms in the host (i.e., asymptomatic disease). A classic example is Typhoid Mary, the infamous cook and *carrier* of typhoid fever. Typhoid Mary is believed to have infected as many as 53 people with typhoid fever over a period of 15 years.[10] The total number of infections that resulted from her presence could number in the thousands (see exhibit 3-1). A **carrier** of a communicable disease is an individual who has no clinical signs or symptoms of the disease but nevertheless harbors the causative agent, which can be transmitted to others.[1] Individuals can be carriers for short periods (e.g., during the incubation period) or for long periods of time (e.g., chronic carriers). Other examples of presymptomatic disease include atherosclerotic plaque buildup in the coronary arteries prior to the manifestation of any coronary heart disease symptoms and precancerous lesions of the cervix evident only from a Pap test.

In the **stage of clinical disease** the condition is clearly apparent, and the host experiences one or more overt signs or symptoms characteristic of the

---

Exhibit 3-1
A Brief Profile of Typhoid Mary

The infamous Typhoid Mary was really Mary Mallon (1869–1938), a New York cook who came to the United States from Ireland in 1883. In the summer of 1906 an outbreak of typhoid fever occurred in the town of Oyster Bay on Long Island, New York. Though typhoid fever caused about 25,000 deaths in the U.S. in 1906, the outbreak in Oyster Bay surprised the three resident physicians, and local investigators were not able to find any obvious sources of contamination. Six of those living in the house where Mary was employed as a cook contracted typhoid fever, and one died. Concerned that they might not be able to rent the house, the owners commissioned George Soper, a sanitary engineer from the New York City Health Department, to investigate. After some initial dead ends, Soper began to focus his investigation on Mary Mallon, who had left unexpectedly about three weeks after the outbreak. Soper suspected she might be a healthy *carrier* of the disease. He later tracked her down in Manhattan where she was serving as a cook for another family. She reportedly threatened him when he sought to test her for the disease. Convinced she was a carrier, Soper looked into her work history and found that in the previous ten years she had worked for eight families, seven of whom contracted typhoid fever. A 1903 outbreak in Ithaca, New York, which claimed 1,300 lives, is believed to have originated with Mary Mallon. In March, 1907, Mary was taken, kicking and screaming, to a city hospital to be tested. Fecal samples showed high levels of *Salmonella typhi*, the bacillus that causes typhoid fever. Mary was given an offer to have her gall bladder removed, which would have ended her carrier state. She adamantly refused, however, claiming vociferously that she was not responsible for the outbreaks. Mary was therefore placed in an isolation cottage at Riverside Hospital on North Brother Island in New York. She remained there a virtual prisoner and an emerging celebrity until she was released three years later, ostensibly due to adverse public opinion regarding her detention. The conditions of her release stated that she would keep in touch with the health department and not work in the food handling profession again. Several years later in 1915, she was found working as a cook in Sloane Maternity Hospital in Manhattan under the assumed name of Mrs. Brown. During her employment at the hospital she is believed to have infected at least 25 of the medical and support staff, two of whom died. She was arrested and taken back to a cottage on North Brother Island where she remained in relative isolation for the remainder of her life. Mary Mallon died in 1938, nearly 70 years of age, from complications of a stroke. According to one source, she still baked and sold cakes while she resided on North Brother Island.

Typhoid fever, which is usually characterized by sudden onset, causes sustained fever, severe headache, anorexia, malaise, splenomegaly, and sometimes rose-colored spots on the body. Although once prominent in the U.S., today less than 500 cases occur each year primarily due to better sanitation measures aimed at water supplies, food, and milk. Untreated, typhoid fever has a case fatality of 10–20 percent.

References: Ochs, R. (no date). Dinner with Typhoid Mary. Available: http://www.lihistory.com/7/hs702a.htm (Access date: February 3, 2000); Alcamo, I. E. (1997). *Fundamentals of Microbiology*, 5th ed. Menlo Park, CA: Benjamin/Cummings; Chin, J., ed. (2000). *Control of Communicable Diseases Manual*, 17th ed. Washington, DC: American Public Health Association.

disease. This stage is where the disease is commonly diagnosed and treated by physicians. Clinical disease may range in degree of severity and advance slowly or rapidly depending upon a variety of host, agent, and environmental factors. As an example, influenza causes fever, headache, muscle aches, coughing, and fatigue in most adults for up to a week,[9] but in some, especially those with weak immune systems, symptoms may continue much longer. In addition, some individuals may appear only moderately upset by the symptoms, while others may find them quite oppressive. Some chronic diseases may be graded during this stage depending on their degree of progression. Cancer, for example, is classified by **stages of cancer.** *Stage one cancers* are localized and have not yet metastasized to other parts of the body. *Stage two cancers* have infiltrated underlying tissues more than stage one cancers, but they have still not metastasized to other parts of the body. *Stage three cancers* have metastasized to surrounding tissues, and *stage four cancers* have spread extensively throughout the body. This latter stage represents advanced cancer for which treatment is often largely palliative.[2]

The final stage in the natural history of disease can be referred to as the **stage of diminished capacity.** It is characterized by a convalescent period or a residual disability. In the case of *convalescence,* there is a period following completion of clinical disease during which the individual has not yet returned to his or her former level of health. For example, though influenza has passed, it may be several days or even weeks before an individual feels enough strength to say he or she is well again. This represents the convalescent period. Many moderate to serious infectious diseases require some convalescence after the disease has run its course. *Residual disability* can result from diseases that produce temporary or protracted complications. Examples are poliomyelitis, which has left some of its victims with permanent physical disabilities, and influenza in the elderly, which can sometimes result in secondary pneumonia. Also, heart attacks and strokes can leave individuals with limited functional capacity. The distinction between the convalescent period and residual disability is not always clear. In summary, the convalescent period represents the time it takes recovered (disease-free) individuals to get back on their feet, while residual disability refers to the development of complications or disability resulting directly from the clinical disease.

Ultimately, the natural history of a disease concludes in either full recovery or death. The number of stages a person passes through or the length of time one stays in a particular stage will vary depending on the specific disease, the overall health of the individual, and other factors. Individuals with chronic diseases, such as emphysema or a severe stroke, will remain in the clinical or diminished capacity stages for life.

LEVELS OF PREVENTION

The definition of epidemiology (chapter 1) encompasses preventing and controlling diseases in human populations (i.e., deterrents). This is usually accomplished using one or more of three **levels of prevention**. **Primary prevention** seeks to prevent *new* cases of disease from occurring by controlling the causes of disease. Thus, it is most appropriately applied to persons who are in the stage of susceptibility. **Secondary prevention** attempts to identify *existing* cases of disease in an early stage, especially subclinical cases, so as to effect a cure or prevent any complications of the disease. Therefore, it is most appropriately aimed at those in the stage of presymptomatic disease or the early stage of clinical disease where treatment is more likely to be effective. **Tertiary prevention** tries to limit disability and improve functioning where clinical disease or its complications are already well established. This is often accomplished through rehabilitation. Therefore, tertiary prevention is most applicable in the late stage of clinical disease or the stage of diminished capacity. As the foregoing discussion demonstrates, the natural history of disease and the levels of prevention are closely linked. Figure 3-5 illustrates where each level of prevention is most appropriately employed in the natural history of disease.

Figure 3-5   Stages in the Natural History of Disease and Corresponding Levels of Prevention

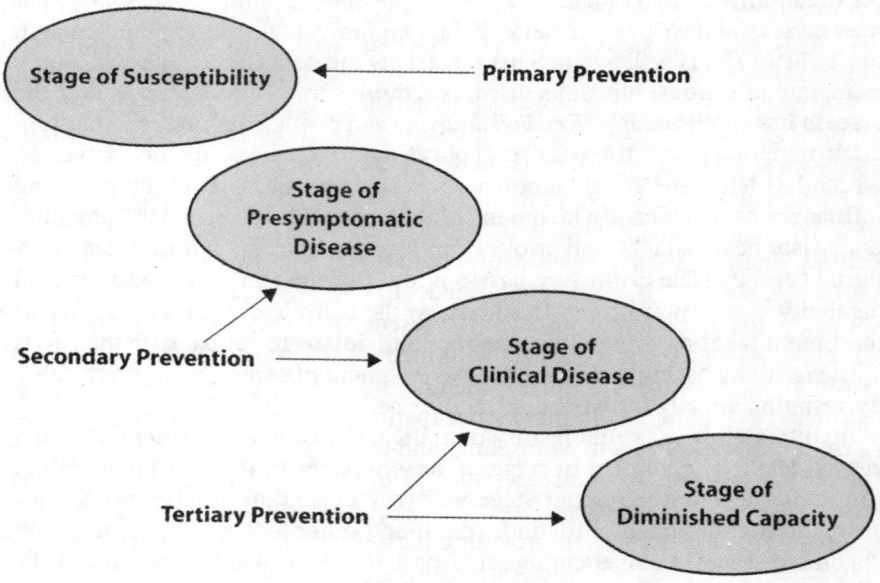

Primary Prevention Strategies

On a community level, primary prevention strategies emphasize general health promotion, risk factor reduction, and other health protective measures. The general methods may include health education and health promotion programs designed to foster healthier lifestyles and environmental health programs designed to improve environmental conditions and safety. Specific examples of primary prevention measures include immunization against communicable diseases; public health education about good nutrition, exercise, stress management, and personal responsibility for health; chlorination and filtration of public water supplies; and legislation requiring child restraints in motor vehicles. Each of these measures is aimed at preventing *new* cases of disease or injury from occurring in a population.

Secondary Prevention Strategies

Secondary prevention focuses on early detection and prompt treatment of disease. Its purpose is to cure *existing* disease, slow its progression, or reduce its impact on individuals or communities. A common strategy of secondary prevention is screening for disease, such as the noninvasive computerized test for the early detection of heart disease. This test uses computerized tomography scans to look for calcium deposition in the arteries, which can signal previously undetected heart disease. Other examples of screening include mammography for breast cancer detection; eye tests for glaucoma; blood tests for lead exposure; tests for colorectal cancer; the Pap test for cervical cancer; the breath test for *Helicobacter pylori*, the bacterium implicated in duodenal and gastric ulcers; and the prostate-specific antigen (PSA) test for prostate cancer. In each case, screening is performed with the goal of detecting disease early so that treatment can be initiated when it is most likely to be successful. Removal of intestinal polyps during a routine colonoscopy and removal of pre-cancerous skin lesions are examples of secondary prevention strategies. Screening is discussed in detail in chapter 13.

Tertiary Prevention Strategies

Tertiary prevention strategies involve both therapeutic and rehabilitative measures once disease is firmly established.[5] Examples include treatment of diabetics to prevent complications of the disease and the ongoing management of chronic heart disease patients with medication, diet, exercise, and regular examinations. Other examples include improving functioning of stroke patients through rehabilitation by occupational and physical therapy, nursing care, speech therapy, and counseling, and treating those suffering from complications of debilitating diseases such as bacterial meningitis, multiple sclerosis, or Parkinson's disease.

On a community level, providing high quality, appropriate, and accessible health care and public health resources is critical to assuring satisfactory primary, secondary, and tertiary prevention. Table 3-2 summarizes the three levels of prevention and provides examples of their applications at the community level.

Table 3-2   Examples of Levels of Prevention

Level of Prevention	Main Purpose	Examples at the Community Level
Primary	To prevent disease before it develops so as to maintain health	Smoking prevention programs, air pollution control enforcement, health education in the schools
Secondary	To diagnose and treat disease in its early stages so as to restore or improve health	Blood pressure screening for hypertension, vision screening in schools, case finding and referral for treatment of sexually transmitted diseases
Tertiary	To reduce complications of well established disease and improve functioning or quality of life where possible	Rehabilitation programs for heart attack victims, hospice programs for dying patients, group counseling for those with chronic fatigue syndrome

IMMUNITY TO DISEASE

Antibodies are involved in producing immunity to disease. When certain foreign substances, such as those introduced by pathogenic bacteria or viruses, enter the body, antibodies are typically formed as a defensive response. Antibodies are protein substances or globulins derived from B and T lymphocytes, which originate in the bone marrow. They are generally *specific* to the particular invading substance, known as an **antigen**, and thus provide highly selective protection.[2] Because antigens stimulate antibody production, we often speak of antigen-antibody reactions. Antibody production is important to epidemiology because *titers* (concentrations) of specific antibodies can be measured in individuals and used to indicate the relative immunity of different populations to specific diseases, as well as to identify asymptomatic cases of disease.[1]

Types of Immunity

Disease immunity can be classified as active or passive. **Active immunity** occurs when the body produces antibodies in reaction to an infection or a vaccine.[2] Vaccines typically use attenuated, modified, or killed pathogenic organisms, or their inactive toxins, to achieve active immunity in the host without producing disease.[1] **Passive immunity** can be acquired in three ways:

- By injection of a serum (a refined suspension containing antibodies already produced by another host, e.g., immune globulin)
- By placental transfer (i.e., transfer of a mother's antibodies to her developing fetus during pregnancy)
- By breast-feeding (i.e., transfer of a mother's antibodies to her child through breast milk)

The major differences between active and passive immunity have to do with how rapidly protection against a given disease is conferred and how long the protection lasts. In general, active immunity takes about two to three weeks to confer immunity, while passive immunity is immediate. On the other hand, active immunity usually lasts for a number of years, and often for a life-time,[11] while passive immunity persists about two weeks if received from a serum and up to six months if received by placental transfer or breast-feeding.[2]

Another epidemiologic concept related to disease immunity is **herd immunity**, a type of group immunity. Specifically, it refers to the resistance of a group or population to the spread of a specific disease through the group. This resistance is due to the fact that a high proportion of the group members is immune to the disease, usually due to previous immunizations or infections. The concept is important to epidemiology because it renders populations less susceptible to outbreaks from particular diseases. The reason for this becomes clear when one realizes that:

> *The probability of a communicable disease spreading in a population depends on the number of susceptible people in that population and the likelihood that they will come into contact with an infected person.*

Thus, the higher the proportion of immune individuals in a population, the less chance there is that a susceptible person will come into contact with an infected person. Theoretically, when at least 85–90 percent of a population are immune to a given disease, herd immunity should be expected to protect most of the other 10–15 percent.[10, 12] Therefore, it would seem that the ideal goal of 100 percent immunization is not always necessary to prevent disease outbreaks. One problem with this thinking, however, is that the remaining susceptible people frequently represent a demographic subgroup where the members live in close proximity to each other. If the disease is introduced into the subgroup, a localized outbreak could occur.[12] Therefore, it is important to realize that the concept of herd immunity assumes a relatively well distributed population of immune persons.

Vaccines

Many vaccines are readily available for use in the United States and other countries to prevent potentially serious communicable diseases in individuals as well as disease outbreaks. Common vaccines administered to children in the U.S., their purposes, and general recommendations for their use are delineated in table 3-3. With the exception of the meningococcal vaccine and the recently approved human papillomavirus vaccine (HPV), most childhood immunizations are normally scheduled to begin sometime before the age of two years with any required subsequent doses to be completed no later than age six.[13] It is important to note that these recommendations are subject to change and are updated on a regular basis. Common vaccines for adults, 19 years of age and older, along with their purposes and selected commentary, are shown in table 3-4 starting on p. 49. As with the childhood vaccines, recommendations for adult immunizations are also subject to change.

Table 3-3 Common Vaccines for Children in the United States

Vaccine	Purpose	General Recommendations*
Hepatitis B	To prevent hepatitis B infection	Administer monovalent hepatitis B vaccine (HepB) to all newborns prior to hospital discharge. Subsequent doses should be provided as medically indicated.
Rotavirus	To prevent rotavirus infection (causes severe diarrhea)	Administer first dose of the vaccine (Rota) at age 6–12 weeks. Subsequent doses should be provided as medically indicated.
Diphtheria, Tetanus, Pertussis	To prevent diphtheria, tetanus (lockjaw), and pertussis (whooping cough)	Administer four doses of the vaccine (DTaP) as medically indicated between two and 18 months of age with a final dose between four and six years of age.
Haemophilus influenzae type b	To prevent a type of bacterial meningitis	Administer two doses of the vaccine (Hib) as medically indicated at two months and four months of age, respectively, with subsequent doses as medically indicated.
Pneumococcal	To prevent pneumococcal pneumonia	Administer pneumococcal conjugate vaccine (PCV) starting at two months and as medically indicated thereafter.
Inactivated poliovirus	To prevent poliomyelitis	Administer vaccine starting two months of age and as medically indicated thereafter with the final dose at 4–6 years of age.
Influenza	To prevent influenza	Administer the vaccine annually from 6–59 months of age. Use in children 59 months or older is recommended only for high risk groups.
Measles, Mumps, Rubella	To prevent measles, mumps, and rubella	Administer the vaccine (MMR) starting with the first dose at 12–18 months of age with a second dose at 4–6 years of age.
Varicella	To prevent varicella (chickenpox)	Administer the vaccine at 12–18 months of age with a second dose at 4–6 years of age.
Hepatitis A	To prevent hepatitis A	Administer the vaccine (HepA) at age one. Administer a second dose at least six months later.
Meningococcal	To prevent bacterial meningitis	Administer to high risk children 2–10 years of age.
Human papillomavirus	To prevent cervical cancer, precancerous genital lesions, and genital warts due to certain types of human papillomavirus	Administer first dose of human papillomavirus vaccine (HPV) to females 11–12 years of age. Subsequent doses should be provided as medically indicated.

*The recommendations in this table are generalized and do not constitute medical advice. Individuals seeking immunizations for children in their care should consult a qualified health care professional for specific recommendations, including applicability, scheduling, contraindications, and possible side effects.

Reference: Centers for Disease Control and Prevention (2007). Recommended Immunization Schedule for Persons Aged 0–6 Years—United States, 2007, and Recommended Immunization Schedule for Persons Aged 7–18 Years—United States, 2007. Atlanta: The Centers. Available: http://origin.cdc.gov/nip/recs/child-schedule-bw-press.pdf (Access date: February 5, 2007).

Table 3-4   Common Vaccines for Adults in the United States

Vaccine	Purpose	Selected Comments*
Tetanus, Diphtheria, Pertussis (Td/Tdap)	To prevent tetanus (lock-jaw), diphtheria, and per-tussis (whooping cough)	Adults who have previously completed the vaccine series should receive a booster shot every 10 years.
Human papillomavirus (HPV)	To prevent cervical cancer, precancerous genital lesions, and genital warts due to certain types of human papillomavirus	Women aged less than 26 years who have not previously com-pleted the vaccine series should receive the vaccine except dur-ing pregnancy.
Measles, Mumps, Rubella (MMR)	To prevent measles, mumps, and rubella	Adults born before 1957 are generally considered immune to measles and mumps. The MMR vaccine should not be administered to women who are pregnant or likely to be within four weeks of receiving the vaccine.
Varicella	To prevent varicella (chickenpox)	Adults without evidence of immunity to varicella should receive two doses of the vaccine. It should not be administered to women who are pregnant or likely to be within four weeks of receiving the vaccine.
Influenza	To prevent influenza	Adults at high risk (e.g., chroni-cally ill, pregnant, caregivers for the chronically ill) and others wishing to be vaccinated should receive the vaccine.
Pneumococcal (polysaccharide)	To prevent pneumococcal pneumonia	Adults at high risk (e.g., those with certain chronic illnesses, certain Native American popu-lations, residents of long-term care facilities) should receive the vaccine.
Hepatitis A	To prevent hepatitis A	Adults at high risk (e.g., persons with clotting factor disorders, chronic liver disease, men who have sex with men, users of ille-gal drugs, travelers to certain areas) should receive the vaccine.

(continued)

Table 3-4 *(continued)*

Vaccine	Purpose	Selected Comments*
Hepatitis B	To prevent hepatitis B	Adults at high risk (e.g., hemodialysis patients, patients receiving clotting factor concentrates, workers exposed to blood, injection drug users, persons with multiple sex partners) should receive the vaccine.
Meningococcal	To prevent bacterial meningitis	Adults at high risk (e.g., patients with terminal complement component deficiencies, first-year college students living in dormitories, travelers to certain areas) should receive the vaccine.

*The comments in this table are selective and do not constitute medical advice. Adults seeking immunizations should consult a qualified health care professional for specific recommendations, including applicability, scheduling, contraindications, and possible side effects.
Reference: Centers for Disease Control and Prevention (2006). Recommended Adult Immunization Schedule, United States, October 2006-September 2007. Atlanta: The Centers. Available: http://www.cdc.gov/nip/recs/adult-schedule.pdf (Access date: February 5, 2007).

Since many members of the public have questions or concerns about vaccines, especially those intended for children, exhibit 3-2 presents some common myths and facts about vaccine use in the United States according to the Centers for Disease Control and Prevention. In addition, the Immunization Safety Review Committee of the National Institute of Medicine, rejected the hypothesis that a causal link exists between vaccines, specifically the measles, mumps, and rubella (MMR) vaccine, and autism based on its review of published and unpublished epidemiologic studies. The Committee came to the same conclusion regarding the possible link between the vaccine preservative thimerosal, which contains a form of mercury, and autism.[14] The controversial nature of these topics was an impetus for the study. Autism is a chronic developmental disorder that has no cure. As a precautionary measure, starting in 1999 thimerosal in vaccines routinely recommended for infants started to be eliminated or greatly reduced.[15]

Research and development of new vaccines continues to be of high priority in the U.S. In addition to recently approved vaccines for rotavirus gastroenteritis and human papillomavirus (tables 3-3 and 3-4), a new vaccine to reduce the risk of shingles was licensed by the Food and Drug Administration in late May, 2006. This vaccine, which is intended for use in adults 60 years of age and older, has been shown to reduce the occurrence of shingles by about 50 percent in this age group. Shingles is caused by the varicella-zoster virus, which is the same virus that causes chickenpox. It can produce clusters of blisters, which develop on one side of the body and can cause severe pain that may last from weeks to years.[16] Several other vaccines are currently under development.

Exhibit 3-2
Fact and Fiction Regarding Vaccines

Despite some claims to the contrary, on the whole vaccines present a relatively low risk of adverse side effects. Most side effects from vaccine administration are relatively minor and short-lived, such as transient pain at the site of administration or mild fever. Serious side effects are on the order of 1 in 1,000 to 1 in 1,000,000 or more. The benefits of vaccines appear to far outweigh the risks. Consider measles. One complication of infection with measles is encephalitis, which is estimated to occur at a rate of 1 in 2,000. Immunization for measles with the MMR vaccine, however, is believed to be associated with encephalitis or severe allergic reaction at a rate of only 1 in 1,000,000. Also, without the Tetanus, Diphtheria, Pertussis vaccine, pertussis cases would be expected to increase by over 70 times according to the Centers for Disease Control and Prevention. Nonetheless, there is significant misinformation about vaccine safety in the United States and elsewhere. The following myths and facts might help to set the record straight.

Myth	Fact
Diseases were on the decline in the U.S. before vaccines were introduced due to better sanitation and personal hygiene.	While some diseases were on the decline, significant drops in disease prevalence have occurred following routine vaccine use.
Most people in the U.S. who get disease have already been vaccinated.	This may be because so many people have been vaccinated in the U.S. If one compares the attack rates in unvaccinated and vaccinated subgroups, however, one will invariably find that the rate in the vaccinated subgroup is substantially lower than that in the unvaccinated subgroup.
Vaccines are very risky, causing many serious side effects, including death.	Overall, vaccines present considerably smaller risks that the diseases they are designed to prevent.
There is no need for vaccination since most vaccine-preventable diseases have all but been eliminated in the U.S.	While many vaccine-preventable diseases have been greatly reduced in the U.S., some of these diseases are highly prevalent in other parts of the world. Infected travelers could introduce them into the U.S. Without a highly immunized population, this could lead to large scale epidemics.
Giving multiple vaccines to children at the same time raises the probability of harmful side effects and can overwhelm the immune system.	Children are exposed to multiple antigens every day without adverse effects. Besides scientific studies have shown that multiple vaccines work well together and do not increase the probability of adverse side effects.

Reference: Centers for Disease Control and Prevention (2002). *Epidemiology and Prevention of Vaccine-Preventable Diseases*, 7th ed. Atlanta: The Centers.

SUMMARY

- Disease is an important concept in epidemiology because much of the field deals with the distribution, etiology, prevention, and control of communicable and noncommunicable diseases. Communicable diseases follow a well-recognized chain of infection, while noncommunicable diseases are not infectious. Though diseases remain an important focus area of epidemiology, the field has expanded to encompass all types of health-related issues.

- The ecological model is a relatively simple paradigm for explaining disease causation in terms of host, agent, and environmental factors. According to this model, disease occurs when these three factors are not in balance. While useful in explaining infectious diseases, the model seems less applicable to many contemporary health issues and, therefore, has often been replaced by more complex models, including holistic models of health, such as the health field concept and the model of Evans and Stoddart. Health is usually conceived of as a state of well-being and positive functioning and not just the absence of disease.

- Understanding the natural history of disease as manifested in its four stages (susceptibility, presymptomatic disease, clinical disease, and diminished capacity) and the three levels of prevention (primary, secondary, and tertiary) is helpful in developing effective public health interventions.

- Immunity to disease may be due to active immunity, which occurs when the body produces its own antibodies in reaction to an infection or vaccine, or to passive immunity, which occurs when one receives antibodies produced by another host. Herd immunity is group immunity due to a high proportion of immune individuals in a population. It tends to reduce the potential for outbreaks of a given disease when the immune population is well distributed.

- There are many vaccines available in the United States that can be used to prevent potentially serious communicable diseases in children and adults. Vaccine research and development continues to be a high priority in the U.S. Recent advances in vaccine development include the vaccine against the rotavirus, which causes gastroenteritis, and that against the human papillomavirus, which is responsible for most cases of cervical cancer.

New Terms

- active immunity
- antibody
- antigen
- carrier
- chain of infection
- communicable disease
- disease

- ecological model
- health
- herd immunity
- holistic model of health
- incubation period
- induction period
- infectious disease

- latency period
- latent period
- levels of prevention
- natural history of disease
- noncommunicable disease
- noninfectious disease
- passive immunity
- primary prevention

- secondary prevention
- stage of clinical disease
- stage of diminished capacity
- stage of presymptomatic disease
- stage of susceptibility
- stages of cancer
- subclinical disease
- tertiary prevention

Study Questions and Exercises

1. Use the ecological model to explain the occurrence of bubonic plague in medieval Europe. Now use the chain of infection to describe its transmission (Note that chapter 2 discusses plague.)

2. Describe in detail the natural history of coronary heart disease and provide specific examples of prevention strategies that can be applied at the individual and community levels at each stage of the natural history of the disease. Identify the prevention strategies by level of prevention.

3. In school immunization programs, it is usually impossible to achieve a 100% immunization rate due to legitimate objections by parents on the grounds of religion, medical contraindications, or other reasons. Explain why and under what circumstances 100% immunization for a given disease may not be required to protect the students and their families from an outbreak of the disease.

4. Use the health field concept to explain the relatively low prevalence of childhood malnutrition in affluent parts of the United States.

References

1. Last, J. M., ed. (2001). *A Dictionary of Epidemiology*, 4th ed. New York: Oxford University Press.
2. Hurster, M. M. (1997). *Communicable and Non-communicable Disease Basics: A Primer.* Westport, CT: Bergin and Garvey.
3. Page, R. M., Cole, G. E., and Timmreck, T. C. (1995). *Basic Epidemiological Methods and Biostatistics: A Practical Guidebook.* Boston: Jones and Bartlett Publishers.
4. Dever, G. E. A. (1980). *Community Health Analysis: A Holistic Approach.* Germantown, MD: Aspen.
5. Beaglehole, R., Bonita, R., and Kjellström, T. (1993). *Basic Epidemiology.* Geneva: World Health Organization.
6. Lalonde, M. (1975). *A New Perspective on the Health of Canadians: A Working Document.* Ottawa: Information Canada.
7. Evans, R. G., and Stoddart, G. L. (1994). Producing Health, Consuming Health Care. In *Why Are Some People Healthy and Others Not? The Determinants of Health of Populations,* R. G. Evans, M. L. Barer, and T. R. Marmor, eds. New York: Aldine de Gruyter, pp. 27–64.
8. Patel, D. A., Bock, C. H., Schwartz, K., Wenzlaff, A. S., Demers, R. Y., and Severson, R. K. (2005). Sexually Transmitted Diseases and Other Urogenital Conditions as Risk Factors for Prostate Cancer: A Case-control Study in Wayne County, Michigan. *Cancer Causes and Control* 16 (3): 263-273.

9. Chin, J., ed. (2000). *Control of Communicable Diseases Manual*, 17th ed. Washington, DC: American Public Health Association.

10. Timmreck, T. C. (1998). *An Introduction to Epidemiology*, 2nd ed. Boston: Jones and Bartlett Publishers.

11. Centers for Disease Control and Prevention (2002). *Epidemiology and Prevention of Vaccine-preventable Diseases*, 7th ed. Atlanta: The Centers.

12. Centers for Disease Control and Prevention (1992). *Principles of Epidemiology: An Introduction to Applied Epidemiology and Biostatistics*, 2nd ed. Atlanta: The Centers.

13. Centers for Disease Control and Prevention (2007). Recommended Immunization Schedule for Persons Aged 0-6 Years—United States, 2007, and Recommended Immunization Schedule for Persons Aged 7-18 Years—United States, 2007. Atlanta: The Centers. Available: http://origin.cdc.gov/nip/recs/child-schedule-bw-press.pdf (Access date: February 5, 2007).

14. Immunization Safety Review Committee, National Institute of Medicine (2004). *Immunization Safety Review: Vaccines and Autism*. Washington, DC: National Academy of Sciences.

15. U.S. Food and Drug Administration (2004). IOM Report: No Link Between Vaccines and Autism (by Michelle Meadows). Available: http://www.fda.gov/fdac/features/2004/504_iom.html (Access date: February 10, 2007).

16. U.S. Food and Drug Administration (2006). FDA News: FDA Licenses New Vaccine to Reduce Older Americans' Risk of Shingles. Available: http://www.fda.gov/bbs/topics/NEWS/2006/NEW01378.html (Access date: February 5, 2007).

CHAPTER FOUR

An Overview of Epidemiologic Study Designs

This chapter describes the basic designs of the major types of descriptive, analytic, and experimental studies in epidemiology.

Learning Objectives

- Distinguish between observational and experimental studies.
- Explain the differences between descriptive and analytic studies.
- Identify differences and uses for case studies and case series.
- Classify descriptions of epidemiologic studies as to their correct study designs.
- Describe three types of ecological studies.
- Distinguish among the various types of hybrid studies.
- Identify important differences between randomized controlled trials and group randomized trials.
- Describe the selection of the study population in a randomized controlled trial.
- Distinguish between preventive and therapeutic trials.
- Define *a priori* hypothesis, clinical trial, cohort, ecological fallacy, ecological unit, exploratory study, exposure and outcome status, longitudinal study, natural experiment, primary and secondary sources, quasi-experimental study, randomization, study population, and unit of analysis.

INTRODUCTION

This chapter introduces study designs frequently employed in epidemiology. Since many of these designs are referred to in subsequent chapters, it is important that you have a working knowledge of them before proceeding. Chapters 9–12 provide additional details on specific types of studies, including a discussion of potential sources of error and basic methods of analysis.

Before we begin discussing epidemiologic study designs some terms need to be clarified. **Exposure status** is a term referring to how individuals or groups are classified with regard to an **exposure**, which is defined as a potential risk factor, whether the factor represents an actual exposure (e.g., environmental tobacco smoke), a specific behavior (e.g., sedentary lifestyle), or an individual attribute (e.g., age). **Outcome status** refers to how individuals or groups are classified with regard to an **outcome**, which refers to a disease or another health-related occurrence. Both exposure status and outcome status can be dichotomous (e.g., exposed or unexposed; outcome present or outcome absent) or represent several levels (e.g., high exposure, moderate exposure, low exposure; severe outcome, moderate outcome, mild outcome, no outcome). Unless otherwise indicated, we will describe studies where both exposure and outcome status are dichotomous.

The application of the above terms can be illustrated by a **longitudinal study*** designed to assess whether or not obesity increases the risk of stroke. Subjects might be classified as obese (the exposed group) or not obese (the unexposed group) at the start of the study and followed over time to see if those in the exposed group develop stroke at a greater frequency than those in the unexposed group. In this example, exposure status refers to how the subjects are classified with regard to the exposure (i.e., as obese or not), and outcome status refers to how the subjects are classified with regard to the outcome (i.e., as having developed a stroke or not).

CATEGORIES OF EPIDEMIOLOGIC STUDIES

There are two broad categories into which epidemiologic studies can be classified. These categories are:

- Observational studies

- Experimental studies

Observational studies are epidemiologic studies where the investigators collect, record, and analyze data on subjects *without* controlling exposure status or the conditions of the study. The investigators simply observe the subjects as they naturally divide themselves by potentially significant variables or exposures.[1] By contrast, in **experimental studies** the investigators control the conditions of the experiment, including the subjects' exposure status. Experimental studies can be recognized by a planned intervention, which involves the introduction of an investigational treatment, procedure, program, or service so as to determine its efficacy or effectiveness (see chapter 1) with regard to a given outcome. To illustrate this difference, consider two possible ways of studying the effect of vitamin C supplementation on the prevention of the common cold. In an *observational study*, investigators might select a

---

*A longitudinal study is one in which subjects are studied over time. It is a general term applied to several types of epidemiologic studies in which data on study subjects are collected during successive time periods

sample of individuals, query them about their use of vitamin C, and then follow the sample over time to see if those who routinely take a certain amount of vitamin C on their own develop fewer colds than those who do not. In an *experimental study*, the investigators might randomly assign volunteers to take either a prescribed amount of vitamin C or an inactive substance (i.e., a placebo; chapter 12), and then follow up to see if those taking the vitamin C develop fewer colds than those taking the placebo. In the first example, there was no intervention or control by the investigators (e.g., the subjects were not asked to change their exposure status). The investigators simply observed what occurred in the exposed and unexposed groups and recorded their findings. In the second example, the investigators intervened by controlling the subjects' exposure status (i.e., the investigators determined that some subjects would receive the vitamin and that some would receive a placebo). The efficacy or effectiveness of vitamin C was determined by comparing the rate at which colds developed in the experimental group (those taking vitamin C) to that in the control group (those not taking vitamin C). Clearly, the second study went beyond simple observation.

Descriptive and *analytic epidemiology* (chapter 1) are dimensions of epidemiology that utilize observational studies. Specifically, descriptive epidemiology makes use of **descriptive studies**, and analytic epidemiology makes use of **analytic studies**. Both of these study types are considered observational studies and are discussed in the following sections. *Experimental studies* encompass a third dimension of epidemiology, *experimental epidemiology*, which was also discussed in chapter 1.

To recapitulate briefly, epidemiologic studies may be classified as observational or experimental. Observational studies include both descriptive studies and analytic studies, while experimental studies exist in a category by themselves. This is illustrated in figure 4-1.

Figure 4-1   Classification of Epidemiologic Studies

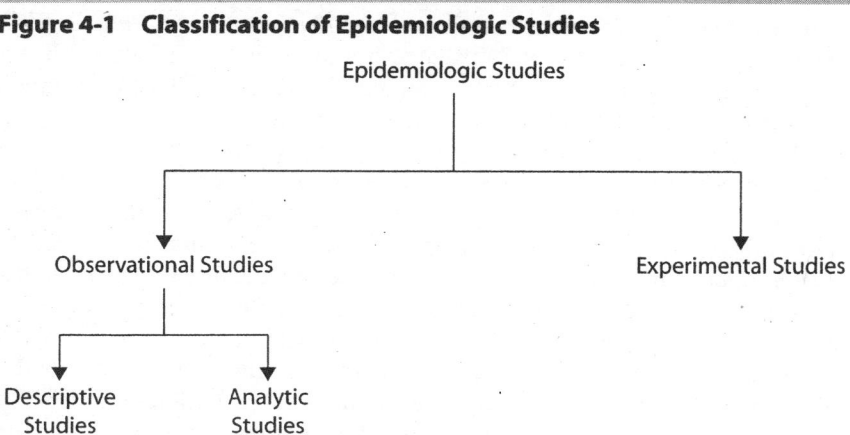

DESCRIPTIVE STUDIES

Descriptive epidemiologic studies are a class of epidemiologic studies that focus on characterizing health-related occurrences by person, place, or time variables and that have *no* specified *a priori* **hypotheses** to test. That is, they are not designed to test preconceived expectations about relationships between specified exposures and outcomes. Instead, their focus is on describing *what exists*. For example, an investigator may study the frequency and quantity of alcohol consumption among college students according to various demographic factors, such as age, sex, race/ethnicity, socioeconomic background, and academic level. In this example, the investigator is simply observing what exists in a defined population in order to discover patterns that may later turn out to have some predictive value. The investigator may find, for instance, that male college students drink significantly more alcohol on a weekly basis than female college students of the same age, race, and academic level. It is important to keep in mind that while descriptive studies may be used to identify statistical associations between various exposures and outcomes in a population, they are not designed to test *a priori* hypotheses. Any associations found in a descriptive study represent *non-hypothesized* relationships that will need to be confirmed by more advanced epidemiologic studies before one can even consider the possibility of cause and effect. In fact, sometimes descriptive studies are conducted as **exploratory studies** where the investigators literally search for any relationships that might be potentially important. Later, if they choose to, they can test any hypotheses they develop using analytic or experimental designs. In essence, descriptive studies with the specific objective of identifying associations between various exposures and outcomes that are not predetermined are "hypothesis-seeking" studies versus "hypothesis-testing" studies. Thus, one advantage of descriptive studies is that they can be helpful in generating hypotheses about disease causation. Descriptive studies are also useful in demonstrating temporal trends, such as the secular trend in the U.S. infant mortality rate for all races, which has been characterized by a marked, sustained decline of over 70 percent since 1965.[2] In addition, descriptive studies may be valuable to health professionals by providing a profile of susceptible populations that can aid diagnosis and assist in planning and allocating scarce health care resources in communities.[3]

Two types of epidemiologic studies that are commonly descriptive in nature are **ecological studies** and **cross-sectional studies**. Sometimes they are referred to as *descriptive ecological studies* and *descriptive cross-sectional studies*, respectively, to distinguish them from their analytic counterparts—*analytic ecological studies* and *analytic cross-sectional studies*. Generally, no such distinction is made. The studies are simply referred to as either ecological or cross-sectional studies regardless of whether the focus is descriptive or analytic. One has to examine the context the terms are used in to determine how the studies are best classified. Because of similarities in design between the descriptive and analytic versions of these studies, they are discussed in the section on analytic studies so as to avoid unnecessary repetition.

Descriptive ecological and cross-sectional studies may or may not involve original data collection. In fact, most ecological studies, and a fair number of cross-sectional studies, use data previously collected by other sources (e.g., federal or state agencies, private health insurers, school systems) to describe specific health-related occurrences. In addition to descriptive ecological and cross-sectional studies, there are two types of descriptive studies commonly used in clinical epidemiology (chapter 1). These are:

- Case reports
- Case series

A **case report** is a detailed description about an individual patient. Published case reports provide a valuable service by bringing unusual conditions or novel treatments to the attention of other clinicians. This in turn can lead to speculation about possible causes of the condition or potential therapies. At the same time, case reports often stimulate further epidemiologic investigation. Birth defects resulting from thalidomide, a drug widely used in Europe during the 1960s for morning sickness, and the condition fetal alcohol syndrome were first described in case reports.[4] A more recent example is the case report of a 15-year old Wisconsin girl,[5] who is the only person known to have survived rabies infection without receiving some form of prophylaxis before development of the disease.[6] Normally, rabies is 100 percent fatal unless one receives the rabies vaccine before clinical signs and symptoms develop. This landmark case represents an exception.

Though common in clinical epidemiology, case reports are not in the strictest sense true epidemiologic studies. For one thing, there is no appropriate comparison group, a hallmark of epidemiologic studies. For another thing, case reports are not population-based, another characteristic of epidemiologic studies.

A **case series** is an extension of the case report that describes the characteristics of a group or cluster of individuals with the same condition. Case series attempt to quantify various aspects of the group so as to present a relatively complete profile of the illness or its treatment, which may generate hypotheses for further study. It was a case series, for example, that first identified toxic shock syndrome, which was later determined by analytic epidemiologic studies to be strongly associated with the use of Rely brand tampons.[7] Today, we know that this rare but severe condition is associated with strains of *Staphylococcus aureus*, a toxin-producing bacterium.[8] Like case reports, case series are not true epidemiologic studies because there is no appropriate comparison group (i.e., similar individuals without the condition). Nevertheless, as was true for toxic shock syndrome, a case series may suggest hypotheses that can be followed up using controlled epidemiologic studies.

ANALYTIC STUDIES

Unlike descriptive studies, *analytic studies* are designed to test *a priori* hypotheses about associations between specified exposures and outcomes.

Like descriptive studies, however, they are *observational* and not experimental (see figure 4-1). There are several common types of analytic studies employed in epidemiology. These include:

- Ecological studies
- Cross-sectional studies
- Case-control studies
- Cohort studies
- Hybrid studies

As discussed in the previous section, ecological and cross-sectional studies may descriptive or analytic in design. The major difference is the *intent* of the study. If the intent is simply to *describe* a health-related occurrence by person, place, or time variables, whether or not statistical associations are identified, then the study is descriptive. On the other hand, if the intent is to *test* one or more *a priori* hypotheses, even in a preliminary way, then the study is analytic. This is also true for the other types of study designs discussed in this section (e.g., an exploratory case-control study is best classified as a descriptive study). The following discussion, however, focuses on analytic designs.

Ecological Studies

In order to understand ecological studies, it is important to know what is meant by **unit of analysis**. Unit of analysis refers to that which is being studied.[9] In most epidemiologic studies the unit of analysis is the individual. In other words, epidemiologists typically study individuals in order to draw conclusions about groups or populations. To say, for example, that smokers are at a significantly higher risk of lung cancer than nonsmokers is to draw a conclusion about a group (smokers) presumably based on a study of individuals, some of whom smoke and some of whom do not. Unlike most epidemiologic studies, the unit of analysis in an ecological study is the *group* versus the individual. The group, or **ecological unit**, as it has been traditionally referred to in epidemiology, represents an aggregate of individuals, such a country, state, county, city, census tract, hospital, or school. As discussed in chapter 9, ecological units can also represent time periods, such as a country in 2007 and 2008, respectively.

Because the unit of analysis is the group in ecological studies, investigators have some *overall* or *summary* measure of exposure and some *overall* or *summary* measure of outcome for each group being compared.[10] Exposure measures may represent mean values or proportions, for example, and outcome measures may be population rates. It is important to note that data on exposure and outcome for individuals have not been collected. For example, an analytic ecological study conducted in Taiwan examined the association between water chlorination (the exposure) and cancer mortality (the outcome) among 28 municipalities (the ecological units).[11] "Chlorinating municipalities" were defined as those in which more than 90 percent of the population was offered chlorinated drinking water, and "nonchlorinating municipalities" were those in which less than five percent of the population was offered chlorinated drinking water. The investigators found a positive correlation between water chlorination and mortality rates from rectal, lung, bladder, and kidney cancers. It is crucial to understand, however, that only municipalities as a whole were studied. The investigators had no comparable data for the individuals within the municipalities. Therefore, the only associations identified by the investigators were at the *group level*. One cannot know what associations, if any, exist at the individual level due to the study design. In other words, it was the chlorinating municipalities that showed the higher rates of cancer mortality when compared to the nonchlorinating municipalities. The association between chlorinated water and cancer mortality among individuals was not examined in this study. If, based on this study, we assume that *individuals* who drink chlorinated water are at a higher risk of dying from these cancers, we commit what is known as an **ecological fallacy**. This is an "error of reasoning" that one makes when group associations are used to draw conclusions about associations at the individual level.[9] The problem with drawing conclusions about individual associations based on group associations can be understood if one considers that it is possible that most of those who died of cancers in the chlorinating municipalities were among the small percentage who were not offered chlorinated drinking water. If so, a positive association between drinking chlorinated water and cancer mortality would probably not exist at the individual level. The problem of an ecological fallacy, however, is not whether a group association also exists at the individual level, it is the inability to know based on the study design. Ecological fallacies are a concern in ecological studies when the real interest is the relationship at the individual level. When the interest is only at the group level, ecological fallacies are not a problem. More is said about this in chapter 9.

Despite some limitations, ecological studies are valuable to epidemiologists. They are relatively quick and inexpensive to perform, and they can reveal potentially important associations between exposures and outcomes at the group level. They are frequently a practical choice for the initial investigation of preliminary hypotheses because they can be completed in a short period of time, often using existing data sources. If positive findings are revealed, they may stimulate studies of similar hypotheses at the individual level. Ecological studies may even be better than individual-level studies in detecting associations when the variability of the exposure is low within populations but high between populations.[12] This is discussed in chapter 9. An example of a research question that might be examined in an ecological study is: do countries with nationalized health care have lower rates of infant mortality than countries without nationalized health care? In this example, the variables, nationalized health care and country-specific infant mortality, are group phenomena that are most appropriately studied at the group level.

Hal Morgenstern has identified three types of ecological study designs commonly used in epidemiology.[13] Each of these designs may be descriptive (Morgenstern calls them exploratory) or analytic. In descriptive (exploratory) ecological studies the primary exposure of potential interest is not measured, only the outcome. Hence, there are no *a priori* hypotheses to test. In *analytic* ecological studies both exposure and outcome are measured, and there are one or more hypotheses. An example of findings from a descriptive ecological study appears in figure 4-2. In this illustration, for each ecological unit only outcomes are described. Specifically, average annual injury death rates for each of 11 different countries are compared. England and Wales have the lowest rate of 31 injury deaths per 100,000 population, while France has the highest rate of 75 injury deaths per 100,000. Scotland is in the middle with an injury death rate of about 50 per 100,000. The data in this example do not appear to suggest any obvious explanations for the pattern. Further analysis, however, may reveal important differences between countries that could serve as a basis for additional studies. Differences in death registration and reporting practices among the countries are possible explanations that have been targeted for further investigation.[14]

Analytic ecological studies are designed to test if exposures of interest are associated with outcomes of interest at the group level. The hypotheses may be preliminary and *non-directional* (i.e., not indicating whether an increase or decrease in outcome is expected based on exposure status), but they are always stated or implied before the study is actually conducted. In other

Figure 4-2   Average Annual Injury Death Rates from a Descriptive Ecological Study

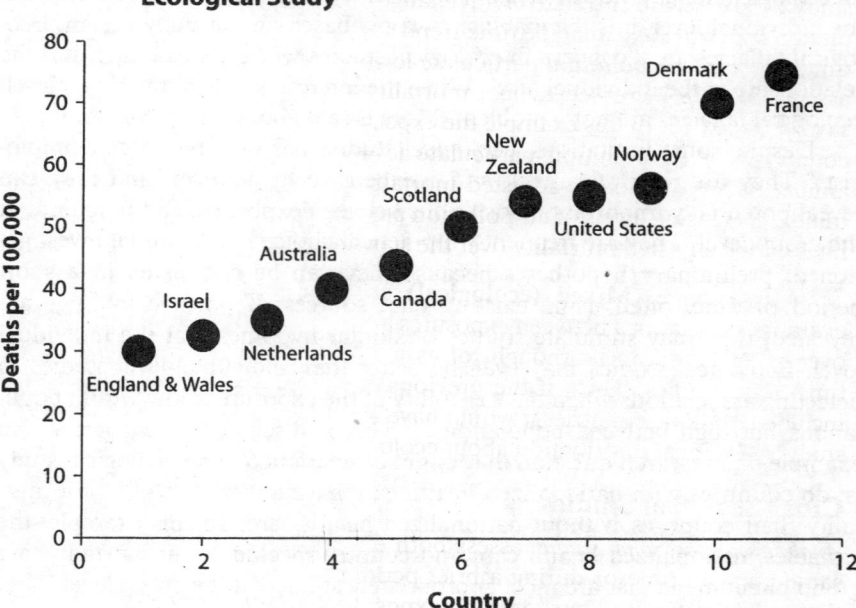

Reference: Fingerhut, L. A., Cox, C. S., Warner, M., et al. (1998). International Comparative Analysis of Injury Mortality: Findings from the ICE on Injury Statistics. *Advance Data from Vital and Health Statistics*, No. 303. Hyattsville, MD: National Center for Health Statistics.

words, they are always predetermined or *a priori* hypotheses. The three types of analytic ecological studies identified by Morgenstern are *multiple-group studies*, *time-trend studies*, and *mixed studies*.[13] These are described below:

Multiple-group studies. **Multiple-group** studies are ecological studies where the ecological units are places (e.g., countries, states, institutions). Generally, several ecological units are examined at the same time to determine if a hypothesized relationship exists between one or more exposures and outcomes. An example of an analytic multiple-group study is one designed test the hypothesis that countries with high levels of dietary fat intake have higher rates of mortality from all causes than countries with low levels of fat intake. To test this hypothesis one might obtain published data on mean dietary fat intake for each of the countries in the **study population** (the sample selected for study)[1] and information on country-specific mortality rates. Of note, these data would likely represent **secondary sources*** that would probably come from different agencies (e.g., the Food and Agricultural Organization and the World Health Organization, respectively). Typically, these data would have been collected independently for other purposes so that linkage at the individual level would not be available.

Time-trend studies. **Time-trend** studies are ecological studies where the ecological units are time periods. They are designed to determine if changes in study exposures are correlated with changes in study outcomes in a single population over time. An analytic time-trend study could be one designed to determine if annual air pollution particulate levels in a rapidly growing country are associated with increased annual mortality rates over a specific time period, say 2000 to 2010. In this example the exposure measure might be annual mean country-wide air pollution particulate levels and the outcome measure the annual country-wide age-adjusted mortality rates. One would seek to determine if increasing levels of air pollution particulates correlated with increasing rates of age-adjusted mortality over the stated 10-year period.

Mixed studies. **Mixed (ecological)** studies are ecological studies that examine associations between exposures and outcomes for several populations over time. They can be thought of as a combination of multiple-group and time-trend studies. Thus, if the previous example of a time-trend study had included multiple countries it would have been classified as a mixed ecological study. Additional information about ecological studies appears in chapter 9.

Cross-Sectional Studies

Analytic cross-sectional studies assess both exposure and outcome status at the same point in time or during a brief period of time, where the individual is the unit of analysis. Thus, data on exposure and outcome can be said to be

*Secondary sources are sources of data that have not been collected firsthand. Therefore, they represent non-original sources. When investigators use other people's data in their research instead of data they have collected themselves, they are relying on secondary sources. **Primary sources** represent original data collected firsthand.[9]

collected simultaneously. These studies generally survey, interview, or examine a representative sample of individuals from a given population. Figure 4-3 illustrates the basic design of an analytic cross-sectional study. Note that once the sample is selected, both exposure and outcome status are determined during the same time period. Being analytic, there are one or more *a priori* hypotheses about relationships between specified exposures and outcomes that the investigators seek to examine. An example is a study conducted by J. A. Metz and colleagues that sought to determine if blood pressure and dietary intake of calcium (the exposures) were associated with bone mass (the outcome).[15] After identifying a suitable study population, the investigators measured the subjects' blood pressure, assessed their dietary intake, and tested their bone mass all in the same time frame. They found that blood pressure levels showed an inverse association, and calcium intake a positive association, with regional measures of bone mass, factors associated with the likelihood of developing osteoporosis. Because the time sequence in which exposure and outcome occurred was not clear, the authors were careful not to suggest that the associations were causal. In order for an exposure to be classified as a cause of an outcome it must, among other things, *precede* the outcome. This, by the way, is one of the limitations of most cross-sectional studies. It is often impossible to establish a clear time sequence between exposure and outcome because these attributes are assessed at the same time. Thus, one cannot always be sure whether the exposure preceded the outcome, the outcome preceded the exposure, or both occurred at the same time.

Figure 4-3 Cross-Sectional Study Design

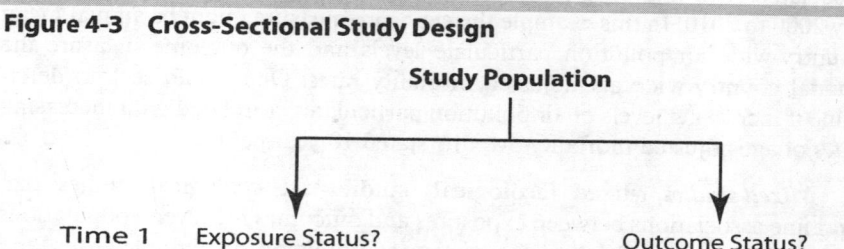

In a *descriptive* cross-sectional study, there are no *a priori* hypotheses; the study is designed simply to uncover patterns of distribution by person, place, or time variables that may suggest hypotheses for further study. In some descriptive cross-sectional studies, only exposure or only outcome is assessed. A study designed to determine HIV prevalence,* that is, the number of those infected with HIV, in a specific community at a specific time among various

*Prevalence, which is discussed in chapter 5, is the usual measure of disease occurrence in cross-sectional studies. Generally, when studies employ prevalence, one may suspect that they are descriptive or analytic versions of cross-sectional studies. In fact, some epidemiologists refer to cross-sectional studies as prevalence studies.

age and racial/ethnic groups, is an example of a descriptive cross-sectional study as long as there are no *a priori* hypotheses to test. Cross-sectional studies need to be well designed if the results are to be meaningful. Additional details regarding the cross-sectional design and its limitations, interpretation, and analysis can be found in chapter 9.

Case-Control Studies

Traditionally, **case-control studies** have been described as studies where individual subjects are classified according to their outcome status before determining their exposure status. It was taught, more or less, that investigators simply selected a group of subjects with the outcome of interest (the cases) and a comparable group of subjects without the outcome of interest (the controls). The cases and controls were then compared regarding their history with regard to the exposure of interest (see figure 4-4). This simplistic view of the case-control study is no longer accurate. Modern conceptions of the case-control study are of a study in which cases are selected from a well-defined population, known as the *source population* (chapter 8), and controls are selected from the same population so as to represent the exposure frequency of that population. In this way, one determines the relative frequency of exposed and unexposed subjects who developed the disease of interest. Details of case-control design are discussed in chapter 10. Ideally, only *new* cases are included in the study, and only *past* exposures are assessed. This is done to maintain an appropriate temporal (time) sequence between exposure and outcome, which is necessary to establish causal relationships (see chapter 7). A positive association between an exposure and outcome resulting from a case-control study is said to exist when the proportion of cases with the exposure is significantly greater than the proportion of controls with the exposure, all other factors being equal. The case-control method is illustrated in a study of the relationship between environmental tobacco smoke (ETS) and lung cancer. In this study, the researchers interviewed 292 nonsmoking subjects

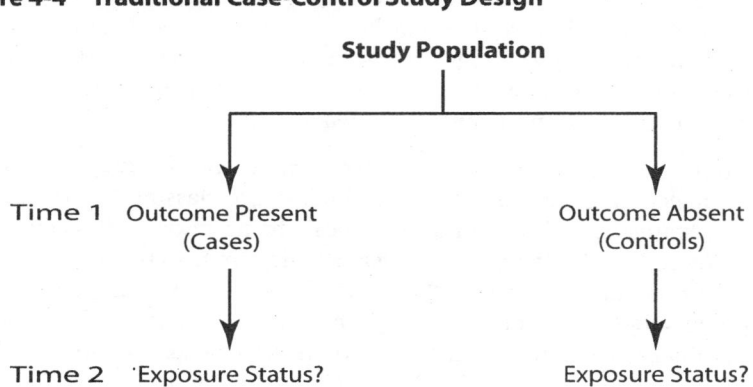

Figure 4-4   Traditional Case-Control Study Design

Study Population

Time 1   Outcome Present   Outcome Absent
          (Cases)   (Controls)

Time 2   Exposure Status?   Exposure Status?

with lung cancer (the cases) and 1,338 nonsmoking subjects without lung cancer (the controls) about prior exposure to ETS. Among the findings was an elevated risk of lung cancer among those who were exposed to the highest levels of ETS in their transportation vehicles compared to those who were not.[16] Although usually analytic in design, case-control studies can also be descriptive (exploratory) when there is no explicit or implied intent to test *a priori* hypotheses between exposures and outcomes.

Cohort Studies

Cohort studies involve initially classifying members of the study population by exposure status and then following them longitudinally to determine their subsequent outcome status (see figure 4-5). Differences in the occurrences of outcomes among the exposed and unexposed groups provide a basis for determining if there is an association between the exposure and outcome as originally hypothesized. Although conceptually the modern case-control study can be considered a type of cohort study (see chapter 10 for details), to the casual observer they may appear to be design opposites. They are not, however, nor should they be viewed as such.

Figure 4-5   Basic Cohort Study Design

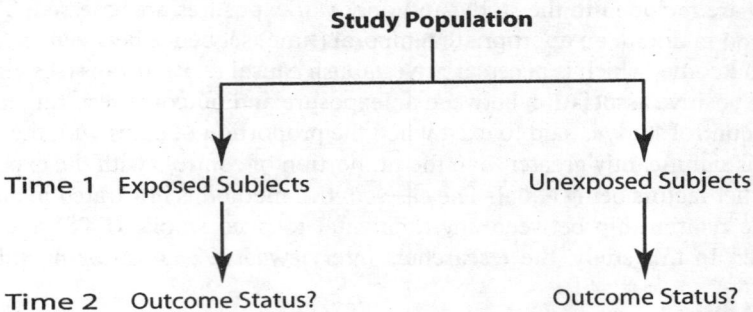

The design of cohort studies may be *prospective, retrospective,* or *mixed.* Prospective and retrospective designs are described briefly in this section. A more detailed discussion of cohort studies, including pertinent aspects of design, analysis, and interpretation, appears in chapter 11.

Prospective cohort studies.   In a **prospective cohort study** (PCS) individual subjects without the outcome of interest are classified on the basis of exposure status according to the hypothesis being tested. The subjects are then followed longitudinally into the *future* to determine if the development of the study outcome is significantly greater in the exposed compared to the unexposed subjects. A finding that the incidence (see chapter 5) of the outcome is materially different in the exposed versus the unexposed subjects implies that the exposure is associated with the outcome, all other factors being equal. Prospective cohort studies, especially those investigating chronic diseases, typically take a long time to complete. The investigators must provide sufficient time for the study outcome to develop, which may take many years if the disease has a long induction or latency period (chapter 3). The fact that the disease has already occurred in case-control studies removes the need to wait for disease development during a follow-up period.

The Framingham Heart Study, which was referred to in chapter 1, is an example of a PCS. Another example is a study conducted by E. J. Jacobs, M. J. Thun, and L. F. Apicella.[17] This was a U.S.-based study, which ran from 1982 to 1991 and examined the relationship between cigar smoking (the study exposure) and death from coronary heart disease (the study outcome). The study population included 121,278 men 30 years of age and older. Each subject completed a baseline questionnaire in 1982 designed to assess smoking history and determine the presence of other risk factors. Only subjects who were free of heart disease at baseline were included in the study. The results showed that males less than 75 years old who smoked cigars from the beginning of the study had a 30 percent higher risk of dying from coronary heart disease by the end of the study compared to those who did not smoke cigars. It is important to note that this investigation excluded subjects who already had heart disease at the beginning of the study. This is critical if the findings are to be attributed to the observed exposure. It is also important in PCSs to reassess the exposure at regular intervals if it can change over time. In this way, subject exposure can be reclassified where necessary and the change accounted for in the analysis. These and other relevant design issues are examined in chapter 11.

Retrospective cohort studies. The **retrospective cohort study** (RCS) is a variation of the basic cohort study design shown in figure 4-5. In an RCS an *historical cohort** is reconstructed from existing data sources before the study begins. The cohort is considered historical because it represents individual subjects as they once were in the past. For example, researchers conducting an RCS on the effects of pesticide exposure on cancer mortality could reconstruct a cohort of factory workers who were employed by a particular pesticide manufacturer from 1970 to 1975 using personnel records supplied by the company. Because of the time element, we would expect few of the members of this cohort to be working for the company today. In fact, many may even be deceased. Nevertheless, the attempt is to assemble *on paper*, so to speak, a cohort that would have existed between 1970 and 1975. Once the cohort has been identified, the next step is to classify each member of the cohort by exposure status. This can be difficult unless adequate records are available to identify exposed and unexposed subjects. One might classify the exposed subjects, for instance, as those who worked with pesticides on a routine basis and the unexposed subjects as those who did not. This information may be available

---

*A cohort, formally defined in chapter 11, is a group of individuals who are followed over time.

from archived company records indicating past job classifications. Other records (e.g., company medical records) would also need to be reviewed to identify factors that could distort the association or otherwise invalidate the findings. These factors, known as *confounding factors*, are discussed specifically in chapter 8 and elsewhere in the text. Assuming this information was available, the final step would be to see what happened to each of the subjects. This would involve following up the cohort members from the 1970-75 period to the present time. This might be done by contacting the subjects themselves, their families or relatives, or by consulting cancer registries (chapter 10), death certificates, or other applicable data sources. We would want to know whether the exposed subjects had a higher mortality rate from cancer than the unexposed subjects, and if so, to what degree. In other words, the pertinent question is: To what extent is pesticide exposure associated with cancer mortality?

Both RCSs and PCSs assess exposure status *first* and outcome status *second*; however, this is done in different time frames. Prospective cohort studies assess exposure status in the *present* (at the beginning of the study) and outcome status in the *future* (sometime after the beginning of the study). In contrast, RCSs assess exposure in the *past* (at the time the cohort actually existed) and outcome status up to the *present* (up to the time of the beginning of the study). Thus, RCSs follow the cohort from the past up to the present, and PCSs follow the cohort from the present into the future. This difference in time frames is illustrated in figure 4-6. As mentioned earlier, in addition to prospective and retrospective cohort studies, there are also mixed studies, which involve aspects of both the prospective and retrospective designs. More detail is provided in chapter 11.

Figure 4-6   Retrospective versus Prospective Cohort Study Designs

Retrospective Cohort

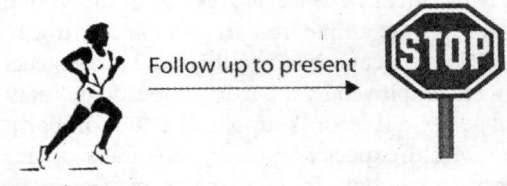

Follow up to present

Start in Past

Prospective Cohort

Follow into future

Start in Present

Hybrid Studies

Not all analytic epidemiologic studies fit neatly into the above categories. Some studies combine features of two or more types. These studies can be referred to as **hybrid studies**.[18] While a complete discussion of the possible designs is beyond the scope of this book, it should be helpful to highlight a few of the more common types.

Nested case-control studies.   The popular **nested case-control study** is a case-control study embedded (nested) within an existing, defined cohort. The cohort may be part of a prospective or retrospective cohort study, randomized controlled trial, or another source. The cases normally consist of all, or a representative sample of, the cases generated in the cohort during a specified follow-up period.[12] Typically, for each case, one or more controls is selected randomly from all non-cases in the cohort that are present at the time the case occurs. In most instances, the controls are matched to the cases with regard to the length of follow-up time. This way the cases and controls will have been observed for the same amount of time. This offers certain statistical advantages in the analysis of the findings, but other sampling schemes for control selection are sometimes used.[19, 20]

An example of a nested case-control study is one where the investigators examined whether selected blood cholesterol and triglyceride levels increased the risk of ischemic stroke in a cohort of male physicians. The subjects were drawn the first Physicians' Health Study, a large randomized controlled trial with over 22,000 participants. Specifically, 296 cases of ischemic stroke for whom blood samples had been collected at the beginning of the study were matched with an equal number of controls based on age, tobacco use, and follow-up time. Potential controls included all participants free of stroke at the time each stroke case occurred and for whom baseline blood samples were also available. Overall, no significant association between the measures examined and ischemic stroke was found in this study.[21] Taking blood samples at the beginning of a prospective longitudinal study and storing them for later analysis has become a relatively common practice in recent years and has facilitated the use of the nested case-control design.

One reason nested case-control studies are appealing is because of the increasing number of large, well-established cohorts that can serve as data sources.[12] Another reason is because the cases and controls are more likely to be comparable than in many traditional case-control studies since they both come from the same, usually well-defined, cohort. In many traditional case-control studies the cases and controls are selected from different populations so that they are not always strictly comparable. Thus, nested case-control studies have the effect of minimizing potential *selection bias* and *confounding* (chapter 8) that can be problematic in traditional case-control studies.[1, 12, 18] Finally, nested case-control studies are economical compared to many cohort studies or randomized controlled trials. For example, if a large cohort study failed to collect certain information necessary to address a pertinent research question, a nested case-control study could be conducted and would not require the data to be collected on all subjects in the cohort but just on the cases and a sample of the controls.[12] In the example cited above, the research question addressed in the nested case-control study required data on only a fraction of the 22,000 plus subjects in the original cohort. Though classified as hybrid studies because they are embedded in a cohort, these studies are also properly regarded as a special type of case-control study. Therefore, they are often discussed in connection with case-control studies.

Case-cohort studies. The **case-cohort study** can also be classified as a hybrid study or a special type of case-control study. It is a variation of the nested case-control study. The cases are selected in the same manner as in the nested case-control study, but instead of randomly selecting controls from cohort members who have not developed the outcome at the time each case occurs, a sample is randomly selected from *all* members of the cohort before the cases develop, typically at the *beginning* of the study. This is done even though some of the controls may later become cases. In addition to many of the advantages of the nested case-control study, the case-cohort study provides a convenient way of identifying controls for subsequent case-control studies and can also provide data on the prevalence of various risk factors among the cohort.[12, 22]

Panel studies. A **panel study** is a type of hybrid study that combines features of the cross-sectional and prospective cohort designs. It can be viewed as a series of cross-sectional studies conducted on the *same* subjects (the panel) at successive time intervals, sometimes referred to as *waves*. This longitudinal design allows investigators to relate changes in one variable to changes in other variables over time.[1, 10] For example, a California study identified the employment and depression status of a group at the first wave of a two-wave panel study. At the second wave, the investigators found that those who were not depressed at the first wave but who subsequently lost their jobs were over twice as likely to suffer depressive symptoms as those who were still employed.[23] In other words, the investigators were able to link changes in employment status to changes in depression status at the individual level. An example of a nationally-based panel study is the Health and Retirement Study sponsored by the National Institute on Aging. The purpose of this study is to provide researchers and policy makers with a database for the study of interrelationships of health, retirement, and other factors.[24]

The typical unit of analysis for panel studies is the individual or individual household. Though panel studies can reveal important changes in a group over time, they can be affected by significant attrition among the respondents, especially if there are several waves in the study. Respondents may become weary of repeated participation or may otherwise be lost to follow up due to address changes, death, or other factors. The most common methods of data collection are questionnaires, interviews, and examinations. Unlike cohort studies, there is no requirement that the subjects be free of the study outcome at the beginning of a panel study. Depending on research intent, panel studies may be descriptive or analytic. Analytic panel studies test *a priori* hypotheses.

Repeated surveys. **Repeated surveys** (sometimes referred to as *repeated cross-sectional studies, serial surveys, sequential cross-sectional studies,* or *trend studies*) are hybrid studies in which successive cross-sectional studies are performed over time on the same study population, but each sample is selected independently. Therefore, unlike panel studies, the actual subjects will differ somewhat from one survey to the next, although the samples can be expected to be representative of the study population as a whole. Since panel studies follow the *same individuals* from survey to survey, investigators can link individual exposures to individual outcomes over time. This is not possible with repeated surveys. Repeated surveys are useful, however, in identifying overall trends in health status and factors that may help to explain them.[18] Several large repeated surveys are conducted by the National Center for Health Statistics. Examples are the Health and Nutrition Examination Surveys (NHANES; see appendix B) and certain studies derived from them. For example, researchers at the University of Chicago used data from NHANES conducted in 1971-1974, 1976-1980, 1988-1994, and 1999-2000 to examine trends in the relationship between obesity and socioeconomic status (SES) among U.S. adults over time. The researchers found that the disparity in obesity across SES has declined over the past three decades. Interestingly, this has occurred during a period when obesity has been increasing significantly.[25] Unlike panel studies, repeated surveys show no cumulative losses to follow up since new samples are taken with each successive survey. Otherwise, like panel studies, questionnaires, interviews, and examinations are common methods of data gathering, and the studies can be considered descriptive or analytic depending on whether or not *a priori* hypotheses are being tested. Also, like panel studies, repeated surveys are considered longitudinal studies, and the unit of analysis is typically the individual or the individual household. A summary of the differences in panel studies and repeated surveys appears in table 4-1.

EXPERIMENTAL STUDIES

Like analytic studies, experimental studies are designed to test *a priori* hypotheses about associations between specific exposures and outcomes. The major difference is that in experimental studies the investigators have direct control over the study conditions.[1] Of particular significance, the investigators control the exposure (i.e., the intervention). Though very important, these studies are employed less frequently in epidemiology than observational studies due in part to ethical concerns. Experimental studies on people are only feasible under conditions of uncertainty about the value of the intervention. This is especially true if serious side effects from the intervention are

Table 4-1 A Quick Comparison of Panel Studies and Repeated Surveys

Panel Study	Repeated Surveys
Longitudinal in design	Longitudinal in design
Uses the same subjects during each wave of the study	Uses a new representative sample of the targeted population during each phase of the study
Unit of analysis is usually the individual or the individual household	Unit of analysis is usually the individual or the individual household
Affected by cumulative attrition of subjects during the course of the study	Not affected by cumulative attrition of subjects during the course of the study
Can relate trends to changes in individuals	Cannot relate trends to changes in individuals
May be descriptive or analytic in design	May be descriptive or analytic in design
Commonly employs questionnaires, interviews, or examinations to gather data	Commonly employs questionnaires, interviews, or examinations to gather data

possible. In general, the investigators must show that the intervention has enough promise to justify exposing some individuals but not so much as to justify denying others of the potential benefits.[26]

There are two major types of experimental studies in epidemiology:

- Randomized controlled trials
- Group randomized trials

Randomized controlled trials (RCTs) are often referred to generically as **clinical trials** probably because of their historical and frequent use with patients in clinical care facilities. This design, however, has applications that go beyond the clinical setting. Therefore, RCTs better reflect this broader use. In addition, not all clinical trials involve randomization, so the term clinical trials is not always a good substitute for RCTs. Other common names for RCTs appear in table 4-2. **Group randomized trials** (GRTs) are also known as **cluster randomized trials** or sometimes **randomized community trials**, which is more appropriately applied to GRTs where entire communities are the units of interest.[27] Other common designations, which are often slight variations of the foregoing terms, are provided in table 4-2. An important distinction between RCTs and GRTs regards who is assigned to the experimental and control groups. In RCTs *individuals* are randomly assigned, while in GRTs *clusters of individuals* (i.e., intact groups) are randomly assigned. A brief description of these designs is presented below. More detail appears in chapter 12.

Table 4-2 Typical Characteristics of the Most Common Analytic and Experimental Epidemiologic Study Designs

Type of Epidemiologic Study	Typical Exposure-Outcome Assessment Sequence	Key Identifying Characteristics	Some Alternative Designations
Analytic Designs			
Ecological Study	Outcome and exposure status usually assessed during the same time period	• Unit of analysis is the group • Conclusions are usually tentative	Ecologic study, correlational study
Cross-Sectional Study	Outcome and exposure status assessed during the same time period	• Unit of analysis is the individual • Conclusions are usually tentative	Prevalence study, prevalence survey
Case-Control Study	Outcome status assessed before exposure status	• Unit of analysis is the individual • Ideally, exposure precedes outcome	Retrospective study, case-referent study, case-comparison study
Prospective Cohort Study	Exposure status assessed before outcome status	• Unit of analysis is the individual • Follow up proceeds from study initiation forward in time	Prospective study, concurrent cohort study, cohort study, longitudinal study, follow-up study, incidence study
Retrospective Cohort Study	Exposure status assessed before outcome status	• Unit of analysis is the individual • Follow up proceeds from an earlier period up to time of study initiation	Historical cohort study, nonconcurrent cohort study, historical prospective study
Experimental Designs			
Randomized Controlled Trial	Exposure status assessed before outcome status	• Unit of analysis is the individual • Investigator controls exposure status	Clinical trial, randomized clinical trial, randomized controlled clinical trial
Group Randomized Trial	Exposure status assessed before outcome status	• Unit of assignment is the group • Unit of analysis is usually the individual • Investigator controls exposure status	Cluster randomized trial, clustered randomization trial, randomized community trial, community randomized trial, community trial, community intervention trial

Randomized Controlled Trials

Randomized controlled trials involve at least three fundamental steps:

1. Selection of an appropriate study population
2. Randomization of subjects into experimental and control groups
3. Follow up and outcome assessment

Traditionally, the selection of the study population was considered a three-step process (see figure 4-7). First, a *reference population* was selected. This was to represent the population to which the investigator hoped to generalize the study findings. Next, an *experimental population* was defined. This was to be a practical representation of the reference population. Finally, volunteers from the experimental population who met the eligibility criteria for the study were selected for inclusion in the study population.[26] Contemporary epidemiologic thinking, however, discounts the need for a reference population. Instead, the focus is on establishing the efficacy or effectiveness of an intervention and worrying about generalizing the findings later. Therefore, like all analytic studies, RCTs start with the identification of a *source population* (defined in chapter 8) from which the study population is derived. The study population for an RCT will have strict eligibility requirements aimed at improving the integrity of the study design rather than promoting its generalizability to other populations.

One of the most important aspects of RCTs is **randomization** (also called *random allocation, random assignment*, etc.). Randomization is the random distribution of study subjects into the experimental and control groups. This helps assure that all subjects have the same probability of being assigned to an experimental group, which receives the intervention, or to a control group, which usually receives the standard regimen or no regimen at all.[28] If properly applied, randomization eliminates *selection bias* (chapter 8) in the assign-

Figure 4-7   Traditional Design of a Basic Randomized Controlled Trial

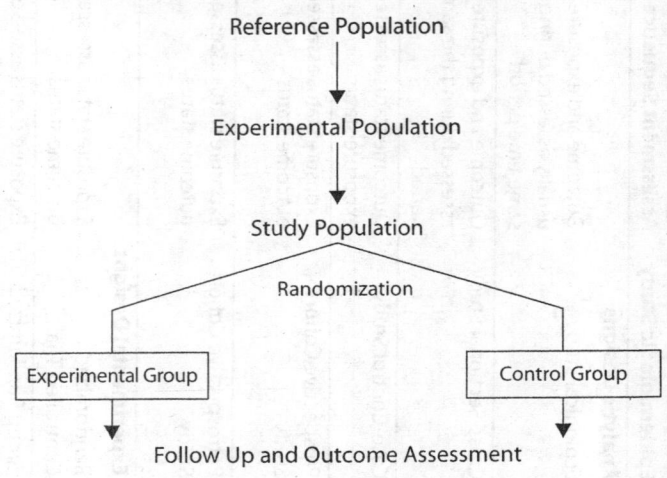

ment of subjects and minimizes *confounding* (chapter 8), which can result because of differences between the experimental and control groups. Randomization thus increases study *validity* (chapter 8), making the RCT the most powerful research design in epidemiology. Randomization tends to work best when the study population is large.

There are two basic types of RCTs:

- Preventive trials
- Therapeutic trials

Preventive trials are also known as **prophylactic trials**. In general, these RCTs focus on individuals *without clinical manifestations of the disease of interest.* Their purpose is to determine if a particular intervention reduces the clinical occurrence of the disease. For example, a large preventive trial, the Women's Health Initiative Dietary Modification Trial, was conducted to assess the effects of a low-fat eating pattern on the occurrence of invasive colorectal cancer in postmenopausal women.[29] Over 48,000 postmenopausal women, 50-79 years of age, were randomized to the dietary modification intervention (the experimental group) or a control group, which consisted of subjects who continued their usual eating patterns. The investigators did not find any significant difference in the incidence of invasive colorectal cancer between the experimental and control groups during an approximate eight-year follow-up period. Since the women did not have colorectal cancer to begin with and since the study was designed to determine if a low-fat diet reduced the occurrence of colorectal cancer, this study can be classified as a preventive or prophylactic trial.

Therapeutic trials focus on patients *with the disease of interest.* The objective is to test interventions that might cure the disease, prevent recurrences, or improve the patients' quality of life. Therapeutic trials are commonly used in testing the efficacy of new drugs and medical or surgical procedures. Clinical trials are examples. The titles of the following published studies illustrate the variety of possible therapeutic trials:

"A Randomized, Controlled Trial of the Effects of Remote, Intercessory Prayer on Outcomes in Patients Admitted to the Coronary Care Unit"[30]

"Effectiveness of Manual Physical Therapy and Exercise in Osteoarthritis of the Knee. A Randomized, Controlled Trial"[31]

In general, preventive trials focus primarily on primary prevention, while therapeutic trials focus primarily on tertiary prevention. Levels of prevention were discussed in chapter 3. Preventive and therapeutic trials are discussed again briefly in chapter 12.

Group Randomized Trials

While RCTs involve the random assignment of *individuals* to experimental and control groups, GRTs involve the random assignment of *groups of individuals* (e.g., schools, hospitals, entire communities) to intervention and control conditions. For example, eight schools may be randomly assigned to either receive an intervention or to serve as controls such that four of the schools end up in the intervention group and four in the control group.

Group randomized trials involve at least four important steps:

1. Selection of the participating groups
2. Collection of baseline data on the study outcomes and other factors
3. Randomization of groups to intervention and control conditions
4. Follow up, outcome assessment, and evaluation

An example of a GRT involving entire communities is Communities Mobilizing for Change on Alcohol (CMCA).[32] This experimental study involved 15 communities that were randomly assigned to either a community organizing intervention designed to reduce the accessibility of alcohol to adolescents under the legal drinking age or a control condition. The results showed that the CMCA intervention had some significant and beneficial effects on the personal behaviors of 18–20 year olds and on the practices of some of the alcohol establishments, based on data collected before and after the intervention. Another example involved a study of 20 preschools conducted by University of Texas researchers at the M. D. Anderson Cancer Center in Houston. In this GRT the preschools were randomly assigned to intervention or control conditions in order to evaluate the effectiveness of a strategy to improve parents' practices relating to the protection of their pre-school children from the effects of sun exposure.[33] As mentioned earlier, GRTs are discussed in more detail in chapter 12.

Quasi-Experimental Studies

A **quasi-experimental study** is one where the investigators do not have full control over the assignment or timing of the intervention but where the study is still conducted as if it were an experiment.[1] Trials where subjects are not randomly assigned to experimental and control groups are examples of quasi-experimental studies. In many group trials, for example, randomization is not always feasible. Sometimes practical matters dictate whether or not random assignment is possible, or even desirable. For example, perhaps only one school, hospital, or community will agree to an intervention, or perhaps one of the groups has resources that will make the intervention easier to implement, such as a local television station for broadcasting health promotion messages. Where possible, random assignment of groups to experimental and control conditions is the ideal since it guards against unconscious or conscious preferences on the part of the investigators that could bias study results. Technically, trials that do not involve random allocation cannot be termed RCTs or GRTs since by definition no randomization is involved.

A classic example of a non-randomized group trial is the Newburgh-Kingston Caries-Fluoride Study that began about 1944.[34] Two cities in New York, Newburgh and Kingston, agreed to participate in the "experiment." Both cities had populations of about 30,000 and were approximately 35 miles from each other on the West Bank of the Hudson River. Both cities were also using fluoride-deficient water. After collecting baseline data on the number of decayed, missing, and filled (DMF) teeth in the two cities, Newburgh's water supply was subjected to continuous fluoridation beginning in 1945. The fluoride content of Kingston's water was not altered. After ten years of follow up, child and adolescent rates of DMF teeth were substantially lower in Newburgh than in Kingston. In the youngest-age group reported, the rate of DMF teeth after 10 years was 58 percent lower in the experimental versus the control community. In a published article of their findings the authors stated that the analysis "demonstrates conclusively two important facts—fluoridation is effective in reducing dental caries and it is a safe public health practice."[34(p235)]

Another type of study that some have classified as a quasi-experimental study is the **natural experiment**.[35] This design was briefly referred to in chapter 2 in connection with Dr. John Snow and one of his famous studies of cholera deaths in London during the 1850s. It is also referred to briefly in chapter 12. Technically speaking, a natural experiment is an observational study that *appears* as an "experiment of opportunity." In other words, it represents a situation in nature that *mimics* an experimental study. It is not a true experiment, however, because it is unplanned, and it is also not a quasi-experimental study since there is no actual intervention.[1] Kenneth J. Rothman refers to it as "a cohort study that simulates what would occur in an experiment."[36(p60)]

IDENTIFYING EPIDEMIOLOGIC STUDY DESIGNS

By now you should have a good idea of the basic epidemiologic study designs and should be able to identify them in the public health and biomedical literature. To assist you in this task, exhibit 4-1 presents an algorithm for identify-

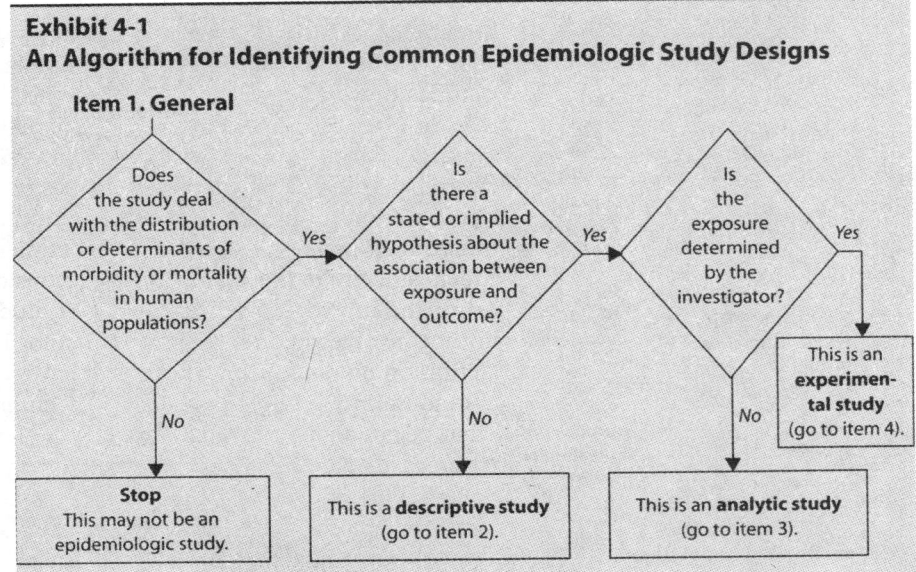

Exhibit 4-1
An Algorithm for Identifying Common Epidemiologic Study Designs

Item 1. General

Does the study deal with the distribution or determinants of morbidity or mortality in human populations? — Yes → Is there a stated or implied hypothesis about the association between exposure and outcome? — Yes → Is the exposure determined by the investigator? — Yes → This is an **experimental study** (go to item 4).

No → **Stop** This may not be an epidemiologic study.

No → This is a **descriptive study** (go to item 2).

No → This is an **analytic study** (go to item 3).

(continued)

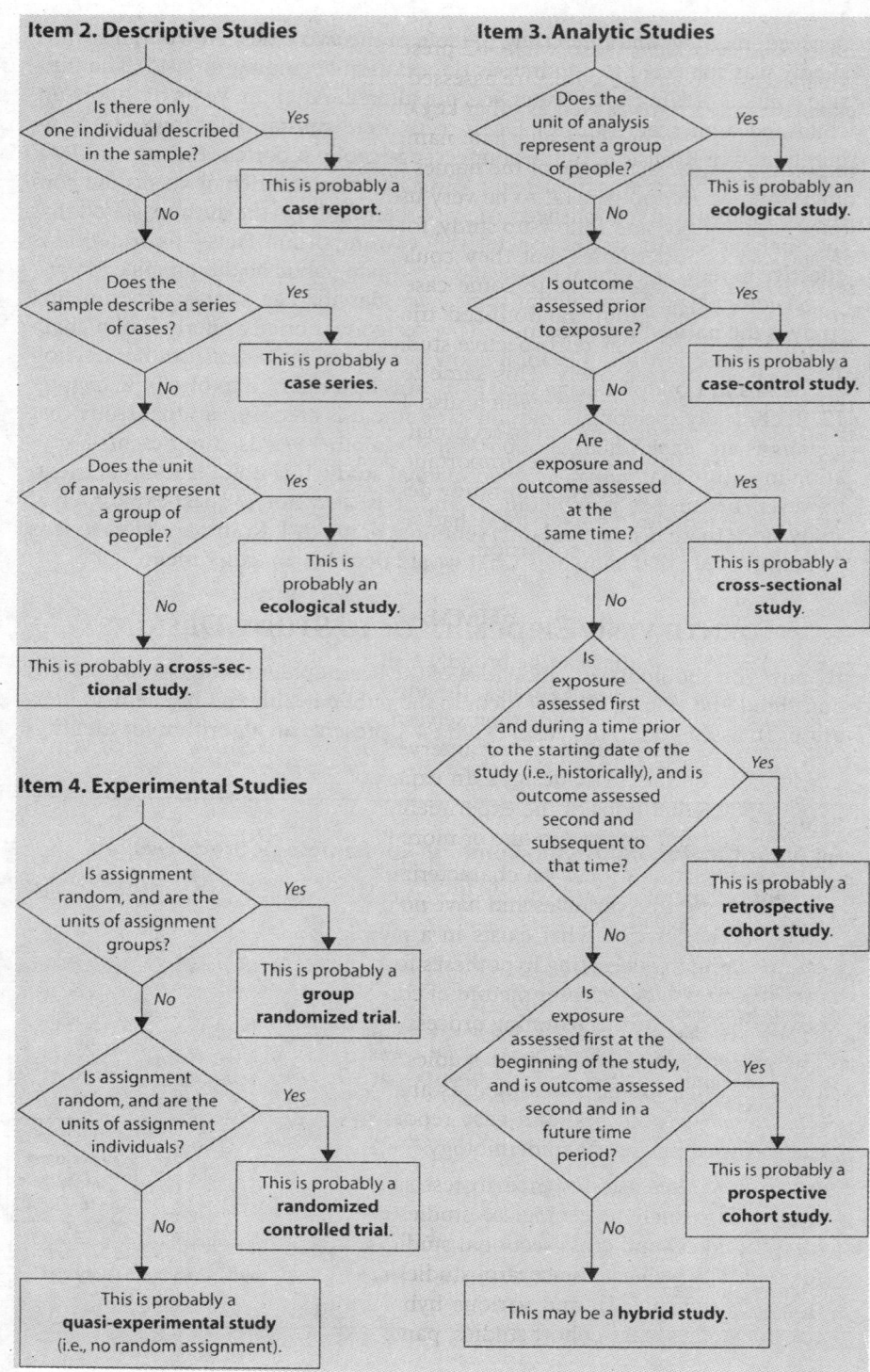

Item 2. Descriptive Studies

Is there only one individual described in the sample? — Yes → This is probably a **case report**.

No ↓

Does the sample describe a series of cases? — Yes → This is probably a **case series**.

No ↓

Does the unit of analysis represent a group of people? — Yes → This is probably an **ecological study**.

No ↓

This is probably a **cross-sectional study**.

Item 4. Experimental Studies

Is assignment random, and are the units of assignment groups? — Yes → This is probably a **group randomized trial**.

No ↓

Is assignment random, and are the units of assignment individuals? — Yes → This is probably a **randomized controlled trial**.

No ↓

This is probably a **quasi-experimental study** (i.e., no random assignment).

Item 3. Analytic Studies

Does the unit of analysis represent a group of people? — Yes → This is probably an **ecological study**.

No ↓

Is outcome assessed prior to exposure? — Yes → This is probably a **case-control study**.

No ↓

Are exposure and outcome assessed at the same time? — Yes → This is probably a **cross-sectional study**.

No ↓

Is exposure assessed first and during a time prior to the starting date of the study (i.e., historically), and is outcome assessed second and subsequent to that time? — Yes → This is probably a **retrospective cohort study**.

No ↓

Is exposure assessed first at the beginning of the study, and is outcome assessed second and in a future time period? — Yes → This is probably a **prospective cohort study**.

No ↓

This may be a **hybrid study**.

ing the major designs. Also, table 4-2 presents a summary of the sequence in which exposure and outcome are assessed in the most common analytic and experimental designs as well as other key characteristics.

Table 4-2 also presents alternate names for each major study type. It is important to note that some of the names that have been applied to epidemiologic studies are too general to be very useful. The terms prospective study, longitudinal study, and follow-up study, for example, have all been applied to prospective cohort studies, but they could also apply to panel studies and repeated surveys, as well as to some case-control studies, randomized controlled trials, and group randomized trials. Likewise, case-control studies have been referred to as retrospective studies because exposure status is usually assessed retrospectively. This same term, however, has been applied to retrospective cohort studies, which also look at exposure status retrospectively. Some ecological and cross-sectional studies may also involve retrospective assessment. It is, therefore, important not to rely on these general terms as a sole method for determining study designs. The titles used for epidemiologic studies in this chapter have had wide acceptance and use and are unlikely to be a source of confusion.

SUMMARY

- Epidemiologic studies can be broadly classified as observational or experimental. In observational studies, the investigators simply observe the subjects as they naturally divide themselves by potentially significant variables or exposures. There is no direct intervention. These studies include both descriptive and analytic designs. In experimental studies, the investigators control the conditions of the experiment, including the subjects' exposure, by selecting and employing one or more interventions.

- Descriptive studies focus on characterizing morbidity or mortality by person, place, or time variables and have no *a priori* hypotheses to test. Instead, they simply describe what exists in a population. Descriptive studies are often helpful in generating hypotheses for further study or providing health professionals with a clearer picture of community health problems that can be useful in the health planning process.

- The major types of descriptive studies are ecological and cross-sectional studies, which are also classified as analytic studies when the intent is to test *a priori* hypotheses, and case reports and case series, which are frequently used in clinical epidemiology.

- Analytic studies are designed to test specified *a priori* hypotheses. These studies also include ecological studies (multiple-group, time-trend, and mixed studies) and cross-sectional studies when there are *a priori* hypotheses to test as well as case-control studies, cohort studies (prospective, retrospective, and mixed), and various hybrid designs, including nested case-control studies, case-cohort studies, panel studies, and repeated surveys.

- Experimental studies are also designed to test *a priori* hypotheses. The two major types of experimental studies in epidemiology are randomized controlled trials and group randomized trials. A major difference between the two is who is assigned to the experimental and control groups. In randomized controlled trials, individual subjects are assigned; in group randomized trials, groups of individuals are assigned. Randomized controlled trials include two basic types—preventive (or prophylactic) and therapeutic trials.

- In addition to experimental studies there are quasi-experimental studies. These generally do not include randomization of subjects. Natural experiments, which are related, are situations in nature that mimic experimental studies. Technically speaking, however, they are not experimental or quasi-experimental studies since they are unplanned and do not involve actual interventions. They are best classified as observational studies, specifically cohort studies.

New Terms

- *a priori* hypothesis
- analytic study
- case-cohort study
- case-control study
- case report
- case series
- clinical trial
- cluster randomized trial
- cohort study
- cross-sectional study
- descriptive study
- ecological fallacy
- ecological study
- ecological unit
- experimental study
- exploratory study
- exposure
- exposure status
- group randomized trial
- hybrid study
- longitudinal study
- mixed (ecological) study
- multiple-group study
- natural experiment
- nested case-control study
- observational study
- outcome
- outcome status
- panel study
- preventive trial
- primary source
- prophylactic trial
- prospective cohort study
- quasi-experimental study
- randomization
- randomized community trial
- randomized controlled trial
- repeated surveys
- retrospective cohort study
- secondary source
- study population
- therapeutic trial
- time-trend study
- unit of analysis

Study Questions and Exercises

Using the key below, classify each of the following descriptions of epidemiologic studies according to study type. Also give reasons for your selections.

A. Descriptive Study
B. Analytic Ecological Study
C. Analytic Cross-Sectional Study
D. Case-Control Study

E. Retrospective Cohort Study
F. Prospective Cohort Study
G. Randomized Controlled Trial
H. Group Randomized Trial

_____ 1. A total of 825 insulation workers employed between 1951 and 1955 was identified from the personnel records of three large insulation manufacturing plants in the southeastern U.S. in 1995. During the period 1951–1995, 26 deaths from lung cancer were discovered among the workers. Only six lung cancer deaths, however, were reported among a comparable group of 700 coworkers who did not work with insulation during the same time period. The investigators had postulated that exposure to the insulation material increases the risk of lung cancer.

_____ 2. To see if hypnosis could reduce chronic pain, investigators randomly assigned 120 volunteers with osteoarthritis to either hypnosis therapy or standard treatment. Pain levels were checked among the subjects every three months during the 12-month study using validated pain measures. Those assigned to the hypnosis group reported reduced pain compared to those in the standard treatment group after three and six months, but not after nine and 12 months, of follow up.

_____ 3. The prevalence of type 2 diabetes was determined from a randomly selected sample of 3,000 adults over 50 years of age in a large city in the Southwest. Based on clinical examinations and testing, the prevalence of diabetes was 7.5% in men and 6.2% in women. The prevalence of diabetes increased with age more among the women than the men. Also, the rates in both men and women were higher than they had been in past years.

_____ 4. A study was undertaken to test the hypothesis that chewing tobacco increases the risk of stomach cancer. Detailed historical data on chewing tobacco use were collected from 400 subjects with newly diagnosed stomach cancer and 400 subjects without stomach cancer. The results revealed that chewing tobacco was not a significant risk factor for stomach cancer.

_____ 5. Two hundred babies were followed from birth to age five to determine if those whose mothers smoked during pregnancy were more likely to have respiratory infections in the first five years of life than those whose mothers did not smoke during pregnancy. The findings supported the investigators' assumption that smoking during pregnancy increases the frequency of respiratory infections in young children.

_____ 6. To study a presumed inverse relationship between black tea consumption and cardiovascular disease, investigators randomly selected a sample of 13,500 subjects, 50–64 years of age, and queried them about tea consumption and current treatment for cardiovascular disease. No significant association was found between drinking black tea and having cardiovascular disease.

_____ 7. To find out if drug prevention classes conducted by local community leaders would reduce the frequency of drug use in high schools in Detroit, 10 high schools in the city were assigned randomly to receive either a weekly drug prevention program led by a community leader or the standard messages on drug prevention that were part of the existing school curriculum. After two years, the frequency of drug use among students in the schools using the program with local community leaders was less than that among those in the schools using the existing curriculum, although the difference was not statistically significant.

_____ 8. A sample of residents of Grover County (population 43,000) was invited to participate in a survey to determine the prevalence of *Helicobacter pylori*, a bacterium that causes ulcers. Five thousand residents participated and were given diagnostic blood tests. The results revealed that *H. pylori* was about two times more common among men than women in the county. The overall proportion of positive tests was 58%.

_____ 9. Fifty patients recently diagnosed with hepatitis A were selected along with another 50 patients without hepatitis A from among those attending a local clinic. The subjects in the two groups were then interviewed to determine if they had had any body piercing within the last two months. To assure the subjects in the groups were comparable, they were matched for age, sex, and race. The findings revealed that body piercing was more likely among the those with hepatitis A than those without the disease after controlling for other factors.

_____ 10. In order to determine if vitamin D (the "sunshine" vitamin) is associated with reduced levels of ovarian cancer, an epidemiologist identified 12 geographic regions in Sweden and obtained data on the average annual number of days of sunlight and ovarian cancer rates for each region. The findings indicated that those regions with the highest average days of sunlight per year had significantly lower rates of ovarian cancer than those regions with the fewest average days of sunlight per year. The epidemiologist reported her findings at the Scandinavian Conference on Cancer.

References

1. Last, J. M., ed. (2001). *A Dictionary of Epidemiology*, 4th ed. New York: Oxford University Press.
2. Hoyert, D. L., Kochanek, K. D., and Murphy, S. L. (1999). Deaths: Final Data for 1997. *National Vital Statistics Reports* 47 (19). Hyattsville, MD: National Center for Health Statistics.
3. Friedman, G. D. (2004). *Primer of Epidemiology*, 5th ed. New York: McGraw-Hill Companies, Inc.

4. Fletcher, R. H., Fletcher, S. W., and Wagner, E. H. (1988). *Clinical Epidemiology: The Essentials*, 2nd ed. Baltimore: Williams and Wilkins.
5. Willoughby, R. E., Jr., Tieves, K. S., Hoffman, G. M., Ghanayem, N. S., Amlie-Lefond, C. M., Schwabe, M. J., Chusid, M. J., and Rupprecht, C. E. (2005). Survival After Treatment of Rabies with Induction of Coma. *New England Journal of Medicine* 352 (24): 2508–2514.
6. North Dakota Department of Health, Division of Disease Control (2005). Rabies Survival Case. *The Pump Handle*. Available: http://www.health.state.nd.us/disease/Documents/pump%20handle/02-05.pdf (Access date: June 30, 2005).
7. Centers for Disease Control (1992). *Tampons and Toxic Shock Syndrome*. 1992 EIS Course (available from the Association of Teachers of Preventive Medicine, Washington, DC). Atlanta: The Centers.
8. Chin, J., ed. (2000). *Control of Communicable Diseases Manual*, 17th ed. Washington, DC: American Public Health Association.
9. Vogt, W. P. (1999). *Dictionary of Statistics and Methodology: A Nontechnical Guide for the Social Sciences*, 2nd ed. Thousand Oaks, CA: Sage Publications.
10. Kelsey, J. L., Thompson, W. D., and Evans, A. S. (1986). *Methods in Observational Epidemiology*. New York: Oxford University Press.
11. Yang, C. Y., Chiu, H. F., Cheng, M. F., and Tsai, S. S. (1998). Chlorination of Drinking Water and Cancer in Taiwan. *Environmental Research* 78 (1): 1–6.
12. Szklo, M., and Nieto, F. J. (2000). *Epidemiology: Beyond the Basics*. Gaithersburg, MD: Aspen.
13. Morgenstern, H. (1995). Uses of Ecologic Studies in Epidemiology: Concepts, Principles, and Methods. *Annual Review of Public Health* 16: 61–81.
14. Fingerhut, L. A., Cox, C. S., Warner, M., et al. (1998). International Comparative Analysis of Injury Mortality: Findings from the ICE on Injury Statistics. *Advance Data from Vital and Health Statistics*, No. 303. Hyattsville, MD: National Center for Health Statistics.
15. Metz, J. A., Morris, C. D., Roberts, L. A., McClung, M. R., and McCarron, D. A. (1999). Blood Pressure and Calcium Intake Are Related to Bone Density in Adult Males. *British Journal of Nutrition* 81 (5): 383–388.
16. Kreuzer, M., Krauss, M., Kreienbrock, L., Jockel, K. H., and Wichmann, H. E. (2000). Environmental Tobacco Smoke and Lung Cancer: A Case-control Study in Germany. *American Journal of Epidemiology* 151 (3): 241–250.
17. Jacobs, E. J., Thun, M. J., and Apicella, L. F. (1999). Cigar Smoking and Death from Coronary Heart Disease in a Prospective Study of U.S. Men. *Archives of Internal Medicine* 159 (20): 2413–2418.
18. Kleinbaum, D. G., Kupper, L. L., and Morgenstern, H. (1982). *Epidemiologic Research: Principles and Quantitative Methods*. Belmont, CA: Lifetime Learning Publications.
19. MacMahon, B., and Trichopoulos, D. (1996). *Epidemiology: Principles and Methods*, 2nd ed. Boston: Little, Brown and Company.
20. Checkoway, H., Pearce, N., and Crawford-Brown, D. J. (1989). *Research Methods in Occupational Epidemiology*. New York: Oxford University Press.
21. Bowman, T. S., Sesso, H. D., Ma, J., Kurth, T., Kase, C. S., Stampfer, M. J., and Gaziano, J. M. (2003). Cholesterol and the Risk of Ischemic Stroke. *Stroke* 34 (12): 2930–2934.
22. Hulley, S. B., Cummings, S. R., Browner, W. S., Grady, D., Hearst, N., and Newman, T. B. (2001). *Designing Clinical Research: An Epidemiologic Approach*, 2nd ed. Philadelphia: Lippincott Williams & Wilkins.
23. Dooley, D., Catalano, R., and Wilson, G. (1994). Depression and Unemployment: Panel Findings from the Epidemiologic Catchment Area Study. *American Journal of Community Psychology* 22 (6): 745–765.
24. University of Michigan, Institute for Social Research (2004). *The Health and Retirement Study*. Available: http://hrsonline.irs.umich.edu (Access date: July 7, 2005).
25. Zhang, Q., and Wang, Y. (2004). Trends in the Association Between Obesity and Socioeconomic Status in U.S. Adults: 1971 to 2000. *Obesity Research* 12 (10): 1622–1632.
26. Hennekens, C. H., and Buring, J. E. (1987). *Epidemiology in Medicine*. Boston: Little, Brown and Company.

27. Medical Research Council (2002). Cluster Randomised Trials: Methodological and Ethical Considerations. Available: http://www.mrc.ac.uk/index/publications/pdf-cluster_randomised_trials-link (Access date: July 11, 2005).

28. Streiner, D. L., Norman, G. R., and Blum, H. M. (1989). *PDQ Epidemiology.* Toronto: B.C. Decker.

29. Beresford, S. A., Johnson, K. C., and Ritenbaugh, C. et al. (2006). Low-fat Dietary Pattern and Risk of Colorectal Cancer: The Women's Health Initiative Randomized Controlled Dietary Modification Trial. *Journal of the American Medical Association* 295 (6): 643–654.

30. Harris, W. S., Gowda, M., Kolb, J. W., Strychaez, C. P., Vacek, J. L., Jones, P. G., Forker, A., O'Keefe, J. H., and McCallister, B. D. (1999). A Randomized, Controlled Trial of the Effects of Remote, Intercessory Prayer on Outcomes in Patients Admitted to the Coronary Care Unit. *Archives of Internal Medicine* 159 (19): 2273–2278.

31. Deyle, G. D., Henderson, N. E., Matckel, R. I., Ryder, M. G., Garber, M. B., and Allison, S. C. (2000). Effectiveness of Manual Physical Therapy and Exercise in Osteoarthritis of the Knee. A Randomized, Controlled Trial. *Annals of Internal Medicine* 132 (3): 173–181.

32. Wagenaar, A. C., Murray, D. M., Gehan, J. P., Wolfson, M., Forster, J. L., Toomey, T. L., Perry, C. L., and Jones-Webb, R. (2000). Communities Mobilizing for Change on Alcohol: Outcomes from a Randomized Community Trial. *Journal of Studies on Alcohol:* 61 (1): 85–94.

33. Gritz, E. R., Tripp, M. K., James, A. S., Carvajal, S. C., Harrist, R. B., Mueller, N. H., Chamberlain, R. M., and Parcel, G. S. (2005). An Intervention for Parents to Promote Preschool Children's Sun Protection: Effects of Sun Protection is Fun! *Preventive Medicine* 41 (2): 357–366.

34. Ast, D. B., and Schlesinger, E. R. (1956). The Conclusion of a Ten-year Study of Water Fluoridation. *American Journal of Public Health* 46 (3): 265–271.

35. Moon, G., Gould, M., and colleagues (2000). *Epidemiology: An Introduction.* Buckingham, England: Open University Press.

36. Rothman, K. J. (2002). *Epidemiology: An Introduction.* New York: Oxford University Press.

CHAPTER FIVE

Basic Measures of Occurrence in Epidemiology

This chapter covers measures of incidence, prevalence, mortality, and various other measures, as well as confidence intervals for prevalence and incidence.

Learning Objectives

- Compare and contrast cumulative incidence, incidence density, and incidence odds.
- Calculate and interpret cumulative incidence, incidence density, and incidence odds.
- Compare and contrast point prevalence, period prevalence, and prevalence odds.
- Calculate and interpret point prevalence, period prevalence, and prevalence odds.
- Describe the interrelationships between incidence and prevalence.
- Calculate and interpret crude death rate, cause-specific mortality rate, proportionate mortality ratio, infant mortality rate, neonatal mortality rate, maternal mortality rate, perinatal mortality rate, fetal death rate, case fatality, simple survival rate, years of potential life lost, years of potential life lost rate, crude birth rate, and fertility rate.
- Describe the use and limitations of the relative survival rate.
- Explain the rationale, calculation, and interpretation of confidence intervals for measures of occurrence.
- Define count, ratio, proportion, rate, population base, population at risk, risk, competing risks, censored observations, attack rate, person-time units, person-years, lifetime prevalence, stable population, nosocomial infections, steady-state conditions, survival analysis, random selection, point estimate, sampling variation, haphazard or convenience sample, confidence level, and confidence limits.

INTRODUCTION

In epidemiology, **measures of occurrence** are quantitative measures of disease, death, or other attributes. They are usually expressed as *counts, ratios,* *proportions*, or *rates*. As shown in table 5-1, a **count** is simply the number of occurrences. A **ratio** is the relationship of one quantity (the numerator) to another quantity (the denominator) where the quantities are not necessarily measured in the same units. A **proportion** is a type of ratio in which the numerator is always included in the denominator. Because the numerator and denominator have the same measurement units they cancel out, and the proportion itself has no units. A **rate** is a type of ratio where time is expressed or implied in the denominator. It is a measure of change per unit of time. Many measures of occurrence in epidemiology are referred to as rates when in fact they are really ratios or proportions. This usage is long-standing and is not discussed further in this text except where it helps to clarify a particular concept. This chapter discusses the most commonly used measures of occurrence in epidemiology, including incidence, prevalence, and mortality measures.

Table 5-1 Basic Measurements Used in Epidemiology

Measure	Expressed as	Description	Example
Count	a	Number of occurrences	Number of cases of measles in a given community
Ratio	a / b or a : b	Fraction represented by one quantity to another (not necessarily related)	Number of cases of measles in males to the number of cases of measles in females in a given community
Proportion	a / a + b	Ratio where the numerator is included in the denominator	Number of cases of measles per 1,000 residents in a given community
Rate	a / t	Ratio where time is included in the denominator	Number of new cases of measles per day in a given community

MEASURES OF INCIDENCE

One of the most common and versatile measures of occurrence in epidemiology is incidence. **Incidence** deals with what is *new*. Traditionally, it is the number of new occurrences (e.g., cases of a given disease) in a defined population during a specified period of time. When we say that 15 new cases of HIV infection occurred in a given community during a given time period we are talking about incidence. Incidence can refer to specific or general types of morbidity, mortality, or other occurrences, such as the incidence of cigarette smoking among teenagers or high cholesterol levels among adults. When combined with an appropriate denominator, the resulting *incidence measure* takes on added meaning.* There are three basic types of incidence measures, which are described in the following sections. These measures are:

- Cumulative incidence
- Incidence density
- Incidence odds

Cumulative Incidence

One common measure of incidence is **cumulative incidence**, also known as **incidence proportion** or the **cumulative incidence rate**.[†] Typically, cumulative incidence is calculated in epidemiologic studies where the subjects are followed over time, such as in prospective or retrospective cohort studies. By definition, cumulative incidence is the proportion of the initial population at risk that develops a given occurrence or outcome (used interchangeably with occurrence) in a given period of time. It is calculated as follows:

(5.1)
$$CI = \frac{\text{Number of new occurrences during a specified time period}}{\text{Population at risk}} \times 10^n$$

The notation CI refers to cumulative incidence, and 10^n is the **population base**. The population base is 10 raised to a power of two or more. Since the exponent n is a whole number, the population base will have a value of 100, 1,000, 10,000, 100,000, etc. Its sole purpose is to avoid reporting decimal fractions (e.g., 0.012). Usually, the population base is chosen so that the resulting incidence measure is expressed as a number equal to or greater than one for the selected population base. For example, a cumulative incidence of 0.012 would normally be expressed as 1.2 per 100 using a population base of 10^2. The calculation of cumulative incidence will be illustrated shortly in problem 5-1. First, we need to define **population at risk**, the denominator in cumulative incidence. In this context, population at risk (PAR) refers to those in a defined population or cohort who are *at risk* of a given occurrence (outcome) at the *beginning* of the specified time period. This means they are susceptible to the outcome before follow up begins. Sometimes in large

---

*Technically, the term incidence, which refers to the number of new events in a given population during a given period of time, is a count. Incidence measures, like cumulative incidence and incidence density, which are discussed in this chapter, are derivatives of incidence after an appropriate denominator has been applied to the count, which serves as the numerator. Although the resulting measures have unique meanings and applications, terms like incidence, cumulative incidence, incidence rate, etc. are sometimes used interchangeably in the epidemiologic literature. It is therefore important to look at the context in which the terms are used to avoid any confusion or improper interpretation. In most cases, when incidence is mentioned, it is the incidence measure that is of interest.

[†]The term cumulative incidence rate is actually a misnomer since cumulative incidence is a proportion and not a rate as defined earlier in this chapter. Although time is used when expressing cumulative incidence, it is not part of the denominator of the cumulative incidence measure.

populations information on susceptibility is either unknown or known for only a small fraction of the population. If the incidence of the occurrence is relatively low, such as with many chronic diseases, the PAR can be approximated using the average or mid-interval population during the specified time period. This may also be done if the population is changing significantly. Inevitably, when one first begins calculating cumulative incidence, questions arise about who to include or exclude from the numerator and denominator. Exhibit 5-1 addresses these issues.

Exhibit 5-1
Guidelines for Determining the Correct Numerator and Denominator in Cumulative Incidence

One issue that frequently arises when one begins calculating cumulative incidence for the first time is who to include or exclude from the numerator and denominator. Before addressing this issue, it is important to note that *all those who are included in the numerator of cumulative incidence must come from the denominator*, the population at risk. Unless an estimate of the population at risk is being used, all occurrences in the numerator must also be part of the denominator. Confusion about this may come from the fact that the numerator and denominator are determined in different time periods. The denominator is determined at the beginning of follow up, and the numerator is determined after follow up is completed. The numerator includes those who develop the outcome or condition of interest during the follow-up period. The denominator includes those who are at risk of the outcome or condition just prior to the follow-up period. In most cases, it is easier to determine the correct numerator than the correct denominator.

Who is Included in the Numerator?
Some wonder whether or not recurrent events during a specified time period should be included in the numerator of cumulative incidence. If, for example, one person in a population at risk has two incidents of skin cancer during the follow-up period, should both incidents be counted in the numerator? The general answer to this question is *no*, since by definition, *occurrences* in the numerator of cumulative incidence refer to *people* who develop the outcome or condition of interest and not to individual incidents. If all incidents of skin cancer are counted, it would be possible theoretically to have a cumulative incidence that exceeds 100 percent. While the general rule is that the numerator represents *first occurrences only*, there may be some instances where it makes sense to include all occurrences during a specified time period. However, this is not the usual definition of cumulative incidence and not one used in this text.

Who is Included in the Denominator?
Determining who to include or exclude from the denominator in cumulative incidence is not as easy as it may first appear. By definition, the population at risk (PAR) includes only those in the defined population who are *at risk* of the occurrence at the *beginning* of the specified time period. *In practice, this usually means excluding* those who have had the outcome or condition of interest in the past and those who have it at the start of the specified time period. This is based on the assumption that

these individuals are no longer at risk of becoming new cases. This works fairly well for those who have diseases that confer lifetime immunity, such as measles, mumps, or chickenpox. It also works well for many chronic diseases, such as diabetes, multiple sclerosis, or Parkinson's disease. But, what about occurrences like injuries, strokes, or the common cold that can reoccur? Should individuals with these and similar conditions be excluded from the PAR? The answer lies in what is being investigated. If one is concerned with *entirely new* (first-time ever) occurrences, then anyone who *has* or *has had* the occurrence before should be excluded from the PAR. On the other hand, if one is only concerned with occurrences that are new *for the specified time period*, then previous cases that are still susceptible to the outcome or condition of interest should be included. For example, if one wanted to know the cumulative incidence of first-time ever strokes in a given cohort during a given year, one should exclude from the population at risk anyone who has had a stroke any time prior to initiation of the follow-up period. However, if one wanted to know how many new stroke cases occurred in the cohort during the year, whether or not they were first-time ever strokes, then it would be necessary to include survivors with a history of stroke in the population at risk. Usually, for chronic diseases, new cases mean *first-time ever* cases. For acute diseases where recovery is possible and recurrences can occur (e.g., influenza), new occurrences typically refer to cases among those who do not have the given outcome or condition at the beginning of the specified time period *and* who are not immune to the occurrence regardless of whether or not they have had it in the past. Those with the outcome or condition or those who have immunity to it, however, should be excluded from the denominator since they are not at risk of the occurrence at the beginning of the specified time period.

Cumulative incidence is useful in cohort studies because it measures a subject's *average* **risk** (probability) of developing the study occurrence during the follow-up period. There is one important qualification, however. *The length of follow-up for all subjects not developing the study outcome must be the same.*[1] Assuming all subjects begin a study at the same time, this means that those who do not develop the study outcome must be followed for the entire duration of the study. Deaths due to **competing risks** (causes other than the study outcome) and losses to follow up will affect the measure of risk, which depends on this qualification. For example, if deaths occur in a cohort study due to competing risks, the cumulative incidence will generally be *understated*. This is because those dying from competing risks are not included in the numerator of cumulative incidence even though some might have developed the study outcome had they lived. They are, however, included in the denominator since they were initially at risk. Losses to follow up, whether due to voluntary withdrawal from the study, relocation of participants, or other reasons, will have the same effect on cumulative incidence, and hence, the measurement of risk. Because of these problems, cumulative incidence is best used in studies were membership is fixed at the outset (in a fixed population or *closed cohort*; see chapter 11) and where deaths and losses to follow up are likely to be minimal. This may mean studies where the follow-up period is relatively short or the population is relatively young and stable. An example might be a study of a communicable disease outbreak in a secondary school. When it is not possible to avoid a significant number of competing risks or losses to follow up, or when subjects can enter a study at different times (in a dynamic population or *open cohort*; see chapter 11), more sophisticated procedures for estimating cumulative incidence are available.[2] One method is based on actuarial life tables (used in **survival analysis**; see exhibit 5-2) and is given in formula 5.2.

(5.2)
$$CI = \frac{\text{Number of new occurrences during a specified time period}}{\text{Population at risk} - (C/2)} \times 10^n$$

In this expression, C is the number of **censored observations**, which in this context refers to measurements on those subjects who do not complete the entire study period for reasons other than developing the study outcome. Specifically, these censored observations relate to subjects: (a) who die due to competing risks, (b) who are lost to follow up, or (c) whose follow-up time is shortened due to late entry into the study.[2] Thus, formula 5.2 can be used to estimate cumulative incidence for a given time period, and hence the average risk, for cohorts that do not meet the qualification for formula 5.1 (i.e., that the length of follow up is the same for all subjects not developing the study outcome). Half of the censored observations (C / 2) is subtracted from the PAR because the method is based on the assumption that censoring occurs, on average, at the midpoint of the study period.[1] There are a few other assumptions, which are not discussed here. For a relatively concise explanation of these refer to the texts by Moyses Szklo and F. Javier Nieto[2] or Harold A. Kahn and Christopher T. Sempos.[3]

It is very important to keep in mind that cumulative incidence, whether calculated by formula 5.1 or 5.2, is affected by the length of the specified time period. Obviously, cumulative incidence for a given chronic disease calculated over a ten-year period would be expected to be greater than that calculated over a one-year period. It is therefore imperative to report the time period for which cumulative incidence is calculated regardless of whether formula 5.1 or 5.2 is used.

Finally, it is worth noting a special type of cumulative incidence known as the **attack rate**. The attack rate is a measure of cumulative incidence applied to a narrowly but well-defined population being observed over a limited time period.[4] Attacks rates are usually calculated in connection with outbreaks (or epidemics) of disease, such as a foodborne disease outbreak in a local community (see chapter 14). Attack rates, which are really proportions, are calculated in the same manner as cumulative incidence (formula 5.1), but the actual time period may not be precisely specified. It is usually considered the time from the first to the last case in the outbreak (i.e., the duration of the outbreak). Because of the limited time period over which most attack rates are calculated the estimate of risk should be fairly accurate.

Exhibit 5-2
A Brief Overview of Survival Analysis

What is survival analysis?
Survival analysis is a set of statistical techniques used to characterize *survival time* in one or more groups. **Survival time** is the *time to occurrence* of a specific outcome from a defined starting point. A commonly used synonym for survival analysis is **time-to-event analysis**, where event refers to the outcome of interest. While epidemiologists have traditionally used survival analysis to study time to death, contemporary use also includes a variety of other response variables. Hence, it is common to see survival time expressed as time to a specific disease, time to recovery, time to hospital discharge, time to childbirth, time to relapse, and so on. A typical study employing survival analysis might examine the survival time of a group of cancer patients undergoing a specific drug therapy or the time until relapse in a group of newly diagnosed alcoholics. Survival analysis is most frequently associated with follow-up studies (i.e., cohort studies and randomized controlled trials). One important product of survival analysis is the **survival curve**, which is a graphic presentation of the proportion of subjects surviving to successive points in time. To the extent to which the sample is representative of a larger defined population, a survival curve has broader prognostic value. Nevertheless, one should be cautious in interpreting survival curves when some of the data points are based on small numbers. It is also a good idea to develop confidence limits for a survival curve. Survival curves may be presented for one group or compared between two or more groups based on exposure variables of interest, such as age, sex, or race/ethnicity. In addition, certain multivariable statistical methods may be used to examine multiple potential risk or prognostic factors for time-dependent variables. The value of survival analysis is indicated by its wide use in a variety of disciplines, including medicine, public health, sociology, marketing, economics, biology, engineering, and astronomy.

Why is survival analysis used?
Survival analysis is used primarily because traditional statistical procedures are not appropriate for analyzing time-to-event data unless all the subjects develop the study outcome prior to the end of the study. This situation is highly unlikely, for example, in open cohort studies (chapter 11) where subjects can enter or leave the cohort at different times. The data on subjects where survival time is incomplete are referred to as *censored observations*. In general, censored observations occur for three main reasons: (a) losses to follow up, (b) study termination prior to development of the outcome, and (c) deaths due to competing risks. In situations a and b, we do not know if the subjects will go on to develop the study outcome, and if so, when. Therefore, the exact survival times are unknown. *Competing risks* are causes other than the study outcome. As in situations a and b, we do not know if those who die due to competing risks would have developed the study outcome had they lived, and if so, when. Of course, if the study outcome is death from all causes, competing risks will not be relevant. Survival analysis is used instead of other statistical methods chiefly because it can accommodate censored observations. Another reason is that time-to-event data are positively skewed since survival time is always non-negative. Therefore, the distribution of survival time may not be normal.

(continued)

What methods are commonly used in survival analysis?

There are several approaches to survival analysis, and new techniques continue to be developed. The methods described here produce practical data that can be used, for example, to construct a survival curve, ascertain the median survival time, and determine the risk of the outcome for a given time period. One approach is the **life table method** (also called the **actuarial method** because of its use in estimating life expectancy in the insurance industry). In this approach survival times are divided into a number of small time intervals, not necessarily equal, but usually spanning a period of a year or less. A basic assumption is that the outcomes, as well as the entry of new subjects or losses, are uniform in each time interval. Another is that subjects who are censored have the same risk of the study outcome as the non-censored subjects. These assumptions are usually reasonable if the time intervals are kept small. The proportion of subjects surviving to a given interval is estimated by the product of the proportions surviving each prior interval. These data are then used to construct a survival curve. The life table method, though historically the oldest method of survival analysis, is used less frequently today because of the availability of other more precise methods. One of the most commonly used methods of survival analysis is the **Kaplan-Meier product limit method**. This is a non-parametric method where each "failure" (death, disease, relapse, or other study outcome) defines the start of an interval. The proportion of failures is equal to the number of failures divided by those still surviving at the start of the interval. This approach estimates the probability of surviving longer than a specified time, usually denoted as $S(t)$. In general, the Kaplan-Meier method requires a smaller sample size than the life table method since it uses each subject's exact survival time rather than estimates based on the uniformity assumption. As with the life table method, the Kaplan-Meier method is based on the assumption that subjects who are censored prior to developing the study outcome have the same risk of the outcome as those continuing in the study. In addition, it is assumed in both methods that time of entry into the study is independent of the risk of the study outcome. In the sample survival curve depicted to the left, note that at time zero the survival proportion is equivalent to 100 percent as expected. It decreases thereafter until it plateaus starting at about three and a half years from the beginning of follow up. The rate of decrease will depend on the specific outcome and the characteristics of the study population. Each downward step in the curve indicates a failure (i.e., an outcome). Also note that the median survival time is 1.6 years, which can be derived directly from the curve. Another approach used in survival analysis, and a very popular one, is the *Cox proportional hazards model*, which is a multiple regression technique used with time-to-event (survival) data. It is described briefly in chapter 11 (exhibit 11-3). Comprehensive descriptions of survival analysis can be found in several specialized references, and more detailed summaries are available in a number of biostatistical or epidemiologic texts.

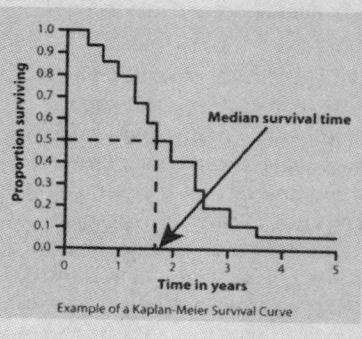

Example of a Kaplan-Meier Survival Curve

References: Lee, E. T., and Go, O. T. (1997). Survival Analysis in Public Health Research. *Annual Review of Public Health* 18: 105–134; Morton, R. F., Hebel, J. R., and McCarter, R. J. (2001). *A Study Guide to Epidemiology and Biostatistics*, 5th ed. Gaithersburg, MD: Aspen Publishers, Inc.

Problem 5-1: Cumulative Incidence

Imagine that exactly five years ago, a team of epidemiologists identified a study population of 4,500 men, 65–74 years of age, in Cedar Rapids, Iowa, to determine the incidence of prostate cancer. Initial testing indicated that seven percent of the men already had prostate cancer and, therefore, were not at risk of developing the disease. The remaining men were followed prospectively to the present time to determine the cumulative incidence of prostate cancer. By the end of the five years of follow-up, 156 men had developed prostate cancer. Based on this information, what was the five-year cumulative incidence of prostate cancer in this population?

Solution:
Use formula 5.1 to calculate the cumulative incidence.

$$CI = \frac{\text{Number of new occurrences during a specified time period}}{\text{Population at risk}} \times 10^n$$

For convenience, let's represent the above formula as $CI = (X / Y) \times 10^n$, where $X =$ the number of new occurrences during a specified time period, $Y =$ the population at risk, and $10^n =$ the population base.

Step 1: Determine the numerator or X. The 156 men who developed prostate cancer in the sample were *new* occurrences that developed during the specified five-year follow-up period. Therefore,

$$X = 156$$

Step 2: Determine the denominator or Y.

$$Y = 4,500 - (4,500 \times 0.07) = 4,500 - 315 = 4,185$$

Because seven percent of the men were not initially at risk, they are not are included in the denominator (i.e., they were not followed up). Therefore, they have been subtracted from the original sample of 4,500. It is important to realize that the remaining 4,185 men include the 156 who subsequently developed prostate cancer. This is because the 156 men were initially at risk; it is only after the follow up began that they developed prostate cancer. In cumulative incidence the new occurrences (the numerator) always arise from the population at risk (the denominator).

Step 3: Complete the calculation of cumulative incidence (CI) using a population base that will produce a result that is at least one for the selected population base. In this problem, 10^2 or 100 is the smallest population base that will produce a result of at least one per 100.

$$CI = (X / Y) \times 10^n = (156 / 4,185) \times 10^n = 0.037 \times 10^2 = 3.7 \text{ cases per 100 men}$$

Answer: The five-year cumulative incidence of prostate cancer in Cedar Rapids, Iowa, was 3.7 cases per 100 men, initially aged 65–74 years, during the specified follow-up period.

Comments:
1. The population base is a convention in epidemiology that is used for the convenience of not having to report decimal fractions. In actuality, 0.037 is the cumulative incidence, and it is the same as 3.7 per 100, 37 per 1,000, 370 per 10,000, etc. Usually, we select the smallest population base to achieve its purpose since larger population bases make the cumulative incidence appear less precise. Exceptions are made when we want to maintain a common population base when comparing several different measures or when we select a larger population base because that

is the way a particular measure is commonly reported in the literature. A convenient way to determine the appropriate population base is to divide X by Y and then determine what population base is needed to produce a measure that is at least one per the selected population base.

2. Since cumulative incidence measures the average risk of an outcome, we can say, based on the results of this study, that, on average, a subject's risk of developing prostate cancer in this population during the specified time period is 3.7 per 100.

3. It is important to note that the results of this problem represent findings among a particular subgroup, at a particular place, and during particular time period. Unless this information is clear from the context, one should specify the relevant person, place, and time factors. *Since cumulative incidence can be expected to increase with time of observation,* it is especially important to indicate the period the cumulative incidence encompasses. For example, the five-year cumulative incidence of prostate cancer would be expected to be greater than the one-year cumulative incidence in the same population.

Incidence Density

A second type of incidence measure is **incidence density**, also known as the **incidence rate** or sometimes the **person-time incidence rate**. Like cumulative incidence, this measure is usually calculated in follow-up studies (e.g., cohort studies). Unlike cumulative incidence, which is a proportion, incidence density is a *rate* (a measure of change per unit of time). Incidence density (ID) can be calculated as shown in formula 5.3.

(5.3)
$$ID = \frac{\text{Number of new occurrences during a specified time period}}{\text{Total person-time units observed}} \times 10^n$$

While the numerator and population base for incidence density are the same as those for cumulative incidence, the denominator differs significantly. *Total person-time units observed* is the sum of every cohort member's time at risk, which is defined as the time until he or she develops the study outcome, dies from competing risks, is lost to follow up, or completes the follow-up period without developing the study outcome. Thus, the denominator is the sum of known outcome-free time contributed by each of the subjects. **Person-time units** are defined as combined measures of the number of persons at risk of the study occurrence and the actual time they were at risk. The most common person-time units are **person-years**,[5] although person-months, person-days, or other person-time units may be used, usually depending on the length of the study. A person-year represents one person at risk for one year, two persons each at risk for half a year, or any other combination of persons and years whose ultimate product is one. Similarly, five person-years can mean one person at risk for one year plus two persons at risk for two years, and so on. A point to keep in mind is that person-time units represent time at risk even though time is linked to the experience of individual persons. This is important because having time in the denominator makes incidence density a rate, specifically the *rate* at which new cases of the study occurrence are taking place in a defined population or cohort. It can be thought of as a measure of the rate of disease movement in a population at any particular moment and can be likened to the speed of an automobile in miles (or kilometers) per hour. At any given point, the automobile (or disease) is moving at a given rate of speed. The term *force of morbidity*, sometimes used to describe incidence density, is a expressive term that captures the essence of this measure. The calculation of incidence density (formula 5.3) is based on assumptions which are similar to some of those made for cumulative incidence using actuarial life tables (formula 5.2). These can be summarized as follows: (a) the risk of the outcome is relatively constant during the specified time period; (b) censored observations do not differ from non-censored observations regarding risk of the outcome; and (c) there are no secular trends operating where subjects are added to the study over a relatively long period of time.[2] For a discussion of the rationale for these assumptions one should consult a more advanced text on epidemiology.

Incidence Density Versus Cumulative Incidence

Incidence density can be thought of as an alternative way to measure incidence when follow-up times vary due, for example, to competing risks or losses to follow up. Thus, unlike cumulative incidence (formula 5.1), incidence density is well suited to dynamic populations (open cohorts; chapter 11) where subjects may enter or leave the cohort at different times. It is also important to emphasize that while incidence density measures the *rate* of disease development, cumulative incidence measures the *risk* of disease development. Thus, these are two distinct incidence measures, although they approximate each other in certain circumstances (see problem 5-3). Table 5-2 summarizes some of the major differences between cumulative incidence and

Table 5-2   Comparison of Cumulative Incidence and Incidence Density

Cumulative Incidence	Incidence Density
• Simple proportion with no units	• Rate expressed per person-time units
• Ranges from 0 to 1 without a population base (e.g., 0.15 without a population base = 15 per 100 with a population base of 100)	• Has a lower boundary of 0 but no upper boundary; magnitude depends on person-time units used (e.g., 20 per 100 person-months = 240 per 100 person-years)
• Measures average risk of disease development	• Measures rate of disease development
• Appropriate with fixed populations or closed cohorts where follow-up times are uniform	• Appropriate with dynamic populations or open cohorts where follow-up times vary
• Assumes no deaths due to competing risks or losses to follow up	• Accounts for deaths due to competing risks and losses to follow up
• Easily interpreted	• Not easily interpreted

incidence density. Problem 5-2 illustrates the calculation of incidence density using a hypothetical study.

Problem 5-2: Incidence Density

Assume another study of prostate cancer was initiated, this time in Des Moines, Iowa. A total of 1,000 men, 55–64 years of age, with no prior evidence of prostate cancer were enrolled in the study. The men were then followed by the investigators for four years. Each year during the study, the men being observed were examined and tested for the presence of prostate cancer. The results of the annual examinations revealed the following:

10 cases were confirmed at the first examination

15 additional cases were confirmed at the second examination

20 additional cases were confirmed at the third examination

25 additional cases were confirmed at the fourth, and final, examination

What is the incidence density of prostate cancer in this group?

Solution:
Use formula 5.3 to calculate the incidence density.

$$ID = \frac{\text{Number of new occurrences during a specified time period}}{\text{Total person-time units observed}} \times 10^n$$

For convenience, let us represent the formula for incidence density as: $ID = (X / T) \times 10^n$, where X = the number of new occurrences during a specified time period, T = the total person-time units observed, and 10^n = the population base.

Step 1: Determine the numerator or X, which in this problem is the number of those who developed prostate cancer anytime during the four-year follow-up period. Note that all subjects were initially free of prostate cancer. Therefore,

$$X = 10 + 15 + 20 + 25 = 70$$

Step 2: Determine the denominator or T. The denominator of incidence density is the sum of each individual's time at risk, whether or not the subject subsequently developed prostate cancer. *For those who developed prostate cancer* we can calculate their *portion* of T as follows:

10 cases confirmed at first exam: 10 persons × 1 year = 10 person-years observed

15 cases confirmed at second exam: 15 persons × 2 years = 30 person-years observed

20 cases confirmed at third exam: 20 persons × 3 years = 60 person-years observed

25 cases confirmed at fourth exam: 25 persons × 4 years = 100 person-years observed

Thus, the total person-time units contributed by the 70 cases is:

$$10 + 30 + 60 + 100 = 200 \text{ person-years}$$

After we have accounted for the person-time units contributed by the 70 cases, we must then account for the person-time units contributed by the remaining sample, which consists of *those who did not develop prostate cancer.* Even though these individuals did not develop prostate cancer, they were at risk of prostate cancer during the four years of follow up and, therefore, must be included in the denominator of incidence density. Since 70 subjects developed prostate cancer, there were 930 (i.e., 1,000 – 70 = 930) who did not. These individuals were followed for the entire four years of the study. Therefore, the total person-time units contributed by the 930 subjects *who did not develop prostate cancer* is:

$$930 \text{ persons} \times 4 \text{ years} = 3,720 \text{ person-years}$$

As a final step, we add the person-time units contributed by those who did and those who did not develop prostate cancer. The calculation of the total person-time units observed (T) is thus:

$$T = 200 \text{ person-years} + 3,720 \text{ person-years} = 3,920 \text{ person-years}$$

The entire calculation of T can be represented in one step as follows:

$$T = (10 \times 1) + (15 \times 2) + (20 \times 3) + (25 \times 4) + [(1,000 - 70) \times 4] = 3,920 \text{ person-years}$$

Step 3: Calculate the ID using a population base that will produce a rate that is at least one for the selected population base.

$$ID = (X / T) \times 10^n = (70 / 3,920) \times 10^n = 0.018 \times 10^2 = 1.8 \text{ cases per 100 person-years}$$

Answer: The incidence density of prostate cancer is 1.8 cases per 100 person-years among men, initially 55–64 years of age, in Des Moines, Iowa, during the stated period.

Comments:

1. When calculating incidence density, once a subject develops the study outcome that subject is no longer at risk and, hence, no longer contributes any additional person-time to the denominator. Similarly, *subjects who die due to competing risks (causes other than the study outcome) or who are lost to follow up are only counted for the time they were actually observed to be at risk of the outcome.* Once these subjects are no longer observed to be at risk they cease to be followed. In this problem, the only reason some subjects were not observed for the entire four-year follow-up period was because they had contracted prostate cancer. In most studies there will also be losses to follow up or deaths due to competing risks that must be taken into account in calculating the denominator. In addition, subjects who are added after a study commences may be at risk for less than the specified time period.

2. The population base is selected in the same manner as with cumulative incidence. Since the rate is technically 0.018 cases per person-year, a population base of 10^2 allows us to express this as 1.8 cases per 100 person-years, a statement more agreeable to many health professionals, although either rate is correct.

3. Since time is already represented in incidence density, it would be inappropriate to indicate that this is a four-year incidence rate. It is proper, however, to indicate the observation period along with person and place information if these are not clear from the context.

4. Ideally, investigators should count the *actual* time each subject is observed until the subject is no longer at risk (i.e., died due to competing risks, contracted the study outcome, lost to follow up). In this problem, it was assumed that subjects diagnosed with prostate cancer at each examination period had been at risk for the entire time prior to the examination. In reality, the disease likely began sometime before the examination, thus reducing the real time at risk. For example, 20 new cases were identified at the third examination. It was assumed that all 20 had been at risk for exactly three years; however, most, if not all, of these 20 cases probably developed prostate cancer sometime between two and three years (on average, two and a half years). In most cases, disease onset is assumed to be the time of diagnosis or the midpoint between the previous examination and the examination at which diagnosis is made.[1] Some epidemiologists use estimates of total person-time

units observed rather than counting each individual's time at risk, which can be very tedious in a large study. This is discussed in the next section.

Estimating Total Person-Time Units

In large populations or cohorts it can be very time consuming to calculate the total person-time units observed, the denominator of incidence density (see formula 5.3). For this reason, instead of counting each subject's time at risk, some epidemiologists make estimates based on certain assumptions. Formula 5.4, for example, can be used to estimate the incidence density by approximating the total person-time units observed. Use of this formula assumes that cases of the study outcome and censored observations are uniformly distributed over the course of the specified time period and occur on average at the midpoint of this period. This assumption is likely to be met if the sample is large and the specified time period is relatively short.[2]

(5.4)
$$ID = \frac{\text{Number of new occurrences during a specified time period}}{(\text{Population at risk} - Z/2) \times \text{the specified time period}} \times 10^n$$

The value Z is the number of cases plus the number of censored observations. The population at risk is the number of subjects initially at risk of the outcome, and the specified time period is the duration of the study. Using formula 5.4 with the data from problem 5-2, we obtain the same result as in the problem: $70 / [1,000 - (70 / 2) \times 4] = 70 / 3,860 = 0.018$ per person-year or $0.018 \times 10^2 = 1.8$ cases per 100 person-years. In this example, there were 70 cases and no censored observations. The parenthetical portion of the denominator in formula 5.4 is equivalent to the average population at risk, which can be calculated by averaging the beginning and ending populations at risk during the specified time period.[2]

If the outcome is relatively uncommon, and the population is stable in size and composition, one can substitute the size of the entire population for the parenthetical portion in the denominator to estimate incidence density. In this case the estimated incidence density using the data in problem 5-2 is: $70 / (1,000 \times 4) = 0.018$ per person-year or $0.018 \times 10^2 = 1.8$ cases per 100 person-years.

Estimating Cumulative Incidence from Incidence Density

Because risk is an important concept in epidemiology and because of the difficulty in estimating risk accurately in dynamic populations (i.e., open cohorts; chapter 11), incidence density is sometimes used to estimate cumulative incidence and, hence, the average risk of a study occurrence. A simple formula for doing this is offered by J. H. Abramson. Use of the formula assumes that incidence density is constant during the stated time period.[6]

(5.5)
$$CI = \frac{ID \times t}{(ID \times t/2) + 1}$$

In this equation, CI is cumulative incidence, ID is incidence density, and t is the study period (or time of interest). Both CI and ID *must be stated as decimal fractions* for this expression to make sense. Use of formula 5.5 is demonstrated in problem 5-3 below.

Problem 5-3: Relationship between Cumulative Incidence and Incidence Density

On January 1, 2006, 5,000 healthy men beginning highly stressful jobs in Los Angeles County, California, were enrolled in a follow-up study of the relationship between job stress and hypertension. Medical histories and physical examinations revealed that all subjects were normotensive at the time. The study was concluded on December 31, 2007. The authors reported the following statistics at the conclusion of the study:

10 men developed hypertension after 6 months

15 additional men developed hypertension after 1 year

20 additional men developed hypertension after 18 months

100 men who had not developed hypertension withdrew from the study after 1 year

Based on this information, calculate the incidence density and cumulative incidence for hypertension and compare the two measures. Also, use formula 5.5 to estimate the cumulative incidence of hypertension from the incidence density.

Solution:
Step 1: Calculate the incidence density of hypertension in the group using formula 5.3.

$$ID = \frac{\text{Number of new occurrences during a specified time period}}{\text{Total person-time units observed}} \times 10^n$$

The number of new occurrences of hypertension during the two-year study period is:

$$10 + 15 + 20 = 45$$

Next, we need to calculate the total person-time units observed, which is the sum of each individual's person-time units observed. Based on the information provided, this can be calculated as follows:

10 cases after 6 months:	10 persons × 0.5 year =	5 person-years
15 cases after 1 year:	15 persons × 1 year =	15 person-years
20 cases after 18 months:	20 persons × 1.5 years =	30 person-years
100 withdrawals after 1 year:	100 persons × 1 year =	100 person-years
145 (cases + withdrawals)		150 person-years

The 145 subjects who either developed hypertension or withdrew from the study contributed 150 person-years to the denominator of the incidence density. In addition, we must account for the remaining subjects in the study. These were the subjects who did not develop hypertension and did not withdraw from the study.

$$5,000 - 145 = 4,855$$

Since these subjects were followed for two years, their total contribution in person-time units is:

$$4,855 \text{ persons} \times 2 \text{ years} = 9,710 \text{ person-years}$$

Consequently, the total number of person-years observed is:

$$145 + 9,710 = 9,860 \text{ person-years}$$

The incidence density (ID) of hypertension, therefore, is:

$$ID = (45 / 9,860) \times 10^n = 0.0046 \times 10^3 = 4.6 \text{ cases per } 1,000 \text{ person-years}$$

Step 2: Calculate the cumulative incidence using formula 5.1.

$$CI = \frac{\text{Number of new occurrences during a specified time period}}{\text{Population at risk}} \times 10^n$$

Because all individuals were free of the study outcome at the beginning of the study, the population at risk is 5,000. Also, as shown in step one, there were 45 cases. Therefore,

$$CI = (45 / 5,000) \times 10^n = 0.0090 \times 10^3 = 9.0 \text{ cases per } 1,000 \text{ population}$$

Step 3: Compare the two measures.

Although the value of the cumulative incidence appears to be nearly twice that of the incidence density (9.0 per 1000 vs. 4.6 per 1000 person-years), it is necessary to remember that the cumulative incidence is based on a two-year period. On an annual basis the values of the measures are very similar (see comment number 3 below for details).

Step 4: Estimate the cumulative incidence using formula 5.5.

This formula is based on the assumption that the incidence density is relatively constant. It also requires that the incidence density be stated on a per-person-time basis.

$$CI = \frac{ID \times t}{(ID \times t / 2) + 1}$$

$$CI = (0.0046 \times 2) / [(0.0046)(2 / 2) + 1] = 0.0092 / 1.0046 = 0.0092 \times 10^3 = 9.2 \text{ per } 1,000$$

Answer: The incidence density of hypertension in the study population is 4.6 cases per 1,000 person-years, and the two-year cumulative incidence of hypertension is 9.0 cases per 1,000 population. The estimated cumulative incidence using formula 5.5 is 9.2 cases per 1,000 population. (See comment number 3 below regarding a comparison of the two measures.)

Comments:
1. The total person-years observed for all subjects in the study was included in the denominator of the incidence density measure. The 45 subjects who developed hypertension contributed 50 person-years to the denominator, and the 100 subjects who withdrew from the study prior to developing hypertension contributed 100 person-years. The remaining 4,855 subjects who completed the study without developing hypertension contributed the majority of the person-years to the denominator, which amounted to 9,710 person-years. This suggests that a relatively small percentage of the subjects did not complete the entire follow-up period ($145 / 5,000 \times 100 = 2.9$ percent).

2. The denominator for the cumulative incidence consisted of all subjects who were at risk of hypertension at the beginning of the study. This included all 5,000 subjects since none had clinical evidence of hypertension prior to the start of the study.

3. Though the measures are not directly comparable because cumulative incidence has no units and incidence density is measured in units of time (see table 5-2), it is interesting to note that the measures are similar numerically. The two-year cumulative incidence was 9.0 cases per 1,000 population, or on average 4.5 cases per 1,000

population per year, while the incidence density was 4.6 cases per 1,000 person-years (or 4.6 cases per 1,000 persons per year).

4. Since the cumulative incidence is a measure of the average risk of developing hypertension, we can say that the two-year probability (risk) is 9.0 cases per 1,000 population based on the direct calculation using formula 5.1 or about 9.2 cases per 1,000 population based on the estimate using formula 5.5. The small withdrawal rate in the study ($100 / 5,000 \times 100 = 2.0$ percent) means that the qualification for using formula 5.1 (that the follow-up times be the same for those developing and not developing the study outcome) was generally met.

Incidence Odds

A third but less commonly used incidence measure is **incidence odds**. It can be defined as the ratio of the number of people who develop a new occurrence to the number of people who do not develop the occurrence in a given population during a specified period of time. The formula for incidence odds is given in formula 5.6.

(5.6)

$$\text{Incidence Odds} = \frac{\text{No. who develop a new occurrence during a specified time period}}{\text{No. who do not develop the occurrence in same time period}}$$

As with cumulative incidence, incidence odds has no units, but the time period should always be specified since its value can be expected to increase with time of observation. The term *odds* refers to the probability of an outcome occurring to the probability of it not occurring. Outside of epidemiology, odds are most commonly used in gambling such as at racetracks where bettors put their money on horses based on the odds of winning a race. Say, for example, that Lucky Pony is favored in the third race because its odds are 4:1. This means that the probability of Lucky Pony winning the race is four times its probability of losing the race. These are pretty good odds. The *probability* of winning, however, is 4 / 5 or 80 percent, which is also a good bet. Probability is equivalent to the odds of occurrence / (the odds of occurrence + 1). Thus, if the odds are 4 / 1, which is the same as 4:1, the probability of the occurrence is 4 / (4 + 1) or 4 / 5, which is equal to 80 percent. These odds would be considered unusual in epidemiologic applications, except perhaps in a disease outbreak, since the probability of *not* developing a particular disease is usually greater than the probability of developing it in any given population. Theoretically, odds can range from zero to a value that has no specific upper limit. Probabilities, on the other hand, can only range from zero to one.

A brief example of the calculation of incidence odds should be illustrative. Imagine that a cohort of 450 children in the same age group were followed for three years to determine the incidence of acute bronchitis. Twenty-two of the children developed acute bronchitis for the first time during the follow-up period. The incidence odds for the three-year period is therefore:

$$22 / (450 - 22) = 22 / 428 = 0.051$$

This means that the odds of developing acute bronchitis in the cohort during the three-year study period is 0.051. In epidemiology, this odds would usually be stated as 0.051 rather than 0.051: 1. A denominator of one is assumed and therefore not expressed. The probability (risk) of developing acute bronchitis is 22 / 450 = 0.049, which is the same as the cumulative incidence expressed as a decimal fraction. When the frequency of the outcome is relatively rare (say, less than 0.10), the incidence odds approximates the cumulative incidence relatively well as it did in this example. While incidence odds and cumulative incidence both have lower bounds of zero, as stated before, incidence odds has no specific upper limit. Cumulative incidence, stated as a decimal fraction, however, has an upper limit of one since it is a proportion (see table 5-2).

MEASURES OF PREVALENCE

Whereas incidence deals with what is new, **prevalence** deals with what *exists*, whether new or old. Technically, prevalence is the number of existing occurrences (i.e., a given disease or attribute) in a defined population at a designated time. Unlike incidence, prevalence does not include mortality, which always represents *new* occurrences. It can, however, be used to refer to all types of morbidity or other types of occurrences, such as drug use, cigarette smoking, blood type, or blue eyes. To say there are 10 cases of leukemia in a particular community at a given time is to make a statement about prevalence. When combined with an appropriate denominator, the resulting prevalence measure is a proportion, although it is sometimes referred to as a *prevalence rate.** Specifically, it is the *proportion* of a defined population that has a specific occurrence at a designated time. It is expressed in a manner similar to cumulative incidence, although, unlike cumulative incidence, it is an unreliable estimate of risk. More will be said about this later in the chapter.

There are three basic types of prevalence measures used in epidemiology. These are:

• Point prevalence
• Period prevalence
• Prevalence odds

Point Prevalence

The most common prevalence measure is **point prevalence**, which is usually referred to as just *prevalence* and sometimes **prevalence proportion**. It is calculated as follows:

---

*The term prevalence rate, although commonly used in epidemiology, is a misnomer since prevalence does not represent a change per unit of time, which is the common definition of a rate. A more appropriate term is *prevalence proportion;* however, most refer to a measure of prevalence simply as prevalence. To distinguish whether one is referring to a count or a proportion, it is necessary to look at the context in which the term is being used. In most studies, when prevalence is mentioned, it is the proportion that is of interest.

(5.7) $$P = \frac{\text{Number of existing occurrences at a specific point in time}}{\text{Total defined population at the same point in time}} \times 10^n$$

The P in this expression refers to point prevalence, and 10^n is the population base, which was defined earlier in reference to incidence. Typically, when epidemiologists refer to prevalence, they are referring to point prevalence. Point prevalence can be conceived as an instantaneous *snapshot* of the proportion of a defined population with a given disease or other attribute. The defined population is generally considered to be the entire population being investigated. Although the "point in time" in formula 5.7 is theoretically instantaneous, in practice it usually represents a particular day or a specific date. It can also be an event in time, such as the prevalence of cleft palate *at birth*.

Point prevalence is most commonly measured in cross-sectional studies and repeated surveys. It is also used in screening for disease and in health planning because it represents the *disease burden* of a community at any given time. Alexander Walker[7] refers to prevalence as a "status report" since it represents the status of a population with regard to any given occurrence.

Period Prevalence

Another prevalence measure is **period prevalence** (Pd P), which is calculated as shown in formula 5.8.

(5.8)

$$Pd\ P = \frac{\text{Number of occurrences existing anytime during a specified time period}}{\text{Total defined population during the specified time period}} \times 10^n$$

While point prevalence can be viewed as a snapshot of the proportion of a defined population that has a given outcome or condition, period prevalence can be thought of as a video of the specified time period. It shows what has existed in a defined population over a stated period of time. Conceptually, period prevalence is the sum of point prevalence at the beginning of a specified time period *plus* cumulative incidence for the remainder of the time period. In period prevalence, all occurrences (e.g., cases of a given disease) that existed *anytime* during the stated time period are included in the numerator regardless of what happens to the cases. Hence, even if a case dies during the specified time period that case is still included in the numerator. The denominator for period prevalence is generally the average or mid-interval population for the specified time period. In the epidemiologic literature period prevalence may be referred to simply as prevalence. Therefore, it is important to look at the context to know whether the authors are referring to point or period prevalence. Some epidemiologists do not consider period prevalence to be a useful measure in epidemiology,[8] and its use in the epidemiologic literature has declined in recent years.

A variant of period prevalence is **lifetime prevalence**. This term refers to the proportion of individuals in a defined population who *have had* a given occurrence (e.g., disease) at *any time* during their lives. Thus, the time period for lifetime prevalence is the collective lifetimes of the individuals in the population. We can expect lifetime prevalence for a given disease to be greater than point prevalence and "less than lifetime" period prevalence in the same population. In fact, since period or lifetime prevalence may give the impression that the magnitude of a particular problem is greater than other problems that are represented by point prevalence, it is important to know what type of prevalence is being reported in epidemiologic studies. Many common health problems (e.g., headaches, injuries) have lifetime prevalences in adults at or near 100 percent. The relationship between incidence and prevalence is discussed in a subsequent section. The calculation of point and period prevalence is shown in problems 5-4 and 5-5, respectively.

Problem 5-4: Point Prevalence

Assume 3,465 women, 60–74 years of age, were screened for the presence of osteoporosis at a major women's health fair held in Phoenix, Arizona, from January 3rd to January 10th of last year. A total of 974 cases of osteoporosis were identified at the screening. What was the prevalence of osteoporosis in this group?

Solution:
We can use formula 5.7 to determine the prevalence.

$$P = \frac{\text{Number of occurrences existing at a specific point in time}}{\text{Total defined population at the same point in time}} \times 10^n$$

For convenience, let us represent this formula as: $P = (X / Y) \times 10^n$, where $X =$ the number of occurrences existing at a specific point in time, $Y =$ the total defined population at the same point in time, and $10^n =$ the population base. Therefore,

$$X = 974 \text{ cases of osteoporosis}$$
$$Y = 3,465 \text{ women, 60–74 years of age}$$
$$P = (974 / 3,465) \times 10^n = 0.281 \times 10^2 = 28.1 \text{ cases per 100 women}$$

Answer: The prevalence of osteoporosis is 28.1 cases per 100 women, 60–74 years of age, based on the findings at the women's health fair in Phoenix, Arizona, held last year from January 3 to January 10.

Comments:
1. Although not specifically indicated in the problem, it is implied that the prevalence to be calculated is point prevalence. The cases of osteoporosis were those that existed at a point in time (i.e., at the time of screening). That the health fair ran for eight days does not alter the fact that the implied point in time is the time of screening.

2. The defined population includes all women in the specified age group who were screened. As with cumulative incidence, the numerator of prevalence arises from the denominator, which can be considered the reference group. The reference group, therefore, refers to those women who were screened for osteoporosis.

3. The population base is selected in the same manner as that for incidence measures. A population base of 10^2 (or 100) is the smallest population base that will make the prevalence at least one per the selected population base.

4. As with incidence measures, it is important to note that the result is indicative of particular persons at a particular time and place. Unless this information is clear from the context, it is important to specify the relevant person, place, and time factors.

Problem 5-5: Period Prevalence

From January 1 to March 14 of the previous year, 112 cases of salmonellosis were reported to health officials in Shelby County, a county with a population of 210,000 at the time. An additional 10 cases were reported March 15–30. On March 31, six new cases of salmonellosis were reported. Routine surveillance in the county indicated that four of the above reported cases in Shelby County died due to complications. Based on this information, what was the prevalence of salmonellosis in Shelby County during the first quarter of last year?

Solution:
We can use formula 5.8 to calculate the period prevalence of salmonellosis in this county.

$$Pd\ P = \frac{\text{Number of occurrences existing anytime during a specified time period}}{\text{Total defined population during the specified time period}} \times 10^n$$

For convenience, let us represent the formula for period prevalence as: $Pd\ P = (X\ /\ Y) \times 10^n$, where X = the number of occurrences existing anytime during a specified time period, Y = the total defined population during the specified time period, and 10^n = the population base. Since, by definition, period prevalence includes all cases that existed anytime during the specified time period, the four cases that died from salmonellosis must be included in the numerator. They were cases at some time during the first quarter of last year, and, therefore, they should not be excluded. Thus,

$$X = 112 + 10 + 6 = 128 \text{ cases of salmonellosis}$$

The total defined population includes everyone in Shelby County last year since no restrictions are placed on the population by demographic or other factors. Thus,

$$Y = 210,000 \text{ people}$$

$$Pd\ P = (128\ /\ 210,000) \times 10^n = 0.00061 \times 10^4 = 6.1 \text{ cases per } 10,000 \text{ population}$$

Answer: The period prevalence of salmonellosis was 6.1 cases per 10,000 population in Shelby County during the first quarter of last year.

Comments:
1. Period prevalence is the appropriate measure to use in solving this problem. The problem requests the prevalence over a period of time (i.e., the first quarter of last year), which is what period prevalence measures.

2. The population base is selected as in the previous problem. In this problem, a population base of 10^4 (or 10,000) is the smallest population base that will produce a prevalence of at least one per the selected population base.

3. As in the other previous problems, it is important to indicate the relevant person, place, and time factors unless this information is clear from the context of the problem.

Relationship between Incidence and Prevalence

Intuitively, it makes sense that incidence and prevalence are related. If there is an increase in the incidence of a nonfatal, non-curable disease in a *stable* community, the prevalence of the disease would also increase. In other words, if many new cases of the disease are developing in a community, and these cases continue to live with the disease, then unless there is significant migration of healthy individuals into the community or individuals with the disease out of the community, we would expect the prevalence of the disease to rise. Such is the case with type 2 diabetes. An increase in the incidence of type 2 diabetes in a **stable population** (one where there is little migration into or out of the population) would be accompanied by an increase in the prevalence of this disease since it is chronic and not rapidly fatal. On the other hand, if the disease is either rapidly fatal or curable, we would not expect an increase in incidence to be associated with an increase in prevalence of the disease. Such is the case with some **nosocomial infections** (hospital-acquired infections).

The relationship between incidence and prevalence is illustrated in figure 5-1 where incidence is depicted by the rate at which water flows from a faucet into a basin, and prevalence is represented by the water level in the basin. When the rate of inflow is heavy (high incidence), the basin fills readily (high prevalence). The process, however, is mediated by another factor, which is represented by the basin drain. This factor is *disease resolution* or duration of the disease. If, for example, the disease resolves quickly by recovery or death (short duration), this will have the effect of reducing the prevalence unless the

Figure 5-1   Relationship between Incidence and Prevalence

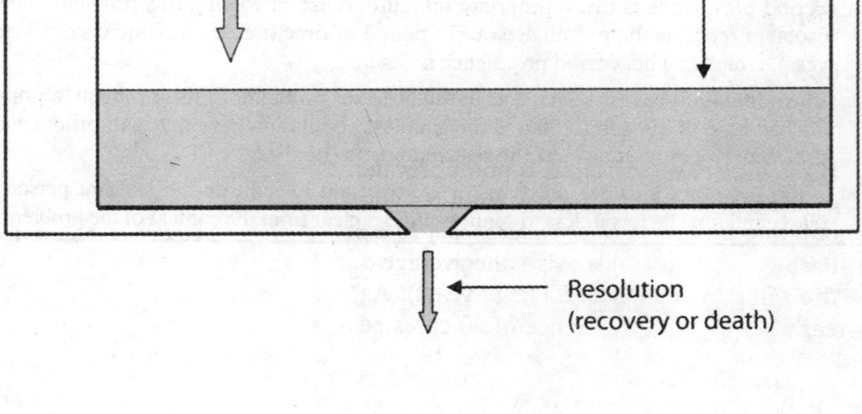

inflow is heavy enough to sustain the water level in the basin. A number of scenarios representing incidence, prevalence, and disease resolution can be inferred from the illustration. Some are these are summarized in figure 5-2. It seems like a paradox that advances in medical treatment that increase the life expectancy of patients without curing their diseases actually increase the prevalence of the diseases. This has been the case with AIDS, diabetes, and certain cancers.

Figure 5-2   Some Factors Affecting Prevalence in a Population

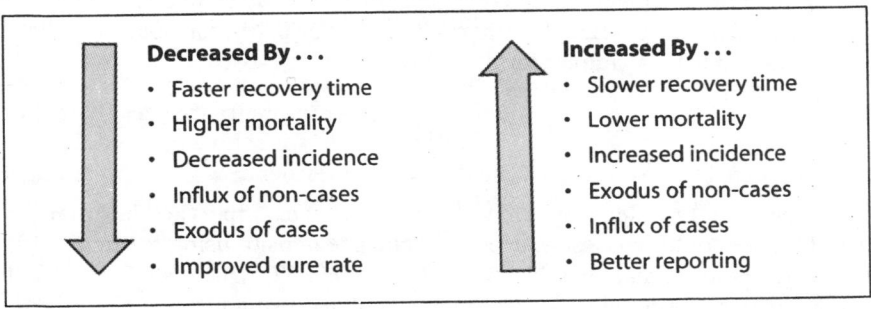

Decreased By...	Increased By...
• Faster recovery time	• Slower recovery time
• Higher mortality	• Lower mortality
• Decreased incidence	• Increased incidence
• Influx of non-cases	• Exodus of non-cases
• Exodus of cases	• Influx of cases
• Improved cure rate	• Better reporting

Incidence Density and Point Prevalence

When a population is stable and incidence and prevalence are unchanging, we have what are known as **steady-state conditions**. Under these conditions we can easily predict incidence density if we know the point prevalence. This can be very useful because point prevalence tends to be easier to obtain than incidence density. While prevalence can be attained in a one-time assessment of disease status in a population, incidence requires at least two assessments. First, to determine who does not have the disease and second to determine who develops the disease during follow up. Therefore, incidence studies tend to be more costly and time consuming than prevalence studies.

Assuming steady-state conditions, incidence density can be estimated from point prevalence using the following formula:

(5.9)

$$ID = \frac{P}{(1-P) \times D}$$

ID is incidence density, P is point prevalence, and D is the average duration of the disease from diagnosis until resolution (i.e., recovery or death). In calculating formula 5.9, *the rates should be expressed as decimal fractions* (e.g., P = 0.05 versus 5 per 100). Also, the average duration (D) should be expressed in the same time units as ID (e.g., years). As a simple example, say a given disease has a point prevalence of 20 cases per 1,000 population and an average duration of three years from diagnosis to resolution. The incidence density would be estimated as follows:

$$ID = 0.020 / [(1 - 0.020) \times 3] = 0.020 / 2.94 = 0.0068$$

Using a population base of 10^3, the estimated incidence density is $0.0068 \times 10^3 = 6.8$ per 1,000 person-years assuming steady-state conditions. Note that 0.020, a decimal fraction, is equivalent to 20 per 1,000. Using decimal fractions avoids the problem of what to do with the population bases during the arithmetic procedures. This formula works best if the duration of the disease shows little variance.

If in addition to meeting the requirement for steady-state conditions, the point prevalence is low (i.e., less than 10 per 100 or 0.10), formula 5.9 can be approximated from a simpler formula (5.10).

(5.10)

$$ID = \frac{P}{D}$$

Since the point prevalence was low in the previous example (i.e., less than 10 per 100), we could have estimated the incidence density using formula 5.10. In this case the estimate would be $0.020 / 3 = 0.0067$, which is 6.7 per 1,000 person-years and very close to what was calculated using formula 5.9.

Cumulative Incidence, Point Prevalence, and Risk

While cumulative incidence is generally a reliable estimate of the average risk of disease development, point prevalence is not. This is due to the fact that the magnitude of point prevalence is influenced by both the probability (risk) of disease development and the duration of the disease. Cumulative incidence, on the other hand, is affected by the probability of disease development but not disease duration. That is, whether cases recover or die has no bearing on the number of *new* cases developing in a defined population, but it does have an influence on the number of cases that *exist* in a population. Stated succinctly, cumulative incidence reflects the *risk* of disease development, while point prevalence reflects both *risk* and *disease duration*. These latter two elements can be difficult to untangle when trying to determine the causes of disease. For this reason prevalence should not be used to estimate risk. The problem is illustrated by early results from the Framingham Heart Study (chapter 1). Initial examinations of the 30–44-year age group revealed the same prevalence of coronary heart disease (CHD) in males and females (each 5 per 1,000). Eight years of follow up, however, revealed something unexpected. The cumulative incidence of CHD for males was 24 per 1,000 versus only 1 per 1,000 for females. Had prevalence been used to estimate the risk of CHD, one would have concluded incorrectly that there is no difference in the risk of CHD between males and females in the this age group when in fact the risk in males was apparently over 20 times that in females. The reason for the different findings between the sexes had to do with the duration of

CHD. The males tended to develop more fatal myocardial infarctions than the females, while the females tended to develop more nonfatal cases of angina pectoris than the males.[9] Thus, CHD in the males tended to be of shorter duration, resulting in a relatively low prevalence compared to cumulative incidence, and CHD in the females tended to be of longer duration resulting in a relatively high prevalence compared to cumulative incidence. In other words, prevalence of CHD was affected by duration of the disease, while cumulative incidence was not. Table 5-3 compares the measures of cumulative incidence and point prevalence.

Table 5-3   General Characteristics of Incidence and Prevalence

Cumulative Incidence	Point Prevalence
• Dynamic concept indicating change in disease status over time	• Static concept indicating existing disease status at a particular time
• A good estimate of the risk of disease	• An unreliable estimate of the risk of disease
• Unaffected by recovery or death	• Affected by recovery or death

Prevalence Odds

A third prevalence measure, **prevalence odds**, is analogous to incidence odds except that it is the ratio of the number of people who *have* a given occurrence (e.g., disease) to the number of people who do *not have* the occurrence at a point in time. The prevalence odds reflect prevalence of the disease (what exists), while the incidence odds reflect incidence of the disease (what develops). The equation for calculating prevalence odds is given in formula 5.11.

(5.11)

$$\text{Prevalence Odds} = \frac{\text{No. who have a given occurrence at a specific point in time}}{\text{No. who do not have the occurrence at the same point in time}}$$

Under steady state conditions (described earlier), the prevalence odds estimate the incidence density times the average duration of the disease (i.e., Prevalence Odds = ID x D). This is a simple transformation of formula 5.9 since the expression $P / (1 - P)$ is equivalent to the prevalence odds when P is expressed as a decimal fraction. For example, if there are 35 people with a given disease in a population of 500 on a given day, the prevalence odds using formula 5.11 is:

$$35 / (500 - 35) = 35 / 465 = 0.075$$

This means that the odds of *having* the disease in this population is 0.075. This is equivalent to what we would get using $P / (1 - P)$, where P is the point prevalence stated as a decimal fraction. This calculation is:

$$(35 / 500) / [1 - (35 / 500)] = 0.07 / 0.93 = 0.075$$

It should be clear from the above example that prevalence odds can be calculated in two ways: (a) using formula 5.11, or (b) by the expression $P / (1 - P)$, where P is the point prevalence stated as a decimal fraction. Prevalence odds may also be used to estimate incidence density under steady state conditions (i.e., ID = Prevalence Odds / D, based on formula 5.9). Moreover, just as the incidence odds approximate cumulative incidence when the disease is rare, prevalence odds approximate point prevalence when the disease is rare. In the example cited above, the prevalence odds were 0.075, and the point prevalence (P) was 0.07. These values (0.075 and 0.07) are close because the disease is relatively rare (i.e., it has prevalence of less than 0.10). Figure 5-3 briefly summarizes the basic measures of incidence and prevalence discussed in this chapter.

Figure 5-3   Basic Measures of Incidence and Prevalence

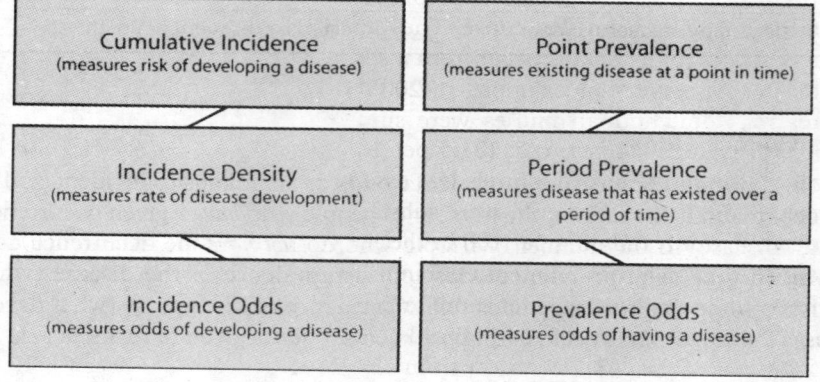

GENERAL HEALTH AND POPULATION INDICES

There are a number of measures of occurrence used in epidemiology as general indicators or indices of the health status of a population. Many of these measures relate to mortality since these data are generally more readily available than data on morbidity. In addition, there are several indicators of population dynamics (e.g., the **crude birth rate** and the **fertility rate**), which indicate changes in population growth. Appendix C lists some of the more common indices reported in epidemiology. The population bases shown are those most frequently reported in the U.S. As should be clear from the preceding discussion, other population bases may be used in specific circumstances.

The **crude death rate** (CDR) is actually a type of cumulative incidence and, hence, a proportion, even though it is commonly referred to as a rate.

The occurrence being measured is death, and since everyone is at risk of dying, the population at risk is the entire defined population. The CDR in the United States in 2003 was reported to be 841.9 deaths per 100,000 population.[10] Like cumulative incidence, it is important to indicate the time period for which the CDR and other proportions are reported since they generally can be expected to increase with time of observation.

Another common index is the **cause-specific mortality rate**, which measures the risk of death in a defined population due to a specific cause. It also is a proportion, though commonly referred to as a rate. In 2003, the reported U.S. cause-specific mortality rate for diseases of the heart was 235.6 per 100,000, which was over four times that reported for cerebrovascular diseases (54.2 per 100,000) and 38 times that reported for Parkinson's disease (6.2 per 100,000).[10]

The **proportionate mortality ratio** (PMR) appears similar to the cause-specific mortality rate but is actually quite different. Instead of measuring the *risk* of dying from a specific cause of death, it measures how important a particular cause of death is in relation to all deaths occurring in a defined population. A high PMR means that a certain cause of death contributes substantially to all deaths in a particular group, but it tells us nothing about the risk of dying from that cause. The PMR, which is a ratio, depends not only on how many deaths occur from a specific cause but also on how many total deaths occur. For example, in 2003, the U.S. cause-specific mortality rates for unintentional injuries were similar in 55–64 year olds (32.9 per 100,000) and 25–34 year olds (31.5 per 100,000),[10] implying that the risk of dying from unintentional injuries was essentially the same between these age groups. The PMRs, however, were substantially different (3.5 per 100 in the older age group and 30.4 per 100 in the younger age group). Thus, although the risks of dying from unintentional injuries were similar in both age groups, unintentional injuries were far more important as a cause of death in the 25–34 year olds than in the 55–64 year olds. The explanation is in the math. Only 3.5 percent of the 262,519 deaths from all causes in the older age group were due to unintentional injuries, while 30.4 percent of the 41,300 deaths from all causes in the younger age group were due to unintentional injuries.[10] The PMR is often used to determine leading causes of death.

Other common health status indices include the **infant mortality rate**, the **neonatal mortality rate**, the **maternal mortality rate**, the **perinatal mortality rate**, and the **fetal death rate** (see appendix C). Note that the first three of these "rates" have the number of live births in the denominator. This is not the exact population at risk, but it is a convenient estimate, and one that is reliably reported and readily available. The population at risk for the maternal mortality rate, for example, should be the number of pregnancies during the specific time interval, but as this is virtually impossible to obtain in a population, the number of live births provides a convenient estimate. The denominators for the perinatal mortality rate and the fetal death rate are also denominators of convenience. With regard to the infant and neonatal mortality rates, which are usually reported on a calendar year basis, some of the infant deaths in one year may be from births that occurred in the previous year. For example, some deaths that occurred in January of a particular calendar year may represent births that occurred in December of the previous year. Nevertheless, these routinely reported measures of occurrence are good indices of the health status of a population and are valuable in identifying potential public health problems, establishing trends, and making comparisons to other populations or periods of time. We would be very concerned, for example, about the quality of health care and public health services in a population if the infant mortality rate was increasing or high compared to similar populations.

OTHER MEASURES OF OCCURRENCE

Case Fatality

One special type of mortality measure that deserves mention is **case fatality**. Case fatality is a proportion, although it is usually referred to as the **case fatality rate** or **case fatality ratio**. Specifically, it is the proportion of cases of a given disease that die from that disease in a specified period of time. Hence, it is a measure of the *deadliness* of a given disease. In clinical epidemiology (chapter 1) case fatality is used as a measure of prognosis among those diagnosed with a given disease. In outbreak investigations (chapter 14) it is often used to measure the severity of a disease. In health care applications it can be used as an indication of the quality of care or the benefits of medical treatment.

Ideally, case fatality is calculated by following a specific group of patients with a common diagnosis for a specific period of time to determine the proportion of the patients that die from the disease.[11] For example, assume that on January 1 of a given year 40 cases of a particular disease are diagnosed at a major hospital at the time of admission. By the end of the year, 12 of these cases have died from the disease. The case fatality (CF) for that year would be calculated as follows:

$$CF = (12 / 40) \times 10^n = 0.30 \times 10^2 = 30 \text{ percent}$$

Following up individual patients and confirming the cause of death in each case can be very expensive and time consuming, especially when it involves a large group dispersed over a wide area. More commonly case fatality is estimated using formula 5.12.

(5.12)

$$CF = \frac{\text{Number of deaths from a specific disease during a specified time period}}{\text{Number of cases of the disease during the same time period}} \times 10^n$$

In this equation, CF refers to case fatality, 10^n is the population base, which is usually 10^2 (or 100), but can be larger if the CF is very small (i.e., less than one per 100). As an example, assume that 120 human cases of West Nile disease are reported in Illinois from June 1 until August 31 during a given year. Also assume that 10 cases die from West Nile disease during the same time period. Using formula 5.12, the estimated case fatality is calculated as:

$$CF = (10 / 120) \times 10^n = 0.83 \times 10^2 = 8.3 \text{ percent}$$

Note that this is the *three-month* case fatality for West Nile disease in Illinois and that it is stated as a *percent*. It is important to report the time period the case fatality represents (just as it was for cumulative incidence) since case fatality can be expected to increase with time. Also, most case fatalities are expressed as percents, although as mentioned earlier, if the case fatality is very small, a population base greater than 10^2 may be used.

There are some potential problems with case fatalities reported in the literature. First, the time period is not always specified as it should be. For example, the case fatality for untreated bubonic plague is reported to be about 55 percent.[12] While this tells us on average the percent of diagnosed cases that die from the disease, it does not give us a very precise indication of how long after diagnosis death is likely to occur. This is more problematic for chronic diseases such as prostate cancer or diabetes. Consequently, case fatality can be difficult to interpret, particularly if the normal time from diagnosis to death is relatively long. For one thing, case fatality may increase with time of observation, and for another, a longer time period may mean that more of the deaths are due to factors other than the disease (e.g., automobile crashes, homicides). Therefore, case fatality-may be best suited as a measure of prognosis for diseases where the period of risk is relatively short.[13] Another problem can arise when the denominator is estimated using incident cases during the specified time period. Since the deaths and the cases would not necessarily be linked, some deaths could be due to cases that occurred in a previous time period and not to those in the denominator. Unless the incidence and mortality of the disease are relatively stable, this could affect the accuracy of the measure.[14]

Survival Rates

A measure of occurrence related to case fatality can be referred to as the **simple survival rate** (SSR). It is also called the *survival rate*. Like case fatality, it is an indication of disease severity and patient prognosis and, therefore, useful in applications of clinical epidemiology. The simple survival rate, which is actually a proportion, measures the probability of surviving from a given disease for a specified period of time,[15] generally five years for cancers. The SSR is usually expressed as a percent and can be calculated as shown in formula 5.13. As with case fatality and cumulative incidence, it is imperative to report the time period represented by the SSR since it is affected by time.

(5.13)

$$SSR = \frac{\begin{array}{c}\text{Number of newly diagnosed patients with a given disease} - \\ \text{Number of deaths among the patients during a specified time period}\end{array}}{\text{Number of newly diagnosed patients with the disease}} \times 10^n$$

For example, say one wanted to calculate the five-year simple survival rate for breast cancer. Suppose there were 150 newly diagnosed breast cancer cases in a sample population served by a major metropolitan medical clinic, and the investigators followed each patient for five years. During the five years of follow up, 35 of the cases died from breast cancer. The simple survival rate would be calculated in the following manner:

$$\text{SSR} = [(150 - 35) / 150] = (115 / 150) \times 10^n = 0.767 \times 10^2 = 76.7 \text{ percent}$$

Thus, 76.7 percent of the patients survived five years after diagnosis with breast cancer. The SSR assumes that death due to the disease is the only reason that patients do not complete the prescribed follow-up period. It does not account for censored observations. Life table analysis and other methods of survival analysis (exhibit 5-2) have been developed to handle these situations and are discussed succinctly by Beth Dawson and Robert G. Trapp[16] and others. The survival rates calculated using these methods are more useful than the SSR, which is unrealistic in dynamic populations where some follow-up times may be relatively long.

Conceptually, the simple survival rate is the complement of the "ideal" case fatality referred to in the previous section. You will recall in the example that 12 deaths occurred among 40 cases in a year's time (CF = 30 percent). The one-year SSR for this group is therefore: $[(40 - 12) / 40] \times 10^2 = 70$ percent. Thus, when all cases are observed for the duration of the stated time period except for those that die, the sum of case fatality and the simple survival rate will always equal 100 percent. This situation, however, rarely exists except perhaps in certain disease outbreaks.

A popular variation of the survival rate calculated using survival analysis is the **relative survival rate**. This rate (actually a ratio) compares the survival rate for a group of patients with a given disease (i.e., the observed rate) to the survival rate in a general population sample that has similar characteristics, such as age, sex, race/ethnicity, and calendar year of observation (i.e., the expected rate).[17] The relative survival rate is then multiplied by 100 and expressed as a percent. The purpose of the relative survival rate is to control for other common causes of death that could affect the accuracy of the observed rate. For example, the observed rate might be influenced by the age of the sample. If the patients in the group are elderly, they may be more likely to die from age-related conditions not associated with the study disease than younger age groups. By comparing the observed rate to a population rate with a similar age distribution one in effect controls for the influence of age on mortality. In other words, any difference in the ratio of the observed to expected rates should not be due to age since the populations have similar age distributions. Therefore, differences in survival rates are likely to be due to the study disease.

The relative survival rate can be expected to be higher than the observed rate because it has been adjusted for deaths unrelated to the study disease (see example 1 in exhibit 5-3). The relative survival rate may be underestimated, however, for diseases like lung cancer. This is because groups of lung cancer patients tend to have more smokers compared to general population samples from which the expected rate is calculated. Smokers tend to be at higher risks for deaths from other diseases, as well as lung cancer, lowering their survival rate. The expected rate, however, will not be affected to the same degree by these unrelated deaths because of fewer smokers in the population. Thus, the

Exhibit 5-3
Issues with Relative Survival Rates

Relative Survival Rate = (Observed Rate / Expected Rate) x 100

Example 1:   Assume there is a cohort of 1,000 patients with colon cancer in which 300 die in a given year. This cohort is compared to a population of 1,000 people with a similar age, sex, and race/ethnicity distribution in which 50 deaths occur from all causes in the same year.

The observed rate = (1,000 − 300) / 1,000 = 700 / 1,000 = 0.70
The expected rate = (1,000 − 50) / 1,000 = 950 / 1000 = 0.95

Therefore, the one-year relative survival rate is:

Relative Survival Rate = (0.70 / 0.95) x 100 = 73.7%

Notice that the relative survival rate for colon cancer is *greater* than the observed rate. This is because the relative survival rate has been adjusted for deaths unrelated to colon cancer. Had these unrelated deaths not occurred in the patient cohort the observed rate would have been higher than 0.70 (70 percent). This is why the relative survival rate gives a better indication of the survival rate due to colon cancer than the observed rate.

Example 2:   Assume there is a cohort of 1,000 patients with lung cancer in which 800 die within a given year (assume 700 from lung cancer and 100 from heart disease). This cohort is compared to a population of 1,000 people with a similar age, sex, and race/ethnicity distribution in which 50 deaths occur from all causes in the same year.

The observed rate = (1,000 − 800) / 1,000 = 200 / 1,000 = 0.20
The expected rate = (1,000 − 50) / 1,000 = 950 / 1,000 = 0.95

Therefore, the one-year relative survival rate is:

Relative Survival Rate = (0.20 / 0.95) x 100 = 21.1%

Notice, however, that the relative survival rate for lung cancer is an *underestimate* of the survival rate for lung cancer alone, which is:

(1,000 − 700) / 1,000 = (300 / 1,000) x 100 = 30.0%

This is because many of the 100 deaths due to heart disease in the patient cohort were probably due to the high percent of cigarette smokers in this group. A high percent of cigarette smokers would be expected in the patient cohort because of the very close relationship between cigarette smoking and lung cancer. The number of smokers in the general population is likely to be much less. Because cigarette smoking is also closely related to death from heart disease, we would expect proportionately less deaths from heart disease in the general population due to the lower prevalence of cigarette smoking. The result is that the relative survival rate underestimates the survival rate for lung cancer alone. This underestimate could be minimized if in addition to controlling for age, sex, race/ethnicity, and calendar year, the investigators were also to control for differences in cigarette smoking.

relative survival rate will be lower than the survival rate for lung cancer alone because of a failure to adjust adequately for smoking-related deaths not related to lung cancer.[18] This is illustrated in example 2 in exhibit 5-3.

The concept of the relative survival rate is illustrated in an analysis of cancer statistics compiled from 1990 to 1999 by researchers at the National Cancer Institute. They found, for example, that the five-year relative survival rate for colon cancer in any stage was 62 percent overall, but 96 percent for patients in stage one of the disease and only six percent for those in stage four (see chapter 3 for definitions of cancer stages).[18] These statistics highlight the importance of early detection of colon cancer.

Years of Potential Life Lost

Years of potential life lost (YPLL) and its variants (e.g., years of productive life lost) measure the relative impact of premature death on society and can be used to establish public health priorities. In contrast to other mortality measures, they are weighted toward deaths at younger ages. Hence, a death of a 10 year old contributes substantially more to the YPLL than the death of a 60 year old.[19] This weighting has a definite economic overtone, but it does dramatize the societal impact of some diseases. The YPLL can be calculated for all premature deaths or only those from specific causes (see figure 5-4).

Figure 5-4   Years of Potential Life Lost before Age 65 by Causes of Death, U. S., 1995

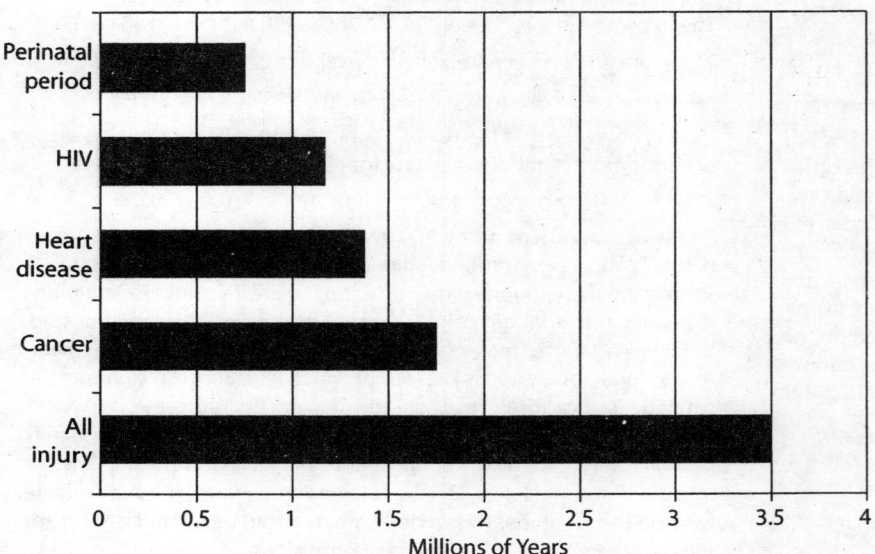

Millions of Years

Reference: National Center for Prevention and Control (1997). Years of Potential Life Lost Before Age 65 Due to Injury. Available: http://www.cdc.gov/ncipc/images/yp1995.gif (Access date: March 3, 2000).

To calculate YPLL, one must first decide upon a suitable *endpoint*. The endpoint represents an age that is considered *not* to constitute premature or untimely death. Typical endpoints are 65, 70, or 75 years or average life expectancy, which is now about 75 years for males and 80 years for females in the U.S. For both sexes combined it is 77.5 years.[20] Once the endpoint has been determined, every death in a population that occurs *before* the endpoint is subtracted from the endpoint to obtain the number of years of potential life lost. This can be represented mathematically as:

(5.14) $$YPLL = \Sigma \, (E - a_i)$$

where Σ = sum of, E = the chosen endpoint (e.g., 75 years), and a_i = the age of an individual who dies *prior* to the endpoint. Thus, this formula represents the sum of the differences between the endpoint and age at premature death for all individuals in the population who have not yet reached the endpoint. When YPLL is calculated from a distribution of deaths by age categories, the *midpoints* of the age categories are used.

The **YPLL rate** is a measure of the number of years of potential life lost in relation to the population *younger* than the selected endpoint in a specified time period. It is calculated as follows:

(5.15)

$$YPLL \; Rate = \frac{YPLL}{Number \; in \; the \; population \; below \; the \; selected \; endpoint} \times 10^n$$

where YPLL is calculated as shown in formula 5.14, the denominator is the population younger than the chosen endpoint (e.g., those under 75 years of age), and 10^n is usually 10^3 or 1,000. The following problems are illustrative.

Problem 5-6: Years of Potential Life Lost before 75 Years

Health officials reported five deaths in the village of Spring Valley during the previous calendar year. Three of these deaths were in persons under the age of 75. One death occurred in a 19-year-old male due to a motorcycle crash. The other two deaths occurred from drowning when a brother and sister went swimming in an abandoned quarry. The boy was 11, and his sister was nine. The estimated population of Spring Valley last year was 5,400, and 65 percent of the population were under the age of 75. Based on these data, calculate the overall years of potential life lost (YPLL) before 75 years and the YPLL for each cause of death in Spring Valley. Also, calculate the overall YPLL rate.

Solution:
Step 1: Calculate the overall YPLL before 75 years using formula 5.14.

$$YPLL = \Sigma \, (E - a_i)$$

where Σ = sum of, E = the endpoint of interest, and a_i = the age of an individual who dies prior to the endpoint. Therefore,

$$\Sigma \, (E - a_i) = (75 - 19) + (75 - 11) + (75 - 9) = 56 + 64 + 66 = 186 \; YPLL$$

Step 2: Calculate YPLL for each cause of death. YPLL due to motorcycle injury is:

$$75 - 19 = 56 \text{ YPLL}$$

YPLL due to drowning is:

$$(75 - 11) + (75 - 9) = 64 + 66 = 130 \text{ YPLL}$$

Step 3: Calculate the overall YPLL rate using formula 5.15.

$$\text{YPLL Rate} = \frac{\text{YPLL}}{\text{Number in the population below the selected endpoint}} \times 10^n$$

For convenience, let's represent the formula as: YPLL rate = $(X / Y) \times 10^n$, where X = YPLL, Y = the population under age 75, and 10^n = the population base. Therefore,

$$X = 186 \text{ YPLL (from step 1)}$$

$$Y = 5,400 \times 0.65 = 3,510 \text{ people under age 75}$$

$$X / Y = 186 / 3,510 = 0.0530$$

$$\text{YPLL rate} = 0.0530 \times 10^3 = 53.0 \text{ YPLL per 1,000 population under age 75}$$

Answer: Last year in Spring Valley 186 years of potential life were lost before age 75. Fifty-six of these due to a motorcycle crash, and 130 were due to drowning. The YPLL rate was 53.0 per 1,000 population under age 75.

Comments:

1. Since age 75 is the endpoint, the two deaths that occurred in those 75 years or older are not considered in calculating YPLL, and the population 75 years or older is not included in the denominator of the YPLL rate.

2. The YPLL before age 75 in Spring Valley last year was 186. This implies that 186 years of life could have been saved if the deaths could have been prevented.

3. Drowning was the most important cause of death in Spring Valley last year in terms of YPLL before age 75. Over twice as many years of potential life were lost before age 75 due to drowning compared to the motorcycle crash (130 years versus 56 years).

4. The sum of YPLL due to the motorcycle crash and drowning is equal to the total YPLL before age 75 because these were the only causes of death in the population among those less than 75 years of age. Had there been other causes of death before age 75, the sum of the YPLL due to the motorcycle crash (56) and drowning (130) in this population would have been less than the total YPLL before age 75.

5. The YPLL rate is the number of years of potential life that were lost for every 1,000 persons in Spring Valley last year who had not yet attained the age of 75. A population base of 1,000 is commonly used with this rate, but any suitable population base may be chosen (e.g., 5.3 per 100).

6. Unless it is clear from the context, it is a good idea to indicate the population, place, and time observed when reporting YPLL or the YPLL rate. In this case it was the population of Spring Valley during the previous calendar year.

Problem 5-7: Years of Potential Life Lost before 70 Years

Assume that the following statistics were reported for Humboldt County in the previous calendar year:

Age Group	Population	Deaths
0–9	3,610	3
10–19	2,500	2
20–39	5,125	3
40–59	4,950	8
60–69	3,945	12
70 and over	2,900	13

Based on these data, calculate the total YPLL before age 70 and the YPLL rate in Humboldt County for the previous calendar year.

Solution:

Step 1: Calculate YPLL using formula 5.14.

$$YPLL = \Sigma \, (E - a_i)$$

where Σ = sum of, E = the endpoint of interest, and a_i = the midpoint of an individual age category where a death occurred prior to the endpoint. *The midpoint is determined by summing the initial and ending age for each age category, adding one, and dividing the sum by two.* Since all deaths in each age category are assumed to have occurred at the midpoint, the number of deaths in a category is multiplied by the difference between age 70 and the midpoint (i.e., $E - a_i$). Based on the data in the above table, YPLL are calculated as follows:

$$\Sigma \, (E - a_i) = [3 \, (70 - 5)] + [2 \, (70 - 15)] + [3 \, (70 - 30)] + [8 \, (70 - 50)] + [12 \, (70 - 65)] =$$
$$195 + 110 + 120 + 160 + 60 = 645 \text{ YPLL}$$

Step 2: Calculate the YPLL rate using formula 5.15.

$$YPLL \ Rate = \frac{YPLL}{\text{Number in the population below the selected endpoint}} \times 10^n$$

For convenience, let's represent the formula as: YPLL rate = $(X / Y) \times 10^n$, where X = YPLL, Y = the population under age 70, and 10^n = the population base. Therefore,

$$X = 645 \text{ YPLL (from step 1)}$$
$$Y = 3,610 + 2,500 + 5,125 + 4,950 + 3,945 = 20,130 \text{ people under age 70}$$
$$X / Y = 645 / 20,130 = 0.0320$$

YPLL rate = 0.0320×10^3 = 32.0 YPLL per 1,000 population under age 70

Answer: Last year in Humboldt County 645 years of potential life were lost before age 70, and the YPLL rate was 32.0 per 1,000 population under age 70.

Comments:

1. Since the age of 70 is chosen as the endpoint, the deaths that occurred in those 70 years and over are *not* considered in calculating YPLL. Also, the population 70 years and over is not included in the denominator of the YPLL rate.

2. To calculate YPLL in this problem, it is first necessary to determine the midpoint for each age category. This is accomplished by summing the beginning and ending age of an age category, adding one, and dividing the result by two (e.g., for the 0–9-year age group, the midpoint = $[0 + 9 + 1] / 2 = 5$). The one is added because the ending age (e.g., nine) is virtually a year long since it actually extends to within a day of the next year (i.e., 10). The midpoint is then subtracted from the endpoint (i.e., 70 years) and multiplied by the number of deaths in that category. In problem

5-6 we had each individual's age at death, which we subtracted from the endpoint. We do not have this information in this problem; therefore, we have assumed that all deaths in a particular age category were on average at the midpoint of the interval. For example, multiplying the difference between the endpoint and the midpoint in the first age category by three is the same as adding 70 − 5 three times, since all deaths in the category are presumed to have occurred at age five, which is the midpoint of the 0–9 age group.

3. The overall YPLL before age 70 is estimated to be 645. This means that based on the chosen endpoint of 70 years, approximately 645 years of life could have been saved in Humboldt County last year if the deaths could have been prevented. The reason this number is approximate is because exact ages at death are not available and were therefore estimated using the midpoints of the age categories. Exact ages may not always be available when secondary data sources are being used.

4. The YPLL rate is the estimated number of years of potential life that were lost for every 1,000 persons in Humboldt County who were not yet 70 years of age. A population base of 1,000 is commonly used, but as in the previous problem any suitable population base may be used.

5. Unless it is clear from the context, it is important to indicate the population, place, and time observed when reporting YPLL or the YPLL rate. In this case it was the population of Humboldt County in the previous calendar year.

CONFIDENCE INTERVALS FOR INCIDENCE AND PREVALENCE

Background

In statistics, when a sample is based on **random selection**, a method where each person in the sampled population has an equal chance of being chosen, the sample value is considered a **point estimate*** of the population parameter. The precision of the point estimate (i.e., how well it estimates the population parameter), however, depends on **sampling variation** (also known as **sampling error**).[21] Sampling variation is due to the fact that any given sample is an imperfect representation of the sampled population since not all possible subjects are included, and those who are included may be more or less like those in the population. The amount of sampling variation will depend on the amount of variability in the population and the size of the sample.[22] Since the amount of sampling variation is dependent on the sample chosen, it cannot be determined directly, although it can be estimated.

One way of estimating the precision of a point estimate is to calculate a **confidence interval**, which is the range of values in which the population

---

*Technically, in order for a point estimate to be an *unbiased* estimate of a population parameter it must be based on a representative sample of the population (e.g., a randomly selected sample). **Convenience** or **haphazard samples**, where subjects are selected on the basis of expediency, are potentially biased and may not be representative of the desired population. Study populations used in epidemiology are rarely randomly selected from a population, except for certain cross-sectional studies, but confidence intervals (described shortly) are nevertheless used to indicate the relative amount of variability in the estimates.[13]

parameter is likely to fall based on statistical probability. The most commonly reported confidence interval in epidemiology is the *95 percent confidence interval*. It may be loosely interpreted as follows:

> *The 95 percent confidence interval means that we are 95 percent certain that the population parameter lies within the range of values indicated by the interval.*

Figure 5-5 provides an example of a 95 percent confidence interval for a point prevalence of 4.8. The 95 percent represents the **confidence level**, that is, how sure we are the population prevalence is in the range indicated. The range represents the *confidence interval*, and the start and end of the range represent the **confidence limits**. The lower prevalence is known as the **lower confidence limit** (LCL), and the upper prevalence is known as the **upper confidence limit** (UCL). With regard to the example in figure 5-5, we can state that we are 95 percent confident that the true value lies between 4.2 per 1,000 and 5.4 per 1,000 based on the sample selected. This implies, of course, that we cannot be 100 percent certain because for every 100 samples drawn randomly from a population, we would expect that five percent would produce point estimates outside the lower and upper confidence limits because of sampling variation. Nevertheless, we have a high degree of confidence about the relative magnitude of the true value.

Figure 5-5   Anatomy of a 95% Confidence Interval (CI)

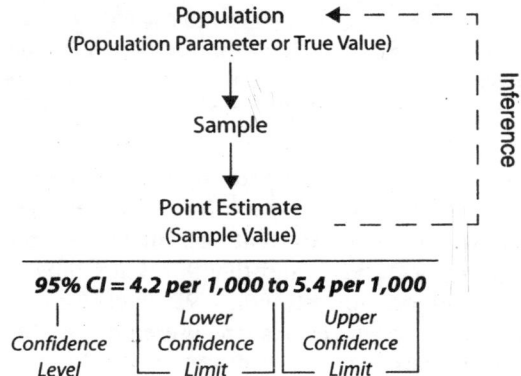

A confidence interval will be affected by sample size, the variance in the population, and the confidence level chosen. Narrow confidence intervals indicate more precision than wide confidence intervals. In general, for a given confidence level, which is usually, though not always 95 percent, the greater the sample size, the more precise the point estimate, and thus the narrower the confidence interval. On a relative basis it is easier to be 50 percent confident about the probable range of a population parameter than to be 99 percent confident. Therefore, the greater the confidence level for a particular sample, the wider the confidence interval, all other factors being equal. Exhibit 5-4 presents the general format of confidence intervals for measures of occurrence based on the assumption that the measures are normally distributed.

Exhibit 5-4
General Format of Confidence Intervals for Measures of Occurrence (Based on the Assumption of Normality)

If we assume that the measure of occurrence (e.g., prevalence, cumulative incidence, incidence density) for a given sample is part of a sampling distribution that is normally distributed, then a confidence interval (CI) can be constructed using the following general format:

$$\% \; CI = \text{point estimate} \pm z \; (S.E.)$$

The point estimate is the sample measure of occurrence. It is the value calculated from a representative sample of the population. The z refers to the **z-score**, which represents the number of standard deviation units from the mean of a standardized normal distribution with a mean of zero and a standard deviation of one. The term S.E. refers to **standard error**, which is a measure of sampling error. A 95% confidence interval, for example, can be written as:

$$95\% \; CI = \text{point estimate} \pm 1.96 \; (S.E.)$$

A z-score of ± 1.96 is used because this represents 95% of the area on either side of the mean value of the measure of occurrence in a standardized normal distribution. A 90% confidence level could be calculated using a z-score of ± 1.65 instead of 1.96; likewise, a 99% confidence interval could be calculated using a z-score of ± 2.58.

For a further explanation of confidence intervals consult any basic statistics textbook. The terms z-score and standard error are defined in more detail in the glossary.

Because of their extensive use and importance in epidemiology, you will be reading more about specific types of confidence intervals in subsequent chapters. For now it is important that you understand their usefulness with sample measures of occurrence and that you know how they are calculated and interpreted. Methods for estimating 95 percent confidence intervals for incidence and prevalence measures are presented in the following section along with relevant examples.

Estimating Confidence Intervals

A 95 percent confidence interval for *either* cumulative incidence (formula 5.1) or prevalence (formula 5.7) can be approximated using formula 5.16 below. This formula is based on the assumption that the measure of occurrence is normally distributed. While "exact" confidence intervals for cumulative incidence or prevalence, which are proportions, can be calculated based on the binomial distribution, the procedure is complex and is not recommended without an appropriate computer program to perform the calculations. An approximation, known as the *Wald confidence interval for a proportion*, is based on a normal distribution and is much easier to use but does not always yield very accurate results, especially when the sample size is small or the population proportion (cumulative incidence or prevalence) is near zero or one.[23, 24] A modification of the Wald interval has been suggested by Alan Agresti and Brent A. Coull.[24] This is the basis for formula 5.16. Although it is approximate, according to the authors, it "behaves adequately for practical application for essentially any *n* regardless of the value of *p*."[24(p124)]

(5.16)
$$95\% \text{ CI} = p \pm 1.96\sqrt{p(1-p)/(n+4)}$$
$$\text{where } p = (x+2)/(n+4)$$

The p in the above expression refers to the adjusted sample proportion (either cumulative incidence or prevalence *stated as a decimal fraction*, e.g., 0.10 vs. 10 per 100). The n is the appropriate denominator of the proportion (i.e., the population at risk for cumulative incidence or the total population for prevalence; see formulas 5.1 and 5.7, respectively), and x is the appropriate numerator of the proportion (new cases for cumulative incidence or existing cases for prevalence; also see formulas 5.1 and 5.7, respectively).

A somewhat different formula may be used to estimate the 95 percent confidence interval for incidence density. This formula also assumes that the measure of occurrence is normally distributed and is easier to use than the exact method, which is based on the Poisson distribution.[25]

(5.17)
$$95\% \text{ CI} = ID \pm 1.96\sqrt{x/T^2}$$

In this expression ID is incidence density *stated as a decimal fraction* (e.g., 0.10 per person-year vs. 10 per 100 person-years), x is the number of new cases (i.e., the numerator for incidence density), and T is the total person-time units observed. The use of formulas 5.16 and 5.17 are illustrated in the following problems.

Problem 5-8: Estimation of the 95% Confidence Interval for Prevalence

A randomly selected sample of 2,000 residents of a large city in Southeast Asia revealed that there were 141 cases of active tuberculosis on January 1, 2007. Based on the sample, what was the prevalence of tuberculosis on this date and its approximate 95 percent confidence interval?

Solution:
Step 1: Calculate the prevalence using formula 5.7.

$$P = \frac{\text{Number of occurrences existing at a specific point in time}}{\text{Total defined population at the same point in time}} \times 10^n$$

$$P = 141 / 2,000 \times 10^n = 0.0705 \times 10^2 = 7.05 \text{ cases per 100 population}$$

Step 2: Calculate the approximate 95 percent confidence interval for the prevalence determined in step 1 using formula 5.16.

$$95\% \ CI = p \pm 1.96\sqrt{p(1-p)/(n+4)} \ \text{where} \ p = (x+2)/(n+4)$$

$$p = (141+2)/(2{,}000+4) = 143/2{,}004 = 0.0714$$

$$95\% \ CI = 0.0714 \pm 1.96\sqrt{0.0714(1-0.0714)/2{,}004}$$

$$0.0714 - (1.96)(0.00575) = 0.0714 - 0.0113 = 0.0601$$
[This is the lower confidence limit.]

$$0.0714 + (1.96)(0.00575) = 0.0714 + 0.0113 = 0.0827$$
[This is the upper confidence limit.]

$$95\% \ CI = 0.0601 \ \text{to} \ 0.0827 \ \text{or} \ 6.01 \ \text{per} \ 100 \ \text{to} \ 8.27 \ \text{per} \ 100$$

Answer: The prevalence of tuberculosis in this Southeast Asian city on January 1, 2007, was 7.05 cases per 100 population (95% CI = 6.01 per 100 to 8.27 per 100).

Comments:

1. The prevalence measure referred to in this problem is point prevalence since it represents existing cases at a point in time (i.e., the prevalence on January 1, 2007). Typically, when one refers to prevalence, one is referring to point prevalence (for a further explanation refer to the earlier section on prevalence in this chapter).

2. Estimating the 95 percent confidence interval using formula 5.16 requires two basic steps. In the first step, the measure of occurrence (p) is adjusted using the formula $p = (x + 2) / (n + 4)$. This value is then used to estimate the 95 percent confidence interval. The quantity to the right of the converted p in the equation for the 95 percent confidence interval (i.e., that following the $\pm$ sign) is first subtracted from the adjusted measure of occurrence to obtain the lower confidence limit (LCL). The same quantity is then added to the adjusted measure of occurrence to obtain the upper confidence limit (UCL). These limits define the range of the 95 percent confidence interval, which is usually reported along with the point estimate of the measure of occurrence as shown in the answer to this problem.

3. The calculated 95 percent confidence interval suggests that we are 95 percent certain that the true prevalence in this city is between 6.01 per 100 and 8.27 per 100. Our best single estimate (i.e., the point estimate) is 7.05 per 100. Note that this lies within the 95 percent confidence limits.

4. Although this problem concerned prevalence, the same formula for the 95 percent confidence interval (formula 5.16) may be used when the measure of interest is cumulative incidence. Thus, *formula 5.16 is applicable to both prevalence and cumulative incidence.*

Problem 5-9: Estimation of the 95% Confidence Interval for Incidence Density

A recent prospective cohort study of adult residents from a northwestern city in the United States revealed that 65 newly diagnosed cases of glaucoma developed during 1,300 person-years of follow up. Based on this information, calculate the incidence density of glaucoma in this sample and its approximate 95 percent confidence interval.

Solution:

Step 1: Calculate the incidence density using formula 5.3.

$$ID = \frac{\text{Number of new occurrences during a specified time period}}{\text{Total person-time units observed}} \times 10^n$$

ID = (65 / 1,300) x 10^n = 0.0500 x 10^2 = 5.00 cases per 100 person-years

Step 2: Calculate the approximate 95 percent confidence interval for the incidence density determined in step 1 using formula 5.17. Note that ID must be stated as a decimal fraction.

$$95\% \text{ CI} = ID \pm 1.96\sqrt{x/T^2}$$

$$95\% \text{ CI} = 0.0500 \pm 1.96\sqrt{65/1,300^2}$$

0.0500 – (1.96) (0.00620) = 0.0500 – 0.0122 = 0.0378
[This is the lower confidence limit.]

0.0500 + (1.96) (0.00620) = 0.0500 + 0.0122 = 0.0622
[This is the upper confidence limit.]

95% CI = 0.0378 to 0.0622 or 3.78 per 100 person-years to 6.22 per 100 person-years

Answer: The incidence density of glaucoma among adults in this northwestern city is 5.00 cases per 100 person-years (95% CI = 3.78 per 100 person-years to 6.22 per 100 person-years).

Comments:
1. Estimating the 95 percent confidence interval using formula 5.17 requires that the measure of occurrence be stated as a decimal fraction. In this problem the decimal fraction (0.0500) was calculated in step 1 prior to applying a population base of 10^2. The quantity to the right of the measure of occurrence in formula 5.17 (i.e., that following the ± sign) is first subtracted from the measure of occurrence to obtain the lower confidence limit (LCL). The same quantity is then added to the measure of occurrence to obtain the upper confidence limit (UCL). These limits define the range of the 95 percent confidence interval, which is usually reported along with the point estimate of the measure of occurrence as shown in the answer to this problem.

2. The calculated 95 percent confidence interval suggests that we are 95 percent certain that the true incidence density in this city is between 3.78 per 100 person-years and 6.22 per 100 person-years. Our best single estimate (i.e., the point estimate) is 5.00 per 100 person-years.

SUMMARY

• Measures of occurrence commonly used in epidemiology are specific types of counts, ratios, proportions, or rates. Incidence is one of the most common and versatile measures of occurrence in epidemiology. While traditionally it refers to a count, most often it is combined with an appropriate denominator and may be designated as an incidence measure. There are three basic types of incidence measures—cumulative incidence, incidence density, and incidence odds. Cumulative incidence is the proportion of the initial population at risk that develops a given outcome during a specified follow-up period. It is an accurate measure of a group member's average risk of developing the study outcome as long as everyone that does not develop the outcome completes the prescribed follow-up period. It is best used in fixed populations or closed cohorts, although it may be estimated in dynamic populations or open cohorts using actuarial life tables or by other more sophisticated procedures. Incidence density is the number of new occurrences in a defined population divided by the total person-time units observed, such as person-years. It is a measure of the rate of disease development in a population and does not require that noncases be followed up for the same time periods. It is useful in dynamic populations or open cohorts where subjects may enter and leave at different times. Under certain circumstances cumulative incidence can be used to estimate incidence density. Incidence odds is an infrequently used measure that measures the odds of developing a specific outcome in a specified time period. It is the ratio of the number of people who develop a new occurrence to the number of people who do not develop the occurrence in a given population during a specified period of time.

- Prevalence is a count of the number of existing cases in a defined population at a specified time. When divided by an appropriate denominator, it is the proportion of the total defined population that has a specific outcome at a specified time. Unlike cumulative incidence, prevalence is an unreliable estimate of risk because it is affected by the duration of the outcome. There are three basic types of prevalence—point prevalence, which is prevalence at a specific point or event in time; period prevalence, which is prevalence over a period of time; and prevalence odds, which are the odds of having an outcome at a point in time. A variant of period prevalence is lifetime prevalence, which the proportion of individuals in a defined population who have had a given outcome at any time during their lives. Under steady-state conditions and when the average disease duration is known, point prevalence and prevalence odds can be used to estimate the incidence density for a given disease. While incidence is a dynamic concept indicating change, prevalence is a static concept indicating the status quo.

- Other common measures of occurrence in epidemiology are used to indicate the health status of a population. These measures include the crude death rate, the cause-specific mortality rate, the proportionate mortality ratio, the infant mortality rate, years of potential life lost (YPLL), and the YPLL rate. In addition, the crude birth rate and the fertility rate can be used as indicators of population growth. Case fatality and the simple survival rate are measures of disease prognosis. The relative survival rate is a ratio that controls for deaths due to causes other than the disease of interest.

- Confidence intervals are commonly used to estimate the probable range in which the true value lies. The 95 percent level is the most common confidence level reported in epidemiology. It tells us with 95 percent confidence the likelihood that a given range of values contains the true value. Sample size, population variance, and the chosen confidence level will affect the range of a confidence interval. In general, for a given point estimate of the measure of occurrence, the narrower the range of a confidence interval, the more precise the point estimate and the wider the range, the less precise the point estimate.

New Terms

- actuarial method
- attack rate
- case fatality
- case fatality rate
- case fatality ratio
- cause-specific mortality rate
- count
- crude birth rate
- crude death rate
- cumulative incidence
- cumulative incidence rate
- fertility rate
- fetal death rate
- haphazard sample
- incidence
- incidence density
- incidence odds
- incidence proportion
- incidence rate
- infant mortality rate
- Kaplan-Meier product limit method
- life table method
- lifetime prevalence
- lower confidence limit
- maternal mortality rate
- measures of occurrence
- neonatal mortality rate
- nosocomial infections
- odds
- perinatal mortality rate
- period prevalence
- person-time incidence rate
- person-time units
- person-years
- censored observations
- competing risks
- confidence interval
- confidence level
- confidence limits
- convenience sample
- point estimate
- point prevalence
- population at risk
- population base
- prevalence
- prevalence odds
- prevalence proportion
- proportion
- proportionate mortality ratio
- random selection
- rate
- ratio
- relative survival rate
- risk
- sampling error
- sampling variation
- simple survival rate
- stable population
- standard error
- steady-state conditions
- survival analysis
- survival curve
- survival time
- time-to-event analysis
- upper confidence limit
- years of potential life lost
- YPLL rate
- z-score

Study Questions and Exercises

1. San Carlos County Health Department reported 17 new cases of tuberculosis in the first half of last year and 18 additional cases during the second half of last year. The population of the county was 204,500 at the beginning of last year and 215,000 at the end of the year. What was the incidence of tuberculosis in San Carlos County last year? Also, what type of incidence measure does this represent?

2. During the period July 1 to December 31, 76 cases of measles were reported among 12–19 year olds in a Russian community of 32,000. Ten percent (3,200) of the residents were 12–19 years old on April 1, and the size and age distribution of the population has remained constant. An investigation of the cases in the 12–19-year age group revealed that 22 of the reported cases were contracted prior to July 1. In addition, another 18 cases developed in April and May but were clinically resolved before July 1. What was the cumulative incidence of measles in 12–19 year olds in this Russian community during the period July 1–December 31 and the associated 95 percent confidence interval?

3. An epidemiologic study of breast cancer among elderly women followed 1,400 women, 65–79 years of age, without evidence of breast cancer over several years. Every two years the investigators examined the women for breast cancer. The results were as follows: 12 new cases at the first evaluation, 11 new cases at the second evaluation, 23 new cases at the third evaluation, and 28 new cases at the fourth (final) evaluation. The investigators also noted that 35 of the women had withdrawn from the study at the third evaluation. Based on this information, calculate and interpret the incidence density of breast cancer in this group and the associated 95 percent confidence interval.

4. Health authorities in Egypt reported that 22 injuries requiring hospitalization occurred in a community of 65,000 on a recent national holiday. Eight additional cases occurred during the following month, and two of these died from their injuries. What was the prevalence of injuries requiring hospitalization on the holiday and for the period as a whole?

5. In Ferguson Junction last year four deaths occurred in males aged 3, 12, 24, and 75 years, and two deaths occurred in females aged 14 and 85 years. The population of Ferguson Junction last year was 24,000, of which 10 percent were 70 years or older. Based on these data, calculate the total years of potential life lost (YPLL) before age 70 and the YPLL rate. Interpret your findings.

6. Each of the following statements suggests a common epidemiologic measure that could be calculated if all the data had been supplied·in the statement. For example, the first statement suggests the crude death rate. The numerator for this rate (82 deaths from all causes) is provided, and the

denominator is the population of Randall County, which could be obtained from census data. For each of the other statements indicate what measure of occurrence is most likely being suggested and indicate the reasons for your answer.

a. In Randall County there were 82 deaths from all causes last year.

b. Twelve cases of rabies were reported for the first time in Asheville this year.

c. Of 10 new cases of ovarian cancer diagnosed in Darrington County, only four were living after five years.

d. Ten percent of all deaths are caused by suffocation in Summit County.

e. Of the 130 babies born in Shannon County last year, 14 died within four weeks.

f. Last year 21 deaths occurred in Culver City from accidental drowning.

g. Sixty percent of the population of Orion has had the flu in the last two years.

h. Of the 45 cases of hemorrhagic stroke admitted to Community Memorial Hospital last year, 12 died within two days of admission.

i. On March 1, 15 students at Gateway Middle School had pertussis while 120 did not.

References

1. Kleinbaum, D. G., Kupper, L. L., and Morgenstern, H. (1982). *Epidemiologic Research: Principles and Quantitative Methods*. Belmont, CA: Lifetime Learning Publications.
2. Szklo, M., and Nieto, F. J. (2000). *Epidemiology: Beyond the Basics*. Gaithersburg, MD: Aspen.
3. Kahn, H. A., and Sempos, C. T. (1989). *Statistical Methods in Epidemiology*. New York: Oxford University Press.
4. Gregg, M. B., ed. (1996). *Field Epidemiology*. New York: Oxford University Press.
5. Last, J. M., ed. (2001). *A Dictionary of Epidemiology*, 4th ed. New York: Oxford University Press.
6. Abramson, J. H. (1988). *Making Sense of Data: A Self-Instruction Manual on the Interpretation of Epidemiologic Data*. New York: Oxford University Press.
7. Walker, A. M. (1991). *Observation and Inference: An Introduction to the Methods of Epidemiology*. Chestnut Hill, MA: Epidemiology Resources, Inc.
8. MacMahon, B., and Trichopoulos, D. (1996). *Epidemiology: Principles and Methods*, 2nd ed. Boston: Little, Brown and Company.
9. Mausner, J. S., and Kramer, S. (1985). *Mausner & Bahn Epidemiology—An Introductory Text*. Philadelphia: W. B. Saunders Company.
10. Hoyert, D. L., Heron, M. P., Murphy, S. L., and Kung, H-C. (2006). Deaths: Final Data for 2003. *National Vital Statistics Reports* 54 (13). Hyattsville, MD: National Center for Health Statistics.
11. Peterson, D. R., and Thomas, D. B. (1978). *Fundamentals of Epidemiology: An Instruction Manual*. Toronto: Lexington Books.
12. Chin, J., ed. (2000). *Control of Communicable Diseases Manual*, 17th ed. Washington, DC: American Public Health Association.
13. Rothman, K. J. (2002). *Epidemiology: An Introduction*. New York: Oxford University Press.
14. Hennekens, C. H., and Buring, J. E. (1987). *Epidemiology in Medicine*. Boston: Little, Brown and Company.
15. Greenberg, R. S., Daniels, S. R., Flanders, W. D., Eley, J. W., and Boring, J. R. III (2001). *Medical Epidemiology*, 3rd ed. New York: Lange Medical Books/McGraw-Hill.

16. Dawson, B., and Trapp, R. G. (2001). *Basic & Clinical Biostatistics*. New York: Lange Medical Books/McGraw-Hill.

17. Centre for Cancer Epidemiology (2001). Appendix 1-Statistical Methods, Relative Survival. Available: http://www.cce.man.ac.uk/statisti.htm (Access date: August 1, 2005).

18. Gloeckler-Ries, L. A., Reichman, M. E., Reidel-Lewis, D., Hankey, B. F., and Edwards, B. K. (2003). Cancer Survival and Incidence from the Surveillance, Epidemiology, and End Results (SEER) Program. *The Oncologist* 8: 541-552.

19. Centers for Disease Control and Prevention (1986). Premature Mortality in the United States: Public Health Issues in the Use of Years of Potential Life Lost. *Morbidity and Mortality Weekly Report* 35 (2S): 1s–11s.

20. Arias, E. (2006). United States Life Tables, 2003. *National Vital Statistics Reports* 54 (14). Hyattsville, MD: National Center for Health Statistics.

21. Vogt, W. P. (1999). *Dictionary of Statistics and Methodology: A Nontechnical Guide for the Social Sciences*, 2nd ed. Thousand Oaks, CA: Sage Publications.

22. Beaglehole, R., Bonita, R., and Kjellstrom, T. (1993). *Basic Epidemiology*. Geneva: World Health Organization.

23. Campbell, M. J. (1999). *Medical Statistics: A Commonsense Approach*, 3rd ed. Chichester: John Wiley & Sons, Ltd.

24. Agresti, A., and Coull, B. A. (1998). Approximate is Better Than "Exact" for Interval Estimation of Binomial Proportions. *The American Statistician* 52 (2): 119-126.

25. Ahlbom, A. (1993). *Biostatistics for Epidemiologists*. Boca Raton: Lewis Publishers.

CHAPTER SIX

Comparing Measures of Occurrence in Epidemiology

This chapter describes basic procedures for rate adjustment, commonly used measures of association in epidemiology, and the fundamentals underlying statistical significance testing.

Learning Objectives

- Compare and contrast crude, specific, and adjusted rates.
- Explain the rationale for rate adjustment or standardization.
- Perform and interpret the results of age adjustment using both the direct and indirect methods.
- Calculate and interpret each of the following measures of association: risk ratio (cumulative incidence ratio), rate ratio (incidence density ratio), odds ratio, prevalence ratio, percent relative effect, risk difference (cumulative incidence difference), rate difference (incidence density difference), prevalence difference, population rate difference, attributable fraction among the exposed, and population attributable fraction.
- Explain the usefulness of measures of association based on relative and absolute comparisons, respectively.
- Describe the process and rationale for hypothesis testing and determining the statistical significance of an association.
- Define 2000 U.S. standard million population and 2000 U.S. standard population; *a posteriori* comparison; absolute risk; alpha level; clinical (or practical) significance; defined population; directional and non-directional hypothesis; disease odds ratio; excess risk, rate, and prevalence; indirectly standardized rate; population risk difference and population prevalence difference; p-value; referent; relative odds; and relative risk.

131

INTRODUCTION

Comparing measures of occurrence between different populations, the same population at different times, or distinct subgroups within a population can provide useful clues to disease etiology and other important information. Say that the infant mortality rate is high in one jurisdiction but low in another with a similar population mix. This suggests that there is something different between the jurisdictions that may be responsible for the different infant mortality rates (e.g., access to health care). Similarly, if those with a particular exposure in a population have a higher cumulative incidence of a given disease than those in the same population without the exposure, it could be that the exposure is responsible for the increased risk of the disease. A first step in uncovering causal factors is to make comparisons of measures of occurrence, which is the subject of this chapter. As will become evident in this and subsequent chapters, comparisons must be made carefully and with due consideration of alternate explanations for the results.

In chapter 5 it was mentioned that the more common measures of occurrence used in epidemiology are specific types of counts, ratios, proportions, and rates. Many measures that are actually ratios or proportions, however, are often loosely referred to as rates. For example, the crude mortality rate reported in most governmental statistics is actually a proportion, specifically the proportion of a **defined population** (i.e., the population of interest) that dies in a given time period. As indicated in chapter 5, the use of the term "rate" for this and other measures is more traditional than accurate. To facilitate a coherent discussion, the term rate is used in its more traditional sense in this chapter. It is important to recognize, however, that not all of the measures referred to as rates are in fact rates; some may be ratios or proportions.

CRUDE AND SPECIFIC RATES

The measures of occurrence referred to in chapter 5 can be classified as either crude or specific rates (using "rates" in the traditional sense as indicated above). **Crude rates** are overall, summary measures of occurrence for a defined population. **Specific rates** are measures of occurrence for distinct subgroups within a defined population. For example, it has been reported that the cause-specific mortality rate for malignant neoplasms in the United States is 193.2 per 100,000. Among males, however, the rate is 203.8 per 100,000, and for females it is 183.0 per 100,000.[1] The cause-specific mortality rate in this example is a *crude rate*. It is an overall, summary measure for the United States as a whole, which is the defined population. The rates for males and females are *specific rates*, however. They are measures for distinct subgroups within the defined population. More precisely, they are *sex-specific rates*.

Specific rates can be calculated for any subgroup of a defined population. The most commonly reported specific rates are those based on age, sex, or race/ethnicity. In determining specific rates, it is essential to know the defined population. If the defined population only includes women, for instance, then sex-specific rates cannot be calculated. Age-specific or race/ethnicity-specific rates, however, could be determined.

Crude rates are useful because with *just a single* measure of occurrence we get an overall summary of the actual experience of a defined population. The crude rate is actually a *weighted average* of the specific rates in a population. For example, if a defined population is 60 percent male and 40 percent female, and if the sex-specific rates are 12 per 100 for males and 16 per 100 for females, then the crude rate is:

$$(12 \text{ per } 100 \times 0.60) + (16 \text{ per } 100 \times 0.40) = 13.6 \text{ per } 100.$$

Crude rates make comparisons between populations relatively simple, but they can be mine fields when it comes to interpreting the comparisons. Consider the following example. The crude death rate in Florida in 2002 was 1,004.1 per 100,000, and the crude death rate in Alaska in the same year was 470.7 per 100,000.[2] Before we conclude that the risk of death due to living in Florida is over twice that due to living in Alaska, we have to be sure that the populations are really comparable. If they differ significantly with regard to factors other than place of residence, and if these factors are related to the risk of death, then we cannot be sure whether the observed difference in the crude death rates is due to place of residence, one or more of these other factors, or a combination of both.

Some common factors that can distort (confound; see chapter 8) comparisons of crude morbidity or mortality measures include differences in population distributions by age, sex, race/ethnicity, and certain lifestyle behaviors, such as cigarette smoking or overeating. Age, for example, is closely related to the overall risk of death. Therefore, if two populations have very different age distributions,* it is possible that the age differences themselves might partially or fully explain any observed difference in the crude death rates. As you are probably aware, Florida has a large proportion of retired individuals, which skews the age distribution of the population toward older age groups. In fact, according to the latest decennial census, about 18 percent of the population of Florida is 65 years or older. Alaska, on the other hand, has a relatively young population. Only about six percent of its residents are 65 or older.[3] Therefore, we would expect Florida to have a higher crude death rate than Alaska simply because it is a relatively older population. In fact, after we adjust for the differences in age distributions between the populations, the death rates in Florida and Alaska are remarkably similar (786.4 per 100,000 and 789.1 per 100,000, respectively, based on age adjustment using the 2000 U.S. population as a standard).[4]

Unlike crude rates, specific rates (e.g., measures in specific age, sex, or racial/ethnic subgroups of a defined population) can generally be compared

---

*Age distribution refers to the proportions or percentages of a population in different age groups. For example, a given population may have 2.0% in the less than 1-year age category, 6.5% in the 1–4-year age category, 17.0% in the 5–14-year age category, etc. The sum of the percentages for all age groups in the population will equal 100%.

between populations *without* fear of distortion by the factor(s) used to categorize the subgroups (e.g., age, sex, or race/ethnicity). This is because specific rates, unlike crude rates, represent subgroups that are the same with regard to the categorizing factor. For example, we can compare the age-specific death rate among 30–34 year olds in Florida with that among 30–34 year olds in Alaska without worrying about the effects of differing age distributions since the age groups are identical. When age-specific rates are compared, however, they should be reliable (e.g., not based on small numbers), and they should represent relatively narrow age groups (i.e., preferably intervals of no more than five or 10 years for most age categories). It the age intervals are too wide, there may be significant differences in risk within the age groups being compared. In general, comparing specific rates between populations provides more detailed information about the differences in the population measures than comparing crude rates, even if the crude rates happen to be unaffected by differences in population distributions. Sometimes, however, when specific rates, especially age-specific rates, are being compared among several populations, the number of comparisons can be very large, and the task becomes unwieldy. To overcome this problem we can use *adjusted rates*.

ADJUSTED RATES

Adjusted rates (also known as **standardized rates**) are overall, summary measures of occurrence that have been modified statistically to remove the distorting (confounding) effect of one or more variables, such as differences in age, sex, or racial/ethnic distributions of the populations being compared. Adjusted rates are statistically derived using a procedure known as **rate adjustment** or **rate standardization**. The rate adjustment procedure is designed to *control statistically* for any distortion in the magnitude of the crude rates due to extraneous variables for which we have no immediate interest. Hence, rate adjustment allows us to make unbiased comparisons of overall, summary measures without the distortion to due differences in the underlying population distributions. For example, when we compared the crude death rates in Florida and Alaska, we wanted to know if Florida was really a riskier place to live than Alaska, which the crude death rates seemed to suggest. The fact that the populations had different age distributions, however, prevented us from finding out since the effect of age differences was mixed in with the effect of place of residence. Adjustment for age differences was a way of removing the effect of differing age distributions so as to get an undistorted look at the effect of place of residence. Had there still been a large difference in the *adjusted death rates* between Florida and Alaska, one may have wanted to investigate further to discover the possible reasons (e.g., different crime rates, environmental factors, quality of health care). The age differences between the states were thus an annoyance in the data that we wanted to control so as to get a fair (undistorted) look at the differences in the risk of death between Florida and Alaska. Of course, there might still be other distorting factors that could influence the risk of death (e.g., differences in race/ethnicity or socioeconomic status). If these were very different between the populations, we might want to adjust for these factors also.

To summarize briefly using the preceding example, the apparent difference in the risk of death between residents of Florida and Alaska as revealed by a comparison the crude death rates was apparently due to differences in age distributions between the two states as revealed by a comparison of the adjusted rates. In other words, the unadjusted crude rates were distorted (confounded) due to age differences between the populations, and rate adjustment removed this distortion thereby providing summary rates that could be fairly compared. This comparison showed virtually no difference in the risk of death between the populations.

It is important to note that adjusted rates are *artificial* rates; they do not reflect the actual rates in the populations since they are statistically derived. In addition, their magnitude is dependent on the **standard population*** used in the rate adjustment procedure. Although it is difficult to interpret adjusted rates on their own, when compared to other rates that have been adjusted using the same standard population, they become meaningful as later examples will illustrate. Table 6-1 provides a summary of the advantages and disadvantages of crude, specific, and adjusted rates. In particular, adjusted rates have the advantage of convenience when it comes to making comparisons of measures of occurrence, but at the same time they may conceal inconsistencies among the specific rates (i.e., where trends are not uniform throughout the subcategories).

AGE ADJUSTMENT

Although crude measures of occurrence can be adjusted (standardized) for any factors that may distort a comparison, the factor most commonly adjusted in epidemiologic analyses is age because of its well known impact on morbidity and mortality. Therefore, for the remainder of this section, we will focus on **age adjustment** (also known as **age standardization**). It should be kept in mind, however, that age adjustment is just one type of rate adjustment, as is adjustment for sex, race/ethnicity, smoking status, and so on. The basic methods of rate adjustment are the same no matter what factors serve as the basis for the adjustment.

The basic reason for age adjustment is to control for possible age differences in the populations being compared. These differences might otherwise distort (confound) the comparison of crude rates. Age adjustment allows us to calculate overall, summary measures of occurrence for defined populations that would exist theoretically if each population being compared had the same age distribution. Although measures of occurrence from several

---

*The standard population is the population that forms the basis for the comparison in rate adjustment. It has a known distribution with regard to the factor(s) being adjusted. This is discussed in subsequent sections.

Table 6-1   Comparison of Crude, Specific, and Adjusted Rates

Type of Rate	Advantages	Disadvantages
Crude	• Represents a convenient overall, summary measure of occurrence • Represents the actual experience of a defined population • Easy to calculate and interpret	• Magnitude may be affected by the underlying population distribution • Comparisons between defined populations may be distorted due to other differences between the populations
Specific	• Permits unbiased comparisons between similar subgroups of the defined populations • Easy to calculate and interpret	• Cumbersome to compare many specific measures between populations • Not representative of an overall measure of occurrence
Adjusted	• Represents a convenient overall measure of occurrence • Permits unbiased comparisons between defined populations	• Hypothetical measure that may vary in magnitude depending on the standard population chosen • Cumbersome to calculate • May mask inconsistencies in trends among the specific rates

References: Mausner, J. S., and Kramer, S. (1985). *Mausner & Bahn Epidemiology: An Introductory Text*. Philadelphia: W.B. Saunders Company; Anderson, R. N., and Rosenberg, H. M. (1998). Age Standardization of Death Rates: Implementation of the Year 2000 Standard. *National Vital Statistics Reports* 47 (3). Hyattsville, MD: National Center for Health Statistics.

populations can be compared at the same time if certain conditions are met, it will be easier to restrict the focus of the following discussion to situations where only two populations are being compared.

Methods of Age Adjustment

There are two common methods of age adjustment, customarily referred to as the **direct method** and the **indirect method**. The type and quality of data available usually determine the method to be used. The *direct method* can be used when the age-specific rates for the populations being compared are available (or can be calculated) and when they are also stable. The *indirect method* can be used when one or more of the age-specific rates in one of the populations being compared is unavailable (due to missing data) or where the age-specific rates are unstable. Age-specific rates may be unstable due to a small number of occurrences (i.e., less than 10) in one or more of the age-specific subgroups or because of unreliable reporting procedures that usually result in an underestimation of the actual number of occurrences.

Both methods of age adjustment permit unbiased comparisons of overall measures of occurrence; however, the procedures are somewhat different. In the *direct method* we determine an adjusted rate for each population being compared after applying the specific rates of each population to the standard population. In the *indirect method* we determine a standardized ratio, which will be described shortly, after applying the specific rates of one population to another.

To illustrate age adjustment let us use the following simple, though imperfect, analogy where two crude rates are different only because of distortion by different age distributions in the populations being compared. Identical twin brothers went to an amusement park, and each looked into a different trick mirror. One brother, Edward, looked tall and thin, and the other, Denison, looked short and fat. When they both looked into a regular mirror together, however, there were no differences in their appearance. In this example, the images of the brothers in the trick mirrors represent the crude rates. When compared, they look quite different. The trick mirrors represent the different age distributions, which distorted the images (i.e., the crude rates). The regular mirror represents the standard population, and the images in the regular mirror are the adjusted rates. Here it is clear that the rates are really the same after the distortion has been controlled. This analogy represents the *direct method* of rate adjustment. Two crude rates (distorted images of the twin bothers) with different age distributions (different trick mirrors) were adjusted using a standard population (the regular mirror) so they could be fairly compared.

Now imagine that Edward moves from his trick mirror over to the other trick mirror into which his twin Denison is looking. Here, though their images are distorted, they both look the same. This analogy exemplifies the *indirect method* of age adjustment. The original images in the trick mirrors represent the crude rates, which appear to be different. The trick mirror Edward looked into represents the population with unavailable or unstable specific rates, and the second trick mirror Denison looked into represents the other population. The images of both brothers in Denison's mirror represent the results of the rate adjustment. Though not representative of their true selves, the twins now appear the same. Now that you have some idea of how these two methods work, we will discuss them in detail so that you can perform age adjustment and interpret your results. After reading the following sections and studying problems 6-1 and 6-2, you may want to reread the above analogies, which should then make more sense.

The Direct Method

The direct method of age adjustment requires that we have or can calculate age-specific rates in the populations being compared and that the age-specific rates are stable. The first step in the direct method is to select a standard population. The standard population is generally: (a) an existing population with a known age distribution that is understood to be stable, or (b) a derived population, that is, one artificially produced. Exhibit 6-1 provides two examples of derived standard populations. The first is based on the **2000 U.S. standard population**, which represents the proportion of the U.S. population in each of

Exhibit 6-1
Examples of Derived Standard Populations for Use in the Direct Method of Age Adjustment

1. This is the 2000 U.S. standard million population, which is based on the age distribution of the projected 2000 census of the U.S. population. Note that the population is arbitrarily set at one million, and the proportions of the projected 2000 population are applied to each age category (e.g., for 1–4 years, the number = 1,000,000 x 0.055317 = 55, 317).

Age	Number	Proportion
All ages	1,000,000	1.000000
Under 1 year	13,818	0.013818
1–4 years	55,317	0.055317
5–14 years	145,565	0.145565
15–24 years	138,646	0.138646
25–34 years	135,573	0.135573
35–44 years	162,613	0.162613
45–54 years	134,834	0.134834
55–64 years	87,247	0.087247
65–74 years	66,037	0.066037
75–84 years	44,842	0.044842
85 years and over	15,508	0.015508

2. This standard population is derived by combining the age-specific groups of two adult populations to form a new population distribution. The age intervals represented are reasonable for an adult population. They would be too broad for very young groups (under five years), however.

Population One		Population Two	
Age (years)	Population	Age (years)	Population
20–29	3,000	20–29	1,000
30–39	2,500	30–39	1,500
40–49	2,500	40–49	2,000
50–59	1,500	50–59	2,000
60–69	900	60–69	1,750
70–79	650	70–79	1,000
80 and over	125	80 and over	250

Standard Population = Population One + Population Two

Age (years)	Combined Population
20–29	3,000 + 1,000 = 4,000
30–39	2,500 + 1,500 = 4,000
40–49	2,500 + 2,000 = 4,500
50–59	1,500 + 2,000 = 3,500
60–69	900 + 1,750 = 2,650
70–79	650 + 1,000 = 1,650
80 and over	125 + 250 = 375
All ages	11,175 + 9,500 = 20,675

Reference: Kochanek, K. D., Murphy, S. L., Anderson, R. N., and Scott, C. (2004). Deaths: Final Data for 2002. *National Vital Statistics Reports* 53 (5). Hyattsville, MD: National Center for Health Statistics.

11 age groups based on the projected year 2000 population of the United States.[5] This standard population is usually represented, as it is in exhibit 6-1, as the **2000 U.S. standard million population**, where the population proportions in each age group from the 2000 U.S. standard population are applied to an arbitrary population of one million. The standard million population can be considered a derived population since it is derived from the U.S. standard population. The second example is another derived standard population that has been artificially produced from the two adult populations being compared. This is a common way of producing a derived population and one that we will use in examples.

The choice of a standard population in the direct method is somewhat arbitrary, but it is generally recommended that the population chosen should have an age distribution roughly similar to the populations being compared.[5, 6] It is also a good idea that the standard population be at least as large as the populations being compared. For example, the age-adjusted rates for Florida and Alaska in the example cited earlier in this chapter were based on the 2000 U.S. standard population. Also, the derived standard population used in the second example in exhibit 6-1 is a reasonable choice since it combines the populations being compared and is therefore similar to those populations but larger. It would also be acceptable to use one of the populations being compared as the standard. While there are no rigid rules, it is important to specify the standard population used in age adjustment. This is because the population chosen as the standard can affect the results. In general, age-adjusted rates will vary depending on the standard population used, and therefore age-adjusted rates should only be compared if they have been calculated using the same standard population. One advantage to using a commonly accepted standard population like the 2000 U.S. standard population is that age-adjusted rates calculated with it can be fairly compared to other age-adjusted rates that have also used this population as the standard.

It is worth reemphasizing that an age-adjusted rate does not represent an actual rate in a population, and it cannot be verified unless one knows the standard population used to produce it. It would be inappropriate to compare one age-adjusted rate using one standard population to another age-adjusted rate using a different standard population. This is another reason why it is important to indicate the specific standard population used when reporting adjusted rates.

Once the standard population has been selected, one is ready to calculate the adjusted rates. Problem 6-1 illustrates the direct method of age adjustment and the interpretation of the results using a step-by-step format. Also, see exhibit 6-2 on p. 143.

Problem 6-1: Direct Method of Age Adjustment

For the two populations described below, calculate and compare the crude death rates. Next, adjust the rates for differences in age distributions using the direct method of age adjustment (standardization). Use a derived population as the standard population by combining populations A and B. Compare your results before and after age adjustment.

Population A

Age (years)	Population	Number of deaths
15–19	1,000	24
20–24	4,000	16
25–29	6,000	121
All ages	11,000	161

Population B

Age (years)	Population	Number of deaths
15–19	5,000	120
20–24	2,000	10
25–29	500	10
All ages	7,500	140

Solution:

Step 1: Calculate the crude death rates for populations A and B using the appropriate formula in appendix C.

$$CDR = \frac{\text{Number of deaths during a specified time period}}{\text{Mid-interval population}} \times 10^n$$

Population A:

Number of deaths = 161; Population = 11,000

$CDR = (161 / 11,000) \times 10^n = 0.0146 \times 10^3 = 14.6$ deaths per 1,000 population

Population B:

Number of deaths = 140; Population = 7,500

$CDR = (140 / 7,500) \times 10^n = 0.0187 \times 10^3 = 18.7$ deaths per 1,000 population

Step 2: Compare the crude death rates.

The crude death rate in Population B is greater than that in Population A. In fact, it is about 1.3 times greater as indicated below. The ratio shown below can be referred to as the ratio of the crude rates (R_C).

$$R_C = CDR_{pop.B} / CDR_{pop.A} = (18.7 \text{ per } 1,000) / (14.6 \text{ per } 1,000) = 1.3$$

Step 3: Determine the standard population for the age adjustment by combining the two populations. This is done by adding populations A and B together as shown below. The result is a derived standard population.

	Population		
Age (years)	A	B	Standard
15–19	1,000 +	5,000 =	6,000
20–24	4,000 +	2,000 =	6,000
25–29	6,000 +	500 =	6,500
All ages	11,000 +	7,500 =	18,500

Step 4: Calculate the age-specific rates *as decimal fractions* for each population being compared.

Population A

Age (years)	Population	Number of deaths	Age-specific rates
15–19	1,000	24	24 / 1,000 = 0.024
20–24	4,000	16	16 / 4,000 = 0.004
25–29	6,000	121	121 / 6,000 = 0.020
All ages	11,000	161	

Population B

Age (years)	Population	Number of deaths	Age-specific rates
15–19	5,000	120	120 / 5,000 = 0.024
20–24	2,000	10	10 / 2,000 = 0.005
25–29	500	10	10 / 500 = 0.020
All ages	7,500	140	

Step 5: Multiply the populations of the respective age groups in the standard population by the age-specific rates for each population to determine the number of expected events in each case.

Standard Population

Age (years)	Population		Specific Rates (Pop. A)		Expected Deaths
15–19	6,000	×	0.024	=	144
20–24	6,000	×	0.004	=	24
25–29	6,500	×	0.020	=	130
All ages	18,500				298

Standard Population

Age (years)	Population		Specific Rates (Pop. B)		Expected Deaths
15–19	6,000	×	0.024	=	144
20–24	6,000	×	0.005	=	30
25–29	6,500	×	0.020	=	130
All ages	18,500				304

Step 6: Divide the total number of expected events in each population by the total standard population to determine the adjusted rates.

Population A: Age-adjusted rate = $(298 / 18,500) \times 10^n = 0.0161 \times 10^3 = 16.1$ per 1,000

Population B: Age-adjusted rate = $(304 / 18,500) \times 10^n = 0.0164 \times 10^3 = 16.4$ per 1,000

Step 7: Compare the adjusted rates visually or by calculating the ratio of the adjusted rates (R_A). R_A for population B to A is:

R_A = Adjusted rate$_{pop.B}$ / Adjusted rate$_{pop.A}$ = (16.4 per 1,000) / (16.1 per 1,000) = 1.0

This indicates that the age-adjusted rate in population B is virtually the same as that in population A. In other words, after age adjustment the rates are effectively the same. Thus, the risk of death is similar in populations A and B after adjusting for age differences between the populations.

Answer: The crude death rates in the two populations were clearly different (population B, 18.7 per 1,000, and population A, 14.6 per 1,000). The ratio of the crude death rates (R_C) was 1.3, indicating that the crude death rate in population B was about 30 percent higher than that in population A. After age adjustment, however, the difference almost disappeared (population B, 16.4 per 1,000, and population A, 16.1 per 1,000). The ratio of adjusted rates (R_A) was 1.0, indicating that the age-adjusted rate in population B was virtually the same as that in population A. In conclusion, the crude rates were significantly distorted (confounded) by age differences between the populations. After adjusting for these differences, however, there was effectively no difference between the rates. Thus, the risks of death in populations A and B are virtually the same after adjusting for age differences.

Comments:
1. In direct age adjustment, when $R_A \neq R_C$, we can say that differences in age distributions between the populations produced distortion (confounding) that affected the magnitude of the crude rates. Age adjustment corrects this distortion and, therefore, represents a more equitable way to make the comparison, assuming all other factors are equal. If there are other suspected confounding factors, these must also be controlled. If $R_A = R_C$, then age adjustment was unnecessary; there is no distortion (confounding) by age differences. The irony here is that it is necessary to perform the adjustment in order to determine if it is really needed (see exhibit 6-2 for more information).

2. When the age-specific rates were calculated for the age adjustment, the rates were computed as *decimal fractions* without a population base. While this is not required, it makes the calculations easier since one never has to worry about what to do with the population base. For example, in population B, the age-specific rate in the 25–29-year age group was determined to be 10 / 500 = 0.020. This could have been reported as 20 per 1,000 using a population base of 1,000. However, when this is multiplied by 6,000 in the standard population, one has to be careful to also divide the product by 1,000. In other words, it is *not* 20 × 6,500 = 130,000 deaths, but (20 per 1,000) × 6,500 = 130 deaths. Although this may seem obvious, the mistake, unfortunately, is not uncommon among beginners. It is highly recommended that specific rates be calculated to at least three places to the right of the decimal point to ensure precise measurements.

3. The population base used in this problem was 1,000. The reason 1,000 was used is because this is one of the conventional population bases used with crude death rates (see appendix C), and the adjusted rates were being compared to the crude rates, so it is desirable to use the same population base. The use of 100 also would have been acceptable, if not conventional, because the resulting rates would still have been greater than one per 100.

The Indirect Method

The so-called indirect method is frequently used in occupational epidemiology (chapter 2) when investigators are trying to assess whether the outcome in a study population is more or less than that expected based on a broader general population.[7] For example, investigators might be interested in whether or not the injury rate among migrant farmers in Indiana exceeds

---

Exhibit 6-2
Interpreting Findings from Rate Adjustment

Direct Method

If $R_A = R_C$, then there is *no* distortion (confounding) by the factor(s) for which adjustment was performed. Hence, adjustment was unnecessary, and the crude rates can be fairly compared.

If $R_A \neq R_C$, then there *is* distortion (confounding) by the factor(s) for which adjustment was performed. Hence, adjustment was necessary, and the crude rates should *not* be compared. The more the ratio, R_A / R_C, departs from 1.0, the greater the degree of distortion. Small differences may be due to random error and are not statistically important. When $R_A \neq R_C$, only the adjusted rates should be compared.

R_A = the ratio of the adjusted rates, and R_C = the ratio of the crude rates. The respective numerators and denominators of these ratios must correspond to the same populations.

Indirect Method

If $SMR = R_C$, then there is no distortion (confounding) by the factor(s) for which adjustment was performed. Hence, adjustment was unnecessary, and the crude rates can be fairly compared.

If $SMR \neq R_C$, then there is distortion (confounding) by the factor(s) for which adjustment was performed. Hence, adjustment was necessary, and the crude rates should *not* be compared. The greater the ratio, SMR / R_C, departs from 1.0, the greater the degree of distortion. Small differences may be due to random error and are not statistically important. When the $SMR \neq R_C$, only the SMR should be used.

SMR = the standardized mortality (or morbidity) ratio, and R_C = the ratio of the crude rates where the numerator is the crude rate in the study population, and the denominator is the crude rate in the reference population.

$SMR = OE / EE$ where OE = the number of observed events in the study population, and EE = the number of expected events in the study population based on the specific rates in the reference population.

---

what would be expected based on injury rates in the general Indiana population. The method is also used in other circumstances where the objective is to control for age differences between the populations being compared. It is particularly appropriate as a method of age adjustment when the direct method cannot be used, specifically when not all of the specific rates are available in one of the populations being compared or when some of the specific rates in this population are unstable. Like the direct method of age adjustment, the indirect method begins with the selection of a "standard population," although it is better to refer to this as a *reference population* for reasons that will become clear shortly. This reference population is usually a general population or the larger, or more stable, of the two populations being compared. The next step is to calculate the age-specific rates in the reference population and then to multiply these rates by the numbers in the respective age-specific groups in the other population so as to arrive at the number of expected events (e.g., deaths) in each age group. The total number of actual or observed events (OE) in the study population (i.e., the non-reference population) is then divided by the total number of expected events (EE) in the same population to obtain the **standardized mortality ratio** if the event of interest is death or the **standardized morbidity ratio*** if the event is not death but a disease or injury. Both ratios are generally referred to as the SMR. The SMR provides an indication of how much the observed and expected rates differ after age adjustment. In essence, the SMR compares the crude rate to the expected rate in the study population based on the age-specific rates in the reference population. Mathematically, SMR = [OE / n] / [EE / n], where n is the size of the non-reference population (in persons or person-time units). This formula can be simplified to:

(6.1)
$$SMR = \frac{OE}{EE}$$

where OE is the number of observed events in the study population, and EE is the number of expected events in the study population based on the age-specific rates in the reference population. Some epidemiologists multiply the SMR by 100, although this practice is becoming less common,[8] and therefore will not be discussed here. Sometimes an **indirectly standardized rate** (ISR) is calculated by multiplying the crude rate in the reference population by the SMR (see formula 6.2 and problem 6-2).

(6.2) $ISR = CR_{\text{ref. pop.}} \times SMR$

In this expression, ISR is the indirectly standardized rate, $CDR_{\text{ref. pop.}}$ is the crude rate in the reference population (e.g., crude death rate), and SMR is the standardized mortality or morbidity ratio as applicable. The indirectly standardized rate can be considered the adjusted rate in the study population. It represents what the rate in this population would be if its age distribution were the same as that of the reference population. Hence, the results of indirect adjustment can be interpreted in more than one way.

An SMR of 1.0 implies that there is *no difference* between the observed and expected rates or the number of observed and expected events in the study population based on the age-specific rates in the reference population. Thus, the original comparison is not distorted by differences in age distribution. An SMR less than or greater than 1.0 implies that there is a *difference* between the observed and expected rates (or number of events) after age adjustment. The amount of difference depends on how much the SMR departs from 1.0. An SMR of 2.3, for example, implies that the observed rate is 2.3 times or 130 percent higher than the expected rate, and an SMR of 0.8 indicates that the observed rate is only 0.8 times or 20 percent lower than the expected rate after age adjustment. It could also be said that there were 130 percent more or 20 percent less events than expected in the applicable study (non-reference) population. An ISR can be compared to the crude rate in the

---

*Standardized morbidity ratio is a general term that encompasses other specific measures of morbidity such as the *standardized incidence ratio, standardized prevalence ratio*, etc.[7]

reference population. Any difference would be attributable to differences in age distributions between the reference and study populations.

Often there is a desire to compare multiple SMRs calculated for several populations. Although this is sometimes done in practice, strictly speaking, SMRs should *not* be compared to each other even if they have been calculated using the same reference population. The reason for this is simple. In reality, *the study population is the standard population* in indirect adjustment.[7] Therefore, unless the populations from which the SMRs have been calculated have the same age distributions, the comparisons will not be valid. The same is true for multiple comparisons of ISRs. You might ask why the study population is considered the standard population. Recall that in the direct method the standard population provides the age distribution to which the age-specific rates of the other populations are applied. Similarly, in the indirect method the study population provides the age distribution to which the specific rates in the reference population are applied. For this reason, the term "indirect method" is a misnomer.[9, 10] Instead, it can be viewed as the direct method in disguise. It is always appropriate, of course, to use indirect adjustment when there are just two populations—the reference population to obtain the age-specific rates and a study population to develop the SMR or ISR. Comparing SMRs or ISRs, however, needs to be done with caution recognizing that the study (non-reference) population is the true standard population. A demonstration of indirect adjustment and its interpretation is provided in problem 6-2.

An approximate 95 percent confidence interval for the SMR can be easily estimated if the measure is assumed to be normally distributed. This assumption can be considered reasonable when both the number of observed and expected events are relatively large, say 25 or more.[11] The basic formula is shown below.

(6.3)
$$95\% \; CI = SMR \pm 1.96 \sqrt{SMR / EE}$$

SMR is the standardized mortality or morbidity ratio depending on whether death or disease/injury is being evaluated. EE is the number of expected events in the study (non-reference) population. An example of this calculation is provided in problem 6-2, which illustrates the indirect method of age adjustment.

Problem 6-2: Indirect Method of Age Adjustment

For the two populations below, calculate and compare the crude death rates, then perform age adjustment using the indirect method with one of the two populations serving as the reference population. Report and interpret the standardized mortality ratio (SMR), the indirectly standardized rate (ISR), and the 95 percent confidence interval for the SMR.

Population A

Age (years)	Population	Number of deaths
15–19	1,000	12
20–24	2,000	20
25–29	3,000	91
All ages	6,000	123

Population B

Age (years)	Population	Number of deaths
15–19	4,000	85
20–24	250	Not available
25–29	750	Not available
All ages	5,000	95

Solution:

Step 1: Calculate the crude death rates for the two populations using the appropriate formula in appendix C.

$$CDR = \frac{\text{Number of deaths during a specified time period}}{\text{Mid-interval population}} \times 10^n$$

Population A:

Number of deaths = 123; Population = 6,000

$$CDR = (123 / 6,000) \times 10^n = 0.0205 \times 10^3 = 20.5 \text{ deaths per 1,000 population}$$

Population B:

Number of deaths = 95; Population = 5,000

$$CDR = (95 / 5,000) \times 10^n = 0.0190 \times 10^3 = 19.0 \text{ deaths per 1,000 population}$$

Step 2: Compare the crude death rates. This can be done visually or quantitatively by calculating the ratio of the crude rates (R_C). In the indirect method, *the crude rate for the study (non-reference) population should be in the numerator of R_C.* This means that we must first determine which population is the reference population and which is the study population. Since the age-specific rates can only be calculated from population A in this problem, it must be the reference population. Therefore, population B is the study population.

$$R_C = CDR_{pop.B} / CDR_{pop.A} = (19.0 \text{ per } 1,000) / (20.5 \text{ per } 1,000) = 0.93$$

This means that the crude death rate in population B (the study population) is 93% of that in population A (the reference population). This is the same as saying that the CDR in population B is 7% smaller than that in population A or only 0.93 times that of population A.

Step 3: Calculate the age-specific rates in the reference population.

Reference Population (Population A)

Age (years)	Population	Number of deaths	*Age-specific rates*
15–19	1,000	12	12 / 1,000 = 0.012
20–24	2,000	20	20 / 2,000 = 0.010
25–29	3,000	91	91 / 3,000 = 0.030
All ages	6,000	123	

Step 4: Multiply the numbers in the respective age-specific groups in the study population by the age-specific rates in the reference population to determine the number of expected events (i.e., deaths) in each age group. Sum the expected events in each age group to obtain the total number of expected events (EE) in the study population.

Study Population (Population B)

Age (years)	Population		Specific Rates from Reference Population		*Expected Deaths*
15–19	4,000	×	0.012	=	48.0
20–24	250	×	0.010	=	2.5
25–29	750	×	0.030	=	22.5
All ages	5,000				73.0

Step 5: Calculate the standardized mortality ratio (SMR) using formula 6.1, the indirectly standardized rate (ISR) using formula 6.2, and the 95 percent confidence interval for the SMR using formula 6.3.

$$SMR = \frac{OE}{EE} = 95/73.0 = 1.30$$

$$ISR = CR_{ref.pop.} \times SMR = (20.5 \text{ per } 1,000) \times 1.30 = 26.7 \text{ per } 1,000$$

$$95\% \; CI = SMR \pm 1.96\sqrt{SMR/EE} = 1.30 \pm 1.96\sqrt{1.30/73.0}$$

$$= 1.30 - 0.26 \text{ to } 1.30 + 0.26 = 1.04 \text{ to } 1.56$$

Answer: The SMR is 1.30 (95% CI = 1.04 to 1.56). This implies that 1.30 times (or 30 percent) more deaths were observed in the study population than expected based on the specific rates in the reference population. Furthermore, we are 95 percent confident that the *true* SMR lies between 1.04 and 1.56 (1.30 is the point estimate). The indirectly standardized rate in the study population is 26.7 per 1,000. This is the hypothetical death rate in the study population after the effects of age differences between populations A and B have been controlled. Since the SMR does not equal the ratio of the crude rates (R_C), we can also say that there was distortion (confounding) by age differences that needed to be controlled (see exhibit 6-2).

Comments:
1. Calculating the ratio of the crude rates (R_C) is a simple but convenient way of determining quantitatively how much the crude rates differ. The greater R_C departs from one, the greater the difference in the crude rates. In calculating R_C the crude rate of the study population should always be in the numerator because it may later be compared to the SMR, whose numerator can be considered to be the crude rate of the study population (i.e., the observed rate). This assures an "apples to apples" comparison.

2. The reference population is usually the larger or more stable of the two populations being compared. In the problem, population A is larger, and nothing suggests that it is unstable. If the number of events in one or more of the age categories was very small (i.e., less than 10) or if there were indications that the data were otherwise unstable, then we would not want to select it as a reference population. Also, when there are missing numbers of events in one or more age categories of a population that population cannot be used as the reference population since the indirect method depends on the age-specific rates of the reference population, which are calculated using these events. In this problem, only population A qualifies as a suitable reference population. Population B is not appropriate because of the missing number of deaths in two of the age categories. If neither population qualifies as a reference population, then an external population may be selected for use as the reference population.

3. As in problem 6-1, when the age-specific rates are calculated for the age adjustment, the rates should be computed as *decimal fractions* without a population base. Once again, this makes the calculations easier since one never has to worry about what to do with the population base later on. It is highly recommended that they be calculated to at least three places to the right of the decimal point to ensure precise measurements.

4. The crude death rates in this problem were relatively close (R_C = 19.0 per 1,000 / 20.5 per 1,000 = 0.93). The SMR provides an indication of how much the rates differ after age adjustment. In this problem, the SMR was 1.30. Since this is different than 0.93, we conclude that there was distortion (confounding) by age, and age adjustment was therefore appropriate. In fact, the SMR was not only different; the difference appeared to be in a direction opposite to what was suggested by the crude rates!

5. Any time the SMR differs significantly from R_C, we can say that age adjustment is necessary (see exhibit 6-2). In a sense, the SMR can be thought of as being analogous to the R_A (see problem 6-1). However, as was stated previously, *when the SMR is compared to R_C, the numerator for R_C must always be the crude rate of the study population* (population B in this problem). This is because the numerator for the SMR is based on the study population. Although with the SMR we do not have two age-adjusted rates like we did in the direct method of adjustment, we can calculate the indirectly standardized rate (ISR) if we wish. This can be compared to the crude rate of the reference population. In this problem, the ISR is 26.7 per 1,000. It is 1.30 times greater than the crude rate.

6. As with problem 6-1, the population base used was 1,000, which is one of the conventional population bases used with crude death rates (see appendix C). The use of 100 would also have been acceptable, if not conventional, because the resulting rates would still have been greater than one per 100.

Rationale for Age Adjustment

In the *direct method* of age adjustment, the *undistorted* age-specific rates from each population being compared are multiplied by the numbers in the *same* age-specific groups in the standard population. Therefore, any differences in the resulting age-adjusted rates *must* be due to differences in age-specific rates between the populations (i.e., true differences) and *not* to differences in age distributions between the populations. Remember, both age-adjusted rates are based on the *same* age distribution (i.e., that of the standard population). This assures that directly adjusted rates can be fairly compared to each other without distortion by age differences between the populations being compared.

In the so-called *indirect method* of age adjustment, the *unconfounded* age-specific rates of the reference population are multiplied by the numbers in the age-specific groups in the study population to determine the number of expected events in this population (i.e., those that would have occurred in the study population if there were no differences in the specific rates between the reference and the study populations). The number of expected events is then divided into the number of observed events in the study population to obtain an SMR. Since the number of observed and expected events are based on the *same* age distribution (i.e., that of the study population), any difference between observed and expected events must be due to differences in the age-specific rates between the standard and study populations (i.e., true differences) and *not* to differences in age distributions between the populations. As with the direct method of age adjustment (age standardization), this assures that the SMR (or ISR) is not distorted by age differences between the reference and study populations.

Figure 6-1 illustrates the transformation that takes place in both direct and indirect age adjustment. In the direct method, as illustrated here, differ-

Figure 6-1   Diagrammatic Illustrations of Age Adjustment

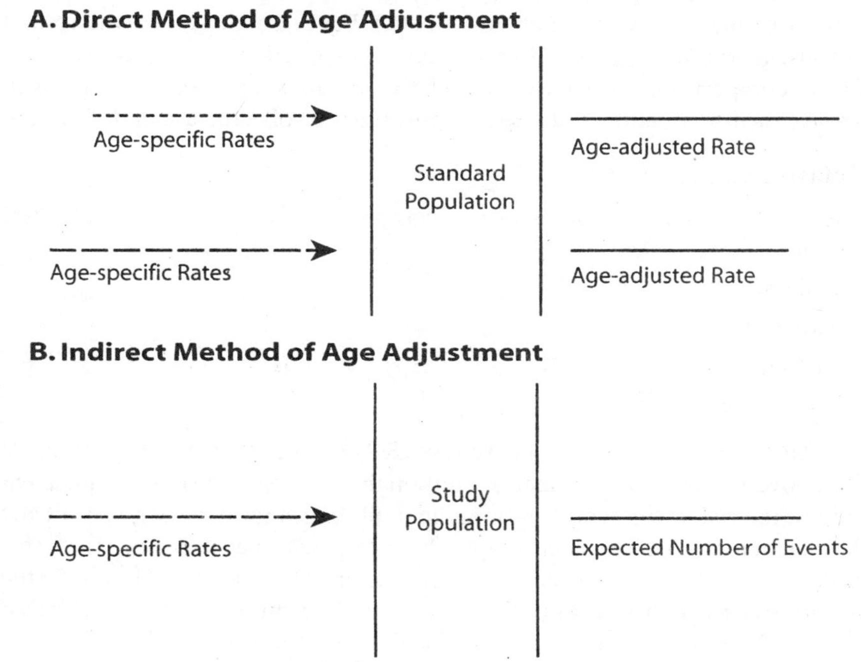

A. Direct Method of Age Adjustment

B. Indirect Method of Age Adjustment

ent age-specific rates from two populations are applied to a common standard population. The result is two different, but comparable, adjusted rates. In the indirect method, the age-specific rates of the reference population are applied to the study population to obtain the expected number of events in the study population, which can then be used to determine the SMR or ISR. The interpretation of the results of age adjustment are summarized in exhibit 6-2.

MEASURES OF ASSOCIATION

A **measure of association** is a quantity that expresses the degree of statistical relationship between an exposure and outcome. An association, if it exists, may be causal or noncausal depending on the circumstances (see chapter 7). In most epidemiologic studies, our interest is in discovering causal associations. Measures of association based on causal associations may also be referred to as **measures of effect**. In general, the term *measure of association* is most appropriately used in reference to statistical relationships discovered in observational studies, while the term *measure of effect* is most appropriately used in reference to statistical relationships discovered in experimental studies. This is not a rigid rule, however, and the terms are often used interchangeably in the epidemiologic literature.

In most cases, measures of association are calculated when we compare a measure of occurrence for a group exposed to a suspected risk factor to that for a similar but unexposed group, which serves as the **referent** (i.e., the comparison or reference group). Comparisons may also be made based on levels of exposure (high to low, moderate to low, etc.). For convenience, we will restrict our discussion to comparisons based only on exposed and unexposed groups. These comparisons may be either relative or absolute. *Relative comparisons* involve the use of ratios, and *absolute comparisons* involve the use of differences.

Relative Comparisons

The most common measures of association based on relative comparisons are the:

- Risk ratio
- Rate ratio
- Odds ratio
- Prevalence ratio

Risk ratio. The term **relative risk** (RR) has been used to refer to all of the above measures of association, although in a strict sense it is equivalent only to the **risk ratio**, which, as it name implies, is a ratio of *risks*, specifically the risk of a given occurrence among those exposed to a suspected risk factor to those who are not exposed. The most commonly reported risk ratio is the **cumulative incidence ratio** (CIR). In practice, it is more commonly referred to as a relative risk or risk ratio. It is calculated as follows:

(6.4)
$$CIR = \frac{CI_e}{CI_{ue}}$$

The expression CI_e refers to the cumulative incidence among the exposed group, and CI_{ue} is the cumulative incidence among the unexposed group. The use of CIR is illustrated in the findings of a retrospective cohort study of 648 workers at an industrial production plant. The study was designed to evaluate the association between direct exposure to pentachlorophenol (PCP; an organic compound used as a product preservative and pesticide) and the occurrence of chloracne, a severe skin condition. The authors reported a CIR of 4.6 (95% CI = 2.6 to 8.1).[12] In other words, workers directly exposed to PCP were purported to be *4.6 times more likely to develop* chloracne than those who were not directly exposed during the 25 years covered by the study.

The following hypothetical example demonstrates the calculation of a cumulative incidence ratio. Assume that many years ago a team of investigators conducted a prospective cohort study to determine if environmental tobacco smoke (ETS) increases the risk of myocardial infarction (MI) in non-smoking spouses of married men. During 15 years of follow up, the investigators identified 120 cases of MI among 20,000 nonsmoking spouses whose husbands smoked (the exposed group) and 100 cases of MI among 22,500 nonsmoking spouses whose husbands did not smoke (the unexposed group). Based on these findings:

$$CI_e = (120 / 20,000) \times 10^n = 0.0060 \times 10^3 = 6.0 \text{ deaths per } 1,000$$
$$CI_{ue} = (100 / 22,500) \times 10^n = 0.0044 \times 10^3 = 4.4 \text{ deaths per } 1,000$$
$$CIR = (6.0 \text{ per } 1,000) / (4.4 \text{ per } 1,000) = 1.4$$

This finding means that the nonsmoking spouses whose husbands smoked *were 1.4 times more likely to develop* an MI than the nonsmoking spouses whose husbands did not smoke, all other factors being equal.* In other words, based on this study, there appears to be an association between exposure to ETS and MI in nonsmoking female spouses. The finding can also be stated by saying that the risk of an MI among the nonsmoking spouses of smoking husbands is *40 percent higher* than that among the non-smoking spouses of nonsmoking husbands. The percent change in a ratio measure of association (e.g., CIR) from a baseline value of 1.0, which represents no association, can be referred to as the **percent relative effect**.[10] It is calculated as shown in formula 6.5.

(6.5)
For a ratio > 1.0
% Increased Change = (Ratio − 1) × 100

For a ratio < 1.0
% Decreased Change = (1 − Ratio) × 100

---

*The phrase, "all other factors being equal" (*ceteris paribus*), which is used throughout this text, is a shorthand way of saying that the results are contingent upon the study being valid; that is, not distorted by confounding or bias. The findings may still be subject to random error (see chapter 8).

Percent relative effect for a risk ratio is interpreted as the percent increased or decreased *risk* of occurrence as noted above. When applied to other ratio measures of association the interpretations are somewhat different as subsequent examples will demonstrate.

Some points to keep in mind regarding risk ratios are: (a) they have a lower limit of zero, but, theoretically, they have no upper boundary; (b) their magnitude is dependent on the length of the observation period; and (c) a high risk ratio is not necessarily associated with a high **absolute risk**, which is the probability of an outcome, usually measured by cumulative incidence and generally referred to simply as risk. With regard to the first point, while the maximum value of a risk ratio is theoretically unlimited, the upper limit in any given situation will depend on the risk in the unexposed group, which serves as the referent. For example, using decimal fractions, if $CI_{ue} = 0.50$, then even if $CI_e = 1.0$, its maximum possible value, the CIR would only equal 2.0. As indicated in the second point, the value of a risk ratio depends on the length of the observation period. The longer susceptible people are observed in a population, the more likely they are to develop the outcome of interest regardless of their exposure status. Thus, a risk ratio will tend to move closer to a value of one as time of observation increases. Hence, the observation period should always be indicated when reporting risk ratios (e.g., in one of the previous examples the CIR was based on 25 years of observation and in the other it was based on 15 years of observation). The final point can be illustrated with a simple example. Say the CIR = 10.0. This value could result if $CI_e = 90.0$ per 100 and $CI_{ue} = 9.0$ per 100 or if $CI_e = 10.0$ per 1,000,000 and $CI_{ue} = 1.0$ per 1,000,000. In the former case, the *absolute risk* of occurrence among the exposed group is very high. In the latter case, it is very small. Thus, a large risk ratio does not necessarily imply that the exposed group has a large absolute risk.

From a public health perspective, one also needs to consider the severity of the outcome and the prevalence of the exposure when interpreting a risk ratio. If, for example, the outcome is life threatening and the exposure is very prevalent in the population, then even a risk ratio slightly above one could be a cause for concern. On the other hand, even a large risk ratio for a serious disease may not garner much attention if the prevalence of exposed individuals is very small. Malignant mesothelioma, for example, is a rare type of terminal cancer that is very closely associated with occupational exposure to asbestos. Nonoccupational exposures to asbestos tend to be very low, however; hence, mesothelioma is not considered a significant health issue for the general public. It is a concern, however, for those working with asbestos-containing materials and for certain other groups that may be indirectly exposed to elevated levels (e.g., those living near asbestos mines or spouses of asbestos workers).

Rate ratio.   The **rate ratio** is a ratio of *rates* of occurrence, specifically the rate of occurrence in the exposed group to that in the unexposed group. Rate ratios are commonly reported in cohort or other longitudinal studies where person-time data have been collected. The most commonly reported rate ratio is the **incidence density ratio** (IDR), also known as the **incidence rate ratio**. In practice, it may also be referred to as a relative risk or rate ratio. It is calculated as shown in formula 6.6.

(6.6)

$$IDR = \frac{ID_e}{ID_{ue}}$$

In this expression. the incidence density in the exposed group (ID_e) is divided by the incidence density in the unexposed group (ID_{ue}). To illustrate, consider the following observation reported during an analysis of national injury data sets for 18–64 year olds: "overall injury mortality rates . . . for men were almost 3 times higher than those for women (overall rate: 68.7 vs. 23.7 per 100,000 person-years). . . ."[13(p71)] This observation is based on a *rate ratio* (i.e., 68.7 per 100,000 person-years / 23.7 per 100,000 person-years = 2.93). Since men are the exposed group in this example, women are the referents. Also note that the injury mortality rates referred to are cause-specific mortality rates measured using person-time units. These can be considered incidence density measures where the outcome is death due to injuries. Since death always represents new cases, the cause-specific mortality rate is a type of incidence measure. Therefore, the ratio of cause-specific mortality rates using person-time units can be considered a type of incidence density ratio (formula 6.6).

The calculation and interpretation of a rate ratio is analogous to that of a risk ratio except that technically reference is made to *rates* versus *risks* of occurrence as inferred from the above quotation. Alternatively, we might have said, the *rate* at which men die of injuries is almost three times greater than the *rate* at which women die of injuries or that the rate is about *200 percent* higher in men than women (see formula 6.5). Since time is incorporated into the denominators of the incidence densities used to calculate a rate ratio, it is not necessary to indicate the period of observation for a rate ratio as it is with a risk ratio. It is still a good idea, however, to indicate person, place, and time factors when reporting any ratios if this information is not clear from the context of the study or report. As with risk ratios, rate ratios have a lower limit of zero but no upper limit. If the incidence densities are constant over time and the period of observation is short, the rate ratio will approximate the risk ratio.[10]

Before proceeding, let us cite one more example where a rate ratio was used. A group randomized trial was conducted by researchers from Columbia University Medical Center in New York. The purpose was to evaluate the effect of antibacterial cleaning and handwashing products on the occurrence of infectious disease symptoms in households. Overall, the authors found virtually no difference in infectious disease symptoms between households using antibacterial products and those not using antibacterial products (IDR = 0.96; 95% CI = 0.82 to 1.12).[14] In other words, the *rates* of infectious disease symptoms were similar in the exposed and unexposed groups.

Odds ratio. A third measure of association involving a relative comparison is the *odds ratio*, also sometimes referred to as the **relative odds**. This measure is most often used in case-control studies, although it is frequently employed in cohort, cross-sectional, and other study designs as well. To facilitate the present discussion, we will focus primarily on its use in case-control studies. As its name indicates, the **odds ratio** is a ratio of odds (defined in chapter 5). Depending on the design of the study, these may be incidence or prevalence odds (chapter 5). Quite often, the odds ratio is measured as the odds of the outcome among the exposed group to the odds of the outcome among the unexposed group. This is called the **disease odds ratio**. There is also an *exposure odds ratio*, which is defined and discussed in chapter 10. For now, we will focus only on the disease odds ratio. In most case-control studies, we can construct a 2 × 2 contingency table like the one presented below.

	Outcome Status	
Exposure Status	Cases	Controls
Exposed	a	b
Unexposed	c	d

The values a through d in the above table represent the frequencies of cases and controls according to their exposure status. These frequencies are used to calculate the odds ratio (OR) as shown in formula 6.7.

(6.7)
$$OR = \frac{odds_e}{odds_{ue}} = \frac{a/b}{c/d} = \frac{ad}{bc}$$

The expression $odds_e$ refers to the odds of the outcome among the *exposed* group, and $odds_{ue}$ is the odds of the outcome among the *unexposed* group. Based on the above 2 × 2 table, this is equivalent to (a / b) / (c / d), since a / b is the odds of the outcome (i.e., being a case) among the exposed group, and c / d is the odds of the outcome among the unexposed group. Mathematically, the odds ratio is the same as ad / bc, as long as the data are set up as in the above table. To illustrate, over 20 years ago, Ruth Bonita and her colleagues conducted a case-control study to determine if cigarette smoking is associated with the incidence of premature stroke.[15] The exposure in the study was cigarette smoking (cigarette smokers versus non-cigarette smokers), and the outcome of interest was premature stroke. The overall study findings are presented in the following 2 × 2 contingency table, which is organized based on the template shown above.

Outcome Status

Exposure Status	Cases	Controls
Exposed	66	424
Unexposed	66	1,162

Based on these results, and using formula 6.7, the odds ratio is calculated as follows:

$$OR = ad \ / \ bc = (66 \times 1{,}162) \ / \ (424 \times 66) = 76{,}692 \ / \ 27{,}984 = 2.7$$

This odds ratio, which is based on incidence odds (chapter 5), can be interpreted by saying, the odds of *developing* a stroke are 2.7 times greater among cigarette smokers than non-cigarette smokers, all other factors being equal. In other words, based on this study, the odds of developing a stroke are 170 percent higher among cigarette smokers compared to non-cigarette smokers (formula 6.5).

The odds ratio found in the study by Bonita and her colleagues was based on *incidence odds*. The same procedures are followed if *prevalence odds* are used to calculate the odds ratio.* The only difference is in the interpretation of the findings, which is illustrated in the following example. Investigators from the University of Texas School of Public Health performed a cross-sectional study using data from 3,689 subjects based on the National Health and Nutrition Examination Survey (see appendix B) to determine if current smoking is associated with the presence of *Helicobacter pylori* infection. They found a positive association as indicated by the *prevalence odds ratio* after controlling for other possible factors (OR = 1.9; 95% CI = 1.4 to 2.5).[16] The interpretation is that the odds of *having* an *H. pylori* infection are 1.9 times greater (or 90 percent higher; formula 6.5) among current cigarette smokers than among current non-cigarette smokers. Notice that in the previous example the interpretation was about *developing* an outcome, while in this example, the interpretation is about *having* an outcome. This is the basic difference in interpretation between an incidence and prevalence odds ratio. One is based on incident cases and prior exposure; the other is based on prevalent cases and concurrent exposure (see chapter 9). Normally, one has to infer from the context whether the OR is a prevalence or incidence odds ratio since it is usually not stated.

*If the study is not a case-control study, the 2 × 2 table used to calculate the odds ratio should not use the terms "cases" and "controls" as the column headings. Instead, outcome status should be labeled "present" or "absent" or equivalent terms. Otherwise, the analysis is the same.

When the risk of an occurrence is small (i.e., less than 0.10), the incidence odds ratio approximates the risk ratio reasonably well. In these cases, the OR is sometimes stated as a risk ratio or relative risk, since more people are familiar with the concept of risk than odds. In general, one should not use the odds ratio to estimate the risk ratio when the risk of the outcome is not small since the values may deviate substantially. There are exceptions to this rule that depend on the way controls are sampled.[9] These are discussed in chapter 10.

Prevalence ratio.   A final measure of association based on relative comparisons is the **prevalence ratio**. This measure is usually used in cross-sectional studies. It can be considered a type of risk ratio, but it has a different interpretation than the cumulative incidence ratio since it is based on prevalence of the occurrence versus cumulative incidence. It is calculated as shown in formula 6.8.

(6.8)

$$PR = \frac{P_e}{P_{ue}}$$

PR refers to prevalence ratio. P_e is the prevalence of the occurrence in the exposed group, and P_{ue} is the prevalence of the occurrence in the unexposed group. An example of a study employing the prevalence ratio was one designed to determine if dairy food intake during high school was associated with severe acne. The researchers examined data retrospectively on over 47,000 women from the Nurses' Health Study II. Among their findings was a positive but weak association between drinking large amounts of skim milk and severe acne after controlling for age and other relevant variables (PR = 1.44; 95% CI = 1.21 to 1.72). The authors speculated that the association may be the result of hormones and bioactive molecules in the milk.[17] The PR in this study can be interpreted as follows: female high school students who drink large amounts of skim milk are 1.44 times more likely *to have* severe acne than those who do not drink large amounts of skim milk. Notice that the interpretation refers to the *prevalence* of severe acne ("to have") versus the *probability* of developing severe acne. It would also be appropriate to say that the prevalence of severe acne among those drinking large amounts of skim milk is 44 percent higher than that among those not drinking large amounts of skim milk (i.e., the referents) based on formula 6.5. Some epidemiologists have noted that the PR measures the *risk of having* the outcome and, therefore, may be considered a type of risk ratio as mentioned at the beginning of this segment.[18] The prevalence ratio is also discussed in chapter 9.

Figure 6-2 provides a summary of the various measures of association based on relative comparisons. Tables 6-2 and 6-3 provide guidelines for interpreting the values of ratio measures of association. Although the each of the measures of association discussed in this section is interpreted somewhat differently depending on whether it is based on risks, rates, odds, or prevalence, the magnitude of the various measures are interpreted in the same manner. For example, a risk ratio of 3.5 represents a strong, positive association

Figure 6-2 Measures of Association Based on Relative Comparisons

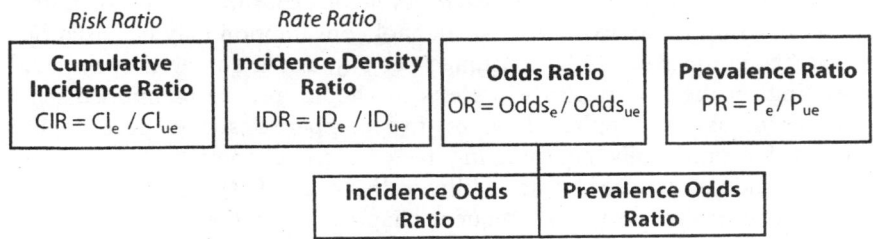

between exposure and outcome, while a risk ratio of 0.3 represents a strong, inverse association between exposure and outcome (see Table 6-2). It would also be appropriate to say that a risk ratio of 3.5 represents a risk that is 250 percent higher in the exposed group compared to the unexposed group and that a risk ratio of 0.3 represents a risk that is 70 percent lower in the exposed versus the unexposed group (see formula 6.5). Similar statements can be made for rate ratios, odds ratios, and prevalence ratios that have the same values.

Table 6-2 Basic Interpretation of Ratio Measures of Association

Value	Interpretation
= 1.0	No increased risk, rate, odds, or prevalence of the outcome due to the exposure (i.e., there is no apparent association between the exposure and outcome).
< 1.0	Decreased risk, rate, odds, or prevalence of the outcome due to the exposure (i.e., the exposure may be protective).
> 1.0	Increased risk, rate, odds, or prevalence of the outcome due to the exposure (i.e., the exposure may be hazardous).

Note: The references to *risk* refer to risk ratios; the references to *rate* refer to rate ratios; the references to *odds* refer to odds ratios; and the references to *prevalence* refer to prevalence ratios.

Table 6-3 General Rules of Thumb for Interpreting the Strength of Ratio Measures of Association

Type of Association		Relative Strength
Inverse	Positive	
0.7 – 0.9	1.1 – 1.5	Weak Association
0.4 – 0.6	1.6 – 3.0	Moderate Association
0.0 – 0.3	3.1 or more	Strong Association

Adapted from Monson, R. R. (1980). *Occupational Epidemiology*. Boca Raton: CRC Press. (Reprinted with permission from Monson, R. R. (1980). *Occupational Epidemiology*. CRC Press, Boca Raton, FL. Copyright CRC Press, Boca Raton, Florida).

Although the measures of association discussed in this section were based on dichotomous levels of exposure (i.e., exposed and unexposed), they can also be applied in situations where levels of exposure are not dichotomous. For example, an exposure like alcohol consumption may be based on the average number of drinks consumed per day, and the referent may vary depending on the investigator's interests. It should also be mentioned that measures of association based on relative comparisons may need to be adjusted for potentially confounding factors (see chapter 8) just as we adjusted crude death rates for age earlier in this chapter. This and other considerations are discussed in subsequent chapters when these measures are referred to in relation to specific study designs.

Absolute Comparisons

Measures of association based on relative comparisons assess the *strength of an association* between an exposure and outcome, which is helpful in determining disease etiology. An alternative is to use measures based *absolute comparisons*. These measures seek to determine the *amount* of a particular outcome that may be associated with a given exposure. While measures of association based on relative comparisons employ ratios, those based on absolute comparisons use differences. The most common measures of association based on absolute comparisons are:

- Risk difference
- Rate difference
- Prevalence difference
- Population-based differences

Risk difference.   As with risk ratio, **risk difference** is a generic term. The most common risk difference is the **cumulative incidence difference**. It is simply the arithmetic difference between the cumulative incidence of an occurrence among those exposed to a suspected risk factor and those who are not exposed. It is calculated as follows:

(6.9) $$CID = CI_e - CI_{ue}$$

In this expression CID stands for cumulative incidence difference. CI_e is the cumulative incidence of the occurrence in the exposed group, and CI_{ue} is the cumulative incidence in the unexposed group. For example, researchers from Finland investigated the changes in white-finger syndrome (a muscle disorder related to the frequent use of vibrating machinery) among lumberjacks (the exposed group), who frequently use vibrating machinery at work, and unexposed referents over a seven-year period. They reported a seven-year cumulative incidence of white-finger syndrome of 14.7 per 100 among the lumberjacks and 2.3 per 100 among the referents.[19] The cumulative incidence difference is therefore:

$$CID = 14.7 \text{ per } 100 - 2.3 \text{ per } 100 = 12.4 \text{ per } 100$$

This value represents the cumulative incidence (risk) of white-finger syndrome among the lumberjacks that is associated with being a lumberjack (i.e., frequently using vibrating machinery at work) over the seven-year period, all other factors being equal. Conceptually, the total risk of white-finger syndrome among the lumberjacks (14.7 cases per 100 lumberjacks) includes the risk associated with frequent use of vibrating machinery at work *plus* the risk associated with *other* factors (e.g., non-occupational use of vibrating machinery, presence of other diseases). When the risk associated with other factors (i.e., the risk among the referents) is subtracted from the total risk among the lumberjacks what is left is the risk associated with being a lumberjack. In generic terms, this represents the **excess risk** of the occurrence in the *exposed group* that is associated with the exposure over a given time period, all other factors being equal. Assuming a study is valid, this can also be conceived as the excess *number of occurrences* in the exposed group that is associated with the exposure over a given time period. A positive risk difference indicates a positive association between the excess risk (or number of occurrences) and the exposure; a negative risk difference indicates an inverse association; and an excess risk of zero represents no association, all other factors being equal.

CID can also be calculated from the cumulative incidence ratio (CIR) using formula 6.10.

(6.10) $$CID = (CIR - 1) \times CI_{ue}$$

Using the figures in the above example, this formula produces an identical result to that obtained using formula 6.9.

$$CIR = (14.7 \text{ per } 100) / (2.3 \text{ per } 100) = 6.4$$
$$CID = (6.4 - 1) \times 2.3 \text{ per } 100 = 12.4 \text{ per } 100$$

Rate difference.   The **rate difference**, which represents the difference between rates of occurrence in exposed and unexposed groups, is typified by the **incidence density difference** (IDD), which is calculated as shown in formula 6.11.

(6.11) $$IDD = ID_e - ID_{ue}$$

The expressions ID_e and ID_{ue} represent the incidence density of the occurrence in the exposed and unexposed groups, respectively. The incidence density difference may also be calculated from the incidence density ratio (IDR) in a manner similar to that for the cumulative incidence difference.

(6.12) $$IDD = (IDR - 1) \times ID_{ue}$$

IDD represents the **excess rate**, which is the rate of occurrence in the *exposed group* associated with the exposure, all other factors being equal. For example, investigators with the Center for Cardiovascular Disease Prevention in Boston found that after treatment with statin drugs heart patients whose low density lipoprotein (LDL) levels were above 70 mg. per deciliter (the exposed group) had 4.0 recurrent coronary events per 100 person-years of observation, and those whose LDL levels were below 70 mg. per deciliter (the referents) had only 2.7 events per 100 person-years of observation.[20] The incidence density ratio was therefore 1.48 (i.e., 4.0 / 2.7). Based on these findings, the incidence density difference can be calculated in either of the following ways:

Formula 6.11:
$$IDD = 4.0 \text{ per } 100 \text{ person-years} - 2.7 \text{ per } 100 \text{ person-years} = 1.3 \text{ per } 100 \text{ person-years}$$

Formula 6.12:
$$IDD = (1.48 - 1) \times 2.7 \text{ per } 100 \text{ person-years} = 1.3 \text{ per } 100 \text{ person-years}$$

The results indicate that 1.3 cases per 100 person-years is the *excess rate* of recurrent coronary events *in the exposed group* that is associated with the exposure, all other factors being equal. The implication is that the remainder of the total rate among the exposed group (2.7 per 100 person-years) is not associated with the exposure but with other risk factors. Note that the time period is not an essential element of the rate difference as it is with the risk difference. This is because time is already incorporated in the rate measures. Similar to the risk difference and assuming all other factors are equal, a positive rate difference indicates a positive association between the excess rate and the exposure, and a negative rate difference indicates an inverse association. A difference of zero implies no association.

Prevalence difference. The **prevalence difference** (PD) is calculated as shown in either formula 6.13 or 6.14.

(6.13) $$PD = P_e - P_{ue}$$

where P_e is the prevalence of the occurrence among the exposed group, and P_{ue} is the prevalence among the unexposed group.

(6.14) $$PD = (PR - 1) \times P_{ue}$$

where PR is the prevalence ratio (see formula 6.8).

The prevalence difference provides an indication of the amount of the prevalence *in the exposed group* that is associated with the exposure, all other factors being equal. This amount is known as the **excess prevalence**. For instance, in a study using a national data base, researchers affiliated with the University of Minnesota School of Medicine found that the prevalence of metabolic syndrome* was 258 per 1,000 for adults with a history of cancer and 184 per 1,000 for adults without a history of cancer (PD = 74 per 1,000; 95% CI = 38 per 1,000 to 110 per 1,000).[21] Thus, the excess prevalence was 74 per 1,000, which is the same as the prevalence difference. Like the prevalence ratio, some consider the prevalence difference to be a type of risk difference (i.e., the risk of *having* the outcome). Its interpretation is parallel to that

---

*Metabolic syndrome is characterized by a cluster of disorders that collectively increase one's risk of heart disease. The syndrome includes conditions such as type 2 diabetes or prediabetes, hypertension, obesity, and elevated blood lipids.

for the risk and rate differences in that a positive prevalence difference implies a positive association, etc. Like the rate difference, time is not an essential element of the prevalence difference since prevalence is conceptually instantaneous (i.e., point prevalence). Nevertheless, it is important to indicate person, place, and time factors when reporting risk, rate, or prevalence differences unless these are clear from the context of a given study or report. Figure 6-3 summarizes the calculation and interpretation of the three basic measures of association based on absolute comparisons.

Figure 6-3   Measures of Association Based on Absolute Comparisons

Risk Difference   *Rate Difference*

Cumulative Incidence Difference	**Incidence Density Difference**	**Prevalence Difference**
$CID = CI_e - CI_{ue}$ or $CID = (CIR - 1) \times CI_{ue}$	$IDD = ID_e - ID_{ue}$ or $IDD = (IDR - 1) \times ID_{ue}$	$PD = P_e - P_{ue}$ or $PD = (PR - 1) \times P_{ue}$

Interpretation: If the risk, rate, or prevalence difference is greater than zero, the association between the exposure and outcome is positive. If the difference is less than zero, the association is negative (i.e., represents an inverse association). If the difference is zero, there is no association. This assumes all other factors are equal. Random error can account for deviations from these guidelines (e.g., a small positive association may be due to random error and not represent a true association between exposure and outcome). Also, the size of the risk, rate, or prevalence difference does not necessarily tell us the strength of the association, which is best measured by a ratio measure of association.

Example: An incidence density difference (IDD) of 2.5 cases per 100 person-years suggests that this is the excess rate of the occurrence among the exposed group that is associated with the exposure. This represents a positive association between the exposure and the occurrence since the difference is greater than one.

Population-based differences. Corresponding difference measures based on an entire defined population can also be calculated. In general, these measures represent the excess risk, rate, or prevalence of the occurrence *in the population as a whole* that is associated with the exposure, all other factors being equal. The basic formula is the risk, rate, or prevalence of the occurrence in the population minus the respective risk, rate, or prevalence of the occurrence in the unexposed group. These measures can also be calculated by multiplying the risk, rate, or prevalence difference by the proportion of the population that is exposed. For example, the **population rate difference** using incidence density measures is:

(6.15) $PRD = ID_p - ID_{ue}$ or $PRD = IDD \times p_e$

PRD represents the population rate difference; ID_p is the incidence density of the occurrence in the *entire defined population*; and ID_{ue} is the incidence density for the unexposed portion of the population. In the alternate expression, IDD is the incidence density difference (formula 6.11), and p_e is the proportion of the population that is exposed to the factor of interest. For example, for a given population, assume $ID_p = 10$ cases per 100 person-years, $ID_e = 18$ cases per 100 person-years, $ID_{ue} = 2$ cases per 100 person-years, and $p_e = 0.5$. Thus,

PRD = 10 per 100 person-years − 2 per 100 person years =
8 per 100 person-years

PRD could also be calculated as follows:

PRD = (18 per 100 person-years − 2 per 100 person-years) × 0.5 =
8 per 100 person-years

The result in either case is the *excess rate* of occurrence *in the population* that is associated with the exposure, all other factors being equal.

Analogous formulas may be constructed for the **population risk difference** or the **population prevalence difference**. The caveats are similar to those for the risk and prevalence differences discussed earlier except that the excess risk or prevalence applies to the *entire population* versus only the exposed group. Unless everyone is exposed to the factor of interest in the defined population, the risk, rate, or prevalence difference will always be greater than the respective population risk, rate, or prevalence difference. For example, using the above figures, the rate difference (incidence density difference) is 16 per 100 person-years, while the population rate difference is only 8 per 100 person-years. This large disparity reflects the fact that the occurrence is closely associated with the exposure, and half of those in the population as a whole are unexposed.

Relative versus Absolute Comparisons

Measures of association based on relative and absolute comparisons must be interpreted differently because they measure different things. As mentioned previously, those based on relative comparisons reflect the *strength of the association* between an exposure and outcome and are useful in discovering causative factors. Measures of association based on absolute comparisons, on the other hand, indicate *how much* of the outcome in the exposed group (or population as a whole) is associated with the exposure. Therefore, a large absolute difference may indicate a potentially important public health problem. Absolute differences, however, cannot be used alone to predict ratio measures of association and vice versa. Together, however, they may provide a more comprehensive picture of the relationship between an exposure and outcome.

In analytic and experimental epidemiology (chapter 1), measures of association based on relative comparisons are often considered more useful than those based on absolute comparisons. This is because they help to identify potential causes of an outcome and because they have a common reference point of one, which indicates no deviation between the measures of occurrence being compared. For example, a risk ratio of three tells us instantly that the risk of the outcome in the exposed group is three times greater than that in the unexposed group, all other factors being equal. Similarly, a risk ratio of one implies no difference in risk between the exposed and unexposed groups. With measures of association based on absolute comparisons, the magnitude of the difference does not necessarily indicate the strength of the association between the exposure and outcome because it is largely influenced by the size of the measure of occurrence in the unexposed group. If this measure is large, then even a small, positive association between exposure and outcome can result in a large risk, rate, or prevalence difference. If the measure of occurrence in the unexposed group is small, however, it will take a substantial association between the exposure and outcome to produce a large difference. Problem 6-3 illustrates the calculation of measures of association based on relative and absolute comparisons.

Attributable Fractions

Risk, rate, and prevalence differences make no assumptions about causality between exposure and outcome. If we have evidence that the exposure is a cause of the outcome (see chapter 7), we can calculate the proportion of the risk that is attributable to the exposure provided that the exposure-outcome relationship is valid and not confounded by other factors.* This can be done for the exposed group alone or for the defined population as a whole using measures known as *attributable fractions*. The importance of attributable fractions lies in the fact that they tend to indicate the *impact* of a given exposure, that is, the proportion of occurrences that might be reduced if the exposure were to be eliminated. There are two major types of attributable fractions. These are:

- Attributable fraction among the exposed
- Population attributable fraction

   Attributable fraction among the exposed.   **Attributable fraction among the exposed** can be expressed mathematically as:

(6.16)
$$AF_e = \frac{CI_e - CI_{ue}}{CI_e}$$

where AF_e refers to the attributable fraction among the exposed, and CI_e and CI_{ue} refer to the cumulative incidence of the occurrence among the exposed and unexposed groups, respectively. Attributable fraction among the exposed is often stated as a percentage and indicates the *proportion* of the risk of a

*It is also possible to calculate the rate or prevalence attributable to the exposure using parallel measures, but we will focus on risk measurements to avoid redundancy and because they may be easier to explain and understand.

given outcome *among the exposed group* over a given time period that is attributable to the exposure of interest. Attributable fraction among the exposed can also be calculated using formula 6.17.

(6.17)
$$AF_e = \frac{RR - 1}{RR}$$

In this case, RR refers to risk ratio, although in other applications it may refer to another type of relative risk. To illustrate the use of formula 6.17, consider the previously cited study of the relationship between direct exposure to pentachlorophenol (PCP) and chloracne among workers.[12] In this study the investigators found a *risk ratio* of 4.6 based on 25 years of follow up. Assuming that the relationship is causal, attributable fraction among the exposed is calculated as:

$$AF_e = (4.6 - 1) / 4.6 = 0.783 \text{ or } 78.3\%$$

This indicates that 78.3 percent of the risk of chloracne *among workers directly exposed to PCP* is attributable to direct PCP exposure during the stated time period, all other factors being equal. The practical implication is that if direct exposure to PCP could be eliminated we would expect 78.3 percent fewer cases of chloracne to occur over the stated time period. Because the cumulative incidence, and hence the risk ratio, are directly affected by the length of the observation period, this period should always be reported for attributable fractions among the exposed that are based on these measures. The same is true for the risk difference.

When the frequency of the outcome is low (i.e., less than 0.10) and in certain other situations (see chapter 10), the odds ratio may be used to estimate the risk ratio in formula 6.17. Thus, in these cases attributable fraction among the exposed may be estimated from the results of a case-control study.

Population attributable fraction. **Population attributable fraction** is a related concept that has significant appeal to public health policy makers and administrators. It has been aptly defined as, "the proportional reduction in average disease risk over a specified time interval that would be achieved by eliminating the exposure(s) of interest from the population while distributions of other risk factors in the population remain unchanged."[22(p15)] The major difference between *attributable fraction among the exposed* (AF_e) and *population attributable fraction* (PAF) is that the object of AF_e is the exposed group, while for PAF it is the entire defined population. Therefore, AF_e measures the proportion of the risk of an occurrence *among the exposed group* due to the exposure, and PAF measures the proportion of the risk of an occurrence *among the entire defined population* due to the exposure. Both measures are based on assumptions that the exposure is a cause of the outcome of interest, and the relationship between the exposure and outcome is not confounded by other factors or biased in any way.

Population attributable fraction is commonly calculated using cumulative incidence measures[22] as shown in formula 6.18, although it can also be calculated using measures of incidence density or prevalence with somewhat different interpretations. The basic calculation using cumulative incidence is as follows:

(6.18)
$$PAF = \frac{CI_p - CI_{ue}}{CI_p}$$

PAF is the population attributable fraction; CI_p is the cumulative incidence of the occurrence in the *entire defined population* regardless of exposure status; and CI_{ue} is the cumulative incidence in the unexposed group. As with AF_e, this measure can be expressed as a decimal fraction or as a percent. For example, Japanese investigators studying stroke reported the following PAFs among those 40-64 years of age in a given community: 14.9 percent for smoking, 13.5 percent for untreated hypertension, 8.6 percent for uncontrolled hypertension, and 3.6 percent for atrial fibrillation based on a 20-year follow-up period.[23]

Population attributable fraction can also be calculated using formula 6.19 if one knows the proportion of exposed individuals in the defined population or if it can be accurately estimated from a sample of the defined population.[22]

(6.19)
$$PAF = \frac{p_e(RR-1)}{p_e(RR-1)+1}$$

In this expression, p_e is the proportion of the defined population with the exposure, and RR is the risk ratio. In the study referred to above, the authors recorded a risk ratio for stroke of 3.61 among residents, 40-64 years of age, with untreated hypertension during 20 years of follow up.[23] Approximately six percent of the population in this age group had untreated hypertension. Therefore, the PAF is calculated as follows:

$$PAF = [0.06\,(3.61 - 1)] / [0.06\,(3.61 - 1) + 1] = 0.135 \text{ or } 13.5\%$$

This is equivalent to the PAF reported by the authors (see above). It implies that 13.5 percent of the risk of stroke *in the defined population* during the follow-up period is attributable to untreated hypertension, all other factors being equal. Assuming untreated hypertension is a cause of stroke (a well established fact), we would expect that if all hypertension were treated in the defined population, the number of cases of stroke would decrease by 13.5 percent over a 20-year period, all other factors being equal.

As with risk differences and attributable fractions among the exposed, the period of observation should always be stated when reporting a PAF that is based on risk measures.* The population attributable fraction may be estimated from an odds ratio using formula 6.19 if one can assume that the odds ratio is a reliable estimate of the risk ratio and if one can accurately estimate

---

*Those based on incidence densities or prevalence do not need to state the period of observation since they are based on rates or prevalence, respectively, at a point in time.

the proportion of the exposed in the defined population. As with population-based differences, the PAF can also be calculated using formula 6.20.

$$(6.20) \qquad\qquad PAF = AF_e \times p_e$$

where AF_e is the attributable fraction among the exposed, and p_e is the proportion of the population that is exposed to the factor of interest. Similar to that for population-based differences, the PAF will always be smaller than the AF_e unless the proportion of the exposed in the population is one.

Final comments. Unfortunately, the use and interpretation of attributable fractions have not always been consistent in the epidemiologic literature.[22, 24, 25] One point of confusion is the many different terms that have been used to describe these concepts, several incorrectly (see table 6-4 for a sampling of terms that have been used).* In fact, about two decades ago, Sander Greenland and James M. Robins stated, "The number of terms for attributable fractions is perhaps the largest of any concept in epidemiology."[24(p1195)] There are also a number of other well established concepts (e.g., prevented fractions) and proposed concepts, such as the case impact number and exposed cases impact number,[26] that attempt to measure related phenomena. Nevertheless, attributable fractions should continue to be important concepts in epidemiology, especially population attributable fraction. Robert A. Spasoff states that population attributable fraction "is the most important epidemiologic indicator for policy purposes, because it illustrates the impact of a hazardous exposure on a whole population. . . ."[27(p50)] When used appropriately, it provides us with an indication of the public health impact of an exposure and optimally what we might expect in a population if the exposure is successfully eliminated. It can also be used to establish public health priorities, that is, determine the potential benefits of controlling different hazardous exposures in a population, as long as they can be considered causal factors for the outcome of interest. If one exposure is associated with a much higher population attributable fraction than another, for example, then public health administrators might decide to extend more resources toward the removal of that exposure than the other because of greater potential benefits to the population. The relative cost of controlling any given exposure would be another consideration, however.

Because the potential benefit measured by population attributable fraction depends on removing the exposure (or reducing it to the level of the referent), the measure is most appropriately cited where an effective intervention exists. One also has to take into account the nature of the disease process. Removal of an exposure may not always coincide with a timely reduction in the risk of occurrence of a given disease or other condition. Consider cigarette smoking, for example. While smoking cessation reduces the

---

*In addition, measures of association based on absolute comparisons have often been referred to as *attributable risk, population attributable risk, attributable rate,* etc. without providing any evidence of a cause-effect relationship between the exposure and outcome. Without such evidence, it is better to refer to differences as we have done in this chapter.

risk of lung cancer, it takes many years for the risk to reach its lowest level. Problem 6-3 illustrates the use of attributable fractions in addition to related measures of association.

Table 6-4   Some Terms Used to Indicate Attributable Fractions

Attributable Fraction among the Exposed (AF$_e$)	Population Attributable Fraction (PAF)
• Attributable fraction	• Attributable fraction
• Attributable fraction (exposed)	• Attributable fraction (population)
• Attributable fraction for the exposed	• Attributable fraction for the population
• Attributable fraction in the exposed	• Attributable fraction in the population
• Attributable proportion	• Attributable proportion
• Attributable proportion among the exposed	• Attributable proportion (population)
• Attributable proportion in exposed subjects	• Attributable proportion among the population
	• Attributable proportion in the population
• Attributable risk	• Attributable risk
• Attributable risk (exposed)	• Attributable risk (population)
• Attributable risk for the exposed group	• Attributable risk for the total population
• Attributable risk in exposed population	• Attributable risk in the total population
• Attributable risk in the exposed group	• Attributable risk in total population
• Attributable risk percent	• Attributable risk percent (population)
• Attributable risk percent (exposed)	• Attributable risk percent for the population
• Attributable risk percent for the exposed	• Etiologic fraction
• Attributable risk percent in the exposed	• Etiologic fraction (population)
• Attributable risk percentage	• Excess fraction
• Attributable risk proportion	• Percent population attributable risk
• Etiologic fraction	• Population attributable risk
• Etiologic fraction among the exposed	• Population attributable risk fraction
• Etiological fraction (exposed)	• Population attributable risk percent
• Excess fraction	• Population attributable risk percentage
• Exposed attributable fraction	• Population attributable risk proportion
• Exposed attributable risk percent	• Population etiologic fraction
• Percent attributable risk in exposed individuals	
• Percentage risk reduction	
• Protective efficacy rate	

Problem 6-3: Use and Interpretation of Measures of Association

According to the U.S. Surgeon General, cigarette smoking is a cause of both lung cancer (LC) and coronary heart disease (CHD). Epidemiologic investigators at a major university conducted a five-year prospective cohort study among a representative sample of residents, 60–64 years of age, in a large northeastern portion of the United States. The investigators reported the cumulative incidences for both LC and CHD in the table below. For both LC and CHD, calculate the appropriate measures of association based on relative and absolute comparisons as well as the attributable fraction among the exposed and the population attributable fraction. Interpret your results.

	Cumulative Incidence	
Population	LC	CHD
Overall	60 per 100,000	240 per 100,000
Cigarette smokers	180 per 100,000	420 per 100,000
Non-cigarette smokers	20 per 100,000	180 per 100,000

Solution:
Step 1: Since the data in this problem represent cumulative incidence measures, the appropriate measure of association based on relative comparisons is the cumulative incidence ratio (CIR; formula 6.4), which is a type of risk ratio. The applicable exposure is cigarette smoking.

$$CIR = \frac{CI_e}{CI_{ue}}$$

LC: CIR = 180 per 100,000 / 20 per 100,000 = 9.00

CHD: CIR = 420 per 100,000 / 180 per 100,000 = 2.33

Step 2: Again, since the data in the problem represent cumulative incidence measures, the appropriate measure of association based on absolute comparisons is the cumulative incidence difference (CID; formula 6.9). Again, the applicable exposure is cigarette smoking.

$$CID = CI_e - CI_{ue}$$

LC: CID = 180 per 100,000 – 20 per 100,000 = 160 per 100,000

CHD: CID = 420 per 100,000 – 180 per 100,000 = 240 per 100,000

Step 3: Use formula 6.16 to calculate the attributable fractions among the exposed.

$$AF_e = \frac{CI_e - CI_{ue}}{CI_e}$$

LC: AF_e = 160 per 100,000 / 180 per 100,000 = 0.889 or 88.9%

CHD: AF_e = 240 per 100,000 / 420 per 100,000 = 0.571 or 57.1%

Note: The numerators for the AF_es were already calculated in step 2.

Step 4: Use formula 6.18 to calculate the population attributable fractions.

$$PAF = \frac{CI_p - CI_{ue}}{CI_p}$$

LC: PAF = [(60 per 100,000) – (20 per 100,000)] / 60 per 100,000 = 0.667 or 66.7%

CHD: PAF = [(240 per 100,000) – (180 per 100,000)] / 240 per 100,000 = 0.250 or 25.0%

Answer: Based on the defined population, the five-year risk ratios for LC and CHD are 9.00 and 2.33, respectively. This means that the risk of developing LC is 9.00 times greater for cigarette smokers than non-cigarette smokers, and the risk of developing CHD is 2.33 times greater for cigarette smokers than non-cigarette smokers. Therefore, cigarette smoking is strongly associated with LC and moderately associated with CHD (see table 6-3), all other factors being equal. The five-year risk differences for LC and CHD are 160 per 100,000 and 240 per 100,000, respectively. These figures represent the excess risk of LC and CHD, respectively, among the cigarette smokers that is associated with cigarette smoking during the five-year study period. The association is greater for CHD than for LC, all other factors being equal. The attributable fractions among the exposed for LC and CHD are 88.9 percent and 57.1 percent, respectively. These are the proportions of the risk of LC and CHD, respectively, among cigarette smokers that are attributable to cigarette smoking during the five-year study period. If the cigarette smokers gave up cigarette smoking, we would expect 88.9 percent fewer cases of LC and 57.1 percent fewer cases of CHD in this group during the stated time period. Finally, the population attributable fractions for LC and CHD are 66.7 percent and 25.0 percent, respectively. These are the proportions of the risk of LC and CHD, respectively, in the population as a whole that are attributable to cigarette smoking during the stated time period. If cigarette smoking could be eliminated from the population, we would expect 66.7 percent fewer cases of LC and 25.0 percent fewer cases of CHD in the population during the five-year study period.

Comments:

1. The answers to this problem may appear somewhat contradictory. However, if we examine each separately we should get a clearer picture of what the answers mean. Let us start with the measure of association based on relative comparisons. The risk ratio (cumulative incidence ratio) tells us the strength of the association between an exposure and outcome. The more the risk ratio departs from one, the stronger the association. Clearly, the association between cigarette smoking and LC is greater than that between cigarette smoking and CHD. In fact, the increased risk of LC for cigarette smokers compared to non-cigarette smokers is 800 percent. That for CHD is only 130 percent (see formula 6.5). A risk ratio, however, only reveals the *relative risk* associated with the exposure (e.g., how many times greater the risk of occurrence is in the exposed group compared to the unexposed group). It does not reveal the *absolute risk* associated with the exposure (i.e., how much greater the risk is in absolute terms in the exposed group compared to the unexposed group). The appropriate measure for determining this is the risk difference. It may be helpful to keep in mind that risk ratios and risk differences measure different aspects of an association.[28]

2. The risk difference (cumulative incidence difference) can be more difficult to explain than the risk ratio. However, there is a simple logic to this measure, which is illustrated here using LC. First, it is important to recognize that even though cigarette smoking is considered a cause of LC, some cigarette smokers may develop LC for reasons other than cigarette smoking (e.g., occupational exposure to toxicants, residential radon exposure, genetics). The risk difference attempts to capture the absolute amount of risk among cigarette smokers that is associated *only* with cigarette smoking. Since the risk of LC among non-cigarette smokers cannot be associated with cigarette smoking (they do not smoke cigarettes), it is subtracted from the total risk among cigarette smokers to determine how much of the risk is associated *only* with cigarette smoking. In essence, we remove the risk associated

with other factors by subtracting that risk from the risk associated with all factors. What is left is the *excess risk* among cigarette smokers that is associated with cigarette smoking. This risk will always be less that the risk of LC among cigarette smokers because cigarette smoking is not the only factor associated with LC. The magnitude of the risk difference does not indicate the strength of an association between an exposure and outcome since it is largely influenced by the size of absolute risk (cumulative incidence) in the unexposed group. The high absolute risk of CHD in the unexposed group, for example, means that even a small increased risk of CHD for cigarette smokers will lead to a high absolute risk among the exposed group. Conversely, the small absolute risk of LC in the unexposed group will mean that even a large increased risk LC for cigarette smokers may not lead to a very high absolute risk among the exposed. This is illustrated by using formula 6.10.

LC: CID = (9.00 − 1) × (20 per 100,000) = 160 per 100,000

CHD: CID = (2.33 − 1) × (180 per 100,000) = 239 per 100,000 ≈ 240 per 100,000

Even though the risk ratio is much greater for LC than CHD, the lower absolute risk of LC compared to CHD among non-cigarette smokers leads to a greater risk difference for CHD than LC. In practical terms, if one smokes cigarettes his or her risk of developing LC is greatly increased, whereas his or her risk of developing CHD is only moderately increased. However, since CHD is a more common occurrence in the population than LC, a cigarette smoker is more likely to develop CHD than LC. Thus, the risk difference depends not only on the strength of the association between the exposure and outcome but also on the frequency of the outcome in the unexposed group.

3. The attributable fraction among the exposed (AF_e) is an extension of the risk difference. Fundamentally, it is the risk difference divided by the risk of the occurrence in the exposed group. Unlike risk difference, however, this measure assumes that the exposure is a cause of the outcome. If it is not, then we cannot determine the proportion of the risk in the exposed group that is *attributable to* the exposure. For LC, the AF_e of 88.9 percent indicates that among cigarette smokers nearly 90 percent of the risk of LC is attributable to cigarette smoking during the five-year study period. It clearly appears to be the most important risk factor for LC among cigarette smokers. For CHD, the AF_e 57.1 percent. Therefore, about 57 percent of the risk of CHD among cigarette smokers is due to cigarette smoking during the study period. This tells us that cigarette smoking appears to be an important cause of CHD but apparently not as important as it is for LC. This may explain the higher cumulative incidence of CHD among *non-cigarette smokers* in the study compared to that for LC.

4. The population attributable fraction (PAF) is an extension of the population risk difference. It is the population risk difference divided by the risk of the occurrence in the population as a whole. It represents the proportion of the risk in the population due to the exposure for the five-year study period. For LC this proportion was 0.667 or 66.7 percent. For CHD it is 0.25 or 25.0 percent. Thus, if cigarette smoking could be eliminated from the population we would expect a higher percentage reduction in the development of LC than CHD, although the expected number of cases reduced by eliminating cigarette smoking in the population would be less for LC than CHD. The reason is the higher absolute risk of CHD compared to LC. This is illustrated below.

Cases of LC potentially eliminated: (60 per 100,000) × 0.667 = 40 per 100,000

Cases of CHD potentially eliminated: (240 per 100,000) × 0.25 = 60 per 100,000

TESTING FOR STATISTICAL SIGNIFICANCE

When two sample measures of occurrence are compared, say by ratios or differences, some may wonder whether the resulting measure of association is **statistically significant**, that is, unlikely due to chance, and therefore potentially representative of a real association. In general, for a given sample size, the more a measure of association departs from its *null value*, the more likely it is statistically significant. The **null value** is that corresponding to no association. For a ratio measure of association it is *one*, and for a difference measure of association it is *zero*. Thus, a statistically significant ratio measure will differ from a value of one to a degree greater than that expected due to chance alone, and a statistically significant difference measure will differ from a value of zero to the same degree.

Statistical significance is rooted in hypothesis testing.* Briefly, an investigator develops a **null hypothesis**, which is one stating that there is no association between an exposure and outcome of interest. At the same time, the investigator develops an **alternative hypothesis** stating there is an association. The alternate hypothesis may be a **non-directional** or **directional hypothesis** (see table 6-5). The investigator then tests the null hypothesis statistically and decides whether or not to reject it. If it is *not* rejected, the investigator concludes that the association is not statistically significant. If it is rejected, the alternative hypothesis is accepted, and the association is considered statistically significant. Statistical significance is measured by a *test of statistical significance*, commonly known as the **test statistic** or **statistical test**. The value of the test statistic is compared to **critical values** that correspond to specific probabilities known as *p-values*. A **p-value** represents the probability of obtaining a measure of association (or other applicable measure) that is at least as extreme as that obtained given that the null hypothesis is true.[29] Typically, an

---

Table 6-5 Examples of Statistical Hypotheses

Hypothesis with a non-directional alternate hypothesis

H_0: OR = 1

H_A: OR ≠ 1

Hypothesis with a directional alternate hypothesis

H_0: OR = 1

H_A: OR > 1

Note: OR refers to the odds ratio. H_0 refers to the null hypothesis, that reflecting no association between the exposure and outcome, and H_A refers to the alternate hypothesis, that reflecting an association between the exposure and outcome.

---

*Statistical significance is often tested in analytic or experimental epidemiologic studies based on one or more *a priori* hypotheses (chapter 4). Statistical significance may also be tested in descriptive epidemiologic studies where no *a priori* hypotheses have been developed. The objective here is to make *a posteriori* comparisons ("after the fact" comparisons) of the findings.

investigator preselects a maximum p-value upon which to make a determination of statistical significance. This is known as the **alpha level** or **significance level** and is usually equivalent to p = 0.05. If the test statistic equals or exceeds the critical value associated with p = 0.05, the observed association is considered statistically significant, and the probability of it being due to chance is said to be p ≤ 0.05. If, on the other hand, the test statistic is less than the critical value associated with p = 0.05, the observed association is considered *not* statistically significant, and the probability of it being due to chance alone is said to be p > 0.05. These decisions are based on the assumption that the null hypothesis is true. In a sense, one is asking how much a measure of association would have to depart from the null hypothesis of no association to be considered a nonrandom departure. Anything less would be considered due to random variation (chance alone). In reality, such decisions are guided by statements of probability, not certainty.

By establishing an alpha level of 0.05, the investigator is protected, on average, from falsely rejecting a null hypothesis more than five percent of the time. An alternative to selecting a specific alpha level is to report simply the particular p-value associated with the value of the test statistic. For example, an investigator may report OR = 2.1, p = 0.02. This means that the odds ratio is 2.1, and the probability that it represents random variation from an odds ratio of 1.0, which represents no association, is only two percent, assuming the null hypothesis is true. In other words, the probability that there is no real association is just two percent, all other factors being equal. In statistics, statistical significance testing is based on the theory that any given sample is an imperfect representation of the sampled population. Therefore, we can never be *entirely sure* that an association observed in a sample also exists in the population. Likewise, the absence of an association in a sample does not mean that one does not exist in the population. The only way one can be certain is to sample the entire population. Statistical significance testing is discussed further in chapter 8 in relation to the topic of random error. Subsequent chapters discuss specific methods for testing statistical significance based on study design.

Finally, it should be pointed out that statistical significance says nothing about the *importance* of a particular association, that is, its **practical** or **clinical significance**. That is best determined by expert opinion. No matter how small a p-value is, it tells us nothing about the strength or meaning of a given association. Likewise, a large p-value does not necessarily mean that the association is weak or unimportant. The purpose of the p-value is to determine the probability that the null hypothesis is true. Measures of association (e.g., risk, rate, prevalence, and odds ratios) tell us about the strength of an association, and experience tells us about its practical or clinical significance to public health.

An alternative to testing for statistical significance is to calculate a confidence interval (chapter 5) for the measure of association. The confidence interval method is generally preferred since it not only provides the probable range for a measure of association, but it also gives us a clue to the magnitude of the association. Furthermore, it can tell us whether or not an apparent association is statistically significant, although this is not a reason it is preferred over statistical significance testing. If a confidence interval for a ratio measure of association contains 1.0, then the association is not statistically significant. If for a difference measure of association it contains 0.0, then it is not statistically significant. In short, a confidence interval for a measure of association can be used to get an idea of the probable magnitude and range of the association in the sampled population. If desired, it can also be used to determine whether or not the association is statistically significant, although those who dislike statistical significance testing will not see this as an advantage.

The use of confidence intervals over significance testing has gained many proponents in epidemiology, and confidence intervals are increasingly the preferred way of reporting results in many epidemiologic, public health, and biomedical journals. Nevertheless, statistical testing is still used and has its adherents. Therefore, it is prudent to be familiar with both methods. More is said about significance testing and confidence intervals in chapter 8 and succeeding chapters.*

SUMMARY

- Crude rates are overall, summary measures of occurrence for defined populations. Specific rates are measures of occurrence for distinct subgroups within a defined population, such as age-specific or sex-specific rates. Crude rates are more convenient to compare between populations than specific rates, especially if there are many specific rates to compare. Unlike specific rates, however, crude rates can be distorted (confounded) by differences in the underlying distributions of the populations being compared, particularly age distributions.

- Adjusted rates, like crude rates, are also overall measures of occurrence, but they have been statistically modified (adjusted) to remove the potential distorting effects of one or more factors like age, sex, or race/ethnicity differences between the populations being compared. Adjusted rates permit fair, unbiased comparisons between overall rates.

- There are two basic methods of rate adjustment—the direct and indirect methods. The direct method uses the specific rates in the populations being compared to develop adjusted rates based on a standard population. The indirect method applies the specific rates in the reference population to the study population to develop a standardized mortality (or morbidity) ratio.

---

*Generally speaking, modern theory in epidemiology holds that study populations do not need to be considered representative samples of some larger general population to provide valid and reliable findings, except in the case of certain cross-sectional studies. This conception, however, can make it difficult to explain the application of confidence intervals and significance testing, which are firmly based on sampling theory. Tools like confidence intervals or tests of significance are used in most epidemiologic studies as relative indicators of the reliability of the findings even if in a technical sense the assumption of random sampling from a normal population is not met.

Unlike the direct method, the indirect method of adjustment can be used even if one or more specific rates in one of the populations being compared is unavailable or unstable.

- Measures of association (or effect) are quantities that express the degree of statistical relationship between a given exposure and outcome. They may be based on relative or absolute comparisons. Those based on relative comparisons (i.e., risk ratios, rate ratios, odds ratios, and prevalence ratios) assess the strength of an association, while those based on absolute comparisons (i.e., risk differences, rate differences, prevalence differences, and population-based differences) assess the quantity of the outcome associated with a given exposure. Measures of association based on relative comparisons tend to be more useful in uncovering causal relationships, while those based on absolute comparisons tend to be more useful in determining the potential burden of an outcome.

- Attributable fractions are based on the assumption that the exposure and outcome are causally related. Attributable fraction among the exposed measures the proportion of the risk of an outcome due to the exposure among the exposed group in a population. Population attributable fraction measures the proportion of the risk due to the exposure in the entire defined population regardless of exposure status. Both measures indicate the proportion of an occurrence that might be eliminated if the exposure is removed. The attributable fraction among the exposed will always be greater than the population attributable fraction unless everyone in the defined population is exposed. Population attributable fraction is commonly used by policy makers and administrators to establish public health priorities.

- Measures of association may be tested for statistical significance (i.e., if they significantly different from 1.0 for measures based on relative comparisons or significantly different from 0.0 for measures based on absolute comparisons). Statistical significance is rooted in hypothesis testing and is measured by the p-value. Generally, $p \leq 0.05$ indicates that an observed measure of association is unlikely to be due to chance alone based on the assumption that there is no real association. Thus, it is considered statistically significant. Conversely, $p > 0.05$ indicates the observed measure of association is probably due to chance alone, and hence, not statistically significant. Statistical significance does not indicate the strength of an association nor does it reveal its practical significance. For a number of reasons, most epidemiologists prefer to use confidence intervals rather than significance testing. For one thing, these provide more information than significance testing.

New Terms

- 2000 U.S. standard million population
- 2000 U.S. standard population
- *a posteriori* comparison
- absolute risk
- adjusted rate
- age adjustment
- age standardization
- alpha level
- alternative hypothesis
- attributable fraction among the exposed
- clinical significance
- critical value
- crude rate
- cumulative incidence difference
- cumulative incidence ratio
- defined population
- direct method
- directional hypothesis
- disease odds ratio
- excess prevalence
- excess rate
- excess risk
- incidence density difference
- incidence density ratio
- incidence rate ratio
- indirect method
- indirectly standardized rate
- measure of association
- measure of effect
- non-directional hypothesis
- null hypothesis
- null value
- odds ratio
- percent relative effect
- population attributable fraction
- population prevalence difference
- population rate difference
- population risk difference
- practical significance
- prevalence difference
- prevalence ratio
- p-value
- rate adjustment
- rate difference
- rate ratio
- rate standardization
- referent
- relative odds
- relative risk
- risk difference
- risk ratio
- significance level
- specific rate
- standard population
- standardized morbidity ratio
- standardized mortality ratio
- standardized rate
- statistical test
- statistically significant
- test statistic

Study Questions and Exercises

1. Meadville and Barton are two small communities in the Northeast. The overall unintentional injury rates among 15–29 year olds are similar in both communities, but the age distributions among the 15–29 year olds are quite different. Use the direct method to age adjust the unintentional injury rates in the two populations based on the data in the table below. The standard population should be derived from a combination of the two populations. Compare and interpret your results.

	Meadville			Barton		
Age	Population	No. Injuries	Age-specific rate	Population	No. Injuries	Age-specific rate
15–19	200	14	0.070	1,000	20	0.020
20–24	1,200	36	0.030	100	14	0.140
25–29	800	12	0.015	400	12	0.030
All ages	2,200	62		1,500	46	

2. Streamland and Castleton represent two relatively young populations in the same state. Both cities are similar economically and culturally. Using the data in the table below, calculate and compare the crude death rates in the two cities. Next, adjust the rates by age. Are the age-adjusted rates different, and why or why not? Was age a distorting (confounding) factor in the comparison of the crude rates, and why or why not?

	Streamland			Castleton		
Age	Population	No. Injuries	Age-specific rate	Population	No. Injuries	Age-specific rate
0–9	2,000	18	0.009	3,000	15	0.005
10–19	3,500	11	0.003	5,500	12	0.002
20–29	4,500	20	0.004	1,000	N.A.*	N.A.
30–39	6,000	12	0.002	3,000	N.A.	N.A.
40–49	1,500	12	0.008	2,500	18	0.007
50–59	1,000	25	0.025	1,500	14	0.009
60 +	1,500	42	0.028	2,500	15	0.006
All ages	20,000	140		19,000	105	

*N.A. = Not available.

3. A prospective cohort study of 18,540 men was designed to determine the relationship of hypertension and cigarette smoking to cardiovascular disease (CVD) deaths. After five years of follow up, the study produced the following results:

Subgroup	Number	CVD Deaths
Cigarette smokers	4,205	339
Non-cigarette smokers	14,335	422
Total	18,540	761
Hypertensives	3,297	305
Nonhypertensives	15,243	456
Total	18,540	761

Based on the data provided, determine: (a) the cumulative incidence ratio of CVD death due to cigarette smoking and hypertension, respectively, (b) the percent relative effect for cigarette smoking and hypertension, respectively, (c) the attributable fraction among the exposed for cigarette smoking and hypertension, respectively, and (d) the population attributable fraction for cigarette smoking and hypertension, respectively. In each case, indicate what your answer means in words. Which factor appears to be more important as a cause of CVD deaths in this population, and why?

4. Epidemiologic researchers from California studied several thousand adult men and women over time. They reported 24 new cases of an unusual disease per 10,000 person-years of observation among the men but only 24 cases of the disease per 100,000 person-years among the women. Based on their findings, calculate the following measures for this unusual disease: (a) incidence density ratio, and (b) incidence density difference. Indicate what your answers mean in words. Are these measures of association likely to be statistically significant? Why or why not? Note that the rates have been reported using different population bases.

References

1. Anderson, R. N., Smith, B. L. (2005). Deaths: Leading Causes for 2002. *National Vital Statistics Reports* 53 (17). Hyattsville, MD: National Center for Health Statistics.
2. Centers for Disease Control and Prevention, National Center for Health Statistics (2004). Worktable 23R: Death Rates by 10-Year Age Groups: United States and Each State, 2002. Available: http://www.cdc.gov/nchs/data/dvs/mortfinal2002_work23r.pdf (Access date: August 15, 2005).
3. U.S. Census Bureau (2005). State and County Quick Facts. Available: http://quickfacts.census.gov/qfd/states/00000.html (Access date: August 15, 2005).
4. Kochanek, K D., Murphy, S. L., Anderson, R. N., and Scott, C. (2004). Deaths: Final Data for 2002. *National Vital Statistics Reports* 53 (5). Hyattsville, MD: National Center for Health Statistics.
5. Anderson, R. N., and Rosenberg, H. M. (1998). Age Standardization of Death Rates: Implementation of the Year 2000 Standard. *National Vital Statistics Reports* 47 (3). Hyattsville, MD: National Center for Health Statistics.
6. Berry, J. G., and Harrison, J. E. (2005). *A Guide to Statistical Methods for Injury Surveillance.* Canberra: Australian Institute of Health and Welfare. Available: http://www.nisu.flinders.edu.au/pubs/reports/2005/injcat72.pdf.
7. Szklo, M., and Nieto, F. J. (2000). *Epidemiology: Beyond the Basics.* Gaithersburg, MD: Aspen.
8. MacMahon, B., and Trichopoulos, D. (1996). *Epidemiology: Principles and Methods,* 2nd ed. Boston: Little, Brown and Company.
9. Rothman, K. J. (2002). *Epidemiology: An Introduction.* New York: Oxford University Press.
10. Rothman, K. J. (1986). *Modern Epidemiology.* Boston: Little, Brown and Company.
11. Kahn, H. A., and Sempos, C. T. (1989). *Statistical Methods in Epidemiology.* New York: Oxford University Press.
12. O'Malley, M. A., Carpenter, A. V., Sweeney, M. H., Fingerhut, M. A., Marlow, D. A., Halperin, W. E., and Mathias, C. G. (1990). Chloracne Associated with Employment in the Production of Pentachlorophenol. *American Journal of Industrial Medicine* 17 (4): 411–421.
13. Cubbin, C., LeClere, F. B., and Smith, G. S. (2000). Socioeconomic Status and the Occurrence of Fatal and Nonfatal Injury in the United States. *American Journal of Public Health* 90 (1): 71–77.

14. Larson, E. L., Lin, S. X., Gomez-Pichardo, C., and Della-Latta, P. (2004). Effect of Antibacterial Home Cleaning and Handwashing Products on Infectious Disease Symptoms: A Randomized, Double Blind Trial. *Annals of Internal Medicine* 140 (5): 321–329.

15. Bonita, R., Scragg, R., Stewart, A., Jackson, R., and Beaglehole, R. (1986). Cigarette Smoking and Risk of Premature Stroke in Men and Women. *British Medical Journal* 293: 6–8.

16. Cardenas, V. M., and Graham, D. Y. (2005). Smoking and *Helicobacter pylori* Infection in a Sample of U.S. Adults. *Epidemiology* 16 (4): 586–590.

17. Adebamowo, C. A., Spiegelman, D., Danby, F. W., Frazier, A. L., Willett, W. C., and Holmes, M. D. (2005). High School Dietary Dairy Intake and Teenage Acne. *Journal of the American Academy of Dermatology* 52 (2): 207–214.

18. Woodward, M. (1999). *Epidemiology: Study Design and Data Analysis*. Boca Raton: Chapman & Hall/CRC.

19. Kivekas, J., Riihimaki, H., Husman, K., Hanninen, K., Harkonen, H., Kuusela, T., Pekkarinen, M., Tola, S., and Zitting, A. J. (1994). Seven-year Follow-up of White-finger Symptoms and Radiographic Wrist Findings in Lumberjacks and Referents. *Scandinavian Journal of Work, Environment & Health* 20 (2): 101–106.

20. Ridker, P. M., Cannon, C. P., Morrow, D., Rifai, N., Rose, L. M., McCabe, C. H., Pfeffer, M. A., and Brauwald, E. (2005). C-reactive Protein Levels and Outcomes After Statin Therapy. *New England Journal of Medicine* 352 (1): 20–28.

21. Ness, K. K., Oakes, J. M., Punyko, J. A., Baker, K. S., and Gurney, J. G. (2005). Prevalence of the Metabolic Syndrome in Relation to Self-reported Cancer History. *Annals of Epidemiology* 15 (3): 202–206.

22. Rockhill, B., Newman, B., and Weinberg, C. (1998). Use and Misuse of Population Attributable Fractions. *American Journal of Public Health*: 88 (1): 15–19.

23. Nakayama, T., Yokoyama, T., Yoshiike, N., Zaman, M. M., Date, C., Tanaka, H., and Detels, R. (2000). Population Attributable Fraction of Stroke Incidence in Middle-aged and Elderly People: Contributions of Hypertension, Smoking and Atrial Fibrillation. *Neuroepidemiology* 19 (4): 217–226.

24. Greenland, S., and Robins, J. M. (1988). Conceptual Problems in the Definitions and Interpretation of Attributable Fractions. *American Journal of Epidemiology* 128 (6): 1185–1197.

25. Goodman, S. (2005). Attributable Risk in Epidemiology: Interpreting and Calculating Population Attributable Fractions. In *Estimating the Contributions of Lifestyle-related Factors to Preventable Death: A Workshop Summary*, Institute of Medicine of the National Academies. Washington, DC: The National Academies Press. Available: http://www.nap.edu (Access date: August 21, 2005).

26. Heller, R. F., Dobson, A. J., Attia, J., and Page, J. (2002). Impact Numbers: Measures of Risk Factor Impact on the Whole Population from Case-control and Cohort Studies. *Journal of Epidemiology and Community Health* 56: 606–610.

27. Spasoff, R. A. (1999). *Epidemiologic Methods for Health Policy*. New York: Oxford University Press.

28. Gerstman, B. B. (1998). *Epidemiology Kept Simple: An Introduction to Classic and Modern Epidemiology*. New York: Wiley-Liss, Inc.

29. Day, S. (1999). *Dictionary for Clinical Trials*. Chichester: John Wiley & Sons, Ltd.

CHAPTER SEVEN

Association and Causation in Epidemiology

This chapter discusses differences among spurious, noncausal, and causal associations, the various types of causes, and common guidelines used in assessing causation in epidemiologic studies.

Learning Objectives

- Describe and give examples of spurious, noncausal, and causal associations in epidemiology.
- State the common reasons for spurious and noncausal associations, respectively.
- Distinguish among necessary, sufficient, necessary and sufficient, necessary but not sufficient, not necessary but sufficient, and not necessary and not sufficient causes and give examples of each type.
- Describe and give examples of direct and indirect causal associations.
- Briefly describe the causal pie model.
- Discuss six guidelines based on Hill's postulates for judging potential causal associations, including the advantages and limitations of each criterion, respectively.
- Explain the importance of finding causal associations in epidemiology.
- Define predisposing or enabling factors, statistical association, and threshold.

INTRODUCTION

As indicated in chapter 1, one of the primary goals of epidemiology is to discover the *causes** of morbidity and mortality in human populations. This goal has immense practical significance for health professionals because a better

---

*There are many terms relating to or derived from the root term *cause*. These include causation, causality, causal, causative, cause-effect, etiology, and so forth. These terms are not defined separately in this chapter, but each refers to something similar.

understanding of the causes of morbidity and mortality often leads to more effective prevention, treatment, and control measures and consequently to a reduction in disease incidence, prevalence, or severity.

A *statistical association* between a given exposure and outcome is the starting point for consideration of a causal relationship in epidemiology. A **statistical association** implies that the exposure is related to a change in the *probability* of the outcome. It does not automatically mean that the exposure *causes* the outcome.[1] Hence, a frequently cited maxim in introductory statistics courses is: "Association does not necessarily imply causation." In short, statistical associations should not be accepted at face value. They should be examined for alternate explanations before any conclusions are drawn. Even a statistically significant association (chapter 6) does not guarantee that a true association exists, much less that the association is causal. A **causal association** between an exposure and outcome means that a change in the frequency of the exposure in a population *will result* in a change in the frequency of the outcome, even though not every individual with the exposure will change. A statistical association only implies that those with the exposure are more or less likely to develop the outcome.

To summarize briefly, a valid statistical association means it is *more or less likely* that the outcome will occur in the presence of the exposure, while a valid causal association means that changes in the frequency of exposure will result in changes in the frequency of the outcome. It should be noted that a causal association may be positive (the exposure increases the outcome) or negative (the exposure decreases the outcome). In the former case, the exposure is *hazardous*; in the latter case it is *protective*. The remainder of this chapter focuses on examining statistical associations to determine whether or not they are likely to represent causal associations. Many factors must be considered, and any conclusions must be based on an overall assessment of the evidence.

TYPES OF ASSOCIATION

Statistical associations found in epidemiologic studies (e.g., OR = 3.4) can be categorized into three types. These categories are mutually exclusive.

- Spurious associations
- Noncausal associations
- Causal associations

Spurious Associations

Spurious associations are literally *false* associations. Though they may be found in a particular study population, they are probably due to other explanations. Spurious associations usually result from *random error* (chance) or *bias*, which are discussed more fully in chapter 8. For example, as mentioned in chapter 6, an association is generally considered statistically significant if p $\leq$ 0.05. This implies that, assuming there is no association, chance is an unlikely explanation for the finding given the sample size and strength of the association. Nonetheless, we would still predict that as many as five times out of 100 the association could be due to chance alone. Thus, even statistically significant associations that result from well-executed epidemiologic studies can sometimes be spurious. Inderjit S. Thind, for instance, conducted an ecological study of the association between dietary intake and cancer using a sample of 60 countries. He found a number of significant statistical associations, including some that were biologically implausible and which he thought to be spurious. In his discussion of the findings, he reiterated a common concern in broad-based studies where large numbers of statistical tests of significance are performed. Specifically, he cautioned the readers by stating, "The . . . large numbers of correlations . . . with [some] significant associations occurring purely by chance, suggest extreme care in assessing the role of specific dietary items as risk factors and using the results as the basis for public policy."[2(p162)]

Spurious associations may also arise from sources of bias. *Bias*, which is discussed in chapter 8, is a type of systematic (nonrandom) error in the design, conduct, or analysis of epidemiologic studies, such as the use of flawed measurement techniques, differential recall among study and comparison groups, or selection of study and comparison groups that are dissimilar. Bias can be quite insidious. Consider a hypothetical case-control study of the relationship between exposure to low-frequency electromagnetic fields, such as those generated by electric power lines, electric blankets, and electric alarm clocks, and the incidence of childhood leukemia. The cases consist of patients from area hospitals newly diagnosed with childhood leukemia, and the controls are those without leukemia of similar age, sex, and racial/ethnic background who have been randomly selected from the communities served by the hospitals. The parents of cases and controls are then queried about their children's exposure to low-frequency electromagnetic fields. The parents of the cases may be more likely to recall their children's exposures than those of the controls since they are probably more motivated to remember past exposures that might help explain their children's leukemia than are the parents of the controls. If this is true, the study could result in a *spurious* association between exposure to low-frequency electromagnetic fields and the incidence of childhood leukemia.

Noncausal Associations

Noncausal associations are real associations, but they are *not* causal associations. That is, a change in the frequency of the exposure in a population does not necessarily result in a change in the frequency of the outcome. Noncausal associations often result from *confounding*, which is discussed in chapter 8. The association exists because the exposure is associated with another factor that in turn is associated with the outcome. A whimsical example is provided by Max Michael III, W. Thomas Boyce, and Allen J. Wilcox.[3] Dr. Al Betzerov conducted a prospective cohort study to test his hypothesis that gambling causes cancer. He chose two neighboring states, one where gambling was legal and the other where it was not. He then followed randomly selected samples of subjects from each state matched by age, sex, urban/rural differences, and family income for 10 years. At the conclusion of the study, he noted a statistically significant positive association between gambling and cancer. Specifically, the residents of Nevada had a higher rate of cancer than those from Utah. The association, although real, was *not* one of cause-effect. Unfortunately for Dr. Betzerov, one of the states he chose was Utah. Utah is a state composed of a large number of Mormons, who have very different lifestyles from typical Nevada residents, who are not Mormons. The fact that the Mormon Church requires its adherents to abstain from tobacco and alcohol explains this association. The apparent causal association between gambling and cancer was due to confounding by alcohol and tobacco use, which are higher in Nevada than in Utah. In other words, alcohol and tobacco use are associated with gambling and are directly linked to cancer. Therefore, although gambling itself does not cause cancer, its association with causes of cancer produces a noncausal association with cancer. This type of association has also been referred to by some as a "spurious association" in that it can lead to an erroneous conclusion about cause and effect.

Risk markers, which were referred to in chapter 1, represent noncausal associations. Although these associations result from confounding with actual risk factors, they are still real associations that have practical significance in screening for disease.[4] For example, calcification in the coronary arteries is a risk marker for coronary heart disease. It does not cause the disease, but it is associated with an increased risk of its occurrence. Its role in coronary heart disease is therefore properly classified as noncausal. Nevertheless, screening for coronary calcium has become an increasingly popular, though controversial, method of detecting possible presymptomatic heart disease (see chapter 13).

Noncausal associations can also result when the defined exposure is a consequence of the outcome instead of the other way around. Hypertension, for example, may result from kidney disease. Thus, one may find a statistical association between hypertension and kidney disease, but in this example, hypertension could not be considered a cause of kidney disease because the exposure does not *precede* the outcome and therefore cannot alter its frequency. In this example, kidney disease is a cause of hypertension. This type of hypertension is generally referred to as secondary hypertension to differentiate it from primary hypertension, which can cause kidney disease.

Causal Associations

Causal associations are those in which changes in the frequency of the exposure in a population produce a change in the frequency of the outcome. In epidemiology, we cannot prove causal associations because it is impossible to account for all the other factors that might play some role in an association, especially in observational studies where there may be many unrecognized, and therefore uncontrolled, variables. Well-designed experimental epidemiologic studies can come much closer to establishing causation than observational studies, but even in these studies there may be other influential factors of which the investigator is unaware. Since no two humans beings are exactly alike in their makeup or reactions to external stimuli, one cannot always be assured that even randomized groups of people are perfectly comparable. Even laboratory experiments with mice rely on well-defined strains to minimize intraspecies differences that can invalidate the results of an experiment.

A given association may not be conclusively spurious, noncausal, or causal. This is because random error can never be completely eliminated as a possible reason for an association in an epidemiologic study, although it can be greatly minimized. Similarly, it would be extremely difficult to discount any possibility of bias in a study. The same can be said for possible confounding. Thus, the job of the epidemiologist is to determine which type of association is more likely, and this is not always an easy task.

Since our main concern is identifying causal relationships when they exist, we need some guidance in determining whether an association is likely or not to be a causal one. In practice, the determination of a causal association is based on a careful review and judgment of all relevant information available, and never on the basis of one or two studies alone, especially observational studies. It is somewhat like trying a criminal case where there are no eyewitnesses to the crime. The prosecutor has to rely on circumstantial evidence to convince a jury beyond a reasonable doubt that the defendant is guilty. It was based on a thorough review of major epidemiologic and non-epidemiologic studies that in 1964 the Surgeon General of the U.S. Public Health Service first concluded that cigarette smoking is a cause of lung cancer.[5] Before discussing some of the guidelines used to assess potential causal associations, it should be worthwhile to first examine the concept of causation in more detail. This is the subject of the following section.

TYPES OF CAUSES

With communicable diseases the concept of causation appears to be relatively straightforward. However, as discussed in chapter 3, this apparent simplicity can be deceiving. Not everyone exposed to *Mycobacterium tuberculosis* (the bacterium implicated in tuberculosis), for example, develops tuberculosis. A number of host and environmental factors must also be considered. Similarly, not everyone exposed to cold germs gets a cold. In fact, the more we learn about causation, the more complex it seems. With many noncommunicable diseases, especially chronic conditions like arthritis, mental illness, Alzheimer's disease, multiple sclerosis, cardiovascular disease, diabetes, and so forth, the causal pathways can be extremely complex. Multifactorial etiology (chapter 2) is the rule rather than the exception for most contemporary health-related problems.

Necessary and Sufficient Causes

To get a better understanding of causation as it is commonly used in epidemiology it is helpful to look at different types of causes.* A **necessary cause** is an exposure that is *required* for a particular outcome to occur. Therefore, it is always associated with the outcome. If the exposure is absent, the outcome cannot occur. A **sufficient cause** is an exposure that by itself will produce a particular outcome, but it may not be the only cause of the outcome. Consequently, the outcome may occur without the exposure if the outcome is also caused by other exposures. These two classifications of causes give rise to four possible combinations,[6] which are shown below in the following 2 × 2 table.

	Necessary	
Sufficient	Yes	No
Yes	A	C
No	B	D

Combination A represents a **necessary and sufficient cause**. This is a cause that is required to produce a particular outcome *and* which is able to cause the outcome by itself. This can be represented by:

$$\text{Exposure X} \rightarrow \text{Outcome Y}$$

where Exposure X is the specified cause, and Outcome Y is the specified outcome.

Necessary and sufficient causes are not very common in the real world. One example of a condition that results from a necessary and sufficient cause is lead poisoning. Exposure to lead is *necessary* to produce lead poisoning, and it is also *sufficient*. The rabies virus might also be considered a necessary and sufficient cause of human rabies. It is *not* essential that a necessary and sufficient cause always produces the outcome. Observations have shown, for example, that not everyone presumably infected with the rabies virus contracts the disease even if they have not been immunized.[7] Nevertheless, anyone who contracts rabies must have the virus (i.e., it is necessary), and no other known cause must be present for the disease to occur (i.e., it is sufficient). It is important to emphasize, however, that as knowledge of disease causation expands, classifications may need to be revised. We may learn in the future, for example,

---

*The types of causes discussed here and subsequently are assumed to be hazardous rather than protective so as to simplify the discussion.

that some causes thought to be necessary and sufficient would be better classified in another way. At one time many believed that cancer was caused by a single factor, still undiscovered. Today we recognize its multifactorial etiology.

Combination B in the above table represents a **necessary but not sufficient cause**. This is a cause that is required to produce a specified outcome *but* is *not* able to cause the outcome by itself. Other causes are necessary for the outcome to occur. This can be represented by:

Exposure X + Other Causes → Outcome Y

Alcoholism is a disease in which alcohol consumption is a necessary but not sufficient cause of the disease. Alcohol consumption is definitely necessary for alcoholism to develop, but other factors, including genetic, social, behavioral, and environmental factors, also appear to be necessary for the disease to manifest itself.

Combination C represents a **not necessary but sufficient cause**. This is a cause that is *not* required to produce a specified outcome *but* when present is able to cause the outcome by itself. This means that there are other causes of the outcome. A not necessary but sufficient cause may be represented by:

Exposure X → Outcome Y and Exposure Z → Outcome Y

where Exposure Z is some other independent cause of Outcome Y. Ionizing radiation at high doses will cause sterility in men. Heavy exposure to certain pesticides will do the same. In this example, Exposure X is ionizing radiation, Exposure Z is a specific pesticide, and Outcome Y is sterility in men. Thus, sterility in men has more than one cause. Both ionizing radiation and certain pesticides are capable of causing sterility in men (at high doses).

Combination D denotes a **not necessary and not sufficient cause**. This is a cause that is *not* required to produce the specified outcome *and* when present is *not* able to cause the outcome by itself. Hence, there are other causes of the specified outcome. A not necessary and not sufficient cause is known as a **contributory cause**. It can be represented by:

Exposure X + Other Causes → Outcome Y and Exposure Z → Outcome Y

where Exposure Z is another independent cause of Outcome Y. Not necessary and not sufficient causes are very common causes of chronic diseases. For example, a sedentary lifestyle is not necessary and not sufficient to cause coronary heart disease (CHD). It is not required for CHD development, nor is it considered sufficient to cause CHD by itself. It is, however, a contributory cause of CHD, and when present with certain other contributory causes, such as high blood cholesterol, family history of heart disease, hypertension, cigarette smoking, and so forth, can lead to the development of CHD. That is, the frequency of CHD will be higher in groups with these factors than in groups without them.

A logical extension of this paradigm is one conceptualized by Kenneth J. Rothman and referred to as the **causal pie model**.[8] One can imagine one or more intact pies neatly divided into several pieces symbolizing what Rothman calls **component causes**. Each pie represents a *sufficient cause* of a particular disease, and each component cause has an essential part in causing that disease. There may be several sufficient causes (pies) made up of various combinations of some of the same and different component causes for any given disease. Whatever the combination, the component causes work together to cause the disease.[8] The causal pie model may remind one of the information asked for on a death certificate regarding the causes of death (see exhibit 2-1 in chapter 2). In a sense, the immediate, antecedent, and underlying causes of death, as well as other significant conditions, seem to parallel the component causes for a particular death.

As intimated earlier, in epidemiology causation is determined by what occurs in populations or groups of people as opposed to what occurs in any particular individual. We know, for example, based on the Framingham Heart Study that people who live certain lifestyles die more frequently from coronary heart disease than those with healthier lifestyles. From the group data, we can make predictions about individuals based on their lifestyle habits, but we cannot expect that the predictions will always be correct. Everyone seems to know someone, for example, who smoked four packs of cigarettes a day, had high blood pressure, and drank like a fish, but lived until 105. Undoubtedly, this person met an "untimely" death when his bungee cord broke after jumping off a bridge. The exception, however, does not make the rule.

Direct and Indirect Causes

Causal associations can also be classified as direct or indirect. A **direct causal association** (or **direct cause**) can be thought of as representing a causal pathway in which there are *no* intermediate variables, while an **indirect causal association** (or **indirect cause**) involves one or more intervening factors.[9] For example, in a direct causal association, X causes Y, where X is the causative exposure, and Y is the outcome. In an indirect causal association, I causes X, which in turn causes Y. While I is a direct cause of X, it is an *indirect* cause of Y. Since I causes X, and X causes Y, it follows that I causes Y based on the definition of a causal association. A change in the frequency of I in a population will result in a change in the frequency of X, which in turn will result in a change in the frequency of Y. Thus, I can be considered an indirect cause of Y.

Indirect causes can include a variety of **predisposing or enabling factors** that precede the direct cause. For example, excessive heat applied to the skin is the direct cause of burns, but the exposure to the heat may be influenced by a dangerous working environment or failure to follow certain safety precautions, which might be considered indirect causes of burns. Also, the human immunodeficiency virus (HIV) is said to be the direct cause of AIDS, but factors that facilitate contracting HIV include sharing syringes and promiscuous sexual behaviors. In practice, controlling the predisposing or enabling factors should result in a decrease in frequency of the outcome. Therefore, *predisposing or enabling factors* are often referred to as risk factors.

Whatever classification scheme is used, most contemporary health-related problems appear to have multiple causes. This multifactorial etiology, which has been referred to often in this text, presents a challenge to epidemiologists who are concerned with unraveling the determinants of morbidity and premature mortality and to those whose efforts are directed toward their prevention and control. As our knowledge of the natural history of health problems expands, the models of causation and the methods of intervention will continue to undergo change. An interesting article dealing with different conceptions of casusation from an epidemiologic and philosophical perspective is one published in the *Journal of Epidemiology and Community Health* by M. Parascandola and D. L. Weed.[10] While their recommendations may be at odds with many epidemiologists, the discussion itself is can be enlightening, especially for those new to this topic.

GUIDELINES FOR ASSESSING CAUSATION

As shown in figure 7-1, determining whether a statistical association is causal, involves a number of considerations. One must ask if the observed association is likely to be spurious. Random error or bias could explain an association found in a study population. On the other hand, the association could be a noncausal association. Noncausal associations may be due to confounding by an extraneous factor or because the outcome is responsible for the exposure instead of vice versa. Of course, another option is that the association is causal. Okay, you may say, we know the options, but how can we tell if the association is likely to be a causal one? The first step is to examine whether the alternate explanations are plausible. Specifically, is the associa-

Figure 7-1   Deciding Whether an Association Is Likely to Be Causal

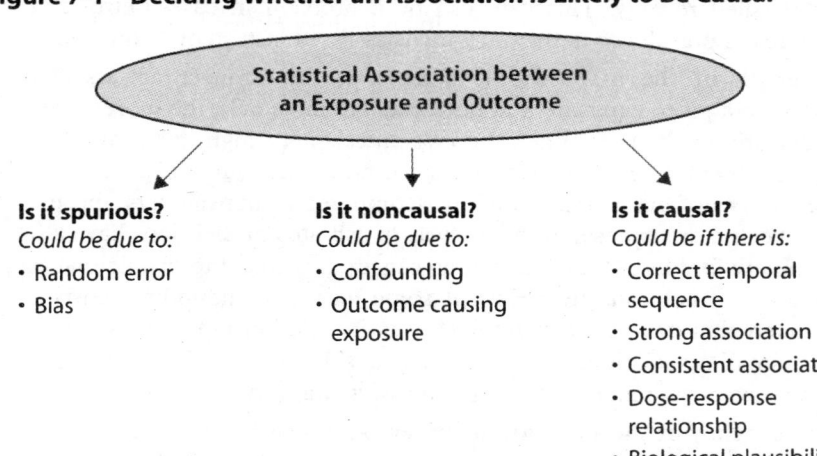

Statistical Association between an Exposure and Outcome

Is it spurious?
Could be due to:
• Random error
• Bias

Is it noncausal?
Could be due to:
• Confounding
• Outcome causing exposure

Is it causal?
Could be if there is:
• Correct temporal sequence
• Strong association
• Consistent association
• Dose-response relationship
• Biological plausibility
• Experimental evidence

tion likely due to random error, bias, confounding, or a reserved causal sequence? This may take some critical thinking, further analysis, or consultation. If these seem to be unlikely explanations, it can be helpful to review some generally accepted guidelines for establishing causation such as those described by Sir Austin Bradford Hill.

In 1965, Sir Austin Bradford Hill, Professor Emeritus of Medical Statistics with the University of London, delivered a landmark address where he outlined nine criteria that could be used to determine if statistical associations were likely to represent causal associations.[11] His reasoning built on the earlier work of others, such as John Stuart Mill, who in 1856 had defined several canons from which causal relationships could be deduced.[6] Over the years many authors have articulated or modified Hill's basic criteria, which have become known as **Hill's postulates**. Using these as a focal point, the following six guidelines should be helpful in deciding whether or not statistical associations are likely to represent causal associations (figure 7-1). In the end, the process of determining causation is largely subjective except for the first guideline, which is actually a requirement.

- **Correct temporal sequence.** In order for an exposure to be considered a cause of an outcome, it must *precede* the outcome. Of all the guidelines used to judge whether an association is causal or not, this is the only one that is considered *absolutely essential*. Exposures that occur concurrently with an outcome or subsequent to an outcome cannot be considered causal because they do not alter the frequency of the outcome. Determining if an exposure precedes an outcome can be problematic in cross-sectional studies where exposure and outcome are assessed concurrently. For example, in a cross-sectional study designed to determine if there is a relationship between the prevalence of excess body weight and osteoarthritis, it may not be clear which factor came first. Thus, the correct temporal sequence cannot be established reliably. This can also be a problem in case-control studies where the prevalence of the outcome is assessed instead of its incidence.

- **Strength of the association.** In general, the stronger an association between a given exposure and outcome (see table 6-3), the more likely the association is causal. When the risk ratio is very high, for example, it is more difficult to explain away the association due to unrecognized or subtle sources of bias or confounding. Compared to nonsmokers, those who smoke and are exposed to high levels of asbestos in their jobs have a fifty- to ninety-fold increased risk of lung cancer. It seems improbable that these factors are not causative. Even if some bias or confounding exists, it is unlikely that it would account for the entire relationship. This is not to say that small associations cannot also be causal in nature. This is one reason why several guidelines are needed to assess causality.

- **Consistency of the association.** When other investigators studying different populations at different times in different places using different methodologies obtain similar findings with regard to a specific association, it increases the probability that the association is causal. In concluding that cigarette smoking is a cause of lung cancer, the Advisory Committee to the Surgeon General of the United States cited diverse epidemiologic and other studies showing a strong relationship between smoking and lung cancer.[5] One way of determining if an apparent association is likely to be due to random error is to replicate the study. If the findings are consistent, it strengthens the case for a causal association, assuming there are no significant sources of bias or confounding in the studies.

- **Dose-response relationship.** In general, if increased levels of exposure lead to greater frequencies of the outcome, then this is suggestive of a causal relationship. Heavy smokers, for example, have been shown to be at a higher risk of lung cancer than light smokers. In fact, a linear dose-response relationship between smoking and lung cancer can be demonstrated based on the number of cigarettes smoked per day. The absence of a dose-response relationship does not necessarily mean that an association is non-causal, however. A threshold may exist. A **threshold** is a level of exposure (dose) that must be reached before effects become apparent. Below the threshold, there are no observed effects. Copper, which may be found in small quantities in drinking water and certain foods, demonstrates a threshold; that is, copper has no adverse effects until it reaches a certain level in the body. In fact, in very small quantities it is an essential mineral needed for proper growth and development. On the other hand, a dose-response relationship could be due to a strong confounding factor that closely follows an exposure.[12] Once again, several guidelines should be considered in assessing causation.

- **Biological plausibility.** The basic question here is, does the association make biological sense? Is the association credible based on our understanding of the natural history of the disease or possible pathogenic mechanisms? When Thind found significant associations for protein, fat, and caloric intake and certain forms of leukemia, he could offer no biological evidence to support the associations, thereby casting doubt on their authenticity.[2] Failure to make biological sense, however, does not necessarily negate the possibility of a causal association. In some cases, our understanding of the biological mechanisms may be incomplete, and what does not make sense today may make sense sometime in the future. From a contemporary vantage point, it seems difficult to understand why the theory of contagion was considered controversial as an explanation for the spread of epidemics during the Middle Ages.

- **Experimental evidence.** Having experimental evidence to support an association between a given exposure and outcome strengthens the case for a causal association. Well-designed randomized controlled trials, for example, can provide strong corroboration of a suspected causal association. This is because this study design, properly implemented, can virtually eliminate selection bias and confounding as alternate explanations for a causal association (see chapters 8 and 12). Of course, the degree of control possible in epidemiologic experiments is not to the same level as that in animal studies. Nevertheless, they can be powerful tools for establishing causation. Evidence from nonepidemiologic experiments can also be used in assessing cause-effect relationships. Because of the limited circumstances in which experimental studies can be conducted with humans, some associations will not be testable in this manner. We would not perform a randomized controlled trial on the effects of microwave radiation on cataract development, for example, because such a study would be unethical even if some were willing to volunteer for the investigation.

Table 7-1 ranks the most common types of epidemiologic studies in descending order of the degree to which identical findings of a statistical association are likely to demonstrate a causal association. The ranking is based on the relative probability of encountering unrecognized bias, confounding, or other errors within the specific study designs. It also assumes that the studies have been planned appropriately and conducted to minimize errors. A poorly designed experimental study can provide less convincing evidence of causality than a well-designed observational study. It should be kept in mind, however, that causality is never determined based on the findings of one study alone. Causation is a judgment based on relevant, cumulative information. Meta-analyses (chapter 12) have provided some hope of reaching more definitive conclusions in epidemiologic studies. Whether they will fulfill this hope depends on the care in which they are designed, implemented, and interpreted.

Table 7-1   Ranking of Common Epidemiologic Studies in Terms of the Relative Probability that the Findings Represent Causal Associations

1. Randomized Controlled Trial	5. Case-Control Study
2. Group Randomized Trial	6. Cross-Sectional Study
3. Prospective Cohort Study	7. Ecological Study
4. Retrospective Cohort Study	8. Descriptive Study

SUMMARY

- Statistical associations found between given exposures and outcomes can be of three types—spurious, noncausal, or causal. Spurious associations are false associations that are usually due to random error or bias. Non-causal associations usually result from confounding, although they can also occur when the exposure is the result of the outcome instead of the other way around. Risk markers represent noncausal associations that have practical value in screening for disease. Causal associations are ones in which a change in the frequency of the exposure results in a change in the frequency of the outcome in a population.

- Causes can be classified as to whether or not they are necessary and/or sufficient and whether they are direct or indirect. A necessary cause is one that is required to produce an outcome, while a sufficient cause is one that can produce the outcome by itself (i.e., in the absence of other known causes). The most common types of causes are those that are not necessary and not sufficient. These are known as contributory causes and are the causes that account for most contemporary health-related problems. The causal pie model expands upon the not necessary and not sufficient causes by considering a constellation of component causes that are sufficient to cause disease. Direct causes do not involve any intermediate factors in the causal pathway. Indirect causes include a variety of predisposing or enabling factors that precede the direct cause of an outcome. Controlling indirect causes can reduce the incidence of particular outcomes and is sometimes easier than controlling the direct causes.

- Because it is not possible to prove causation directly, it is helpful to have reliable guidelines upon which to judge a statistical association in terms of its likelihood of being causal. A final decision regarding causation should be based on all relevant information and not just on the basis of one or two studies, especially observational studies. Six guidelines, derived from Hill's postulates, should help in determining whether an association is likely to be causal. These guidelines are correct temporal sequence, strength of the association, consistency of the association, dose-response relationship, biological plausibility, and experimental evidence. Of these guidelines, only correct temporal sequence is required for an association to be considered causal. The others are highly suggestive of causation, however, especially when all or most of them are met.

New Terms

- biological plausibility
- causal association
- causal pie model
- component causes
- consistency of the association
- contributory cause
- correct temporal sequence
- direct causal association
- direct cause
- dose-response relationship
- experimental evidence
- Hill's postulates
- indirect causal association

- indirect cause
- necessary and sufficient cause
- necessary but not sufficient cause
- necessary cause
- noncausal association
- not necessary and not sufficient cause
- not necessary but sufficient cause
- predisposing or enabling factors
- spurious association
- statistical association
- strength of the association
- sufficient cause
- threshold

Study Questions and Exercises

1. For each of the following statements indicate whether the results are more likely to be due to a spurious association, a noncausal association, or a causal association. Also, explain the reasons for your answers.

   a. A case-control study revealed that there was a moderate to strong association between coffee consumption and deaths from coronary heart disease. Other studies have shown that those who drink coffee are more likely to smoke than those who do not drink coffee.

   b. A prospective cohort study showed that women who exercise regularly were less likely to contract cancer than women who exercised only occasionally or not at all. The exercise group was selected from women attending a fitness center, and the comparison group was selected from women attending a weight-loss clinic.

   c. A large randomized controlled trial showed that folic acid supplementation by prospective mothers significantly reduced the incidence of neural tube defects in their offspring. This finding was confirmed in subsequent studies.

   d. A large exploratory epidemiologic study examined the possible relationship of 25 different lifestyle behaviors to teenage suicide. One of the findings was a positive association between bicycle helmet use and suicide ($p = 0.05$) that had not been previously reported in the literature.

2. On bottles of wine and other alcoholic beverages, it states, "According to the Surgeon General, women should not drink alcoholic beverages during pregnancy because of the risk of birth defects." Discuss the evidence that alcohol consumption causes birth defects using the six guidelines for causation discussed in this chapter. For each guideline, describe the degree to which the evidence supports a conclusion of causation and the reasons for your response. In answering this question it may be necessary to consult a review of epidemiologic literature on alcohol consumption and birth defects.

3. Provide an example other than one used in this chapter of a necessary and sufficient cause, a necessary but not sufficient cause, a not necessary but sufficient cause, and a not necessary and not sufficient cause of disease, respectively. Also indicate why your examples are appropriate.

4. Give two examples, respectively, of direct and indirect causes of disease and justify your choices.

References

1. Vogt, W. P. (1999). *Dictionary of Statistics and Methodology: A Nontechnical Guide for the Social Sciences*, 2nd ed. Thousand Oaks, CA: Sage Publications.
2. Thind, I. S. (1986). Diet and Cancer—An International Study. *International Journal of Epidemiology* 15(2): 160–162.

3. Michael, M. III, Boyce, W. T., and Wilcox, A. J. (1984). *Biomedical Bestiary: An Epidemiologic Guide to Flaws and Fallacies in the Medical Literature*. Boston: Little, Brown, and Company.

4. Szklo, M., and Nieto, F. J. (2000). *Epidemiology: Beyond the Basics*. Gaithersburg, MD.: Aspen Publishers, Inc.

5. U.S. Department of Health, Education, and Welfare (1964). *Smoking and Health: Report of the Advisory Committee to the Surgeon General of the Public Health Service*. USPHS Publication No. 1103. Washington, DC: U.S. Government Printing Office.

6. Last, J. M., ed. (2001). *A Dictionary of Epidemiology*, 4th ed. New York: Oxford University Press.

7. Chin, J., ed. (2000). *Control of Communicable Diseases Manual*, 17th ed. Washington, DC: American Public Health Association.

8. Rothman, K. J. (2002). *Epidemiology: An Introduction*. New York: Oxford University Press.

9. Jekel, J. F., Elmore, J. G., and Katz, D. L. (1996). *Epidemiology, Biostatistics, and Preventive Medicine*. Philadelphia, PA: W. B. Saunders Company.

10. Parascandola, M., and Weed, D. L. (2001). Causation in Epidemiology. *Journal of Epidemiology and Community Health* 55: 905-912.

11. Hill, A. B. (1965). The Environment and Disease: Association or Causation? *Proceedings of the Royal Society of Medicine* 58: 295–300.

12. Brownson, R. C., Remington, P. L., and Davis, J. R. (1998). *Chronic Disease Epidemiology and Control*, 2nd ed. Washington, DC: American Public Health Association.

CHAPTER EIGHT

Assessing the Accuracy of Epidemiologic Studies

This chapter deals with the accuracy of epidemiologic studies,
specifically validity and precision. In particular, threats
to accuracy in the forms of bias, confounding, and
random error are examined.

Learning Objectives

- Define and explain accuracy, validity, and precision.
- Compare and contrast internal and external validity.
- Distinguish between selection and information bias.
- Identify potential types of selection bias based on study descriptions.
- Identify potential types of information bias based on study descriptions.
- Differentiate between differential and nondifferential misclassification and the potential consequences of each.
- Identify basic methods of controlling selection and information biases, respectively.
- Explain the concept of confounding, the requirements for confounding, and the potential consequences of confounding.
- Identify specific methods to minimize confounding.
- Define random error and its major components.
- Describe the major methods of assessing random error, including their relative strengths and weaknesses.
- Explain two methods of reducing random error in a study.
- Define beta level; error; individual, pair, and frequency matching; interval estimation; systematic and nonsystematic error; positive and negative bias; positive and negative confounding; potential confounder; power; probability sample; residual confounding; Simpson's paradox; source population; and type I and type II errors.

The search for truth is always concerned with exposing error
since error obscures the truth and can lead to false conclusions.

INTRODUCTION

In an ideal world, all epidemiologic studies would be designed, conducted, analyzed, and interpreted in a manner that eliminated all sources of error. Although the ideal can never be realized, it must be a goal of epidemiologists to see that errors in epidemiologic studies are minimized to the extent possible. Likewise, those who read and use the epidemiologic literature need to be careful how they interpret or apply the findings. This latter point is especially important when epidemiologic findings are used to support the development or adoption of health-related programs or policies. Though rare, there have been incidents where flawed epidemiologic research has been used to develop expensive programs or establish policies or procedures that have been counterproductive or detrimental to public health.

This chapter deals mainly with threats to the *accuracy* of epidemiologic studies, specifically bias, confounding, and random error. For the sake of continuity and brevity in the discussion, exposure and outcome are considered dichotomous variables, and measures of association are considered to be based on relative comparisons (i.e., risk ratios, rate ratios, odds ratios, and prevalence ratios) unless otherwise noted.

ACCURACY OF A STUDY

The **accuracy** of an epidemiologic study is determined by the extent to which it is free from errors. In particular, we want to be sure that the study findings are sound. An **error** can be defined as the discrepancy between a measured value and its true value.[1] We can represent this relationship as follows:

Error = Measured Value – True Value

If it were possible to eliminate all errors in a study, the measured values would equal their true values, and the study findings would be deemed completely accurate. Unfortunately, this ideal can never be achieved. This is because it would require perfect study design and execution, including such things as flawless data collection, recording, analysis, and interpretation, as well as complete and unbiased participation by the subjects. Perfection, however, is just not possible even under the best of circumstances. Nevertheless, the accuracy of a study can always be increased by minimizing errors. Errors in an epidemiologic study arise from three major sources—bias, confounding, and random error. The first two have to do with the *validity* of a study, and the third has to do with the *precision* of a study. Therefore, accuracy has the following two major components, which are discussed briefly in the next two sections.

- Validity
- Precision

Validity

The **validity** of a study can be defined as the degree to which inferences are warranted given the methods and study population chosen.[2] There are two major types of validity—internal and external. **Internal validity** represents the degree to which the results of a study, apart from random error, are *true* for the **source population**; that is, the population from which those eligible for the study are chosen. Internal validity is threatened by sources of *systematic error*, namely bias and confounding, which are discussed later in this chapter. **Systematic error** denotes *nonrandom* flaws in study design, conduct, analysis, or interpretation that usually have the effect of uniformly increasing or decreasing the true magnitude of the measure of association between a given exposure and outcome. Therefore, systematic error tends to lead to either artificially elevated or artificially reduced measures of association in a study.

External validity, also known as **generalizability**, represents the degree to which the results of a study are relevant for populations *other than* the study population. For example, can the findings of an epidemiologic study conducted on white males in Vermont be generalized to all males in the U.S.? Similarly, can the findings be applied to all adults in the U.S. regardless of their sex or race/ethnicity? These questions have to do with the external validity of a study. Unfortunately, there is no simple formula for determining external validity. A judgment has to be made as to whether the findings would make sense in other populations. This judgment can always be challenged and may have to be defended. When the authors of a large randomized controlled trial in Scandinavia found that long-term treatment with simvastatin (a cholesterol-lowering drug; trade name Zocor) significantly increased the survival of patients with coronary heart disease, it did not seem like much of a stretch to assume that the findings might also apply to coronary heart disease patients in other parts of the world.[3] It would be questionable, however, on the basis of this study alone, to assume that simvastatin would have the same effect on healthy populations. Additional research on groups free from coronary heart disease would need to be conducted to draw this conclusion.

Of the two types of validity, internal validity is *more important* than external validity, since it does not make sense to generalize findings that are *not* internally valid.[4] As a result, internal validity needs to be evaluated carefully before one even considers the external validity of a study. The findings of the Scandinavian Simvastatin Survival Study discussed above were considered reasonably valid internally, thus permitting generalization of the findings to populations other than the one studied.[3]

Precision

The second major component of accuracy is **precision**, which is a measure of the degree to which *nonsystematic error* is absent in a study.[1] **Nonsystematic error** represents *random error* (or random variation as used in chapter 6). **Random error** can be thought of as variability in a measure due to chance.[2] It represents unexplained error in a study. Thus, a precise finding from an epidemiologic study will be one that is replicable. Random errors tend to dilute a measure of association, making it less likely that one will detect an association in a study.

To understand the difference between precision and validity, consider the following analogy. A salesman has an expensive new watch that he sets five minutes fast to help him get to appointments on time. The watch keeps *precise* time, but at any given moment the time is *not valid*, since it consistently overestimates the actual time of day. The error here is systematic (nonrandom). If it were nonsystematic (random), the watch would sometimes overestimate and sometimes underestimate the true time in a completely arbitrary way. This would be a very *imprecise* watch. Nonsystematic or random errors are not predictable or reproducible. The topic of random error is discussed further in the last section of this chapter following a discussion of bias and confounding. Figure 8-1 summarizes the major threats to the accuracy of an epidemiologic study.

Figure 8-1   Assessing the Findings of Epidemiologic Studies (or "The House Upon Which Accuracy Is Built")

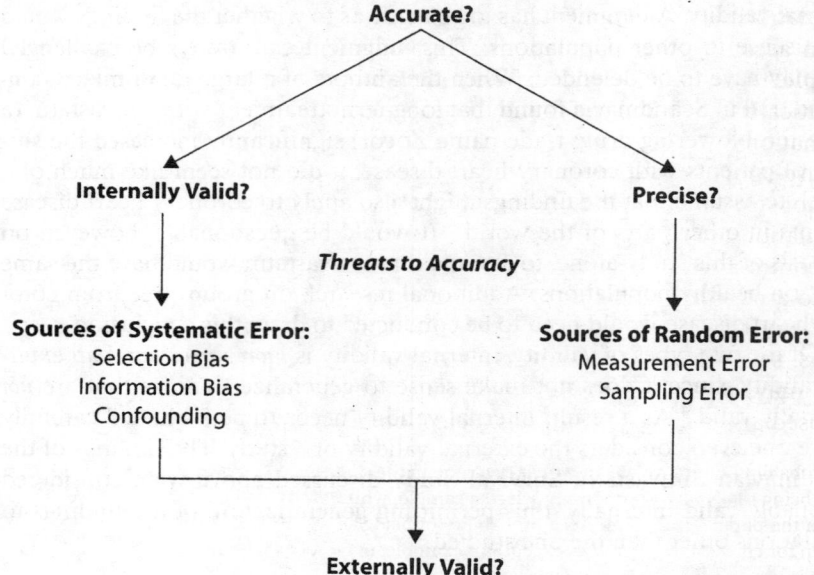

BIAS

Bias is a type of systematic (nonrandom) error in the design or conduct of epidemiologic studies. It affects the internal validity of a study, and hence, its accuracy. Bias is generally divided into two major categories as follows:

- Selection bias

- Information bias

Both of these forms of bias can lead to spurious measures of association (see chapter 7), which can present problems in the interpretation of epidemiologic findings. Although bias cannot be quantified per se, the direction and potential magnitude of the effect can often be discerned.[5] A bias that leads to an overestimate of the true value of the measure of association is referred to as a **positive bias** (e.g., $OR_E = 2$ vs. $OR_T = 1$ or $OR_E = 0.5$ vs. $OR_T = 0.8$, where OR_E is the estimated OR, and OR_T is the true OR). That which leads to an underestimate is termed a **negative bias** (e.g., $OR_E = 1$ vs. $OR_T = 2$ or $OR_E = 0.8$ vs. $OR_T = 0.5$). While bias can occur in all types of epidemiologic studies, it is primarily a concern in observational studies, particularly poorly designed studies.

Selection Bias

Selection bias refers to systematic error resulting from the manner in which subjects are *selected* for a study. This form of bias can occur when the characteristics of the subjects included in a study differ systematically from those in the source population.[6] Fundamentally, selection bias is a consequence of differing distributions of exposure or outcome between the study and source populations. For example, selection bias can occur in a cross-sectional study when a convenience sample (chapter 5) is chosen instead of a **probability sample**.* The frequency of exposure or outcome in the sample may be systematically different from that in the sampled population leading to an overestimation or underestimation of the true value of the measure of association. In case-control studies, selection bias may occur, for instance, when controls are not selected from the population that generated the cases (i.e., the source population; chapter 10). In this scenario, the frequency of exposure among the controls may under- or over-represent the true exposure frequency, leading to a negative or positive bias. Many other scenarios are possible. In general, any time the selection of cases or controls is influenced by exposure status, selection bias is a concern. In retrospective cohort studies, selection bias may occur if knowledge of outcome status influences selection of exposed and unexposed subjects. Selection bias can also occur in prospective

---

*A probability sample is one in which everyone in the sampled population has a *known* probability of being selected. In a randomly selected sample, which is a type of probability sample, everyone in the population has an *equal* probability of being selected.[7] Probability samples are rarely chosen for epidemiologic studies except, for example, in certain cross-sectional studies where the intent is to estimate an exposure or outcome in a larger population that is impractical to study in its entirety.

cohort and other follow-up studies *after* the subjects have been selected due to systematic withdrawals or losses to follow up that alter the original composition (i.e., the original selection) of the sample. Withdrawals or losses to follow-up occur when subjects fail to complete the study for various reasons. In short, selection bias may result any time those selected for study, or those retained in a study, differ systematically (nonrandomly) from all subjects eligible for the study.

Selection bias is problematic because, as stated previously, it can result in an overestimation or underestimation of the true magnitude of the relationship between a given exposure and outcome. In fact, in some situations selection bias produces an apparent association when none really exists, or it conceals a real association. The potential for selection bias is not always easily recognized. To minimize this potential, investigators need to be very careful that the subjects selected for a study are representative of the source population in terms of exposure or outcome, that selection of study and comparison groups is based on comparable criteria, and that subject losses are kept to a minimum. Exhibit 8-1 provides a hypothetical example of selection bias in a case-control study.

Common Types of Selection Bias

Perhaps the easiest way of introducing the topic of selection bias is to examine specific types. Many types of selection bias have been identified in the literature, and the list seems to grow with time. Also, some types overlap because they are rooted in similar design flaws. Some of the more common types of selection bias are described below.

Berkson's bias. Named after Dr. Joseph Berkson, who first described it in 1946, **Berkson's bias** is a type of selection bias that may occur in hospital-based case-control studies (chapter 10). According to Berkson, patients with two medical disorders are more likely to be hospitalized than those with only one. Therefore, an association between two diseases found in a hospital-based case-control study may not exist in the source population from which the patients have been drawn.[8]

Today, we recognize the potential for this type of bias when the *combination* of a study exposure and study outcome increases the probability of admission to a study hospital.[2] The likely scenario is that the exposure among hospitalized patients will be spuriously higher among the cases than the controls leading to an inflated measure of association (e.g., an odds ratio that appears stronger than it really is). This is an example of positive bias since the measure of association is overestimated.

Berkson's bias can be illustrated in the following example. Suppose an investigator wanted to test the hypothesis that unmanageable hypertension is related to transient ischemic attacks (TIAs) at a time before the relationship between hypertension and stroke had been scientifically confirmed. The investigator planned a case-control study in a major community hospital

---

Exhibit 8-1
Example of Selection Bias

An investigator hypothesized that coffee drinking is associated with angina pectoris. To test his hypothesis, he designed a case-control study where the cases were drawn from patients attending a heart clinic staffed by cardiologists. The controls, which had no medical history of angina, were drawn from another clinic in the same community that specialized in the treatment and management of ulcers. The patients were matched by age and sex. The results of the investigation were as follows:

Subjects

Coffee Drinkers	Cases	Controls
Yes (1 or more cups/day)	160	100
No (less than 1 cup/day)	90	150

OR = 2.7, p < 0.001

The odds ratio (OR) appears to indicate that coffee drinking is significantly associated with angina pectoris, all other factors being equal. However, all other factors are probably not equal. Since the controls came from a different clinic than the cases, it is possible that they may have been systematically different from the cases in ways that could affect the study results. Patients attending the ulcer clinic are likely to have reduced or stopped their coffee drinking due to the irritation it can cause when one has an ulcer. Therefore, the controls are less likely to be coffee drinkers than all eligible controls. The OR, then, is probably overstated due to selection bias. In fact, when the study was repeated using patients in general clinics where the controls represented a variety of diagnoses unrelated to angina, no significant association was found between coffee drinking and angina pectoris.

Subjects

Coffee Drinkers	Cases	Controls
Yes (1 or more cups/day)	140	130
No (less than 1 cup/day)	110	120

OR = 1.2, p > 0.05

The selection bias in the original case-control study occurred because the cases and controls were systematically different from each other with regard to a factor related to the study exposure. That is, the presence of ulcers was inversely related to coffee drinking.

---

using newly diagnosed TIA patients as the cases and patients with other diagnoses unrelated to TIA as the controls. If the presence of unmanageable hypertension *and* TIA made hospitalization more likely than TIA alone, perhaps due to physician suspicion of an increased potential for stroke or because of the presence of two serious conditions, we would expect the case group to have a higher proportion of patients with unmanageable hypertension than the control group *due solely to hospital admission practices*. This would lead to an inflated measure of association (a positive bias) between unmanageable hypertension and TIAs in this hospital-based case-control study.

Berkson's bias is a form of the more general selection bias known as **admission rate bias** (or **hospital admission rate bias**) since it results from admission practices to health care facilities. Factors like the severity of an illness and the reputation of a facility for treating a particular disease can affect admission rates for patients, making them unrepresentative of the source population. For example, say a midwestern hospital serving a predominantly Latino community is well known for its skilled treatment of complications of diabetes, leading to referrals from all over the midwest. A case-control study of the relationship between ethnicity and diabetes complications conducted at the hospital would be less likely to show a positive association between being Latino and diabetic complications because of an overrepresentation of Latinos in the control versus the case group. The case group, which includes referrals from outside the area, would likely have a smaller proportion of Latinos than the control group, which is more likely to be from the local community. This would represent a negative bias.

Prevalence-incidence bias.   Another form of selection bias is **prevalence-incidence bias**, also sometimes called **Neyman's bias**. This type of bias is most closely associated with cross-sectional studies and case-control studies in which prevalent cases are used. It can occur when asymptomatic, mild, clinically resolved, or fatal cases are inadvertently excluded from a study because the selected cases are examined some time after the disease has already begun (i.e., looking at prevalent versus incident cases).[6] This bias exists if the association would have been different had the asymptomatic, mild, or transient cases been included in the sample, all other factors being equal. A cross-sectional study of the relationship between early parental loss and clinical depression, for example, could result in a spuriously inflated association (a positive bias) between the two study variables if the causes of undetected depression or severe depression resulting in suicide were not related to early parental loss. Had these subjects been included in the analysis, perhaps no association, or at least a weaker association, would have been found.

Healthy worker effect.   The **healthy worker effect** is a type of selection bias that can arise, for example, in cohort studies when study outcomes among workers are compared to general population samples. Imagine a prospective cohort study testing the hypothesis that exposure to low-level nuclear radiation is associated with increased mortality from all causes. The exposed group is selected from those working near radiation sources at nuclear power plants in northern Illinois, and the comparison group is a randomly selected sample of residents of northern Illinois with similar age, sex, and racial/ethnic characteristics as the nuclear power plant workers. It is likely that the measure of association would *underestimate* the true association between exposure to low-level radiation and mortality, all other factors being equal. The reason is that workers as a group tend to be healthier than the general population. This is because one must have a certain level of health to work and hold a job. The general population, on the other hand, is composed of both healthy and unhealthy individuals, including those whose health problems prevent them from engaging in steady employment. Thus, the exposed group in this example is likely to have a lower mortality rate than the comparison group *independent* of exposure status. The consequence is likely to be a negative bias. To avoid the bias it would have been better to select another occupational group for the comparison (e.g., those working in hydroelectric power plants).

The healthy worker effect is a common example of a broader subcategory of selection bias known as **membership bias**.[9] This bias occurs because those who belong to organized groups (e.g., the military, athletic associations, civic groups, religious organizations) tend to differ systematically from the general population in terms of health status and other factors.[6] For example, they tend to be less prone to morbidity and premature mortality than the general population, which includes the severely ill, for example, who may not be able to sustain active membership in a group. Membership biases can occur in both cohort and case-control studies.[9]

Volunteer bias.   Another type of selection bias is **volunteer bias**. It is due to the fact that those individuals who take part in epidemiologic studies tend to be systematically different from those who do not. For example, one study found that volunteers are likely to be better educated, more active in community affairs, less likely to smoke, and more concerned about health matters than nonvolunteers.[10] If these or other characteristics of volunteers are related to the frequency of the study exposure or susceptibility to the study outcome, they can produce associations that are systematically different from those in the source population. If they are not related to the study exposure or outcome, they will not bias the study, although they may still affect its external validity.

Although volunteer bias is not possible in randomized trials where randomization occurs following subject selection,[11] it can be demonstrated in terms of levels of compliance with the post-randomization protocol. This can be problematic when a *per protocol analysis* (see chapter 12) is conducted. This was revealed by the compliance rates in a randomized controlled trial comparing the efficacy of lipid-lowering drugs to a *placebo* (defined in chapter 12). The five-year mortality rate for those receiving the drug clofibrate was 15.0 per 100 among those judged to be compliant with the study regimen and 24.6 per 100 among those who were considered noncompliant. The death rates among those taking the placebo, however, showed a similar divergence. Among the compliant group, the five-year mortality rate was 15.1 per 100 compared to 28.2 per 100 in the noncompliant group. Apparently, *compliance* itself, as revealed by the results in the placebo group, had a positive effect on the outcome. This was most likely due to the fact that those who *voluntarily* comply tend to be systematically different from those who do not.[10]

Volunteer bias is a type of **non-response bias**[12] (also called **non-respondent bias**). It can occur when those who respond to questionnaires (volunteers) are systematically different from those who do not respond (nonvolunteers).[2]

Descriptive studies of sexual behaviors using preprinted surveys in magazines or on the Internet are notoriously biased since: (a) only readers of the magazine or computer users seeking the Web site are likely to respond, and (b) the respondents are more likely to be those with liberal attitudes toward sex. In general, response rates of less than 80 percent may signal potential selection bias. In these cases it is prudent to try to establish the reasons for nonresponses. If the nonrespondents are systematically different from the respondents, this could mean the study findings are affected by selection bias.[9]

Loss to follow-up bias.   Significant losses to follow up during a longitudinal study can lead to a form of selection bias commonly known as **loss to follow-up bias**. This bias may occur, for example, when there are sizeable subject losses in an ongoing cohort or randomized controlled trial. If the final sample is systematically different from the original study population with regard to exposure *and* outcome status, then spurious associations can result.[12] As a general rule of thumb, losses should be no more than 20 percent to minimize the potential for this selection bias. Also, it is a good idea to compare the study results with those among the losses wherever possible.[9] If there are significant differences between these groups, it suggests that the findings may have been biased. Although loss to follow-up bias is a problem of retention, it is generally considered a selection bias because the original subject selection is altered by the losses.

As an illustration of loss to follow-up bias consider the following hypothetical example. A retrospective cohort study was conducted to see if there was an association between the number of hours of flight time and noise-induced hearing loss in a group of airline pilots. The cohort consisted of 3,000 airline pilots whose flying careers occurred between 1985 and 2000. Using archived employment records from the airline companies, 1,000 of the pilots were traced for personal interviews and hearing tests. A statistically significant association was found between the number of hours flown and noise-induced hearing loss after controlling for other possible sources of hearing loss. Subsequent access to the pilots' medical records, however, revealed that over 75 percent of those who could not be traced had flown the maximum number of hours allowed during their careers but did not have any evidence of noise-induced hearing loss that could be attributed to flying. These findings suggest that the original association was spuriously inflated due to the absence of data from pilots that could not be traced (i.e., who were lost to follow up). Had the data on the pilots who could not be traced been included in the original analysis, the association would have been weaker, all other factors being equal. Thus, the original association was affected by a positive selection bias due to losses to follow up.

There are many other types of selection bias, but they all have in common the basic fact that the study population is not representative of the source population in terms of exposure or outcome due to *nonrandom* errors in subject selection or retention. Some of the aforementioned biases as well as other sources of selection bias are discussed as appropriate in subsequent chapters that relate to specific study designs or procedures.

Information Bias

Information bias is a type of systematic error due to measurement flaws that can result in *misclassification* of subjects with regard to exposure or outcome status.[13] It has also been referred to as **observation bias**, **misclassification bias**, and **measurement bias**. Unlike selection bias, which occurs primarily during study design, information bias occurs during data collection and recording. Misclassification, a consequence of information bias, can be of one of two types—differential or nondifferential.

Differential misclassification is likely to occur when the probability of misclassification is *different* between the study and comparison groups. For example, in a case-control study if a greater or lesser proportion of the cases is *mistakenly* classified as being exposed than controls, then the misclassification is differential. Similarly, in a cohort study if a greater or lesser proportion of the exposed group is *mistakenly* classified as having developed the outcome than the unexposed group, then again the misclassification is differential.

Nondifferential misclassification is likely to occur when the probability of misclassification between the study and comparison groups is uniform, that is, when there is likely to be a similar proportion of incorrect classifications on exposure status among those with and without the outcome or on outcome status among those with and without the exposure. Sometimes nondifferential misclassification occurs when the criteria for exposure or outcome are estimated for practical reasons. For example, the exposure, "passive smoking," can be difficult to measure directly in an epidemiologic study, so a proxy measure, "the time subjects spend with smokers," may be used instead.[1] This measure can lead to errors in assessment of exposure status, however, since some smokers may choose not to smoke in the presence of nonsmokers. The probability of misclassification in this example is unlikely to be different on the basis of outcome status unless the outcome is known by the smokers. Therefore, nondifferential misclassification is the probable result.

Generally speaking, *nondifferential misclassification* arises when measurement errors with regard to exposure status are *independent* of outcome status or when measurement errors with regard to outcome status are *independent* of exposure status.[1] *Differential misclassification* arises when they are *not* independent of each other.

It is important to distinguish between differential and nondifferential misclassification since they tend to produce different effects on measures of association. *Differential misclassification* may lead to either overestimation or underestimation of the true value of the measure of association. If the cases in a case-control study, for example, are more likely to be misclassified as being exposed than the controls, the study will tend to *overestimate* the true odds ratio (i.e., produce a positive bias), all other factors being equal. If, on the other hand, the controls are more likely to be misclassified as being exposed than the cases, the study will likely *underestimate* the true odds ratio (i.e., produce a negative bias). *Nondifferential misclassification* generally results in a *dilution* of the measure of association.* That is, the measure of association is usually biased toward the null value (defined in chapter 6). Therefore, nondifferential misclassification is more likely than differential misclassification to result in no association when in fact an association exists. Exhibit 8-2 provides examples of the consequences of differential and nondifferential misclassification using hypothetical data.

Exhibit 8-2

Examples of Differential and Nondifferential Misclassification Based on the Results of a Hypothetical Cohort Study

Differential Misclassification

100 Exposed Subjects ──────────▶ 20 Cases, 80 Noncases

100 Unexposed Subjects ─────────▶ 10 Cases, 90 Noncases

RR = 2.0

100 Exposed Subjects ──────────▶ 30 Cases, 70 Noncases

100 Unexposed Subjects ─────────▶ 10 Cases, 90 Noncases

RR = 3.0

Note: The first set of figures represents the results of a hypothetical prospective cohort study assuming correct classification of the exposed and unexposed groups with regard to outcome status. The second set of figures shows the effects of differential misclassification. In this example, the exposed subjects were more likely to be mistakenly classified as cases than the unexposed subjects, resulting in an inflated risk ratio (RR).

Nondifferential Misclassification

100 Exposed Subjects ──────────▶ 20 Cases, 80 Noncases

100 Unexposed Subjects ─────────▶ 10 Cases, 90 Noncases

RR = 2.0

100 Exposed Subjects ──────────▶ 30 Cases, 70 Noncases

100 Unexposed Subjects ─────────▶ 20 Cases, 80 Noncases

RR = 1.5

Note: The first set of figures represents the results of a hypothetical prospective cohort study assuming correct classification of the exposed and unexposed groups with regard to outcome status. The second set of figures shows the effects of non-differential misclassification. In this example, the exposed subjects were equally likely to be mistakenly classified as cases as the unexposed subjects, resulting in a dilution of the risk ratio (RR) toward its null value (i.e., 1.0).

---

*There are exceptions to this general rule. For example, when there are more than two exposure categories (e.g., low, moderate, and high exposure), it is possible for the estimate of the measure of association to be either underestimated or overestimated.

Common Types of Information Bias

As is the case for selection bias, there are many possible types of information bias, and a number of these overlap. Some of the more common ones are discussed below. Other types are mentioned as appropriate in subsequent chapters.

Recall bias. A type of information bias that is common in case-control studies is **recall bias**. It often results due to the fact that cases tend to remember past exposures better than controls. This usually happens because cases have a tendency to spend more time reflecting on the possible causes of their disease (i.e., so-called **rumination bias**). It can also occur if cases are more motivated than controls to learn if specific factors increased their risk of getting a particular disease. Recall bias is less likely to occur when both cases and controls are patients (e.g., in hospital-based case-control studies; see chapter 10). This is because the degree of rumination is likely to be at similar levels.

As an example of recall bias, consider the following hypothetical study. An investigator is trying to determine if there is a relationship between the number of childhood episodes of serious sunburn and the risk of malignant melanoma in adulthood. To test her hypothesis, she designs a case-control study using newly diagnosed melanoma cases among middle-aged white males in a major metropolitan area identified from the state cancer registry (chapter 10) and a randomly selected sample of healthy middle-aged white males in the same geographic area. She defines serious sunburn as that resulting in any use of topical or other treatments for sunburn whether at home or by a physician. As part of the study, she asks each subject to estimate the actual number of episodes of serious sunburn during childhood. If the cases tend to recall and report more episodes than the controls *simply because they have reflected more on their childhood experiences*, recall bias could result in a spuriously inflated measure of association (i.e., a positive bias), all other factors being equal.

Recall bias can also occur in other types of epidemiologic studies whenever subjects are asked to recall past exposures. While recall bias is typically defined in terms of differential misclassification, nondifferential misclassification because of faulty recall is almost certainly a more common occurrence. One suggestion for overcoming recall bias is to use nested case-control studies or case-cohort studies (chapter 4) where the data on exposure are collected at baseline before the cases occur.[13]

Reporting bias. A related but broader category than recall bias is **reporting bias**, which can occur in all types of epidemiologic studies.[12] It can result when subjects intentionally or unintentionally underreport or overreport exposures or outcomes for a variety of reasons, including their social undesirability (e.g., illicit drug use) or desirability (e.g., handwashing). If study and comparison groups are equally likely to report exposure or outcome status inaccurately, the result is nondifferential misclassification. If one group is more prone to under- or over-report exposure or outcome, then the result is differential misclassification. Reporting bias can also be due to the way organizations report data. For example, the American Social Health Association has suggested that sexually transmitted diseases (STDs) among racial/ethnic minorities in the United States are probably overreported in STD surveillance statistics in comparison to those for whites. The reasoning offered is that minorities are more likely to seek health care through public versus private providers, and public providers do more complete reporting than private ones.[14] If this is the case, it would represent differential misclassification due to reporting bias.

Interviewer bias.   A type of information bias that can arise in all types of epidemiologic studies is **interviewer bias**. It can occur in case-control studies, for instance, when interviewers are aware of the subjects' outcome status, and this awareness influences how they solicit, record, or interpret information on exposure.[6] The bias may be conscious or unconscious and can occur when investigators probe more intensely for exposure information from cases than controls. Examples include seeking clarification, asking follow-up questions that are not part of the study protocol, providing more time to respond to questions, and emphasizing certain words or phrases for cases compared to controls.[13] Interviewer bias may occur in other types of studies when there are systematic differences in how interviewers obtain data between study and comparison groups.

An example of interviewer bias is illustrated in a hypothetical example of a case-control study designed to determine if frequent use of nonsteroidal anti-inflammatory drugs (NSAIDs) is associated with gastroesophageal reflux disease (GERD). An interviewer working for a research epidemiologist interviewed 100 patients with clinically diagnosed GERD and 100 comparable patients without GERD about their consumption of NSAIDs over the past year. Patients in both groups were given a list of examples of NSAIDs, which included the brand and generic names of prescription medications and over-the-counter drugs. The interviewer also asked each patient whether or not he or she had been diagnosed with GERD. A student intern working for the epidemiologist observed the entire interview process. He noticed that when cases asked for clarification if aspirin, which was not on the list, was considered an NSAID, the interviewer typically shook his head up and down indicating yes, but when controls asked, he simply told the patients to review the list again. Interviewer bias is evident in that the interviewer's practice of informing cases of the correct information but not controls wittingly or unwittingly introduced more errors in the data from the control group, leading to differential misclassification. It was inappropriate for the interviewer to ask about the outcome status of the patients since this knowledge was responsible for the misclassifications. In fact, one of the ways of avoiding interviewer bias is to keep the identity of cases and controls from the interviewers whenever possible until after the data have been analyzed. This is called *blinding* and is discussed in more detail in subsequent chapters.

Exposure suspicion bias.   A type of information bias that has some similarities to interviewer bias is **exposure suspicion bias**. This bias can occur in case-control studies when knowledge of the subjects' outcome status influences how exposure is assessed. For example, if investigators know the subjects' outcome status and think they know the cause of the outcome, this may affect the degree to which they search for the suspected exposure in the case and control groups. They may, for instance, make a more intense search among cases than controls, leading to an overestimation of the measure of association (i.e., a positive bias). Exposure suspicion bias has been demonstrated in studies of thyroid cancer among children where intensive inquiries have led to substantially higher reported rates of exposure to irradiation than more routine inquiries.[9]

As an example, consider the following case-control study. An investigator hypothesized that stress at work increases the incidence of irritable bowel syndrome (IBS). In determining the exposure, the investigator tended to classify cases (those with IBS) as moderately to highly stressed (exposed) if they reported any stress at work. He tended to classify controls (subjects without IBS), however, as not stressed or minimally stressed (unexposed) unless they reported excessive levels of work-related stress. The investigator's knowledge of the outcome status of his subjects and his belief in his hypothesis influenced how he assessed the subjects' exposure status. Thus, he was more likely to find a positive association between work stress and IBS because of his methods, which were influenced by his knowledge of the outcome status of his subjects. Similar to interviewer bias, this bias can be controlled by blinding the investigators to outcome status whenever possible.

Diagnostic suspicion bias.   A form of information bias parallel to exposure suspicion bias that can occur in cohort studies or randomized controlled trials is called **diagnostic suspicion bias**. This bias may take place when knowledge of the subjects' exposure status leads to systematic differences in the procedures for diagnosing the outcome.[9] As an example of this type of bias, consider a prospective cohort study of a group of 15 year olds designed to determine if parental alcohol abuse during childhood is positively associated with adult-onset chronic fatigue syndrome. Chronic fatigue syndrome is a controversial diagnosis for a persistent, noncurable condition that is characterized by extreme fatigue, low-grade fever, muscles aches and pains, and other vague symptoms. Say those 15 year olds who grew up living with an alcoholic parent constitute the exposed group and those who did not comprise the unexposed group. The cohort is followed for ten years. If a clinician believed the research hypothesis was true and was aware of the subjects' exposure status, he or she might be more likely to diagnose chronic fatigue syndrome among those in the exposed versus the unexposed group even if the reported symptoms were similar. This would tend to produce a positive bias, all other factors being equal. Diagnostic suspicion bias is more likely to occur when the outcome is not clear cut and requires some subjective evaluation as is the case for chronic fatigue syndrome. The potential for this bias can be reduced by blinding the clinicians who determine outcome status as to the exposure status of the subjects and the study hypothesis or by using several clinicians to evaluate the outcomes independently so as to arrive at a consensus.[13]

A common thread among the aforementioned information biases is that they can result in misclassification. If significant, this can lead to an exaggerated or diminished measure of association (i.e., risk ratio, rate ratio, odds ratio, or prevalence ratio), all other factors being equal.

Controlling Bias in Epidemiologic Studies

Selection and information biases are best controlled by *prevention* during the design, data collection, and execution phases of a study. This means that potential sources of bias must first be recognized. Once they are recognized, measures must be taken to preclude their possibility or to minimize them to the extent possible. This generally will be easier to accomplish in experimental than observational studies, but the goal must always be to avoid bias since it can be a serious threat to the internal validity of a study. Various procedures have been developed to prevent or minimize different types of bias. Table 8-1 lists some common methods for controlling information bias in observational studies. For example, in a case-control study blinding is a way to keep those responsible for assessing exposure status from treating the cases and controls differently based on their knowledge of outcome status. Blinding on outcome status is not always feasible, however, because of the telltale appearance of some cases (e.g., those with severe Parkinson's disease) or because cases consciously or unconsciously reveal their status. General methods to prevent selection bias were cited earlier in the chapter.

Table 8-1   Some Common Ways of Controlling Information Bias in Observational Studies

- Blind data collectors to subject exposure or outcome status
- Blind data collectors and subjects to the study hypotheses
- Standardize data collection instruments and procedures
- Use objective measures of exposure and outcome status
- Verify subject responses with other reliable sources
- Obtain multiple measurements of exposure or outcome status
- Train data collectors in proper data collection procedures
- Pilot test data collection instruments and methods

Note: Not all methods will be feasible in any given study.

CONFOUNDING

A simple dictionary definition of *confound* is "to mix up."[15(p186)] Synonyms include confuse, puzzle, bewilder, baffle, and perplex. This is what confounding can do to the actual relationship between a study exposure and outcome. In epidemiology, we refer to **confounding** as a distortion in the true magnitude of the effect* of a study exposure on a study outcome due to a mixing of effects between the exposure and an extraneous factor.[16] The extraneous factor is known as the **confounding factor** or **confounder**. Like selection and information biases, confounding represents systematic error and threatens the internal validity of a study. Some epidemiologists consider confounding another type of bias, while some prefer to classify it separately as is done in this text. One reason for the latter classification is that biased associations are spurious and always undesirable, while confounded associations are real and may have some practical value in public health. For instance, they may permit us to identify risk markers (chapter 1) that can help in identifying high risk groups for secondary prevention efforts.[13] Low high density lipoprotein (HDL) levels, for example, *may* confound the apparent effect of high triglycerides on atherosclerosis. Nevertheless, even if the apparent effect is a result of confounding, and therefore does not represent a causal association between high triglycerides and atherosclerosis, identifying individuals with high triglyceride levels and referring them for clinical evaluation should help to reduce the overall incidence of atherosclerosis.[13]

Confounding can result in an overestimate or underestimate of the true effect of a study exposure on a study outcome. When a confounder results in an overestimation it is said to be a **positive confounder**. It distorts the effect in a positive direction. Conversely, when it leads to an underestimation it is said to be a **negative confounder**. It distorts the effect in a negative direction. Depending on the nature of its relationship with the exposure and outcome, a confounder can even alter an effect to such an extent that a true positive effect appears negative, or a true negative effect appears positive. This is known as **Simpson's paradox**, which in reality is not a paradox at all but a logical possibility of uncontrolled confounding.[2] It is also possible that confounding can make a real effect disappear or no effect appear as if a causal association exists.[16] Hence, confounding can be a powerful source of systematic error in an epidemiologic study and is something that must be dealt with in order to reach valid conclusions.

In general, for an extraneous factor to confound an effect between a study exposure and outcome, three conditions must be satisfied.[16] These conditions may be described as follows:

1. The factor must be an independent risk factor (hazardous or protective) for the outcome of interest;

2. The factor must be associated with the exposure of interest in the population from which the outcomes are generated; and

3. The factor must *not* represent an intermediate step in the causal sequence between the exposure and the outcome.

---

*The term effect is used here and subsequently as an indication of a causal association as defined in chapter 7.

Generally speaking, if any of these conditions is not met, the factor cannot be a confounder. A brief explanation is in order. A confounder must increase or decrease the risk of the outcome independent of the exposure *and* be associated with the exposure independent of its association with the outcome in order for a mixing of effects to occur. In this way a confounder can exert its independent effect on the outcome in addition to any effect of the exposure. This cannot happen, however, if the factor is part of the causal sequence of events (i.e., the risk factor causes the confounding factor, which in turn causes the outcome). Figure 8-2 illustrates the relationships that must normally exist for confounding to occur. The dashed arrow represents a possible causal association between a given exposure and outcome. The apparent effect may or may not actually exist, but either way, confounding can distort the truth of the situation. The single-headed arrow represents a causal association between the confounder and the outcome (i.e., the confounder is a risk factor for the outcome). The double-headed arrow indicates an association between the confounder and the exposure, which may be a causal or non-causal association (chapter 7).

Figure 8-2   The Presence of Confounding

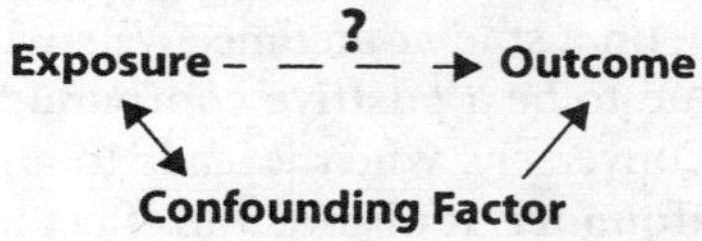

Since we do not know what extraneous factors will actually confound any given effect (including no effect) between an exposure and outcome, it is best to refer to suspected confounding factors as **potential confounders**. Experienced epidemiologists can usually anticipate several potential confounders for a given analysis based on their knowledge of the outcome and then control for them using preventive measures or statistical adjustment (referred to in the following section). Some experts suggest that all known or suspected risk factors for the study outcome, especially if they are also known to be associated with the study exposure, be considered potential confounders. Age, sex, and race/ethnicity are nearly always considered potential confounders because of their close relationship to morbidity and mortality. In any event, as was the case with rate adjustment (chapter 6), it is only after the fact that we learn whether or not confounding was present in a given situation and to what extent. If adjusting the measure of association (e.g., odds ratio) for a potential confounder alters its magnitude appreciably, then the factor must have been a confounder. The extent of confounding is indicated by the degree to which the magnitude of the measure of association is affected, all other factors being equal. As a general rule of thumb, if an adjusted ratio measure of association is more than 10 percent higher or lower than the unadjusted measure, confounding is present (see chapter 11). Conversely, if the difference is less than 10 percent, confounding can generally be considered inconsequential or nonexistent, all other factors being equal.

It is *not* appropriate to assess confounding using statistical tests of significance. For one thing, in observational studies at least, the degree of confounding is not dependent on sample size whereas the results of significance testing are.[16] Thus, in a very large study there may be statistical significance between a potential confounder and the study outcome even when the confounding is negligible (e.g., does not meet the 10 percent rule). In a small study a similar association may not reach statistical significance even when the confounding is considerable.[16]

Because the topic of confounding can itself be confounding in the more common use of the term, it should help to provide an example before we go any further. Several studies have shown a positive association between cigarette smoking and motor vehicle injuries that could be causal in nature.[17] A potential confounder of this association is alcohol consumption. Cigarette smoking and alcohol consumption are associated with each other as any trip to a bar or pub will demonstrate (assuming there is no legislation banning smoking), and alcohol consumption is a well-documented independent risk factor for motor vehicle injuries. Furthermore, it is highly unlikely that alcohol consumption is part of a causal sequence between cigarette smoking and motor vehicle injuries based on current knowledge. Therefore, alcohol consumption is a potential confounder. Now, assume a case-control study finds a positive association between cigarette smoking and motor vehicle injuries. Part or all of the association could be due to a mixing of effects between smoking and alcohol consumption. Even if cigarette smoking is *not* causally associated with motor vehicle injuries, it could appear to be because of its association with alcohol consumption. On the other hand, even if cigarette smoking is causally associated with motor vehicle injuries, the effect could be overstated because of an excess number of drinkers among the exposed group. In fact, when alcohol consumption is controlled in the relationship between cigarette smoking and motor vehicle injuries, the measure of association consistently decreases while remaining statistically significant.[17] Thus, alcohol appears to be a *positive confounder* in these studies (i.e., one that overstates the true measure of association).

Another example concerns a study of coffee consumption and myocardial infarction in women.[18] In this case-control study, the investigators found an elevated risk of myocardial infarction in the heaviest coffee drinkers even after adjusting for cigarette smoking and certain other potential confounders. It seems likely though that women who drink large amounts of coffee on a daily basis probably live highly stressed lives that could increase their risk of myocardial infarction. Stress was not evaluated as a potential confounder in this study; however, it could meet the criteria for confounding, and if a confounder, it could explain all or part of the association between heavy coffee consumption and myocardial infarction.

Controlling Confounding

To assure the validity of epidemiologic studies confounding should be adequately controlled. Whereas selection bias occurs primarily in the design stage of a study and information bias in the data collection and recording stage, confounding takes place mainly in the analysis stage.[4] Confounding can be controlled, however, in either the design or analysis phases of a study. In the design stage, *restriction, matching,* or *randomization* may be used to prevent or reduce the potential for confounding. It is a basic rule that confounding cannot occur if the confounders are *evenly distributed* between the study and comparison groups. In fact, this is the basis for controlling confounding in the design stage.[19] Restriction, matching, and randomization in particular seek to produce study and comparison groups that are similar with regard to potential confounders. In the analysis stage, various statistical procedures can be applied to control or adjust for potential confounding after the fact. These methods commonly involve *stratification* or *multivariable analysis,* which are discussed primarily in chapters 10 and 11 but are also referred to in chapters 9 and 12 as they relate to particular study designs. Stratification and multivariable methods also rely on the fact that confounding cannot exist if the study and comparison groups have the same distribution of confounders. The same is true with *rate adjustment* (*standardization*), which is itself a statistical method of controlling for confounding based on stratification (see chapters 6, 10, and 11). One should note that a combination of methods of preventing or controlling confounding can be used in any given study.

Restriction involves limiting the study subjects to those with certain characteristics. For example, if the study population is limited to women only, then differences in sex cannot confound an effect between a given exposure and outcome. Similarly, if a study of the effect of cigarette smoking on motor vehicle injuries is limited to nondrinkers, then alcohol consumption cannot confound an effect between these variables. Other factors, such as age or not wearing a seat belt may still be confounders, however.[20] Restriction as a method of preventing confounding has its limits. If many potential confounders exist, the study would have to be so restricted that it might be difficult to find a sufficient number of eligible participants. Also, restriction can limit the external validity of a study. A study restricted to women, for example, may not be generalizable to populations including men. On the other hand, restriction is a highly practical, effective, and economical way of preventing confounding. Since it may also be used in combination with other methods of controlling confounding, its potential disadvantages can be minimized. Although usually thought of as a method of controlling confounding in the design stage, restriction can also be applied in the analysis stage by restricting analyses to specific subgroups. More is said about restriction in later chapters.

Matching attempts to produce study and comparison groups that are similar with regard to potential confounders. One form of matching is **individual matching** where individuals in the study group are matched on selected characteristics with individuals in the comparison group. In a cohort study, for example, this entails selecting subjects for the exposed group who are identical or nearly identical to subjects in the unexposed group with regard to one or more potential confounders (e.g., age, sex, smoking status). Like restriction, matching has its limits. Matching on more than four or five characteristics can become very tedious and expensive because many potential subjects may have to be considered to find ones who meet the eligibility criteria. It would be very difficult, for instance, to locate many 85–89 year-old employed males who exercise daily and are not taking any prescription medications.

A specific form of individual matching is **pair matching** where subjects from the study and comparison groups are paired together on a one-to-one basis.[2] Consider a case-control study. For each case chosen for the study a corresponding control is selected with the same characteristics of the matching variables. Thus, if the first case is between 20 and 24 years old, a female, and a nonsmoker, then a control is selected who is also between 20 and 24 years old, a female, and a nonsmoker, and so on. The individually matched cases and controls are then treated as pairs in the analysis phase (see chapter 10). One disadvantage of pair matching is the greater potential for loss of information. For example, if one subject in a matched pair does not respond to a study questionnaire or withdraws from the study, the other paired subject has to be excluded from the analysis.

Another form of matching, known as **frequency matching** (a kind of category or group matching), relies on obtaining similar frequencies of the matched variables in the study and comparison groups. For example, if 25 percent of the subjects in the exposed group of a prospective cohort study are social drinkers, and if social drinking is considered a potential confounder, then the investigator seeks to obtain 25 percent social drinkers in the unexposed group. The goal of frequency matching is to assure that the study and comparison groups are similar with respect to the frequency of potential confounders. Frequency matching, however, does not assure as precise a comparison as individual matching, and some subgroups created during the analysis phase may differ substantially in the frequencies of potential confounders. Therefore, it is still important to adjust statistically for confounding in the analysis phase of those studies relying on frequency matching. In fact, frequency matching is best perceived as a method of increasing *study efficiency* versus controlling confounding.[21] Study efficiency is described later in this chapter in the section, "Reducing Random Error."

As a method of controlling for confounding, matching (i.e., individual matching) generally works well in follow-up studies. It can be very expensive, however, to find a sufficient number of eligible subjects and keep detailed records in what are typically large studies. Therefore, matching is seldom used in follow-up studies.[16] Matching can also be expensive in case-control studies, but there is another more serious concern in these studies when matching is used to control confounding. Making cases and controls similar with regard to potential confounders can have the untoward effect of making them similar with regard to exposure status,* thus biasing estimates of the odds ratio in the direction of the null value (i.e., OR = 1.0). In fact, matching in case-control studies can even create confounding where it never previously existed.[16] This topic and the advantages and disadvantages of matching in case-control studies are discussed further in chapter 10.

Randomization, first defined in chapter 4, can be used in randomized controlled trials and group randomized trials (chapter 12) to reduce confounding during the design stage. Randomization refers to the assignment of study subjects or groups to either experimental or control conditions using random methods. This technique *tends to* eliminate confounding by increasing the probability that the groups being compared are the same with regard to the distribution of extraneous factors that might confound an association. This, of course, assumes that the subjects stay in their assigned groups.

One distinct advantage of randomization is that even unknown or unsuspected confounders are controlled, whereas with restriction and matching one must determine the specific factors to be controlled and collect relevant data on them prior to conducting the study. Of course, randomization does not always achieve its objective since it is subject to laws of probability. However, it is an extremely effective method of controlling confounding if the sample size is relatively large. It is less effective if the number of subjects is small. Randomization is discussed further in chapter 12.

Residual Confounding

One should be aware that controlling for confounding in a study does not necessarily mean that all confounding will be eliminated. Broadly defined, **residual confounding** is confounding that persists in a study even after attempts to control it. Three common reasons for residual confounding are:

• Failure to consider important confounders
• Flawed characterization of confounders
• Misclassification of confounders

With regard to the first reason, *failure to consider important confounders*, there may be unrecognized confounders that were not anticipated or measured in a study; hence, they remain uncontrolled. In the earlier example of the study of coffee consumption and myocardial infarction in women,[18] stress was not considered as a potential confounder, but it probably was a confounder leading to erroneous conclusions about the effect of heavy coffee drinking on myocardial infarction.

Flawed characterization of confounders occurs when the confounders are not precisely defined. For example, a study to determine if cigarette smoking is

---

*This has to do with the unique features of a confounder (i.e., the relationships between the exposure and outcome and between the confounder and the exposure referred to at the beginning of this section). Since matching makes the cases and controls similar with regard to the confounder, and since the confounder is associated with the exposure, the exposures between the cases and controls will also be similar.

linked to breast cancer that controls for alcohol consumption using broad categories like "drinkers" and "nondrinkers" may result in some residual confounding because of differences in risk among drinkers (e.g., light and heavy drinkers). Unless the risk of the outcome is similar within a given category, there may be residual confounding. This can be a problem when continuous variables are collapsed into a small number of categories that are not homogeneous in terms of the risk they pose for the outcome. This is also a problem in age adjustment (chapter 6) when broad categories of age are used in the adjustment procedure. Flawed characterization of confounders may also occur when proxy measures of a confounder are used. If the proxy measure is a poor representation of the intended measure, there may be residual confounding. For instance, using a subject's educational attainment as a proxy for current socioeconomic status is likely to result in incomplete control of confounding (i.e., residual confounding) because it is not a precise measure of the intended construct.

Lastly, residual confounding may result from *misclassification of confounders*. The misclassification can affect the magnitude of the adjusted measure of association, and depending on the pattern of misclassification, it may lead to unpredictable consequences.[13]

RANDOM ERROR

Random error, which was defined earlier in this chapter as variability in a measure due to chance,* can also affect the accuracy of an epidemiologic study. As noted in chapter 7, random error may result in spurious associations between exposures and outcomes. So, what are the sources of random error? Essentially, there are two sources:

- Measurement error
- Sampling variation

Measurement error refers to "an error made in measuring the value of a variable."[22(p109)] This can result from inexact measuring instruments, the subjective nature of some exposures or outcomes, and other factors, including bias. A consequence of measurement error may be misclassification of exposure or outcome status. As long as the measurement errors are random, however, they only tend to dilute a measure of association toward its null value (e.g., CIR = 1.0). One strategy for minimizing *random measurement errors*, a component of random error, is to take multiple measurements and average the values in order to achieve a more stable estimate. For example, if one wanted a precise resting blood pressure for a patient, it would be better to take two or three measurements and average them rather than relying on just one.

---

*Some prefer to call this "ignorance," indicating that chance only means that we have not yet identified the determinants of the so-called random errors. For example, some might say that in tossing dice the result is controlled by factors such as the force of the toss, the density of the table on which the toss takes place, and the weight of the markings on the dice. According to this view, chance is simply unexplained variability.

Sampling variation was defined in chapter 5. Briefly, it arises because samples can be considered point estimates of some hypothetical population.* Therefore, sample estimates will tend to differ from sample to sample. We call this sampling variation, and it is a major source of random error. Assuming no systematic error (i.e., bias or confounding) is present, sampling variation can be represented as follows:

Sample Value = True Value + Sampling Variation

The sample value or estimate represents the true value plus random error due to sampling variation. For example, assume a case-control study of 500 cases and 500 controls was designed to determine if exposure to a certain pesticide increases the risk of liver cancer among men employed in the pest control industry. The investigators reported an overall odds ratio of 1.3. They then replicated the study using a new sample of the same size. The overall odds ratio this time was 1.6. Assuming that systematic errors were adequately controlled in both studies, we would attribute the differences to sampling variation, a source of random error. This example suggests two important characteristics of random error. First, it is unpredictable, and second, it cannot be reproduced. A third sample might reveal an odds ratio of 1.0 or perhaps 2.0. No one knows precisely what to expect since sample estimates can vary. In general, sampling variation can be reduced by increasing sample size.

The concept of sampling variation can be extended to include individual measurements. For example, a radial pulse taken on a patient may be conceived as a sample of all possible radial pulses on that patient. Hence, each measurement may be thought of as being subject to sampling variation. This extended definition of sampling variation incorporates random measurement error and is broad enough to be considered synonymous with random error. Henceforth, sampling variation, when used, will be viewed in this context.

Assessing Random Error Using Statistical Significance Testing

Traditionally, random error has been assessed using statistical significance (hypothesis) testing, which was discussed in chapter 6. P-values are used to determine the relative likelihood that an association as extreme or more extreme than the one observed is due to random error, assuming that the null hypothesis of no association is true. Basically, the p-value measures the compatibility between the null hypothesis and the observed data. A small p-value implies a low degree of compatibility, while a large p-value implies a high degree of compatibility.[16] Normally, the p-value is then used to make a decision regarding whether or not to reject the null hypothesis using an arbitrary cut-off point, usually $p = 0.05$. If $p \le 0.05$, the null hypothesis is rejected in

*Sampling variation is generally assumed to apply to all study populations, whether or not they are randomly selected, and whether or not they represent an actual sample or an entire population. Since populations tend to be dynamic—that is, since they tend to change—measurements based on an entire population can be thought of as being subject to sampling variation.[23]

favor of the alternative hypothesis based on the assumption that random error is an *unlikely* explanation for the finding given that the null hypothesis is true. In this case, the association is declared *statistically significant*. On the other hand, if p > 0.05, the null hypothesis is not rejected on the assumption that random error is a *likely* explanation for the finding, again, assuming that the null hypothesis is true. In this case, the association is declared *not statistically significant*. Some researchers may choose to use a lower p-value (e.g., p = 0.01) to judge statistical significance; rarely is a value greater than 0.05 used.

Statistical significance testing can lead to two common types of errors known as *type I* and *type II errors*. A **type I error** is the probability of finding an association when none really exists. It is the error that results from rejecting the null hypothesis when it is actually true. Type I error is measured by the p-value. For instance, p = 0.25 implies that if the null hypothesis is true (i.e., there is no association between the study exposure and outcome), the probability of making a type I error (rejecting a true null hypothesis) is 25 percent. In other words, the probability of obtaining a result at least as extreme as the one obtained due to random error alone is 25 percent. The lower the p-value, the less likely that random error accounts for an observed association. A p-value of 0.001, for example, indicates that, on average, only one out of 1,000 times would an observed association or a more extreme one be expected to be due to random error, assuming that the null hypothesis is true.

It is important to realize that p-values are affected by sample size and the magnitude of the association. Increasing sample size can reduce random error. Thus, increasing sample size has the effect of decreasing the p-value, thereby increasing the precision of the measurement. Another factor that affects the p-value is the magnitude of the association. When the magnitude of an association is large, the association is less likely to be due to random error. It is important to emphasize, however, that p-values tell us nothing about the strength of an association, just whether an observed association is more or less likely to be due to random error. The strength of an association is determined by a measure of association (e.g., OR).

A **type II error** is the probability of *not* finding an association when one actually exists. It is the error that results from failing to reject the null hypothesis when it is actually false. Type II error is measured by the **beta level** (β). The smaller the beta level, the less chance of a type II error and the greater the **power** of a study, that is, the probability of detecting an association *if* one really exists.[2] Power = $1 - \beta$, or, expressed as a percentage, $(1 - \beta) \times 100$. Thus, beta and power are inversely related. Because power is largely affected by sample size, studies with inadequate sample size have insufficient power to detect real associations (i.e., they are more subject to type II errors). Therefore, if *no* association is found in a study *with small sample size*, it is possible that the result is due solely to a lack of power. This type of result is often regarded as *inconclusive*. In other words, if no statistical association is found, *and* the sample size is small, one should consider the finding inconclusive due to insufficient power. To minimize the chance of a type II error, it is generally recommended that a study have at least 80 percent power or a corresponding beta level of no more than 0.20. Although most epidemiologists are more concerned about making a type I error (finding an association when none exists) than a type II error (not finding an association when one exists), both types of errors are important and need to be minimized if the study results are to be precise. In fact, the two types of error are related, and for fixed sample sizes attempts to decrease type I errors have the effect of increasing type II errors and vice versa. Exhibit 8-3 describes another type of error commonly known as a *type III error*, and exhibit 8-4 on p. 222 summarizes the conclusions that may be drawn from statistical significance testing using an alpha level (chapter 6) of 0.05.

Exhibit 8-3
What Is a Type III Error?

Although many are familiar with type I and type II errors, fewer people have ever heard of a type III error. In fact, this concept is not commonly covered in introductory statistics or epidemiology textbooks. There are at least two different definitions of type III error, which are described briefly in this exhibit.

The First Definition

A. W. Kimball (1957) referred to a type III error as an error of the third kind and defined it as *"the error committed by giving the right answer to the wrong problem"* (p. 134). He was speaking in the context of statistical consulting. The problem as he saw it often results from poor communication between the statistician and the researcher.

More recently, S. Schwartz and K. M. Carpenter (1999) used this concept of a type III error to describe the problem of selecting the wrong method to study a problem. Specifically, they refer to the problem of studying individual differences in the risk of an outcome to answer questions about the causes of the outcome in different populations or the same population over time. For example, in the attempt to understand the causes of homelessness, most studies have focused on individual factors that distinguish homeless people from non-homeless people. The real question of interest, however, is why has homelessness increased over time? According to Schwartz and Carpenter, this question cannot be adequately answered by studies that focus on differences among individuals. This will only tell us which people are more likely to become homeless and not why homelessness occurs. If, for example, homelessness is caused by limited affordable housing, then altering individual risk factors related to homelessness, such as low income, will not change the *rate* of homelessness. Increasing the opportunity for housing for some (i.e., by supplementing their income) will only decrease it for others because the availability of affordable housing is limited. The only way of decreasing the frequency of homelessness then is to increase the amount of affordable housing, which will depend on housing policies, economic conditions, and other community factors. Schwartz and Carpenter state,

> In this way, the particular characteristics of homeless people are simply superficial causes, factors that are related to variation between individuals in risk of homelessness but that have nothing to do with the causes of the incidence of homelessness (p. 1178).

In other words, researchers seeking to understand the causes of homelessness by studying individual risk factors for homelessness are committing a type III error by giving the right answer to the wrong problem.

The Second Definition
Another definition of a type III error has to do with statistical significance or hypothesis testing. Basically, it occurs when one rejects the null hypothesis (H_O), and the alternate hypothesis (H_A) is directional but in the opposite direction of the true association. For example:

$$H_O: OR = 1.0$$

$$H_A: OR > 1.0$$

If one rejects the null hypothesis that the odds ratio equals one in favor of the alternate hypothesis that the odds ratio is greater than one, but in reality the true odds ratio is less than one, then the researcher has committed a type III error. This concept of a type III error is due to sampling variation (i.e., random error). Theoretically, a larger sample should lead to a lower probability of making a type III error. L. Leventhal and C. Huynh (1996) have indicated that this kind of a type III error can also occur when the alternate hypothesis is non-directional as shown below.

$$H_O: OR = 1.0$$

$$H_A: OR \neq 1.0$$

Even though the alternate hypothesis is non-directional, some researchers will assume that the direction of the relationship in their study population is the correct one. If it is not, a type III error has been committed.

References: Kimball, A. W. (1957). Errors of the Third Kind in Statistical Consulting. *Journal of the American Statistical Association* 52 (278): 133–142; Leventhal, L., and Huynh, C. (1996). Directional Decisions for Two-tailed Tests: Power, Error Rates, and Sample Size. *Psychological Methods* 1 (3): 278–292; Schwartz, S., and Carpenter, K. M. (1999). The Right Answer for the Wrong Question: Consequences of Type III Error for Public Health Research. *American Journal of Public Health* 89 (8): 1175–1180.

As implied in chapter 6, statistical significance (hypothesis) testing has a number of limitations and has found disfavor among many epidemiologists. Some common objections are: (a) the cut-off point for determining statistical significance is completely arbitrary; (b) the p-value is confounded by the effects of sample size and strength of the association; and (c) statistical significance is often misinterpreted. With regard to the first point, one can argue convincingly that there is very little difference between $p = 0.04$ and $p = 0.06$. Yet, with an arbitrary cut-off point of $p = 0.05$, two different conclusions would be reached based on these similar values. The second point is important because a p-value will vary simply because of differences in sample size or the strength of the association. For example, a very large sample tends to produce very small p-values, while a very small sample tends to produce large p-values. Thus, even weak associations may be considered statistically significant if the sample size is large enough but not statistically significant if the sample size is smaller. Also, a relatively strong association may be accompa-

Exhibit 8-4

Using P-values to Assess the Potential Effect of Random Error on an Association

Is p ≤ 0.05?	Is p > 0.05?
1. If YES, the association is *statistically significant*. The probability of a type I error is equal to or less than 5%, which is the traditional cut-off point (alpha level).	1. If YES, the association is *not statistically significant*. The probability of a type I error is more than 5%, which is the traditional cut-off point (alpha level).
2. Random error is an *unlikely* explanation for the observed association.	2. Random error is a *reasonable* explanation for the observed association.
3. The *smaller* the p-value, the *less* likely random error explains the association.	3. The *larger* the p-value, the *more* likely random error explains the association.
4. *If* the sample size is *very large*, most associations will be statistically significant, so the association should be judged for its *practical significance*.	4. *If* the sample size is *small*, the association should be considered *inconclusive* due to low power and possible type II error.

Note: This framework assumes that bias and confounding are not responsible for the finding.

nied by a large p-value because of small sample size. In isolation one cannot be sure if a p-value is more a reflection of sample size or strength of the association or both. Finally, "statistically significant" is often misinterpreted as meaning that the null hypothesis is false or that the association is one of cause and effect. Neither can be demonstrated using statistical significance testing, which depends on probabilities. For these and other reasons most epidemiologists prefer using confidence intervals over statistical significance testing when it comes to assessing random error.[16, 24] The basic methods are discussed in the following section.

Assessing Random Error Using Confidence Intervals

Random error can be readily assessed using confidence intervals, which were introduced in chapter 5. This method is referred to as **interval estimation**. Statistically speaking, a confidence interval is constructed around a *point estimate* of the population parameter for a given level of confidence, usually 95 percent. The extent of random error in the estimate is judged by the width of the confidence interval. If the confidence interval is fairly narrow, *and* the confidence level is high, this suggests that there is little random error in the estimate. Therefore, the point estimate can be considered relatively precise. Conversely, if the interval is fairly wide, *and* the confidence level is high, it implies that there is significant random error, and the point estimate can be considered relatively imprecise. Two important caveats need to be kept in mind. First, in assessing the extent of random error it is important to have a high level of confidence since confidence intervals tend to narrow as the confidence level decreases. It is much easier, for example, to be 50 percent confident that a point estimate falls within a relatively narrow range of values than to be 90 or 95 percent confident. Second, confidence intervals tell us nothing about whether or not a measure of association is valid. Bias or confounding may affect a measure of association no matter how precise it may appear based on a confidence interval.

Assuming there is no significant bias or confounding present, if RR = 2.5, and the 95% CI = 2.1 to 2.9, we would be reasonably confident that we have a relatively precise estimate of the measure of association, which in this case happens to be a risk ratio. On the other hand, if RR = 2.5, and the 95% CI = 0.6 to 19.5, we would say that the measure of association appears very imprecise (i.e., subject to substantial random error). These comparisons depend on using the same confidence level, which is usually, but not always, 95 percent. Confidence intervals are best viewed as general indicators of the amount of variability in a measure.[24] If the effects of bias and confounding have been adequately prevented or controlled, however, and if the confidence level is high enough (e.g., 95 percent), then we can be reasonably sure that a narrow confidence interval means that we probably have a relatively accurate measure of association in our study population. Specific methods for calculating confidence intervals for measures of association are discussed in subsequent chapters dealing with specific study designs.

Confidence Intervals and Significance Testing

Primarily for reasons cited in the previous section, many epidemiologists favor interval estimation over statistical significance testing. Confidence intervals can be used to assess statistical significance, but this is not their attraction, since those who favor confidence intervals do not care to do significance testing. For the record, however, a confidence interval for a risk, rate, odds, or prevalence ratio containing a value of one represents a *non-statistically significant* finding, while a confidence interval *not* containing a value of one represents a *statistically significant* finding. Similarly, a confidence interval for a risk, rate, or prevalence difference containing zero is *not statistically significant*, while one *not* containing zero is *statistically significant*. The value of confidence intervals, however, lies in the fact that they provide information not readily available from significance testing. For one thing, confidence intervals give us a range of possible values for the measure of association. RR = 3.4 (95% CI = 0.7 to 15.1) indicates that while the point estimate of the population RR is 3.4, we are 95% confident that the true population RR ranges from 0.7 to 15.1, assuming no systematic errors are present. Furthermore, as stated earlier, we can see from this broad range of values that the estimate is relatively imprecise, and, therefore, we would not want to stake too much on RR really being 3.4. RR = 2.6 (95% CI = 2.1 to 3.0), on the other hand, suggests a relatively precise estimate, and we would be relatively confident using 2.6 as our estimate of the RR knowing that we have probably not under- or overestimated it by too much, assuming again that there are no systematic errors. Of course, on average, there is still a five percent chance that the true value is really outside this range (i.e., we are after all using a 95 percent versus a 100 percent confidence interval, which would be too broad to be useful). Certainty is just not part of the game plan.

Unlike p-values generated from significance testing, confidence intervals provide clues to the magnitude of an association *and* the precision of the point estimate. This information is lost in p-values.[16] Thus, a 95 percent confidence interval of 0.9 to 11.7 tells us much more than a p-value stated as p > 0.05 or even p = 0.07 when the alpha level is 0.05. With the latter information alone, we would be forced to conclude that the finding is not consistent with the null hypothesis without knowing whether the inconsistency is due to small sample size or a weak or nonexistent association. With the former information, however, we could speculate that the association is probably positive and moderate to strong based on the propensity toward high, positive values in the confidence interval. We could also speculate that the sample size that produced the confidence interval is somewhat small given that the interval is relatively wide. The width of a confidence interval is proportional to sample size, which in turn is proportional to the level of precision, all other factors being equal. Thus, the stated confidence interval appears to reflect significant random error and low precision in the estimate based on its width. Of course, like the selection of the alpha level in statistical significance testing, selection of the confidence level is arbitrary. Also, as with statistical significance testing, interval estimation may be influenced by sources of systematic error, and neither is sufficient for establishing causation between an exposure and outcome. Because of the potential for systematic errors, some recommend that bias and confounding be addressed in a study prior to assessing random error.[21]

In conclusion, confidence intervals, and to a lesser extent p-values, can be used to assess random error in study findings. However, because of the potential for uncontrolled systematic errors and for reasons related to the validity of assumptions regarding the statistical model being employed, these methods are best used to make *qualitative* versus *quantitative* decisions about the *relative* amount of random error.[24] Of these two options, confidence intervals have clear advantages over statistical significance (hypothesis) testing. Why then does hypothesis testing persist? Marks R. Nester[25] has suggested some possible explanations: (a) the appearance of objectivity and exactitude; (b) the availability of easy-to-use statistical software; (c) traditional teaching practices; and (d) demands of certain journal editors or thesis directors. Additionally, he seemed to imply that "peer pressure" may be a factor when he included an explanation that "everyone else seems to use them [tests of hypotheses]."[25(p401)]

Reducing Random Error

There are two major methods of reducing random error in a study, one of which has already been mentioned.

- Increasing sample size
- Improving study efficiency

In theory, the easiest way of reducing random error in a study is to increase the size of the study population. Increasing sample size tends to increase the precision of the estimate by reducing sampling variation. This is illustrated in table 8-2. Note that as the sample size increases, the confidence intervals around the point estimate (OR = 4.0) become narrower, indicating increased precision and reduced random error.

Table 8-2   Illustration of the Effect of Sample Size on the Precision of an Estimate

OR = 4.0		
n = 150	n = 300	n = 600
95% CI = 2.0 to 7.9	95% CI = 2.5 to 6.5	95% CI = 2.9 to 5.6

These results are based on a hypothetical case-control study of an equal number of cases and controls where the proportions of exposed and unexposed subjects in the case and control groups, respectively, are fixed. Specifically, two-thirds of the cases are exposed but only one-third of the controls. Sample size differences do not alter these proportions.

Random error can also be reduced by improving study efficiency (also referred to as *statistical efficiency*; see chapter 10). To understand this, consider a prospective cohort study where the cohort consists of 10,000 subjects, but only five percent are exposed to the factor of interest. Thus, there are only 500 exposed subjects and 9,500 unexposed subjects. Now assume that the cumulative incidence of the study outcome is just 1.0 per 100 (1.0 percent) *regardless* of exposure status. Based on these statistics, we would expect only five cases to develop among the exposed portion of the cohort and 95 cases among the unexposed portion. This would yield the following study results: cumulative incidence ratio (CIR) = 1.0, 95% CI = 0.4 to 2.5. The relatively broad confidence interval indicates a rather imprecise estimate and, hence, an inefficient study despite its large sample size. The efficiency would be improved, however, if there was a higher proportion of exposed cases. When there is no association between the study exposure and outcome (i.e., when CIR = 1.0), efficiency is maximized by having an equal number of exposed and unexposed subjects in the study. To illustrate, let us now assume that 50 percent of the cohort is exposed, and 50 percent is not. In this scenario, the results would be: CIR = 1.0, 95% CI = 0.7 to 1.5. Notice that by increasing the study efficiency we have decreased the width of the confidence interval, thereby increasing the precision of the estimate. In other words, we have reduced the amount of random error. When an association exists, particularly when it is a strong association, the optimal apportionment to exposed and unexposed or case and control groups, depending on the study design, may be more or less than 50 percent.[1] In general, the efficiency of a study can be potentially increased to the extent that we have the information necessary to design it in a way that maximizes available data. For example, for a cohort study, if an exposure is known to be rare in the general population (e.g., asbestos exposure), one might consider using a subgroup that is highly exposed (e.g., asbestos workers). Also, if the outcome is rare, one might want to increase the length of the follow-up period to ensure an adequate number of outcomes for comparison purposes.[1]

SUMMARY

- The accuracy of an epidemiologic study is determined by the extent to which it is free from errors. Accuracy has two major components—validity and precision. Validity is the degree to which inferences are warranted given the methods and study population chosen. Validity can be internal or external. Internal validity represents the degree to which study findings, apart from random error, are true for the source population. External validity, also known as generalizability, is the degree to which study findings are relevant for populations other than the study population. Of the two, internal validity is more important since it does not make sense to generalize findings which are not internally valid. Precision is a measure of the degree to which nonsystematic (random) error is absent in a study. While systematic errors tend to increase or decrease the measure of association in a study, nonsystematic errors tend to dilute it toward the null value. Accuracy is threatened by bias, confounding, and random error.

- Bias is a type of systematic error in the design or conduct of a study. It affects a study's internal validity, and hence, its accuracy. There are two major categories of bias—selection bias and information bias. Both can distort the measure of association in a study. Although bias cannot be quantified per se, the direction and relative magnitude of the effect can often be established. Positive bias results in an overestimation of the measure of association, while negative bias results in an underestimation.

- Selection bias can result when the characteristics of the subjects selected for a study differ systematically from those in the source population. It can also result from subject losses or withdrawals that alter the original sample composition. Examples include Berkson's bias, a type of admission rate bias; prevalence-incidence bias; the healthy worker effect, which is a type of membership bias; volunteer bias; and loss to follow-up bias. Methods of preventing selection bias include selecting subjects representative of the source population in terms of exposure or outcome, ensuring that selection of study and comparison groups is based on comparable criteria, and minimizing subject losses.

- Information bias is a type of systematic error due to measurement flaws that can result in misclassification of subjects on exposure or outcome status.

Misclassification may be differential, that is, nonuniform between study and comparison groups, or nondifferential, uniform between study and comparison groups. Differential misclassification can lead to over- or under-estimation of the measure of association, while nondifferential misclassification tends to result in dilution of the measure of association toward the null value. Common types of information bias include recall bias, reporting bias, interviewer bias, exposure suspicion bias, and diagnostic suspicion bias. Methods of preventing information bias include blinding subjects and observers as to study hypotheses, standardizing data collection procedures, training observers, and making multiple measurements on each subject.

- Confounding is systematic error that results from a mixing of effects between an exposure and an extraneous factor or confounder. It can affect the internal validity of a study by distorting the magnitude of the measure of association in a positive or negative direction. In order to be a confounder, the extraneous factor should be an independent risk factor for the outcome of interest, be associated with the exposure of interest in the source population, and not be part of the causal sequence between the exposure and outcome. Potential confounders may include known or suspected risk factors. Confounding may be controlled in the design stage of a study by restricting the study population to exclude potential confounders, matching study and comparison groups by potential confounders, or by randomizing the subjects to study and comparison groups. It may also be controlled in the analysis stage using stratification or multivariable analysis. Residual confounding may still be present, however, if important confounders have not been adequately controlled or have been misclassified.

- Random error affects the precision of a study and hence its accuracy. It includes measurement error (random) and sampling variation. For convenience, sampling variation can be broadly conceived as encompassing both sources of random error. Random error can be assessed using statistical significance (hypothesis) testing or interval estimation using confidence intervals. Statistical significance testing has fallen into disfavor with many epidemiologists for a number of reasons. For one thing, the alpha level is arbitrary, and the p-value is confounded by the effects of sample size and the strength of the association. The results of statistical significance testing are also frequently misinterpreted, and the underlying assumptions may not be met in many epidemiologic studies. Confidence intervals provide more information than p-values, and they do not mix the effects of sample size and strength of the association. In general, when the confidence level is high, a narrow confidence interval implies a relatively precise estimate of the measure of association, indicating little random error. A wide confidence interval, however, implies a relatively imprecise measure of association and a high degree of random error. Random error can usually be reduced by increasing a study's sample size or by improving a study's efficiency.

New Terms

- accuracy
- admission rate bias
- Berkson's bias
- beta level
- bias
- confounder
- confounding
- confounding factor
- diagnostic suspicion bias
- differential misclassification
- error
- exposure suspicion bias
- external validity
- frequency matching
- generalizability
- healthy worker effect
- hospital admission rate bias
- individual matching
- information bias
- internal validity
- interval estimation
- interviewer bias
- loss to follow-up bias
- matching
- measurement bias
- measurement error
- membership bias
- misclassification bias
- negative bias

- negative confounder
- Neyman's bias
- nondifferential misclassification
- non-respondent bias
- non-response bias
- nonsystematic error
- observation bias
- pair matching
- positive bias
- positive confounder
- potential confounder
- power
- precision
- prevalence-incidence bias
- probability sample
- random error
- recall bias
- reporting bias
- residual confounding
- restriction
- rumination bias
- selection bias
- Simpson's paradox
- source population
- systematic error
- type I error
- type II error
- validity (of a study)
- volunteer bias

Study Questions and Exercises

Each of the following problems contains a potential error that could affect the accuracy of the results. Using the key below, indicate the most likely source of error in each problem based solely on the information provided. Also, give a detailed rationale for your answers, including the specific type of selection or information bias, confounding, or random error where possible. If A, B, or C is selected, indicate the likely direction of the bias or confounding (e.g., positive or negative).

A. Selection bias   C. Confounding
B. Information bias   D. Random error

___ 1. The authors of a cross-sectional study hypothesized that lack of regular exercise is associated with obesity in children. Their study of 12 children in Michigan, however, failed to show a statistically significant association between exercise habits and obesity (PR = 1.9, p = 0.11).

___ 2. In a case-control study of the relationship between intravenous drug use and HIV infection, the investigators discovered after the study that the case group had tended to underreport their drug use due to fears arising from previous convictions for drug-related violations. Underreporting was not a problem in the control group, however, which was not under medical supervision at the time.

___ 3. A prospective cohort study followed 8,542 women for 10 years to determine if alcohol consumption increased the risk of breast cancer. No statistically significant association was found. Twelve thousand women had been enrolled in the study at its initiation, but 3,458 had withdrawn during the 10-year period. A follow-up of spouses, friends, and relatives of the women who withdrew revealed that more than 60% of the withdrawals had developed breast cancer and that nearly 84% were regular drinkers.

___ 4. A case-control study was designed to test whether persons exposed to certain types of pesticides during early childhood were more likely to develop neurological problems in later adulthood. The results were statistically significant. The cases consisted of those with severe but treatable neurological disorders, and the controls consisted of those without any diagnosed neurological disorders. Both the cases and controls were asked detailed questions about their pesticide exposures during early childhood.

___ 5. A large epidemiologic study found that elderly adults with dementia were more likely to develop liver cancer than those without dementia. The investigators, however, could offer no plausible biological mechanism for the association between dementia and liver cancer. Many of the subjects reported heavy drinking, however.

___ 6. An epidemiologist reported the following conclusion from a large randomized controlled trial during a national meeting: "Daily use of 500 milligrams of vitamin C for a period of one year was associated with a reduced frequency of upper respiratory infections in children under 10 years of age (RR = 0.9, 95% CI = 0.6 – 1.6)."

___ 7. In a large hospital-based case-control study of smoking and lung cancer, controls consisted of patients with noncancerous chronic pulmonary diseases, such as chronic bronchitis and emphysema. The investigators were surprised to find that the association between smoking and lung cancer was relatively weak (OR = 1.4, p < 0.05).

___ 8. Three hundred cases and 600 controls were selected among mothers for a case-control study to see if maternal coffee consumption was related to low birth weight in the mothers' babies. Data were collected on past coffee consumption patterns for the mothers and on cigarette smoking, a known risk factor for low birth weight. The overall association between maternal coffee consumption and low birth weight was reported to be strong (OR = 3.4). When the data were later reanalyzed and adjusted for cigarette smoking, however, the association was found to be nonexistent (OR = 1.0).

____ 9. The investigators of a prospective cohort study collected blood samples from the participants at the beginning of the study and froze them for later analysis. A subsequent nested case-control study was conducted to determine if blood levels of certain hormones were associated with Alzheimer's disease. The previously stored blood samples were analyzed for the cases and controls. It was later determined that the samples had degenerated during the storage period because of a failure to maintain consistent temperatures.

____10. An epidemiologist examines the association between the use of diet pills and migraine headaches using a case-control study design. His subjects are outpatients at a large community hospital. He finds that those using diet pills are more likely to complain of migraines, but he also discovers that those who have migraine headaches and use diet pills are more likely to be referred to the community hospital for outpatient diagnostic testing than those who have migraines but are not using diet pills.

References

1. Norell, S. E. (1995). *Workbook of Epidemiology*. New York: Oxford University Press.
2. Last, J. M., ed. (2001). *A Dictionary of Epidemiology*, 4th ed. New York: Oxford University Press.
3. The Scandinavian Simvastatin Survival Study Group (1994). Randomised Trial of Cholesterol Lowering in 4444 Patients with Coronary Heart Disease: The Scandinavian Simvastatin Survival Study (4S). *The Lancet* 344 (8934): 1383–1389.
4. Hennekens, C. H., and Buring, J. E. (1987). *Epidemiology in Medicine*. Boston: Little, Brown and Company.
5. Greenberg, R. S., Daniels, S. R., Flanders, W. D., Eley, J. W., and Boring, J. R. III (2001). *Medical Epidemiology*, 3rd ed. New York: Lange Medical Books/McGraw-Hill.
6. Choi, B. C. K., and Noseworthy, A. L. (1992). Classification, Direction, and Prevention of Bias in Epidemiologic Research. *Journal of Occupational Medicine* 34 (3): 265–271.
7. Vogt, W. P. (1999). *Dictionary of Statistics and Methodology: A Nontechnical Guide for the Social Sciences*, 2nd ed. Thousand Oaks, CA: Sage Publications.
8. Berkson, J. (1946). Limitations of the Application of Fourfold Table Analysis to Hospital Data. *Biometrics Bulletin* 2 (3): 47–53.
9. Sackett, D. L. (1979). Bias in Analytic Research. *Journal of Chronic Diseases* 32: 51–63.
10. American Heart Association (1980). The National Diet-Heart Study: Final Report. AHA Monograph No. 18. New York: American Heart Association. (Reported in Streiner, D. L., Norman, G. R., and Blum, H. M. (1989). *PDQ Epidemiology*. Toronto: B. C. Decker).
11. Hernan, M. A., Hernandez-Diaz, S., and Robins, J. M. (2004). A Structural Approach to Selection Bias. *Epidemiology* 15 (5): 615–625.

12. Delgado-Rodriguez, M., and Llorca, J. (2004). Bias. *Journal of Epidemiology and Community Health* 58: 635–641.
13. Szklo, M., and Nieto, F. J. (2000). *Epidemiology: Beyond the Basics.* Gaithersburg, MD: Aspen.
14. American Social Health Association (2005). STD Prevention Partnership Position Statement—Minorities and Sexually Transmitted Diseases. Available: http://www.ashastd.org/involve/involve_adv_minpos.cfm (Access date: October 5, 2005).
15. Merriam-Webster, Inc. (1989). *The New Merriam-Webster Dictionary.* Springfield, MA: Merriam-Webster, Inc., Publishers.
16. Rothman, K. J. (1986). *Modern Epidemiology.* Boston: Little, Brown and Company.
17. Oleckno, W. A. (1988). Is Smoking a Risk Factor for Accidental Injuries? *Health and Hygiene* 9: 56–60.
18. La Vecchia, C., Gentile, A., Negri, E., Parazzini, F., and Franceschi, S. (1989). Coffee Consumption and Myocardial Infarction in Women. *American Journal of Epidemiology* 130 (3): 481–485.
19. Dorak, M. T. (2005). *Bias & Confounding.* Available: http://dorakmt.tripod.com/epi/bc.html (Access date: September 20, 2005).
20. Oleckno, W. A., and Blacconiere, M. J. (1990). Risk-Taking Behaviors and Other Correlates of Seat Belt Use Among University Students. *Public Health* 104: 155–164.
21. Elwood, M. (1998). *Critical Appraisal of Epidemiological Studies and Clinical Trials,* 2nd ed. Oxford: Oxford University Press.
22. Day, S. (1999). *Dictionary for Clinical Trials.* Chichester: John Wiley & Sons, Ltd.
23. MacDorman, M. F., and Atkinson, J. O. (1999). Infant Mortality Statistics from the 1997 Period Linked Birth/Infant Death Data Set. *National Vital Statistics Reports* 47 (23). Hyattsville, MD: National Center for Health Statistics.
24. Rothman, R. J. (2002). *Epidemiology: An Introduction.* New York: Oxford University Press.
25. Nester, M. R. (1996). An Applied Statistician's Creed. *Applied Statistics* 45 (4): 401–410.

CHAPTER NINE

Ecological and Cross-Sectional Studies

*This chapter covers the basic design, analysis, and interpreta-
tion of ecological and cross-sectional studies as well as their
major advantages and disadvantages.*

Learning Objectives

- Describe the basic design and conduct of analytic ecological and cross-sectional studies.
- Summarize the major advantages and disadvantages of analytic ecological and cross-sectional studies.
- Explain the differences between analytic and descriptive ecological studies and analytic and descriptive cross-sectional studies, respectively.
- Interpret the results of analytic ecological studies, including scatter plots, Pearson's correlation coefficient, the coefficient of determination, and regression lines and equations.
- Analyze and interpret the results of analytic cross-sectional studies in terms of crude prevalence, prevalence ratio, prevalence odds ratio, applicable 95% confidence intervals, and the applicable chi-square test for independence.
- Define construct validity, contextual effects, cross-level bias, dependent and independent variables, e or exp, ln, longitudinal study, multicollinearity, multilevel analysis, prevalence study, prevalence survey, r, and r squared (r^2).

INTRODUCTION

The basic design and types of ecological and cross-sectional studies were discussed in chapter 4. In that chapter it was acknowledged that ecological and cross-sectional studies could be classified as descriptive or analytic depending primarily on the investigators' intent. Descriptive studies are designed to *describe* patterns of health-related occurrences by person, place, or time variables. They do not test *a priori* hypotheses, but they may be useful in generating hypotheses for further investigation.* Analytic studies, on the other hand, are concerned with testing predetermined hypotheses about the relationships between specified exposures and outcomes. The modifiers, "analytic" and "descriptive," are used here to differentiate these study approaches. In common practice, they are rarely used in connection with the study names, requiring the reader to infer from the context whether a given ecological or cross-sectional study is descriptive or analytic in nature.

This chapter focuses primarily on analytic ecological and cross-sectional studies. It highlights their key design features, discusses their major advantages and disadvantages, and describes the basic approaches used in analysis and interpretation of study findings. Descriptive ecological and cross-sectional studies are discussed only briefly since they share many features in common with their analytic counterparts, and a prolonged discussion would therefore be repetitive. Chapters 10–12 cover the other major analytic and experimental study designs commonly used in epidemiology. Hybrid designs were discussed in chapter 4.

ANALYTIC ECOLOGICAL STUDIES

Key Design Features

The most fundamental aspect of an **analytic ecological study** is the *ecological unit*. As suggested in chapter 4, an ecological unit is typically a geographical area or time period that depicts a given population or group of people. For example, an ecological unit may be a city, country, or institution or a particular month, year, or decade. For each ecological unit there is an overall or summary measure of exposure and an overall or summary measure of outcome, such as per capita salt consumption and the cause-specific mortality rate for stroke, respectively. It is important to understand that the overall or summary measure is based on the *entire* population or group defined by the ecological unit. That is, it represents the experience of the population or group as a whole and not necessarily the experience any particular individual within the population. Ecological studies are therefore studies of groups of people versus studies of individuals. For convenience, ecological unit and unit of analysis (defined in chapter 4) may be used interchangeably when referring to ecological studies. While the unit of analysis is the group in an ecological study, it is the individual in most other epidemiologic studies (e.g., cross-sectional studies).

Before we go any further it might be helpful to describe briefly how one goes about conducting an analytic ecological study. The typical steps are illustrated in figure 9-1. First, one develops one or more research hypotheses

*When "testing hypotheses" is referred to in this context it does not necessarily imply that statistical significance (hypothesis) testing (chapters 6 and 8) will be used in the analysis. Instead, it simply indicates that the investigators have one or more predetermined research questions that they wish to address in a study.

concerning associations between one or more exposures and outcomes of interest. Next, the ecological units to be compared are defined and selected. After this, overall or summary measures of exposure and outcome are obtained for each ecological unit. Once the data on exposure and outcome have been obtained, the ecological units may be plotted on a graph known as a *scatter plot*. A **scatter plot** is the pattern of points resulting when two variables are plotted on a graph, and each point represents one of the units of analysis formed by the intersection of the values of the two variables.[1] With regard to ecological studies, the intersections represent the ecological units with the x-axis typically representing the exposure levels and the y-axis representing the outcome levels. The data are then analyzed, and the findings are reported and discussed. The analysis, illustrating the use of a scatter plot, will be described later in the chapter. It should be noted that efforts to prevent or control bias and confounding (chapter 8) should also be part of the process.

Exposure and outcome data for each ecological unit are generally obtained from *secondary sources*, that is, from sources that have been collected and recorded by someone else, usually for different reasons (see chapter 4). Also, the information on exposure typically comes from a different source

Figure 9-1   Basic Steps in Conducting an Analytic Ecological Study

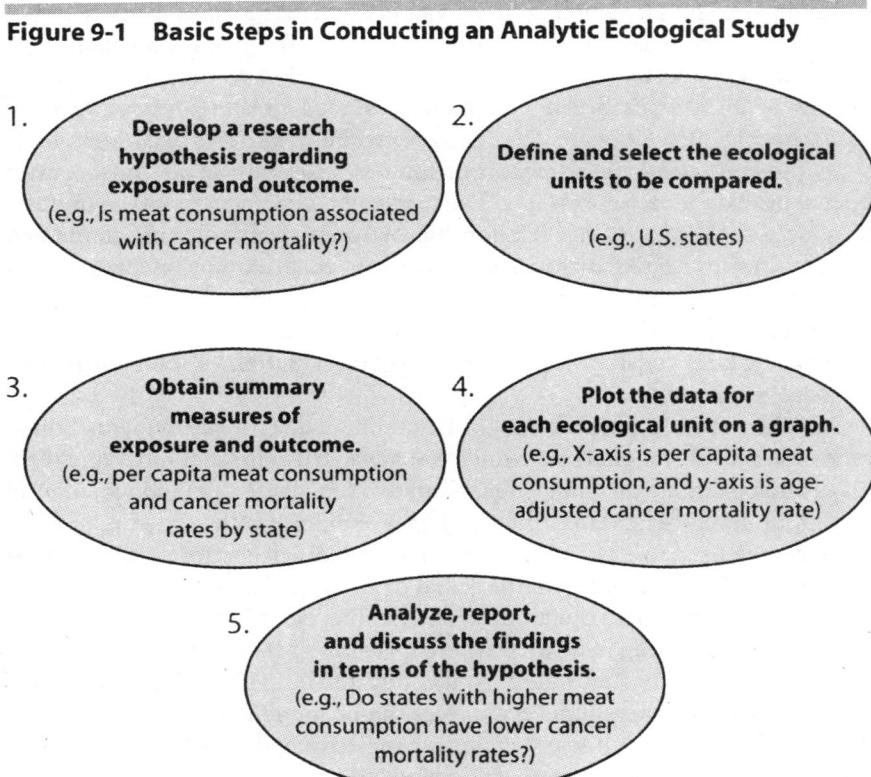

than that on outcome (e.g., per capita salt consumption from a salt trade association based on sales data and stroke mortality from a health organization, such as the World Health Organization).

As indicated in chapter 4, there are three major types of ecological studies. These are *multiple-group studies*, which entail comparisons of many different populations in one study (e.g., multiple countries); *time-trend studies* in which one population is compared at different time periods (e.g., in 2007 and 2008); and *mixed studies*, which combine elements of both multiple-group and time-trend studies.[2] All of these study types can be classified as analytic or descriptive depending primarily on whether or not there are *a priori* hypotheses to be examined.

Use of Ecological Measures in Studies of Individuals

Epidemiologic studies where the unit of analysis is the *individual* sometimes use one or more ecological variables to measure exposure. Although they are not conventional ecological studies, they do have an ecological component. For example, to determine if chronic exposure to high levels of airborne particulates increases the risk of cardiac arrhythmias in sensitive individuals, investigators may find it more convenient to assign average exposure levels based on ambient air sampling in the vicinity where the subjects reside rather than placing particulate monitors on each subject to obtain individual measurements of exposure. Also, sometimes ecological exposures are chosen in studies of individuals because of their presumed greater *construct validity.*[3] **Construct validity** refers to the degree to which a variable accurately measures the theoretical phenomenon of interest.[1] Moyses Szklo and F. Javier Nieto[3] provide a useful example, which may be characterized as follows. A cross-sectional study of the relationship between socioeconomic status and current cardiovascular disease in individuals may employ median family income in the neighborhood to represent socioeconomic status (an ecological measure) as opposed to an individual's income or educational level because the investigators consider it a more valid representation of the construct of socioeconomic status.

Studies that combine ecological and individual measurements sometimes use **multilevel analyses**, which are advanced statistical modeling techniques that examine the independent and combined effects of individual-level and group-level variables in order to better explain health-related outcomes. They can be used to examine contextual and ecological effects.[2] **Contextual effects** refer to the influence of the social or environmental setting on individual risk of health-related outcomes. For example, one might estimate the contextual effects of living in an area where illegal drug trafficking is rampant on the risk of adolescent mortality, controlling for individual drug use. Additional information on multilevel analyses can be found in more advanced epidemiologic texts. Multilevel analysis and contextual effects are often considered in applications of *social epidemiology* (chapter 2).

Major Advantages

A principal advantage of analytic ecological studies is that they can be used to test *a priori* hypotheses relatively quickly and at less expense than more sophisticated epidemiologic study designs. Secondary data on exposure and outcome for ecological studies tend to be readily available from a number of sources, including governmental and non-governmental organizations. These sources can be easily linked at the group level.[2] Increasingly, data sources have also become available online, sometimes even including software that can be used in the analyses. Because ecological studies are relatively quick and inexpensive, they are frequently used to test preliminary hypotheses where the association of interest is at the individual level. Before committing significant resources to undertake a case-control or cohort study, for example, investigators often consider an ecological study when the hypothesis is still relatively undeveloped. Based on the findings of the ecological study, they may then decide if further study appears warranted. Hence, the findings of ecological studies may stimulate additional research by the same or other investigators. When ecological studies in the 1970s began to reveal an inverse relationship between moderate levels of wine consumption and mortality from ischemic heart disease, the findings were intriguing enough to spawn a number of other epidemiologic studies[4-7] involving different populations and different study methods.

Another advantage of ecological studies is that they are the only common type of observational study that is suitable for examining associations between exposures and outcomes at the group level. If we wanted to know if overall levels of illegal drug use are related to overall rates of mortality, it would be appropriate to conduct an ecological study. For example, we might compare several cities in the United States with regard to estimated levels of illegal drug use and age-adjusted mortality rates from all causes. This would be a multiple-group ecological study. Alternatively, we might compare levels of illegal drug use and mortality rates in one city over a given time period, say 2000 to 2005, to determine if there are observable trends in illegal drug use and mortality that correlate with each other. This would be a time-trend ecological study. If we extended this study to include several cities, we would have a mixed ecological study. Of course, such studies would have to be carefully designed to exclude alternate explanations for the findings.

An additional advantage of ecological studies is that they may be more appropriate than individual-based studies when the *intra-group variability* for the exposure of interest is small in the study population. A broader-based ecological study may be able to achieve greater *inter-group variability* across ecological units.[2] For example, consider a study of the effects of dietary fat consumption on cardiovascular disease conducted in Edmonton, Alberta, Canada. The differences in the amount of fat consumed by subjects in Edmonton may be relatively small making it difficult to detect an existing association with cardiovascular disease. An ecological study that correlates mean levels of fat consumption and cardiovascular disease rates across Canadian provinces, however, may show enough variability in fat consumption levels to detect a relationship if it exists.

Also, when the levels of exposure vary significantly *within* individuals, an ecological study may be more likely to detect an existing association than an individual-based study. For example, it can be very difficult to measure accurately the consumption levels of specific dietary factors in individuals (e.g., thiamine, a B vitamin). This is because eating habits, cooking practices, the nutritional content of foods, and portion sizes can vary widely for any given person in a study. Aggregated measures, such as average consumption levels, on the other hand, tend to be more stable and hence more reliable measures.[8]

Major Disadvantages

Historically, the major disadvantage cited for ecological studies has been the possibility of making an *ecological fallacy* (see chapter 4). An ecological fallacy occurs when one uses an association found at the group level to make inferences about the association at the individual level. Since the unit of analysis in an ecological study is the group versus the individual, an association found among groups does not necessarily exist among individuals within the groups. In fact, an ecological fallacy has been described as, "a problem of confusing the group with the members of that group . . ."[9(p821)] For example, the ecological association between wine consumption and mortality from ischemic heart disease implies that countries with moderate levels of wine consumption tend to have below average rates of mortality from ischemic heart disease. This does not necessarily imply, however, that individuals who drink moderate levels of wine will lower their risk of ischemic heart disease. We cannot be sure that an association found at the group level also holds at the individual level based solely on an ecological study. This is because we do not know the joint distribution of the exposure and outcome within individual ecological units.[2] Technically, an ecological fallacy is only an issue when one is interested in individual-level associations. When the interest is strictly at the group level, no such weakness should exist, although in practice the temptation to draw inferences about individuals may be significant.

Why would an association between a given exposure and outcome at the group level be different from that at the individual level? According to Hal Morgenstern, some possible reasons may be within-group bias or confounding, confounding by group, or effect modification (chapter 10) by group.[2] Another possibility has to do with construct validity (defined earlier). A group variable may be measuring a different construct than a similar variable derived from individuals. For example, poverty assessed at the neighborhood level may be measuring something different than poverty assessed at the individual level.[9] Hence, we would not necessarily expect even an internally valid association between poverty and health at the group level to reflect the same association at the individual level. The problem here is similar to that discussed in exhibit 8-3 dealing with type III error. Explanations for the increased rate of homelessness that rely on individual characteristics are unlikely to come to the same conclusions as those based on group measures. Finally, it should be mentioned that the potential bias introduced by an ecological fallacy can also work in reverse. That is, inferences from studies of individuals can be ascribed inappropriately to groups. A term that encompasses both of these errors is **cross-level bias**.

Another disadvantage of ecological studies is that the data on exposure and outcome generally come from secondary sources that have often been collected for different purposes. Thus, the data may not be ideal for testing a given hypothesis. For example, per capita salt consumption may have to be approximated from data on sales of salt. Similarly, estimates of the proportion of smokers in different ecological units may come from data on the collection of tobacco taxes. In both cases, these surrogate measures may not accurately reflect the desired variables.

The use of summary measures poses other potential problems as well. Using summary data (e.g., average levels) for exposure or outcome may lead to imprecise or unstable associations if a high degree of variability exists within the ecological units being examined. Also, some exposure variables in ecological studies, especially social and environmental variables, tend to be more highly correlated with each other than they are on the individual level, making it difficult to isolate their independent effects on the outcome. For example, contaminated drinking water may be associated with cancer mortality based on an ecological study, but it may be difficult to separate the effects of specific contaminants on cancer mortality because of the strong correlations between the contaminants. This problem is often referred to as **multicollinearity**,[10] which technically speaking, "exists when two or more independent variables are highly correlated" in a multiple regression analysis.[1(p180)] When the Environmental Defense Fund released a report in 1974 showing a higher incidence of cancer mortality among white males who derived their drinking water from the Mississippi River compared to a similar group who relied on well water, it was believed that organic compounds in the water were responsible for the effect.[11] It would have been nearly impossible, however, to implicate specific organic contaminants with any degree of accuracy based on the ecological analysis due to multicollinearity, that is, the high degree of correlations among the myriad of organic compounds present in the water.

Other important disadvantages of ecological studies include: (a) difficulty identifying and controlling potential confounders, (b) difficulty in establishing a correct temporal sequence between exposure and outcome, and (c) migration across groups.[2] With regard to confounding, often data on potential confounders is either unavailable or of inconsistent quality among the ecological units being examined. Even if available, it may be difficult to incorporate the appropriate data into the analyses. This, of course, can limit the internal validity of the study results.[12] This is a reason why the findings in some ecological studies may have other logical explanations. For instance, the positive finding in the Taiwanese study of water chlorination and cancer mortality referred to in chapter 4 could be partly due to industrialization. Temporal uncertainty may occur in ecological studies because exposure and outcome are usually assessed simultaneously. For example, an observed positive association between per capita alcohol consumption and unemployment levels across communities in the midwest United States could be due to the fact that increased alcohol consumption tends to follow unemployment and not vice versa. Also, it may be difficult to account for induction or latency periods between exposure and outcome when these periods are unknown or vary significantly. Finally, although migration of individuals across ecological units can cause bias in ecological studies, not much is known how to measure or reduce it.[2] Table 9-1 summarizes the major advantages and disadvantages of analytic ecological studies.

Table 9-1   Major Advantages and Disadvantages of Analytic Ecological Studies

Advantages	Disadvantages
1. They are relatively quick and inexpensive to conduct.	1. Associations among groups may not hold at the individual level; thus, there is a possibility of making an ecological fallacy.
2. Positive findings may stimulate additional epidemiologic research at a relatively early stage of hypothesis development.	2. Readily available secondary sources of exposure or outcome data may not be very accurate.
3. They represent the only common observational study design for uncovering associations at the group level.	3. Summary measures of exposure or outcome may hide wide variability in the data leading to imprecise measures of association.
4. They may be more appropriate than observational studies of individuals when intra-group variability is small but inter-group variability is large.	4. It may be impossible to isolate the independent effects of specific variables on the outcome due to multicollinearity.
5. They may be more appropriate than observational studies of individuals when exposure varies widely within individual subjects.	5. It may be difficult to identify and control potential confounders at the group level.
	6. It may be difficult to establish a correct temporal sequence between exposure and outcome, which is necessary for determining causation.
	7. There may be uncertain effects due to migration of subjects across ecological units.

Analysis and Interpretation

The following discussion gives a general idea of how the results of a conventional *multiple-group study*, the most common type of analytic ecological study, may be analyzed and interpreted. It is assumed that the measures of exposure and outcome are continuous measures, which is typical in ecological studies. A detailed description of the variety of methods that can be used to analyze and interpret the various types of analytic ecological studies is beyond the scope of this text.

The results of multiple-group studies are often analyzed by first looking at the overall association between the exposure and outcome measures for the ecological units being compared. A typical scenario is to first construct a scatter plot. If the scatter plot appears to reveal a linear relationship between exposure and outcome, then the overall **Pearson correlation coefficient (r)** is calculated. The Pearson correlation coefficient measures the degree of linear relationship between two continuous variables (i.e., exposure level and outcome level). *Pearson's r* is a *measure of association* and ranges from −1 to +1, where r = +1 indicates a perfect positive linear relationship, and r = −1 indicates a perfect negative or inverse linear relationship. When r = 0 there is no linear association. Thus, the closer r is to the absolute value of one, the stronger the relationship between exposure and outcome. When one or both of the variables (exposure or outcome) cannot be considered continuous, other statistical procedures are available.

Figure 9-2 illustrates three scatter plots and their respective correlation coefficients for different degrees of association between an exposure and outcome. Note that while the r-values quantify the degree of association between the exposure and outcome, the scatter plots give one a visual sense of the relationship. This can be especially important in identifying nonlinear associations. If the relationship appears to be nonlinear (see figure 9-3 on p. 243), then the Pearson correlation coefficient will not be the appropriate statistic to use.[13] Note also that each point on the scatter plot represents one unit of analysis (e.g., a state or a country). Formulas for calculating r and its 95 percent confidence interval or a test of statistical significance can be found in most standard statistical textbooks.

In addition to producing a scatter plot and calculating the correlation coefficient, the relationship between exposure and outcome is commonly quantified using a form of regression analysis. When there is only one **dependent variable** (the hypothesized effect or outcome) and one **independent variable** (the hypothesized cause of the effect or exposure), *simple linear regression analysis* is used. When there is one dependent variable but more than one independent variable, *multiple linear regression analysis* is the appropriate method.[14, 15]

Let us assume that there is only one dependent and one independent variable represented by the measures of outcome and exposure, respectively. We will also assume there is no bias or confounding present to keep the explanation simple. If the ecological units have been indicated on a scatter plot, *simple*

Figure 9-2   Scatter Plots Representing Various Degrees of Association between Exposure and Outcome

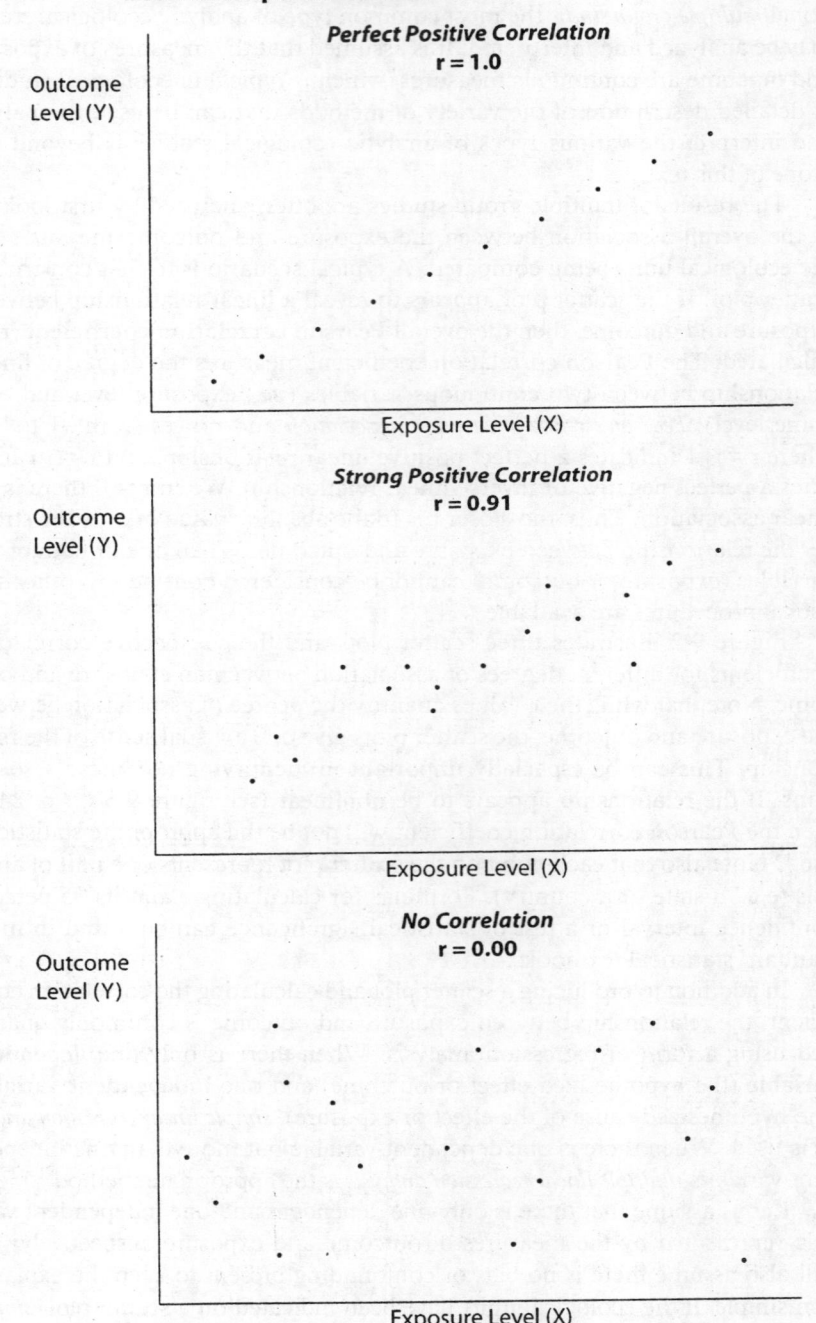

Figure 9-3   Scatter Plot Representing a Nonlinear Association between Exposure and Outcome

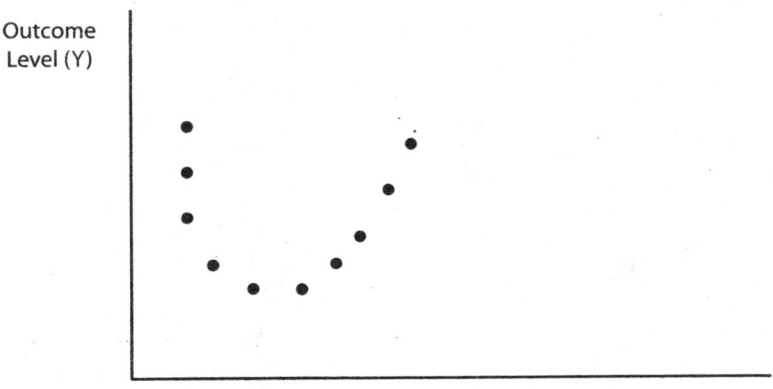

linear regression analysis can be used to develop a **regression line** that best describes the linear relationship between the outcome and exposure values (i.e., a line that best fits the data). The regression line will have the basic formula: Y = a + bX, where Y is the outcome measure; X is the exposure measure; a is the intercept, the point where the regression line crosses the y-axis; and b is the slope of the regression line, which tells us the rate of change in Y for each unit change in X.[15] While we will not actually perform regression analysis here (it is described in most basic statistics textbooks), the important point to remember is that the formula for the regression line (the **regression equation**) represents a *model* that allows epidemiologists to predict the outcome level (Y) based on a knowledge of the exposure level (X), given the estimated intercept and slope of the regression line.[15] Depending on how the data points cluster or scatter, the prediction ability may range from perfect to none (see figure 9-2).

Hal Morgenstern[2, 10] has described how the regression equation (Y = a + bX) can also be used to estimate a rate ratio (RR) at the individual level from an ecological study. This is done by calculating Y assuming all are exposed (X = 1) and then dividing that value by the value of Y assuming none is exposed (X = 0). For simplicity, this can be expressed by the following formula:

(9.1) $$RR = 1 + (b\ /\ a)$$

Note that in this formula a is the intercept, and b is the slope of the regression line. As an example, assume that the following regression equation was produced by an analysis of results from an ecological multiple-group study among 10 countries of the relationship between per capita alcohol consumption and rates of breast cancer in women:

$$Y = 1.2 + 0.6X$$

The estimated rate ratio for individuals in the study is therefore:

$$RR = 1 + (0.6 / 1.2) = 1 + 0.5 = 1.5$$

In other words, we might expect that those women living in the countries with high per capita alcohol consumption develop breast cancer at a rate of about 1.5 times greater than those living in the countries with low per capita alcohol consumption, all other factors being equal. This conclusion assumes that the exposure came before the outcome. This might be a reasonable assumption if alcohol consumption data were determined for a time period that preceded the determination of breast cancer rates by the average induction and latency periods for breast cancer. Using this method of estimating the RR for continuous data depends on being able to dichotomize both exposure and outcome status in a meaningful way. In this example the exposure (alcohol consumption) was dichotomized as high or low, and the outcome (breast cancer) was dichotomized as present or absent. At best, this is a crude way of estimating the individual association between the exposure and outcome assuming that it even exists at the individual level, which in itself represents an ecological fallacy. This method is presented more for intellectual interest than for actual use.

A helpful measure that is often cited when simple regression analysis is performed in an ecological multiple-group study is r^2, which is known as the **coefficient of determination** or simply **r squared**. An analogous measure, *multiple R squared* (R^2) is available when multiple regression is used. The coefficient of determination is a measure of the *magnitude of the effect* of the exposure on the outcome.[16] This measure reveals the proportion of the variance in the dependent variable (i.e., the outcome) that is explained by the independent variable (i.e., the exposure). Before one becomes overly impressed with seemingly high values of r, he or she should calculate r^2. For example, $r = 0.80$ produces $r^2 = 0.64$, which indicates that the exposure (independent variable) only explains 64 percent of the variance in the outcome (dependent variable). This means that 36 percent ($1 - 0.64 = 0.36$) of the variance is due to other factors. An r of 0.50 explains only 25 percent of the variance in the outcome. That means that 75 percent ($1 - 0.25 = 0.75$) of the variance is due to factors other than the exposure.

In summary, many analytic multiple-group ecological studies involve production of a scatter plot, computation of a correlation coefficient, generation of a regression equation, and calculation of the coefficient of determination. Each of these steps reveals something about the linear relationship between the exposure and outcome. When it is expected that the relationship is not linear or when a linear analysis reveals no relationship, other appropriate analytic procedures should be used. Finally, it should be noted that the use of the correlation coefficient as a measure of association is not restricted to the examination of results from ecological studies. In epidemiologic studies of individuals, however, other measures of association are more commonly used when it comes to analytic and experimental approaches. Figure 9-4 illustrates basic results from an analytic multiple-group study of milk and cheese consumption and deaths from coronary heart disease.

Figure 9-4   Ecological Correlation between Milk and Cheese Consumption and Mortality from Coronary Heart Disease for 14 Countries

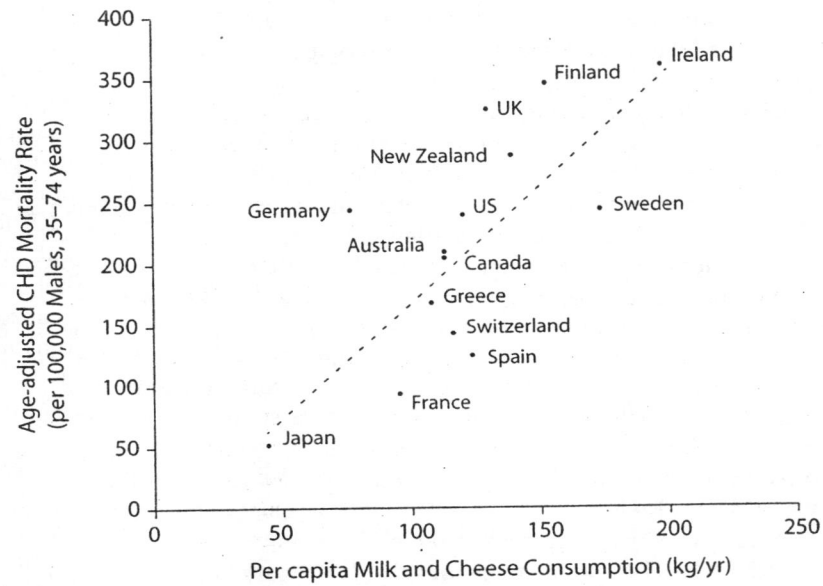

Analysis

r = 0.76

$r^2 = 57.8\%$

Regression Equation: Y = −13.6 + 1.9X

Explanation

The correlation between per capita milk and cheese consumption and the mortality rates in males from coronary heart disease is 0.76 for the 14 countries examined. Thus, those countries that consume higher per capita quantities of milk and cheese have higher rates of mortality from CHD in males than those that consume lower per capita quantities of milk and cheese, all other factors being equal. The regression model for this relationship explains 57.8% of the variability in the CHD mortality rates as indicated by r^2. The regression equation allows us to predict the rate of CHD mortality (Y) from a knowledge of per capita milk and cheese consumption (X). For Ireland, for example, X = 195; therefore, Y = −13.6 + 1.9 (195) = −13.6 + 370.5 = 356.9 deaths per 100,000 males, 35–74 years.

References: British Heart Foundation Health Promotion Research Group (1999). Coronary Heart Disease Statistics. Available: *http://www.dphpc.ox.ac.uk/bhfhprg/99stats* (Access date: February 15, 2000.); United States Department of Agriculture (1998). FAS Online: Fluid Milk and Cheese Consumption Per Capita, Selected Countries. Available: http://ffas.usda.gov/dlp2/circular/1997/97-07-dairy/toc.htm (Access date: February 15, 2000).

DESCRIPTIVE ECOLOGICAL STUDIES

Descriptive ecological studies, which were introduced in chapter 4, usually examine rates of health-related occurrences among one or more ecological units. They are sometimes termed exploratory.[2] Although no *a priori* hypotheses are being investigated in descriptive ecological studies, the findings often suggest hypotheses for further analysis.

Like their analytic counterparts, descriptive ecological studies may be classified as *multiple-group, time-trend,* or *mixed studies.* They may be useful in identifying patterns or trends in morbidity or mortality, including secular trends (chapter 1). An example is a study to determine if there are any differences in skin cancer mortality rates among various countries (a *descriptive multiple-group study*). Another example is a study that looks at changes in the incidence of malignant melanoma in one population over time (a *descriptive time-trend study*). An example of a *descriptive mixed study*, which combines features of the multiple-group and time-trend studies, is one that examined stomach cancer rates in several Asian countries during the last half of the 20th century. The study was designed to observe the pattern of stomach cancer and time trends. The authors reported the highest rates of stomach cancer incidence and mortality in Japan, followed by the Republic of Korea and China. The lowest rate was observed in Thailand. They also noted a decreased trend in stomach cancer mortality rates that was preceded by an increased trend in Japan in the 1950s and in Sri-Lanka in the 1950–60s. The authors recommended further studies of the relationship between host and environmental factors and stomach cancer in Asian countries.[17] Typical of most ecological studies, descriptive and analytic, the data for this study were obtained from secondary sources. Also, it should be clear that no *a priori* hypotheses between exposure and outcome were examined in any of the examples cited here. In fact, only outcome measures were observed.

ANALYTIC CROSS-SECTIONAL STUDIES

Key Design Features

In an **analytic cross-sectional study** one observes a sample of *individuals* from a defined population at a *single point in time*, that is, at a cross-section of the time continuum. Since exposure and outcome status are assessed at the *same* time, they are said to be determined simultaneously. The unit of analysis in a cross-sectional study is the individual, and relevant data are therefore collected for each person in the study population. In terms of methodology, most analytic cross-sectional studies employ population survey methods, such as face-to-face interviews, self-administered questionnaires, physical examinations, or telephone interviews.[18] Cross-sectional studies are sometimes referred to as **prevalence studies** or **prevalence surveys**, since prevalence is the usual measure of occurrence employed in these studies. The major use of analytic cross-sectional studies is testing *preliminary* hypotheses that may provide a basis for more definitive studies in the future. Thus, analytic cross-sectional studies are most appropriately undertaken when relatively little is known about the potential causes of a particular health-related problem.

An investigation by C. A. Mancuso and colleagues illustrates the analytic cross-sectional study design.[19] The purpose of the study was to assess the effects of depressive symptoms on the functional status and health-related quality of life of asthma patients. Two hundred and thirty outpatients with moderate asthma, between 18 and 62 years of age, from a primary care internal medicine practice in New York City were interviewed using appropriate methodology. An association was found between concurrent depressive symptoms and health-related quality of life with depressed patients being more likely to report lower health-related quality of life due to their asthma compared to those who were not depressed. It is important to note that both depression and health-related quality of life were assessed simultaneously in this study.

In the above example and in other analytic cross-sectional studies four basic steps are usually apparent. First, one or more *a priori* hypotheses about the relationships between specified exposures and outcomes is formulated. These are usually preliminary hypotheses, and there may or may not be predictions as to the direction of the relationships (i.e., they may be directional or non-directional hypotheses; see chapter 6). Second, the source population is determined, and the study population is selected, randomly if possible. Third, appropriate measures of exposure and outcome (e.g., prevalence) are determined simultaneously for each individual in the sample. Measures of exposure may be current or historical; measures of outcome are usually current. Primary or secondary data sources may be used. Fourth, the data are collected and analyzed to determine if a valid association exists between the exposure and outcome measures as hypothesized. These basic steps are summarized in figure 9-5.

Figure 9-5   Basic Steps in Conducting an Analytic Cross-Sectional Study

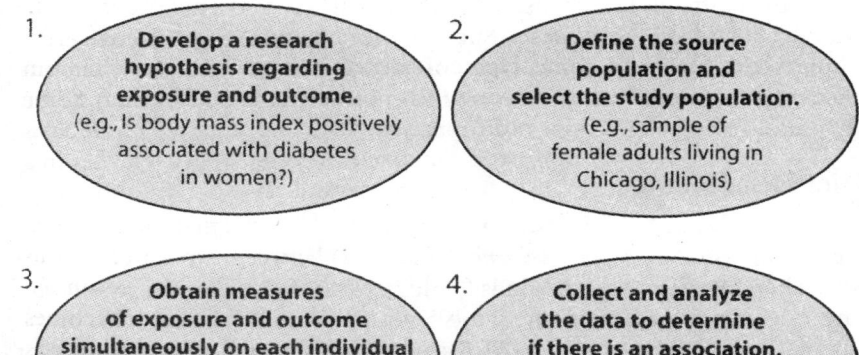

1. Develop a research hypothesis regarding exposure and outcome. (e.g., Is body mass index positively associated with diabetes in women?)

2. Define the source population and select the study population. (e.g., sample of female adults living in Chicago, Illinois)

3. Obtain measures of exposure and outcome simultaneously on each individual in the sample. (e.g., body mass index and diagnosis regarding diabetes)

4. Collect and analyze the data to determine if there is an association. (e.g., Is the prevalence of diabetes higher in those with a large body mass index?)

Major Advantages

Like ecological studies, cross-sectional studies are generally quicker, more economical, and easier to undertake than more sophisticated epidemiologic studies. One reason is that no follow-up time is involved. Cross-sectional studies are essentially *one-time* surveys* in which each participant's exposure and outcome status are assessed during the same time period. Most other types of epidemiologic studies where the unit of analysis is the individual are regarded as *longitudinal studies* (chapter 4). This is because, unlike most cross-sectional studies, exposure status is determined for a time period that *precedes* the development of the outcome.[20] For example, in a prospective cohort study (chapter 11) the investigators assess exposure status at the beginning of the study and follow individuals over time to determine their subsequent outcome status. Most case-control studies (chapter 10) can also be considered longitudinal since exposure status is usually determined for a time period that ostensibly precedes the development of the outcome.

Another advantage of cross-sectional studies is that the findings may be more representative of well-defined general populations than those of other types of epidemiologic studies. This is because general populations are often sought to test the study hypotheses. Other types of analytic and experimental studies frequently rely on subjects that must meet several, sometimes restrictive, eligibility criteria to participate. Also, significant subject losses during follow-up periods in cohort and experimental studies may alter the original composition of the sample. These factors may lead to findings that are not necessarily representative of the source population. In addition, these studies tend to focus on patient samples more often than cross-sectional studies and, thus, are less likely to produce findings which are representative of general populations.

An additional advantage of cross-sectional studies is that they may be the only appropriate design to use when the onset of the study disease (i.e., incidence) is difficult to establish and when health care is only sought in the advanced stages of the disease. Such is the situation with osteoarthritis, chronic bronchitis, and some types of mental illness.[21] In these circumstances, prevalence, which is measured in cross-sectional studies, may be the only useful measure of disease occurrence.

Major Disadvantages

A major disadvantage of analytic cross-sectional studies is that one generally cannot establish the *temporal sequence* (chapter 7) between exposure and outcome. Therefore, if an association is found between a given exposure and outcome, one usually cannot be sure if the exposure preceded the outcome or the outcome preceded the exposure. As discussed in chapter 7, it is essential that exposure precede outcome in order for an association to be considered

---

*Exceptions are the panel study and repeated surveys, which are types of longitudinal cross-sectional studies. These were classified as hybrid studies in chapter 4.

causal. This problem can be illustrated by the association between poverty and mental illness found in many cross-sectional studies. The so-called "Breeder" hypothesis suggests that poverty causes mental illness, while the "Social Drift" hypothesis suggests that mental illness causes poverty. Unfortunately, neither hypothesis can be confirmed by an analytic cross-sectional study. This is due to the simultaneous assessment of exposure and outcome, which is characteristic of this study design. Because of this weakness, one needs to be cautious in interpreting the results of cross-sectional studies. Simply put, *association is not synonymous with causation*. This disadvantage practically vanishes, however, in those occasional instances where the exposure is an inherent factor that does not change over time. For example, if a valid association is found between blood type and colon cancer based on a cross-sectional study, one could state confidently that blood type preceded colon cancer and not the other way around. Thus, it might be possible to conclude that a cause-effect relationship exists between blood type and colon cancer from a cross-sectional study if other important guidelines are also met (see discussion of Hill's postulates in chapter 7).

Another disadvantage of cross-sectional studies is the potential problem of *prevalence-incidence bias* (chapter 8). Because cross-sectional studies typically measure disease prevalence versus incidence, samples tend to overrepresent disease cases of long duration, while underrepresenting those of short duration. This is due to the fact that those cases that tend to recover or die soon after contracting the study outcome have less of a chance of being included in the study population. If the degree of association between exposure and outcome differs significantly for cases of short duration compared to those of long duration, the results could reflect prevalence-incidence bias.

A notable disadvantage of cross-sectional studies is that they are unsuitable for investigating rare exposures or outcomes. For example, if the prevalence of a given outcome is only 2.0 cases per 100,000 population, then on average a sample size of 500,000 participants would be necessary to have reasonable assurance that just 10 cases of the outcome would be detected in the sample. This clearly does not represent a cost-efficient way of testing a hypothesis.

Finally, it is possible that simultaneous assessments of *current* exposure and outcome could lead to erroneous results if exposure status has changed in a significant portion of the sample since the development of the outcome or if a significant portion of exposed persons who had the outcome no longer have it at the time of the study. This problem does not represent an inherent limitation of the cross-sectional study design but underscores the need for careful planning in designing this type of study. It may be necessary, for example, to ask subjects about when exposures occurred and about their duration. Similarly, it may be necessary to test for evidence of past disease.[21] Table 9-2 on the following page summarizes the major advantages and disadvantages of analytic cross-sectional studies.

Table 9-2   Major Advantages and Disadvantages of Analytic Cross-Sectional Studies

Advantages	Disadvantages
1. They are relatively quick, economical, and easy to conduct.	1. Generally, one cannot determine cause-effect relationships since the temporal sequence between exposure and outcome is usually not known.
2. The findings may be more representative of general populations than other epidemiologic studies.	2. There is a potential for prevalence-incidence bias because transitory or fatal cases are likely to be missed.
3. They may be the only appropriate epidemiologic study to use when incidence cannot be measured.	3. They are very inefficient when exposures or outcomes are rare.
	4. Associations based on current exposure or outcome may not be representative of those based on past exposure or outcome.

Analysis and Interpretation

When exposure and outcome status are classified dichotomously, the findings of an analytic cross-sectional study can be analyzed using a simple 2 × 2 contingency table. If the exposure and outcome are measured on more than two levels (e.g., low exposure, moderate exposure, high exposure and no disease, moderate disease, severe disease), then a somewhat more complex table is used (e.g., 3 × 3). For simplicity, the discussion of the analysis of cross-sectional studies will assume that exposure and outcome are each measured dichotomously.

A first step in analyzing the results of an analytic cross-sectional study is to place the frequencies of exposed and unexposed subjects in a contingency table according to whether the outcome is present or absent. The following table is a template for cross-sectional analysis.

Template for Cross-Sectional Studies

	Outcome Status		
Exposure Status	Present	Absent	
Exposed	a	b	a + b
Unexposed	c	d	c + d
	a + c	b + d	n

The frequencies a, b, c, and d represent the number of exposed persons with the outcome, the number of exposed persons without the outcome, the number of unexposed persons with the outcome, and the number of unexposed persons without the outcome, respectively. The sums a + c and b + d represent the number of persons with and without the outcome, respectively, without regard to exposure status. Similarly, a + b and c + d are the number of exposed and unexposed persons, respectively, without regard to outcome status. The total number of subjects in the sample is represented by n, which is the sum of a, b, c, and d.

These frequencies provide the basic information needed to calculate applicable measures of association. Two measures of association commonly calculated in cross-sectional studies are the:

- Prevalence ratio
- Prevalence odds ratio

Both measures were introduced in chapter 6. Also sometimes used, but not discussed here, is the *prevalence difference*, which was also described in chapter 6. From a practical point of view, the choice of which measure of association to use in a cross-sectional study is largely arbitrary, although there are guiding principles based on sampling protocols and analytical methods as well as advocates of one measure over the other.[22, 23] When the outcome is rare (say, a prevalence of less than 0.05), the prevalence ratio and the prevalence odds ratio tend to correspond rather closely.[24] The results can be quite disparate, however, when the outcome is relatively common.

Prevalence ratio.   As indicated in chapter 6, the prevalence ratio (PR) is the ratio of the prevalence of the outcome in the exposed group (P_e) to the prevalence of the outcome in the unexposed group (P_{ue}). Referring to the template presented above, this is equivalent to:

(9.2)

$$PR = \frac{P_e}{P_{ue}} = \frac{a/(a+b)}{c/(c+d)}$$

If desired, one can also calculate the overall prevalence of the outcome in the study population, which is known as the **crude prevalence**. It is calculated as shown in formula 9.3.

(9.3) $$P_c = [(a + c) / n] \times 10^n$$

In this formula, P_c refers to crude prevalence, a + c is the number of those with the outcome of interest, n is the total sample size, and 10^n is the population base (defined in chapter 5). If the sample data represent a *probability sample* (chapter 8), this is a *point estimate* (chapter 5) of the prevalence of the outcome in the sampled population.

As with other ratio measures of association, the size of the PR provides an indication of the strength of the association between a given exposure and outcome (see table 6-3). The PR has a minimum value of zero but no definitive upper limit. A PR of 1.0 indicates no association between exposure and outcome, while a PR of 2.0 indicates that the outcome is twice *as common* in the exposed group compared to the unexposed group. It also depicts a positive association between exposure and outcome. A PR of 0.5 means that the outcome is only half *as common* in the exposed group compared to the unexposed group. It represents a negative or inverse association between exposure and outcome. In summary, the further the PR departs from 1.0, the greater the association, positive or negative, between the exposure and outcome (see table 6-2).

Because the PR is based on prevalence measures (point prevalence to be precise), its interpretation is best restricted to statements about the *frequency or prevalence* of the outcome in the exposed group relative to the unexposed group. Unlike a risk ratio, statements about increased or decreased *risk* are generally not appropriate, since prevalence tends to be a poor estimate of risk (see chapter 5).* The *percent relative effect* (chapter 6) for the PR can be calculated using formula 6.5. It represents the percent increased or decreased *prevalence* instead of risk, however.

Prevalence odds ratio.   The **prevalence odds ratio** (POR), first discussed in chapter 6, is an odds ratio based on prevalent versus incident cases. Sometimes it is simply referred to as an odds ratio (OR) without qualification. It can be calculated as shown in formula 9.4.

(9.4)
$$POR = \frac{a/b}{c/d} = \frac{ad}{bc}$$

In this formula, a / b is the prevalence odds among the exposed group, and c / d is the prevalence odds among the unexposed group based on the frequencies in the 2 × 2 template shown earlier. The actual calculation and interpretation of the POR is illustrated in problem 9-1 along with the other measures referred to in this section.

Confidence intervals and tests of significance.   Approximate confidence intervals for the prevalence ratio and prevalence odds ratio can be determined using an inexpensive scientific calculator. The relevant equations are given in formulas 9.5 and 9.6, respectively.[25, 26]

(9.5) $$95\% \ CI = \exp\left\{\ln(PR) \pm 1.96\sqrt{\left[(b/a)/(a+b)\right] + \left[(d/c)/(c+d)\right]}\right\}$$

(9.6) $$95\% \ CI = \exp\left\{\ln(POR) \pm 1.96\sqrt{(1/a) + (1/b) + (1/c) + (1/d)}\right\}$$

The term **ln** in these expressions refers to the *natural logarithm,* so the expression ln (PR) or ln (POR) is the natural logarithm of the respective measure of

*Some suggest that the prevalence ratio measures the risk of *having* the outcome in the exposed group to that in the unexposed group, whereas the risk ratio measures the risk of *developing* the outcome in the exposed group to that in the unexposed group.

association. The remainder of each expression to the right of the natural logarithm is ± 1.96 times an estimate of the *standard error* of the measure of association. The ± 1.96 corresponds to 95% confidence limits based on a normal distribution. For 99% confidence limits the multiplier is ± 2.58. The term **exp** to left of the braced { } expression refers to *exponential* or e, which is the base of the natural logarithm just as 10 is the base of the common logarithm you probably learned about in high school. It has a value of approximately 2.71828, but like the measure pi (π), it is a irrational constant whose exact value cannot be determined. In the formulas, exp (or e) is being raised by the value of the entire expression in braces. The generic equation for formulas 9.5 and 9.6 is 95% CI = $\exp^x$ where x is everything in the braces. For further explanation of these terms see the glossary at the end of the text.

For those not so mathematically inclined, it may be somewhat comforting to know that you can calculate these confidence intervals in just a few steps using an inexpensive scientific calculator. First, enter your data in a 2 × 2 table using the format in the template provided earlier. Though each calculator is different, the basic steps should be as follows:

1. Calculate the expression under the square root sign, and take its square root.

2. Multiply the square root obtained in step 1 by 1.96. Record this value on a piece of paper or store it in your calculator's memory.

3. Enter the value of the PR or POR in your calculator depending on which formula you are using and strike the key labeled ln. Record or store this value in the calculator's second memory.

4. Subtract the value obtained in step 2 from the value obtained in step 3, and strike the exp or e^x key on your calculator. (Note: you may need to first strike the second function key depending on the model of your calculator). The value you obtain is the 95% *lower* confidence limit (LCL).

5. Add the value obtained in step 2 to the value obtained in step 3, and strike the exp or e^x key on your calculator. (Note: you may need to first strike the second function key depending on the model of your calculator). The value you obtain is the 95% *upper* confidence limit (UCL).

Problem 9-1 includes the calculation and interpretation of confidence intervals for the prevalence ratio and prevalence odds ratio, respectively.

The statistical significance of the PR or POR can be determined using a **chi-square test (χ^2)** for independence *based on a 2 × 2 contingency table with* one degree of freedom.[27] The formula for calculating this specific measure is:

(9.7)
$$\chi^2 = \frac{n(ad - bc)^2}{(a+b)(c+d)(a+c)(b+d)}$$

Note that the values a-d and n are based on the 2 × 2 template described earlier in this section.

If the value of the chi-square test statistic is from 3.84 to 6.62, the association is considered statistically significant at the 0.05 level (i.e., $p \leq 0.05$). If the value is from 6.63 to 10.82, the association is considered statistically significant at the 0.01 level (i.e., p ≤ 0.01), and if the value is equal to or greater than 10.83, the association is regarded as significant at the 0.001 level (p ≤ 0.001). These values, along with examples, appear in table 9-3.

Table 9-3 Common χ^2 Values and Their Associated P-Values*

χ^2	p	Example
0.00 – 3.83	> 0.05	($\chi^2 = 2.92$, p > 0.05)
3.84 – 6.62	≤ 0.05	($\chi^2 = 4.75$, p < 0.05)
6.63 – 10.82	≤ 0.01	($\chi^2 = 6.63$, p = 0.01)
10.83 or more	≤ 0.001	($\chi^2 = 12.91$, p < 0.001)

*Based on one degree of freedom, which applies to chi-square when calculated from a 2 x 2 table.

Problem 9-1: Analysis and Interpretation of Analytic Cross-Sectional Studies

Two epidemiologists wanted to know if heavy cigarette smoking in men (more than two packs per day) is associated with clinical depression. To test their hypothesis, they randomly selected a sample of 149 adult males from Gilford County and initiated an analytic cross-sectional study. The men were queried about current cigarette smoking habits and completed a validated questionnaire designed to measure clinical depression. The results are shown in the following 2 × 2 contingency table. Based on these data, calculate the crude prevalence (P_c) of clinical depression in the sample, the prevalence ratio (PR), and the prevalence odds ratio (POR). Also, calculate the 95% confidence interval and statistical significance for eac' measure of association. Interpret your results.

	Clinical Depression	
Cigarette Smoking	Present	Absent
Exposed	27	34
Unexposed	26	62

Solution:

Warning: Earlier in this section a 2 × 2 template was developed using the letters a–d to represent the frequencies of specific combinations of exposure and outcome status. It is important to note the order in which these letters are used in the table since all the formulas in this section are based on that particular order. If a–d are ordered differently, the formulas provided in this section may no longer be valid.

Step 1: Calculate the *crude prevalence* using formula 9.3 and the data provided in the above contingency table.

$$P_c = [(a + c) / n] \times 10^n = [(27 + 26) / 149] \times 10^n = (53 / 149) \times 10^n$$
$$= 0.356 \times 10^2 = 35.6 \text{ per } 100$$

Step 2: Calculate the *prevalence ratio* using formula 9.2 and the data provided in the contingency table.

$$P_e = [a / (a + b)] = [27 / (27 + 34)] = (27 / 61) = 0.443$$
$$P_{ue} = [c / (c + d)] = [26 / (26 + 62)] = (26 / 88) = 0.295$$
$$PR = P_e / P_{ue} = 0.443 / 0.295 = 1.5$$

Step 3: Calculate the *prevalence odds ratio* using formula 9.4 and the data provided in the above contingency table.

$$POR = ad / bc = (27 \times 62) / (34 \times 26) = 1{,}674 / 884 = 1.9$$

Step 4: Calculate the *95% confidence intervals* for the PR and POR, respectively, using formulas 9.5 and 9.6.

$$95\% \text{ CI} = \exp\left\{\ln(PR) \pm 1.96\sqrt{\left[(b/a)/(a+b)\right] + \left[(d/c)/(c+d)\right]}\right\} =$$
$$\exp\left\{\ln(1.5) \pm 1.96\sqrt{\left[(34/27)/(27+34)\right] + \left[(62/26)/(26+62)\right]}\right\} =$$
$$\exp\{0.405 \pm 0.428\}$$

Thus, LCL = exp {−0.023} = 0.98, and UCL = exp {0.833} = 2.3. Hence, the approximate 95% CI for the PR is 0.98 to 2.3. Note that the LCL is being raised to a negative power. Thus, −0.023, and not 0.023, should be used in calculating this confidence limit.

$$95\% \text{ CI} = \exp\left\{\ln(POR) \pm 1.96\sqrt{(1/a) + (1/b) + (1/c) + (1/d)}\right\} =$$
$$\exp\left\{\ln(1.9) \pm 1.96\sqrt{(1/27) + (1/34) + (1/26) + (1/62)}\right\} =$$
$$\exp\{0.642 \pm 0.682\}$$

Thus, LCL = exp {−0.040} = 0.96, and UCL = exp {1.32} = 3.7. Hence, the approximate 95% CI for the POR = 0.96 to 3.7. Note that the LCL is being raised to a negative power. Thus, −0.040, and not 0.040, should be used in calculating this confidence limit.

Step 5: Calculate *chi-square* (χ^2) for the 2 × 2 contingency table using formula 9.7 to determine if either the PR or POR is statistically significant.

$$\chi^2 = \frac{n(ad - bc)^2}{(a+b)(c+d)(a+c)(b+d)} =$$
$$\frac{149[(26 \times 62) - (34 \times 26)]^2}{(27 + 34)(26 + 62)(27 + 26)(34 + 62)} =$$
$$\frac{149(1{,}674 - 884)^2}{(61)(88)(53)(96)} = 3.40$$

Answer: The *crude prevalence* of clinical depression among adult males in Gilford County is estimated to be 35.6 cases per 100. This implies that slightly more than one-third of the adult males in Gilford County are clinically depressed. The *prevalence ratio* is 1.5 (95% CI = 0.98 to 2.3), indicating that clinical depression appears to be 1.5 times more common among adult men who are heavy cigarette smokers in Gilford County compared to those who are not. We can say that we are 95% confident that the true prevalence ratio is between 0.98 and 2.3. Statistically, the prevalence ratio is not significant at conventional levels, which we can infer from the confidence interval, since it contains 1.0, or from the chi-square test result, which had a value of only 3.40. A chi-square of at least 3.84 is required for an association to be statistically significant at the 0.05 level (see table 9-3). This implies that chance may be a likely explanation for the finding. The *prevalence odds ratio* is 1.9 (95% CI = 0.96 to 3.7). This indicates that the odds of having clinical depression are 1.9 times higher among adult men who are heavy cigarette smokers in Gilford County than those who are not. We can also say that we are 95% confident that the true prevalence odds ratio is between 0.96 and 3.7. The conclusion regarding statistical significance is the same as that for the prevalence ratio.

Comments:

1. The prevalence found in this study indicates that clinical depression is very common among adult males in the county. While the crude prevalence is not required to test the investigators' hypothesis, it is a useful statistic when one is interested in the burden of a particular outcome on a given population. It can also help explain differences between the prevalence ratio and the prevalence odds ratio in cross-sectional studies (see comment 2).

2. The prevalence ratio (PR) of 1.5 implies a relatively weak association between heavy cigarette smoking and clinical depression in the study population (see table 6-3). The 95 percent confidence interval for the PR gives us an idea of the likely range of prevalence ratios we might encounter with continued sampling. We would expect that 95 out of 100 probability samples would reveal a PR somewhere between 0.98 and 2.3. The prevalence odds ratio (POR) of 1.9 implies a moderate association between heavy cigarette smoking and clinical depression in the study population. The likely range of PORs is 0.96 to 3.7. As noted earlier in the chapter, the PR approximates the POR when the prevalence of the outcome is rare (i.e., less than 5.0 per 100). In this problem the prevalence of the outcome was 35.6 per 100. Thus, it is not surprising that the PR and POR are different. It is also important to realize that these two measures of association measure different things. While the PR is a ratio of prevalences, the POR is a ratio of odds. The PR is analogous to the risk ratio often cited in cohort studies, and the POR is analogous to the odds ratio (incidence odds) typically used in case-control studies. Finally, it is helpful to remember that descriptions like "relatively weak" or "moderate" association used here are based on general rules of thumb and not precise scientific criteria. Therefore, not too much weight should be given to the different descriptions.

3. The statistical significance of both the PR and the POR can be determined using the chi-square test for independence based on a 2 × 2 contingency table. This is a test statistic (chapter 6) that employs nominal (categorical) data and is based on the chi-square distribution with one degree of freedom. Although statistical significance testing has found disfavor with many epidemiologists, it continues to be used in health research. One should keep in mind, however, that lack of statistical significance, as found in this problem, may be due to a lack of *power* (chapter 8), which can result if the sample size is too small to detect a given level of association. The power of a study should be estimated before the study is initiated in order to mini-

mize the probability of a type II error. Power can be calculated using various software programs, some of which are free (see appendix A). The lack of statistical significance found for the PR and POR in this study may be due to a type II error. For example, the power to detect a PR of 1.5 is only 39 percent based on power calculations. This is well below the 80 percent traditionally considered the minimally acceptable level. To reach 80 percent power, the sample size would need to be 371 versus 149. Once again, this reiterates the importance of measuring power prior to beginning a study.

4. It is important to realize in this problem that we do not know whether heavy cigarette smoking preceded the development of clinical depression or whether clinical depression preceded heavy cigarette smoking. This is a major disadvantage of most cross-sectional studies. As a consequence, we cannot say whether heavy cigarette smoking is likely to be a cause of clinical depression. This would require a different type of study.

Other Issues in Analysis

The findings of analytic cross-sectional studies, like other epidemiologic studies, may be subject to various sources of selection and information bias as well as confounding. In addition, there may be *interactions* (see chapters 10 and 11) between the study exposures and other factors, such as age, sex, race/ethnicity, and so forth. These need to be examined and explained. To the extent possible, analytic cross-sectional studies should be designed to prevent or minimize sources of bias and confounding. Restriction, matching, and statistical control in the analysis may be used to control confounding as discussed in chapter 8 and subsequent chapters. Matching, however, is rarely used in cross-sectional studies. This is because there is usually no information regarding subject status on potential confounders or study exposures prior to initiating an investigation.[21] With regard to statistical control in the analysis, the methods of controlling confounding are the same as those used in cohort studies (chapter 11). Therefore, they are not discussed here. Random error, which has been described in previous chapters, should also be considered when assessing the findings of cross-sectional studies as well as those of other types of epidemiologic studies. The precision of the findings of a cross-sectional study can be enhanced by having sufficient sample size, which is related to study power (defined in chapter 8). Methods of estimating minimum sample size requirements and power are discussed in chapter 11. These methods can also be applied to cross-sectional studies.

DESCRIPTIVE CROSS-SECTIONAL STUDIES

Descriptive cross-sectional studies typically look at the prevalence of one or more health-related occurrences according to a variety of "categorizing factors" such as age group, sex, or race/ethnicity. There are no *a priori* hypotheses to examine, and the studies may be considered exploratory. For example, a study of over 1,000 college students was conducted at a university in Illinois to determine differences in levels of wellness by gender, race, and academic class standing. The findings indicated in general that female college students showed higher levels of wellness than males, and white students showed higher levels of wellness than nonwhites. Levels of wellness also appeared to increase with academic class standing.[28] None of these associations had been hypothesized prior to the study. Therefore, the study is appropriately classified as descriptive. *Analytic cross-sectional studies*, in contrast, are designed to examine *a priori* hypotheses about associations between specified exposures and outcomes. Well-designed descriptive cross-sectional studies are more likely to use probability samples than their analytic counterparts.

While descriptive cross-sectional studies do not examine *a priori* hypotheses, they are useful in generating hypotheses for additional study. They are also beneficial in measuring the impact of health-related occurrences in a defined population. A relatively recent clinical study, for example, looked at the prevalence and frequency of intimate partner violence (IPV) in the adult inpatient acute care units of a psychiatric hospital. The subjects had suicidal ideation and had been living with an intimate partner for at least six months prior to hospitalization. The authors found that over 90 percent of the subjects reported IPV in the past year. They concluded that psychiatric patients with suicidal ideation or intent would benefit from screening for IPV and available treatment options.[29] Descriptive cross-sectional studies are also sometimes performed at the beginning of prospective cohort studies to determine the initial exposure status of each subject and to assure that only subjects initially free from the study outcome are included in the analysis (see chapter 11).

In terms of statistical analysis, the basic measures used in descriptive cross-sectional studies are frequently the same as those used in their analytic counterparts. These include measures of prevalence and measures of association such as the prevalence difference, the prevalence ratio, and the prevalence odds ratio. A descriptive cross-sectional study of risk-taking behaviors conducted among a sample of 602 adolescents attending nine junior and senior high schools in rural northwestern Illinois, for example, revealed notable differences between males and females with regard to the use of smokeless tobacco (PR = 3.6), cocaine or hard drug use (PR = 2.3), and the use of inhalants (PR = 2.8). In each instance, males were more likely to be using the indicated substances than females. This study was exploratory and looked at the prevalence of a variety of outcomes, including substance use, sexual behaviors, antisocial activities, and mental and emotional health.[30]

SUMMARY

- Analytic ecological studies, which investigate groups of people as a whole versus the individuals comprising the groups, are conducted by first developing a research hypothesis about the association between one or more exposures and one or more outcomes. Next, the ecological units (groups) to be compared are selected, and overall or summary measures of exposure and outcome are obtained for each ecological unit, generally from secondary sources. The data are then typically graphed on a scatter plot with the x-axis typically representing exposure levels and the y-axis outcome levels. Often one looks for a correlation (e.g., Pearson's r) between exposure and outcome and uses linear regression to predict outcome based on exposure. There are three major types of ecological studies—multiple-group studies, time-trend studies, and mixed studies. Sometimes in epidemiologic studies where the units of interest are individuals ecological variables are used to measure one or more exposures either for convenience or because of presumed greater construct validity of the particular measures.

- A principal advantage of analytic ecological studies is that they are relatively quick and inexpensive to perform. In addition, they are the only common type of observational study that is suitable for examining associations between exposures and outcomes at the group level. They are also valuable when the intra-group variability on the exposure variable is small, but the inter-group variability is large across ecological units. Finally, when exposure can vary significantly within individuals, employing an ecological study may provide a more stable measure of the exposure. Major disadvantages include the possibility of making an ecological fallacy, a type of cross-level bias; inaccuracies in available exposure or outcome data; multicollinearity; and other difficulties related to controlling for potential confounders, establishing the correct temporal sequence between exposure and outcome, and migration of individuals across ecological units.

- Analytic cross-sectional studies, where the unit of analysis is the individual, are conducted at a single point in time; that is, exposure and outcome status are assessed simultaneously. Along with their descriptive counterparts, these studies are often referred to as prevalence studies, and they usually employ population survey methods. They are particularly suitable for examining preliminary hypotheses. After forming one or more *a priori* hypotheses about the associations between specified exposures and outcomes, a study population is selected. The subjects are assessed simultaneously with regard to exposure and outcome status to determine if an association exists. Common measures of association used in cross-sectional studies are prevalence ratios and prevalence odds ratios. Prevalence differences may also be used. Statistical significance can be determined using an appropriate chi-square test for independence.

- Like ecological studies, cross-sectional studies are generally quicker, more economical, and easier to undertake than more sophisticated epidemiologic studies. In addition, the findings may be more representative of general populations than other analytic studies since general populations are often sought to test study hypotheses. An additional advantage of cross-sectional studies is that they may be the only appropriate design to use when the incidence of the study outcome is difficult to establish and when health care is only sought in the advanced stages of the disease. In these circumstances, prevalence, which is measured in cross-sectional studies, may be the only useful measure of disease occurrence. A major disadvantage is that one cannot generally establish the correct temporal sequence between exposure and outcome since they are measured simultaneously. This limits the usefulness of cross-sectional studies in uncovering causal factors. Other disadvantages include possible prevalence-incidence bias, unsuitability for studying rare outcomes, and dealing with changes in exposure or outcome status that occurred prior to the study.

- Both ecological and cross-sectional studies are subject to potential sources of bias and confounding, which should be prevented, minimized, or controlled to the extent feasible. Both types of studies may be classified as descriptive or analytic depending primarily on the purpose of the study.

New Terms

- analytic cross-sectional study
- analytic ecological study
- chi-square test
- coefficient of determination
- construct validity
- contextual effects
- cross-level bias
- crude prevalence
- dependent variable
- descriptive cross-sectional study
- descriptive ecological study
- e
- exp

- independent variable
- ln
- multicollinearity
- multilevel analysis
- Pearson correlation coefficient
- prevalence odds ratio
- prevalence study
- prevalence survey
- r
- r squared
- regression equation
- regression line
- scatter plot

Study Questions and Exercises

1. Describe how you would design an analytic ecological study in the United States to examine the hypothesis that consumption of high levels of radium in drinking water are associated with bone cancer. Also, describe how you would design an analytic cross-sectional study to test the same hypothesis. What are the strengths and limitations of your proposed designs?

2. An analytic ecological study was performed among 12 countries to test the hypothesis that beef consumption is associated with gastrointestinal cancers. The following correlation was reported by the investigators: $r = 0.41$. The regression equation for the relationship was $Y = 3.3 + 0.2X$, where X is the per capita level of beef consumption in ounces per day, and Y is the age-adjusted mortality rate from gastrointestinal cancers per 100,000 population. Based on this information, how much of the variability in the gas-

trointestinal cancer mortality rates is explained by beef consumption? Is this a large amount, and why or why not? Also, if a country's estimated per capita beef consumption is 16 ounces per day, what is the estimated gastrointestinal cancer mortality rate in that country based on the study findings? Finally, what is the estimated rate ratio for gastrointestinal cancers due to beef consumption, assuming a cause-effect relationship?

3. Two investigators were interested in testing the hypothesis that high educational attainment is associated with more frequent unintentional injuries in the home. To test their hypothesis the investigators selected a random sample of 5,000 men and women, 21 years of age and older, living in owner-occupied, single-family dwellings in Seattle, Washington. Data were also collected on potential confounders, such as age, sex, income level, and health status. The results of this analytic cross-sectional study were as follows:

- 10% of the sample had high educational attainment (defined as a college degree or higher) and unintentional injuries in the home in the previous 12 months

- 10% of the sample had high educational attainment but no unintentional injuries in the home in the previous 12 months

- 20% of the sample had low educational attainment (defined as having less than a college degree) and unintentional injuries in the home in the previous 12 months

- 60% of the sample had low educational attainment but no unintentional injuries in the home in the previous 12 months

Based on this information, calculate and interpret: (a) the crude prevalence of unintentional injuries in the home, (b) the prevalence ratio and its 95% confidence interval, (c) the prevalence odds ratio and its 95% confidence interval, and (d) the statistical significance of the prevalence and prevalence odds ratios. Assuming that the study was designed to minimize bias and confounding, was the investigators' hypothesis supported, and why or why not?

References

1. Vogt, W. P. (1999). *Dictionary of Statistics and Methodology: A Nontechnical Guide for the Social Sciences*, 2nd ed. Thousand Oaks, CA: Sage Publications.
2. Morgenstern, H. (1995). Uses of Ecologic Studies in Epidemiology: Concepts, Principles, and Methods. *Annual Review of Public Health* 16: 61–81.
3. Szklo, M., and Nieto, F. J. (2000). *Epidemiology: Beyond the Basics*. Gaithersburg, MD: Aspen.
4. St. Leger, A. S., Cochrane, A. L., and Moore, F. (1979). Factors Associated with Cardiac Mortality in Developed Countries with Particular Reference to the Consumption of Wine. *Lancet* 1 (8124): 1017–1020.
5. Nanji, A. A. (1985). Alcohol and Ischemic Heart Disease: Wine, Beer or Both? *International Journal of Cardiology* 8 (4): 487–489.
6. Hennekens, C. H., Willett, W., Rosner, B., Cole, D. S., and Mayrent, S. L. (1979). Effects of Beer, Wine, Liquor in Coronary Deaths. *Journal of the American Medical Association* 242 (18): 1973–1974.

7. Gronbaek, M., Deis, A., Sorensen, T. I., Becker, U., Schnohr, P., and Jensen, G. (1995). Mortality Associated with Moderate Intakes of Wine, Beer, or Spirits. *British Medical Journal* 310 (6988): 1165–1169.

8. Woodward, M. (1999). *Epidemiology: Study Design and Data Analysis.* Boca Raton, FL: Chapman & Hall/CRC.

9. Schwartz, S. (1994). The Fallacy of the Ecological Fallacy: The Potential Misuse of a Concept and the Consequences. *American Journal of Public Health* 84 (5): 819–824.

10. Morgenstern, H. (1982). Uses of Ecologic Analysis in Epidemiologic Research. *American Journal of Public Health* 72 (12): 1336–1344.

11. Oleckno, W. A. (1982). The National Interim Primary Drinking Water Regulations: Part I— Historical Development. *Journal of Environmental Health* 44 (5): 236–239.

12. Rothman, K. J. (1986). *Modern Epidemiology.* Boston: Little, Brown and Company.

13. Dawson, B., and Trapp, R. G. (2001). *Basic & Clinical Biostatistics*, 3rd ed. New York: Lange Medical Books/McGraw-Hill.

14. Jekel, J. F., Elmore, J. G., and Katz, D. L. (1996). *Epidemiology, Biostatistics, and Preventive Medicine.* Philadelphia: W. B. Saunders Company.

15. Wassertheil-Smoller, S. (1990). *Biostatistics and Epidemiology: A Primer for Health Professionals.* New York: Springer-Verlag.

16. Norman, G. R., and Streiner, D. L. (1994). *Biostatistics: The Bare Essentials.* St. Louis: Mosby.

17. Ngoan, L. T., and Yoshimura, T. (2002). Pattern and Time Trends of Stomach Cancer in Asia from 1950–99. *Asian Pacific Journal of Cancer Prevention* 3 (1): 47–54.

18. Last, J. M., ed. (1995). *A Dictionary of Epidemiology*, 3rd ed. New York: Oxford University Press.

19. Mancuso, C. A., Peterson, M. G., and Charlson, M. E. (2000). Effects of Depressive Symptoms on Health-related Quality of Life in Asthma Patients. *Journal of General Internal Medicine* 15 (5): 301–310.

20. Rothman, K. J. (2002). *Epidemiology: An Introduction.* New York: Oxford University Press.

21. Kelsey, J. L., Thompson, W. D., and Evans, A. S. (1986). *Methods in Observational Epidemiology.* New York: Oxford University Press.

22. Pearce, N. (2004). Effect Measures in Prevalence Studies. *Environmental Health Perspectives* 112 (10): 1047–1050.

23. Thompson, M. L., Myers, J. E., and Kriebel, D. (1998). Prevalence Odds Ratio or Prevalence Ratio in the Analysis of Cross Sectional Data: What is to be Done? *Occupational and Environmental Medicine* 55: 272–277.

24. Gerstman, B. B. (1998). *Epidemiology Kept Simple: An Introduction to Classic and Modern Epidemiology.* New York: Wiley-Liss.

25. Katz, D., Baptista, J., Azen, S. P., and Pike, M. C. (1978). Obtaining Confidence Intervals for the Risk Ratio in Cohort Studies. *Biometrics* 34: 469–474.

26. Woolf, B. (1955). On Estimating the Relation between Blood Group and Disease. *Annals of Human Genetics* 19: 251–253.

27. Ferguson, G. A. (1976). *Statistical Analysis in Psychology and Education*, 4th ed. New York: McGraw-Hill Book Company.

28. Oleckno, W. A., and Blacconiere, M. J. (1990). Wellness of College Students and Differences by Gender, Race, and Class Standing. *College Student Journal* 24: 421–429.

29. Heru, A. M., Stuart, G. L., Rainey, S., Eyre, J., and Recupero, P. R. (2006). Prevalence and Severity of Intimate Partner Violence and Associations with Family Functioning and Alcohol Abuse in Psychiatric Inpatients with Suicidal Intent. *Journal of Clinical Psychiatry* 67 (1): 23–29.

30. Oleckno, W. A. (1992). Gender Differences in Adolescent Risk-taking Behaviors. *National Social Science Journal* 4 (2): 40–49.

CHAPTER TEN

Case-Control Studies

*This chapter covers the basic design, analysis, and
interpretation of case-control studies as well as their
major advantages and disadvantages.*

Learning Objectives

- Distinguish between exploratory and analytic case-control studies.
- Describe the conceptual design of the contemporary case-control study.
- Outline the key issues in the design of case-control studies in terms of the research hypothesis, case definition, case selection, use of incident versus prevalent cases, control selection, determination of exposure status, and assurance of adequate study power.
- Compare and contrast the use of population-based and hospital-based case-control studies.
- Determine when to use a matched or unmatched analysis in case-control studies.
- Differentiate among incidence density sampling, case-base sampling, and cumulative incidence sampling in case-control studies. Also, indicate when each sampling method is appropriate.
- Calculate and interpret the crude and Mantel-Haenszel odds ratios in unmatched studies, their 95 percent confidence intervals, and the appropriate chi-square tests of significance for the respective odds ratios.
- Calculate and interpret the matched pairs odds ratio, its 95 percent confidence interval, and McNemar's chi-square test for pair-matched studies.
- Describe how confounding can be controlled in matched and unmatched case-control studies.
- Discuss the advantages and disadvantages of stratification versus multivariable analysis in controlling confounding in case-control studies.
- Describe what is meant by effect measure modification, the factors that affect it, and how it is assessed in case-control studies.
- Differentiate between quantitative and qualitative interaction.
- Compare and contrast the major advantages and disadvantages of case-control studies.

- Describe the design and the advantages and disadvantages of case-crossover studies.
- Define additive and multiplicative effects, additive and multiplicative interaction, additive and multiplicative model, adjusted odds ratio, antagonism, biological interaction, biomarker, concordant pairs, conditional logistic regression, cross-product ratio, discordant pairs, effect modifier, excess odds ratio, exposure odds ratio, hazard period, heterogeneity of effect, hospital controls, interaction, logistic regression, multiple logistic regression, multivariable method, negative and positive interaction, overmatching, pooling, population controls, population-based disease registry, random digit dialing, rare disease assumption, risk set, source population, statistical efficiency, stratification, stratum-specific odds ratio, study base, synergism, and test of heterogeneity or homogeneity.

INTRODUCTION

Case-control studies, which were discussed briefly in chapter 4, represent a popular and important epidemiologic study design. When properly conducted, they can be an efficient way of uncovering possible causal relationships between specified exposures and outcomes. While the early origins of case-control studies can be traced back well over a hundred years, it was not until 1926 that the first "modern" case-control study appeared in the literature.[1] This study of breast cancer was undertaken Janet Lane-Clapon, a physician working for the British Research Council.[2]

Case-control studies have often been referred to as *retrospective studies*, although the term can be confusing since other types of epidemiologic studies may also involve retrospective assessment. As discussed in chapter 4, the term is not recommended as a synonym for case-control studies.

Case-control studies can be *exploratory* (descriptive) or *analytic*. In **exploratory case-control studies** there are no specified *a priori* hypotheses about associations between exposures and outcomes. Cases and controls are selected, and a variety of factors are examined to determine if any are related to the outcomes of interest. Exploratory case-control studies, which are an extension of the case series (chapter 4), have been referred to in a disparaging manner as "fishing expeditions,"[3] but they can be valuable in identifying potential risk factors, especially when they concern an unfamiliar but serious or life-threatening disease. Such was the case when AIDS first emerged in the United States. Exploratory studies are also useful in investigations of disease outbreaks as a means of identifying potential causative factors (see chapter 14). *Analytic case-control studies*, which are the subject of this chapter, are designed to test one or more *a priori* hypotheses about the relationships between specified exposures and outcomes.

This chapter focuses on key design considerations in case-control studies, the basic approaches used in the analysis and interpretation of study findings, and the major advantages and disadvantages of this specific study design. Unless otherwise noted, exposure and outcome variables are assumed to be dichotomous in order to facilitate discussion. We begin our discussion with a brief summary of the conceptual framework for classical and contemporary case-control studies. The remainder of the chapter focuses primarily on the contemporary view of the case-control study.

CONCEPTUAL OVERVIEW

The *classical case-control study* typically involves the selection of a group of newly diagnosed cases of the outcome of interest and a comparable group of controls who do not have the outcome. The groups are then compared regarding the relative frequency of the hypothesized exposure(s) for a time period that presumably precedes the development of the outcome. This retrospective analysis is done to establish a correct temporal sequence between exposure and outcome that is necessary for making statements about risk or possible causation (see chapter 7). If the groups are similar with regard to the distribution of potentially confounding factors, and there are no significant sources of bias, then a difference in the relative frequency of a given exposure among the cases compared to the controls suggests a causal association between exposure and outcome. That is, a study exposure may be considered a risk factor (hazardous or protective) for the study outcome. In the hierarchy of analytic studies, the classical case-control design has been considered "an inferior alternative to the cohort study."[4(p144)] Much of the reasoning for this second-rate evaluation has to do with potential problems of bias resulting mainly from the way cases and controls are selected.

In the late 20th century, the concept of the case-control study changed radically. The *contemporary case-control study* is now envisioned as an efficient sampling technique for measuring exposure-outcome relationships,[5] and it shares elements in common with the cohort design. From this perspective, case-control studies are seen as taking place within a *source population* or **study base**, which in this context refers to the group of persons or the person-time experience from which the cases are generated.[1, 5] The nested case-control study (chapter 4) illustrates this concept well, and may be considered a model for this contemporary view.[6] In a nested case-control study the cases arise from the study cohort, which is the source population or study base, and the controls are randomly selected from members of the cohort who are at risk of the outcome at the time each case is identified. Thus, we can think of the contemporary case-control study as being nested (embedded) within a source population. This contemporary concept presents this design as a method for achieving results similar to those of a cohort study but more efficiently.

The primary challenge of the contemporary case-control study is identifying the appropriate source population (study base) from which to select controls.[5] In a nested case-control study this is easy, but it can be problematic in other situations, which will be discussed shortly. Before proceeding it should be helpful to clarify the purpose of the control group in a case-control study. Its purpose is to determine the relative distribution of exposed and unexposed subjects in the source population for comparison to that in the case group. Any notable difference implies that a causal association may exist between exposure and outcome, all other factors being equal.

To select cases and controls properly, the selection process must be independent of exposure status. Figure 10-1 illustrates the optimal selection process in a case-control study. Ideally, the cases are those generated from the source population during a defined time period, and the controls are those randomly selected from the same source population that generated the cases. Thus, the findings of a carefully designed case-control study should be similar to those of a carefully designed cohort study with the same source population. In other words, a case-control study may be considered a *reasonable alternative* to a cohort study when the source populations are the same. As in cohort and experimental studies, the focus of the comparison in case-control studies is on exposed and unexposed groups in order to determine if a causal association is likely to exist between exposure and outcome status. More is said about this later in the section on analysis and interpretation. As indicated in the introduction to this chapter, the discussion of case-control studies that follows is based primarily on this contemporary view unless otherwise indicated.

Figure 10-1   Selection Process for a Case-Control Study

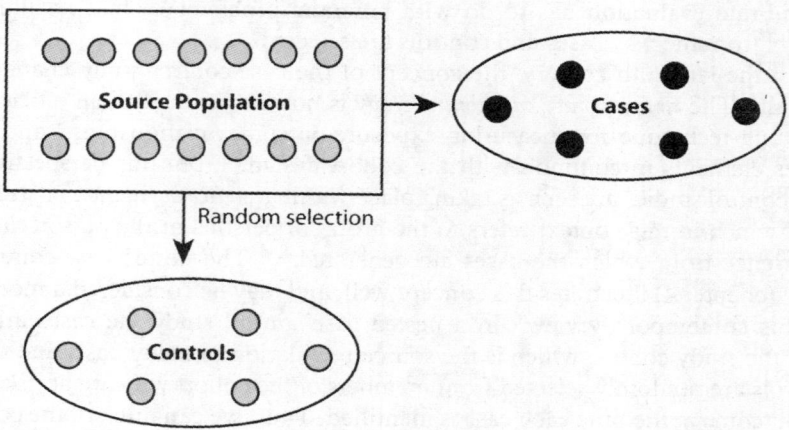

⬤ Newly generated case from source population during a given time period

◯ Subject at risk of the outcome during the given time period

KEY DESIGN FEATURES

The starting point for an analytic case-control study is the development of a research hypothesis about the possible relationship between one or more specified exposures and an outcome of interest. The hypothesis may be stated explicitly or implicitly, but either way, it provides the basic rationale for the study. For example, investigators at the Yale University School of Medicine and Cancer Center examined the hypothesis that the consumption of carbonated soft drinks (CSDs) is a risk factor for esophageal and gastric cancers using a case-control study. Interestingly, they did not find support for their hypothesis; in fact, they found an inverse association between consumption of CSDs and the risk of esophageal adenocarcinoma.[7]

Following the development of a research hypothesis investigators must identify and select cases and controls for analysis. Cases may be all those that developed from a well-defined cohort such as in a nested case-control or case-cohort study (chapter 4), or they may be selected prior to determining what constitutes the appropriate source population. In either instance, once the cases have been identified and enrolled in the study, the next step is the selection of controls. Ideally, they should be chosen from the source population. Some key issues in the selection of cases and controls follows.

Selecting Appropriate Cases

Case definition.   Before selecting cases for a case-control study, a case definition must be developed. Adequate criteria for defining cases are important. If the criteria are not adequate, the case group may be inadvertently diluted with noncases, which can bias study results toward the null value (defined in chapter 6). This can occur when the study outcome is similar to other outcomes that have different etiologies. Let us assume, for example, that a case-control study is being conducted to determine if certain dietary factors are related to the risk of fibromyalgia, a chronic but controversial diagnosis. Because the symptoms of fibromyalgia are similar to many of those associated with Lyme disease (e.g., muscle aches, fatigue, headaches), it is possible that some of the apparent fibromyalgia cases may actually be cases of Lyme disease, which we know is not caused by dietary factors but infected ticks. Unless the case definition of fibromyalgia is strict enough to exclude cases of Lyme disease, any possible effect of dietary factors on fibromyalgia is more likely to be missed or at least understated due to nondifferential misclassification (chapter 8). The best way to avoid this problem is to have reliable and accepted criteria for determining what constitutes a case and to apply these criteria when selecting subjects for the case group.

The criteria for selecting cases should include evidence that the study outcome is actually present. This may come from several sources, including patient medical histories, clinical examinations, and appropriate diagnostic tests where possible. Sometimes diagnosis is relatively straightforward, and other times it can be more complicated. A case-control study of the relationship between alcohol consumption and the incidence of stroke, for example, used the World Health Organization (WHO) criteria for defining stroke cases.[8] If the authors had differentiated each of the various subcategories of stroke, however, the process of defining cases would have been much more complicated. According to WHO, there are 10 types of strokes, not including transient ischemic attacks.[9]

Having strict criteria for case inclusion sometimes may need to be tempered by practical considerations. For example, if there is missing information for a number of potential subjects, it may be necessary to relax the criteria somewhat. Sometimes investigators will initially classify cases as suspect, probable, and definite depending on how many of the criteria in the case definition they satisfy. As additional information becomes available, the classifications can be changed accordingly. Also, the costs of performing expensive or possibly dangerous diagnostic tests on every potential case may need to be taken into account. Sometimes the best methods are impractical and have to compromised somewhat as long as potential bias can still be minimized. Overly strict criteria can also result in the untoward effect of missing actual cases, especially when there are no definitive diagnostic tests available. This can happen when the selected case definition requires the presence of several specific signs and symptoms, not all of which are relevant to every authentic case of the disease. For example, not all patients with gastroesophageal reflux disease (GERD) report burning, bloating, or nausea.[10] The key is to strike a balance between overly strict and overly general criteria with the objective of including the cases while excluding the noncases for the outcome of interest.

As a consumer of epidemiologic research, one should always look closely at case definitions so as to evaluate their suitability for any particular investigation. Epidemiologists may sometimes restrict case definitions, for example, to severe or fatal cases, or apply other restrictions by person, place, or time variables (e.g., men only). These restrictions can affect the *external* validity of the findings, but they will not affect the *internal* validity as long as the study is otherwise properly conducted (e.g., restrictions of cases by person, place, or time variables are also applied to the controls). In some circumstances case restrictions may improve study efficiency and internal validity.

Case selection.   The ideal way of choosing cases for a case-control study is to select all cases generated from a well-defined source population during a specified time period. A close alternative would be to select a probability sample of cases from the population. If sampling is employed, however, it is critical that case selection be independent of exposure status so that the case group is representative of the actual exposure distribution of cases in the population otherwise a selection bias is introduced (see chapter 8).

In reality, selecting cases from a well-defined population, such as a city, school, or state or region, is not always feasible due to the time and expense involved in identifying and enrolling the cases, nor is it always necessary. In fact, the majority of case-control studies are conducted at one or more hospitals or other treatment facilities for which the source population is not precisely known. When feasible, however, **population-based case-control studies**, those where both cases and controls are selected from a well-defined population, can provide findings with a high degree of credibility. In recent years, population-based studies have been facilitated by the expansion of **population-based disease registries**, which are ongoing systems that collect relevant data and register all cases of a particular disease or class of diseases as they develop in a defined population. For example, the New York State Department of Health maintains three population-based chronic disease registries—the Cancer Registry, the Alzheimer's and Other Dementias Registry, and the Congenital Malformations Registry—as well as some communicable disease registries.[11] Also, the Surveillance, Epidemiology, and End Results (SEER) Program of the National Cancer Institute collects and publishes cancer incidence and survival data from population-based cancer registries that cover about 26 percent of the population of the United States.[12] Not all disease registries are population-based, however, and thus some may only represent disease incidence within certain clinical facilities. Though not suitable for population-based studies, these registries may be used in connection with **hospital-based case-control studies**, those in which the cases and controls are selected from one or more hospitals, or with case-control studies involving other types of treatment centers such as clinics, long-term care facilities, or surgical centers.

With regard to case selection from hospitals (or other treatment facilities), while selecting cases is generally straightforward, the cases are not usually representative of all possible cases of the study outcome due to differences in factors related to hospitalization, such as disease severity, comorbidity, and socioeconomic status. As indicated earlier, this can affect the external validity of a study, but it will not affect its internal validity as long as the controls are representative of the same source population. The appropriate source population for hospital-based studies includes those individuals who *would have been cases* at the study hospital(s) had they developed the study outcome during the time of the investigation.[5] In practice, it may be difficult to determine who belongs to this hypothetical source population. More is said about this in the next section on control selection.

Up until this point we have not specified precisely whether the cases selected for a case-control study should be incident or prevalent cases. In general, incident cases are preferred, especially if the study is analytic. Exhibit 10-1 addresses this important issue and should be reviewed carefully before proceeding.

Cases for a case-control study may be selected retrospectively or prospectively. For example, in retrospective case selection one might identify all cases of leukemia at a medical center that were diagnosed for the first time between 2000 and 2005. In prospective case selection one might identify new cases of leukemia as they are diagnosed during a forthcoming period. In both instances, controls would be selected during the same respective time periods.

Exhibit 10-1
Should Incident or Prevalent Cases Be Used in a Case-Control Study?

Having the proper temporal sequence between exposure and outcome maximizes the value of case-control studies. In order to determine causal associations, the study exposure(s) must precede the study outcome. The clearest way to accomplish this is to use *incident* (new) cases and assess *prior* exposure (i.e., exposure that occurred during a time period before the outcome developed). Using prevalent (existing) cases or concurrent exposure does not invalidate a case-control study, but it limits the interpretation of the findings because in these circumstances one cannot be sure whether the exposure preceded the outcome, the outcome preceded the exposure, or the exposure and outcome occurred simultaneously. Thus, one cannot establish causal associations. This is one of the limitations of most cross-sectional studies, which generally rely on prevalence data. Also, prevalence is affected by both incidence and duration of the outcome. Therefore, when prevalent cases are employed in a case-control study one cannot always be sure of the extent to which an exposure is related more to disease prognosis than disease development.

Although desirable, determining incident cases for a case-control study is not as easy as it may first appear. For one thing, it is not always clear when new cases begin. Therefore, for pragmatic purposes, incident cases are usually defined as *newly diagnosed cases*, and the date of diagnosis is used as a proxy for when the disease began. With most acute conditions requiring prompt medical treatment (e.g., automobile-related injuries, botulism), the date of diagnosis approximates the actual date of the outcome quite well. This is not true for most chronic diseases (e.g., multiple sclerosis, emphysema), however. The date of diagnosis may be many years after the disease developed. Unfortunately, this fact can still lead to problems in ascertaining whether the study exposure preceded or followed disease initiation.

When diagnosis occurs long after disease initiation it may be important to assure that the exposure at least preceded the onset of *symptoms* of the disease, since in this situation it would be unlikely that one would have altered exposure because of the disease. As illustrated in the figure below, the original exposure is less likely to be changed before initial symptoms appear than after the symptoms, especially if they are troublesome. If exposure status is determined during the period between initial symptoms and diagnosis, and if this period is long, the true association between the study exposure and outcome might be missed. For example, changes in diet are less likely to be made by someone with stomach cancer prior to any symptoms of the disease than when early symptoms of heartburn and abdominal discomfort begin. By the time someone is diagnosed with stomach cancer his or her dietary habits may be quite different than they were prior to cancer initiation. Furthermore, when prevalent cases are used in case-control studies there is a greater probability that exposure has been modified *after* disease diagnosis. Patients with type 2 diabetes, for example, may have controlled their weight since their diagnosis, making it more likely that investigators would understate the role of obesity as a potential risk factor for diabetes when prevalent cases are examined sometime after diagnosis.

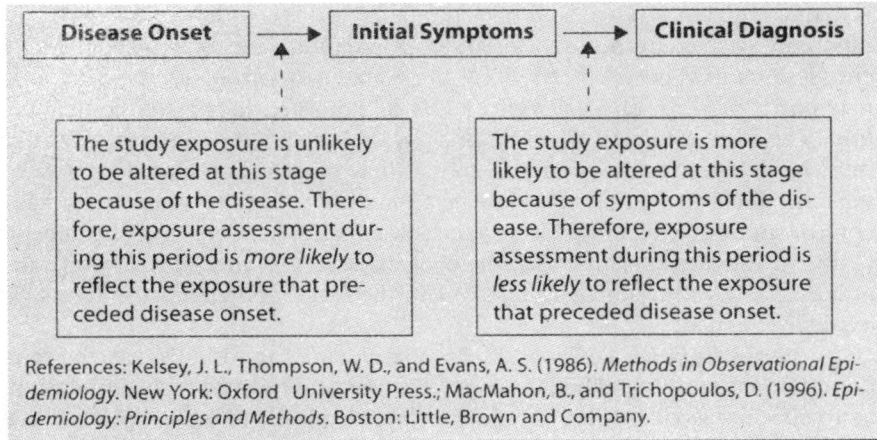

| Disease Onset | → | Initial Symptoms | → | Clinical Diagnosis |

The study exposure is unlikely to be altered at this stage because of the disease. Therefore, exposure assessment during this period is *more likely* to reflect the exposure that preceded disease onset.

The study exposure is more likely to be altered at this stage because of symptoms of the disease. Therefore, exposure assessment during this period is *less likely* to reflect the exposure that preceded disease onset.

References: Kelsey, J. L., Thompson, W. D., and Evans, A. S. (1986). *Methods in Observational Epidemiology.* New York: Oxford University Press.; MacMahon, B., and Trichopoulos, D. (1996). *Epidemiology: Principles and Methods.* Boston: Little, Brown and Company.

One advantage to selecting cases and controls retrospectively is that the investigator can go back as far as needed to get a sufficient number of subjects to maintain a desired level of power in a study. The usefulness of retrospective selection depends, however, on having an accurate database that also contains relevant information on exposure status. Hospital records, for example, may have diagnoses on all admissions or discharges going back many years, but exposure data on intake forms may be incomplete or unreliable. Also, diagnostic methods or disease classifications may have changed during or after the specified time period. Selecting subjects prospectively may also be subject to problems. Better diagnostic procedures may be developed during the course of case selection, and the definition of the disease may change over time.

Selecting Appropriate Controls

Without controls there can be no case-control studies,
but with the wrong controls there can only be regrettable case-control studies.

It is difficult to underestimate the importance of selecting appropriate controls in a case-control study. Put simply, failure to select proper controls can invalidate study results. As implied earlier, a control group is important because it provides a basis for comparison by representing what is "normal" or "expected." If a study exposure in a case-control study is not related to the study outcome, then we would expect the odds of the exposure in the case group to equal that in the control group, all other factors being equal.[3] In fact, all analytic and experimental studies in epidemiology have control or comparison groups. For example, in cross-sectional studies (chapter 9) those who are unexposed to the factor under investigation represent the control group as they do in cohort studies and randomized controlled trials.

In order to avoid selection bias, the controls for a case-control study should be representative of the source population, that is, the population that generated the cases. This is perhaps best achieved when the control group is randomly selected from the entire source population. The main objective is to choose a control group that reflects the actual proportions of exposed and unexposed persons, or the various levels of exposure, in the source population. Therefore, as in the selection of cases, the selection process for controls must be independent of exposure status[6] to avoid selection bias. In practice, the desired control group may only be approximated in the majority of case-control studies, which could introduce some bias. Therefore, it is incumbent on the investigators to show that the controls used in a case-control study are at least likely to be similar to controls in the source population in terms of exposure frequency.

Controls from *population-based case-control studies* are usually selected randomly from the source population and are typically referred to as **population controls**. If selection is truly random, these controls should represent the actual exposure distribution of the subjects in the source population and would therefore exemplify an ideal control group. One popular way of selecting controls in some case-control studies is **random digit dialing**, where telephone numbers are dialed randomly within given telephone exchanges for the selected area. Typical problems with population controls include potential selection bias due to low rates of participation and possible information bias due to poor recall of prior exposures. Sometimes controls are selected from neighbors, family members, friends, or coworkers from the source population. These types of controls may improve participation and reduce the potential for recall bias, but they may also introduce a negative bias in the study results because the controls may be too similar to the cases with regard to exposure status; that is, they may not represent the true range of exposures that exists in the source population because of their similarity to the cases.

An example of a population-based case-control study is one that examined the role of loud noise in the etiology of acoustic neuroma, a benign tumor of the vestibular division of the eighth cranial nerve. Eligible cases were all patients diagnosed with acoustic neuroma between September 1, 1999, and August 31, 2002, and residing in one of three geographic regions in Sweden covered by regional cancer registries. Controls were randomly selected from the source population based on the Swedish population registry. The authors found an increased risk of acoustic neuroma among those reporting exposure to loud noises from any source.[13]

Hospital-based case-control studies normally rely on **hospital controls**, that is, patients admitted to same hospital(s) as cases but for reasons other than the study outcome. As stated previously, the hypothetical source population for a hospital-based study is defined as those who *would have been cases* at the study hospital(s) had they developed the study outcome during the time period covered by the investigation.[5] Some studies that use cases from selected hospitals may employ a control series from the general population or from neighbors, family members, or other associates of the cases. Hospital controls, however, are usually more convenient than other sources, especially population controls, and tend to result in greater participation with less recall bias since patients generally have had time to reflect about past exposures and events and may be more motivated to participate in a study. Cases and controls from the same medical facilities are also more likely to resemble each other with regard to those selective factors that led to the use of the facilities (e.g., socioeconomic status). This may not hold, however, for hospitals where patients with certain conditions (e.g., spinal cord injuries) are likely to be referred from a wider geographic area and be more affluent than those patients without the conditions. Also, hospital controls in general may not represent the exposure distribution in the source population because they represent ill people who may be more likely to have an unfavorable risk profile than healthy people in the source population. Depending on what exposure is being studied, erroneous conclusions could result if the exposure is more *or* less common in hospital controls than it would be in the source population.

An example of a hospital-based case-control study is one that was undertaken to evaluate the role of coffee, decaffeinated coffee, and black tea in breast cancer etiology. Cases were patients hospitalized with primary, incident breast cancer, and controls were other patients hospitalized with non-neoplastic conditions. The study findings supported a protective effect of coffee consumption for premenopausal but not postmenopausal women with regard to the risk of breast cancer.[14]

A question that is frequently asked in selecting a hospital control group is, what diagnostic categories should be included? It is often, but not universally, recommended that patients with a variety of diagnoses be chosen to comprise the control group with the important caveat that those patients with diagnoses that are known or likely to be related to the study exposure should *not be included*.[15] If they are, this could result in an overestimation or underestimation of the true effect of the exposure on the study outcome depending on whether the diagnoses are positively or negatively related to the exposure. It would not be appropriate, for example, to include patients with emphysema or chronic bronchitis in the control group when testing the hypothesis that cigarette smoking causes lung cancer because we know that these diseases are also associated with cigarette smoking. Therefore, the magnitude of the relationship between smoking and lung cancer would be underestimated since the controls would be expected to have a higher proportion of prior smokers than the source population as a whole. In theory, choosing from a variety of diagnoses tends to minimize the impact of this error if any particular disease is unknowingly associated with the study exposure.

In summary, one must be careful when selecting a control group from hospitalized (or other clinical) subjects. While there are some advantages in terms of convenience, better recall, and comparability on potential confounders between cases and controls from the same hospital(s), the chief disadvantage is that the exposure frequency may be different from that in the actual source population. This could lead to erroneous conclusions about the relationship between a study exposure and outcome, thus weakening the internal validity of the study due to selection bias. Also, it should be mentioned that many otherwise eligible controls may be too sick to participate in a hospital-based case-control study. The same can be said for some cases. This can lead to select groups that are unrepresentative of eligible cases or controls. Table 10-1 lists some of the basic questions to ask when one selects a control group for a case-control study.

Table 10-1   Some Basic Questions to Ask When Selecting a Control Group for a Case-Control Study

- Does the control group come from the same source population that generated the cases?
- Is the control group representative of the source population, especially in terms of the exposure distribution?
- Is the control group similar to the case group with regard to potentially confounding factors?
- Have any restrictions or exclusions applied to the case group also been applied to control group?
- Have hospital controls from diagnostic categories known to be associated with the study exposure been excluded from the control group?

Accurately Determining Exposure Status

Exposure status in case-control studies needs to be determined accurately in order to minimize potential sources of information bias, which can lead to exposure misclassification. Two common types of information bias that may result from the way exposure status is assessed in case-control studies are *interviewer bias* and *recall bias* (see chapter 8).

Interviewer bias can result when cases are interviewed more thoroughly than controls regarding their exposure status. This bias is most likely to occur when interviews are conducted in person, and the interviewers are able to identify the cases and controls and also know the study exposure(s). Therefore, keeping the interviewers unaware (i.e., *blinding* the interviewers*) as to subject outcome status and the study hypothesis are ways of controlling this error. Unfortunately, blinding interviewers to outcome status is often difficult. Interviewers may be able to recognize cases due to obvious signs or symptoms of a disorder, or the subjects may inadvertently reveal their outcome status before or during the interview. Interviewers, however, if different from the investigators, can usually be blinded to the specific hypothesis under investigation. This should reduce the usually unconscious tendency to search more thoroughly for a particular exposure among cases than controls during

---

*Blinding is defined formally and explained further in chapter 12 in the context of randomized controlled trials.

an interview. A similar bias can occur when medical records are being examined to determine exposure status. In this case, it is also best to blind the person gathering the information from the study hypothesis, and outcome status, if possible. The fundamental point to remember is that exposure status should be assessed in the same manner for both cases and controls to the point of when, where, and how the assessments take place. In addition, wherever feasible, exposure and other relevant data collected from subjects should be verified using other reliable sources, such as laboratory tests, official records, and information from spouses, relatives, friends, or employers, in order to reduce further the probability of interviewer (or "data gatherer") bias. It is also a good idea to standardize procedures, train interviewers, and monitor the interview process. Other means of data collection may involve survey questionnaires; review of existing medical, employment, or other records; and the use of **biomarkers**, which are cellular or molecular indicators of exposure, such as elevated enzyme levels, metabolites, or toxic residues that may be found in the blood, saliva, urine, hair, or other biological specimens.[1] Each of these methods has its own advantages and disadvantages.

Recall bias can occur in case-control studies because cases often remember past exposures better than controls resulting in a positive bias in the association between study exposures and outcome. This form of information bias results from a natural tendency among those with serious disorders to want to know *why* their disorders developed. The introspection that takes place makes cases more likely than healthy controls to recall past exposures accurately since controls generally have less, if any, vested interest in the findings. Recall bias can be reduced by blinding the subjects to the specific study hypothesis and by consulting objective sources of data on past exposures that do not depend on subject memory. Such is the case when medical or employment records or biomarkers are used to determine exposure status. A well-known biomarker for recent cigarette smoking, for example, is cotinine, a metabolite of nicotine. It can be found in blood several days after smoking. It is also detectable in urine and saliva. Environmental and occupational studies frequently rely on biomarkers to establish or verify exposure status. Methods for assessing biomarkers should be appropriate, standardized, and administered by trained personnel to avoid potential misclassifications. They should also be reliable, acceptable to the subjects, and cost effective.

Assuring Adequate Study Power

Even with the best efforts to minimize systematic errors, the results of a study may be inconclusive if the study has insufficient power (defined in chapter 8). To a large degree, power is related to sample size. Therefore, a case-control study needs to have adequate sample size, and this should be determined before the study begins. Fortunately, various software applications are available that allow one to estimate the sample size needed to obtain a desired level of power. Alternatively, one can also estimate power based on the desired sample size. For brief descriptions of relevant software applications see appendix A. With OpenEpi, for example, one can estimate the minimum sample size needed for an unmatched case-control study (see next section) given the following inputs:

- The confidence level desired (usually 95% corresponding to a p-value of 0.05),
- The level of power desired (usually between 80 and 95%),
- The ratio of controls to cases (may be 1:1, 2:1, 3:1, etc.),
- The expected frequency of the exposure in the control group (usually esti-mated from previous surveys in the source population), and
- The smallest odds ratio one would like to be able to detect (based on practi-cal or clinical significance).

As an example, assuming 95 percent confidence, 90 percent power, a control to case ratio of 1.0 (i.e., 1:1), and an expected exposure frequency of 10 percent in the control group, it would take 1,265 cases and 1,265 controls for a total sample size of 2,530 to detect an overall odds ratio as small as 1.50. The total sample size drops to 806 if one is content with detecting an odds ratio of 2.00, but jumps to 49,958 if one needs to detect an odds ratio as small as 1.10. It is important to note that these figures apply to the overall analysis. The power of any particular subgroup analysis (e.g., by age, sex, or race/eth-nicity) can be expected to be lower due to smaller sample size. Hence, one may need a larger number of cases and controls than initially calculated if one wants to maintain a reasonable level of power in the subgroup analyses.

Using multiple controls per case will lower sample size requirements for the *case group* but will increase the *total* sample size needed. For example, using three controls per case to detect an odds ratio of 1.50 for the parameters stated above will result in a 34.5 percent reduction in the number of cases required (from 1,265 to 829) but a 31.0 percent increase in the total sample size needed (2,530 to 3,315). This may be advantageous where the study out-come is relatively rare, and cases are more difficult to obtain than controls. The value added, however, begins to diminish after awhile. Using four instead of three controls per case in the above example reduces the number of required cases by only 6.6 percent (from 829 to 774) but increases the total sample size needed by 16.7 percent (from 3,315 to 3,869). Going from six to seven controls per case reduces the number of cases needed by only 2.2 per-cent but increases the total sample size required by 11.8 percent.

A rough estimate of the number of cases needed when multiple controls are used for any given set of parameters is provided by the following formula.[3]

(10.1)   Number of cases $\cong$ [k (c + 1)] / 2c

Here, k = the original number of cases required based on a 1:1 control to case ratio, and c = the number of controls per case one plans to use. For example, if 1,265 cases are required based on a 1:1 ratio of controls to cases, and if one wants to see how many cases would be required if three controls were used per case, the estimate would be:

$$[1{,}265\ (3 + 1)]\ /\ (2 \times 3) \cong 5{,}060\ /\ 6 = 843 \text{ cases}$$

This is close to the value of 829 calculated using OpenEpi (see appendix A). Formula 10.1 applies to both unmatched and matched analyses (see next section).

ANALYSIS AND INTERPRETATION OF CASE-CONTROL STUDIES

Typical steps in the analysis and interpretation of case-control studies are outlined in figure 10-2. Following an overall analysis of the findings, attempts are frequently made to determine if effect measure modification (defined later) or confounding is present, and if so, to explain the effect measure modification and control the confounding. The chief means of achieving these ends involve: (a) *stratification*, or (b) *multivariable analysis*, which are explained in a subsequent section. First, we will consider the approach to overall analysis. This depends on whether or not *matching* (chapter 8) has been used in the design stage. Matching is a procedure for making study and comparison groups similar with regard to selected variables, and it has implications for the procedures used in the analysis.

Matched case-control studies are those in which *individual matching* (chapter 8) is used. Basically, for each case enrolled one or more controls is selected to be identical, or nearly identical, to the case with regard to the matched variable(s). The simplest application of individual matching is *pair matching* (chapter 8) in which each case is paired with just one control forming a new unit of analysis—the case-control pair. While there are some advantages, the implications of matching in case-control studies are more complex than might first be imagined. These are discussed in the section on controlling confounding.

Figure 10-2   Typical Steps in the Analysis of Data from a Case-Control Study

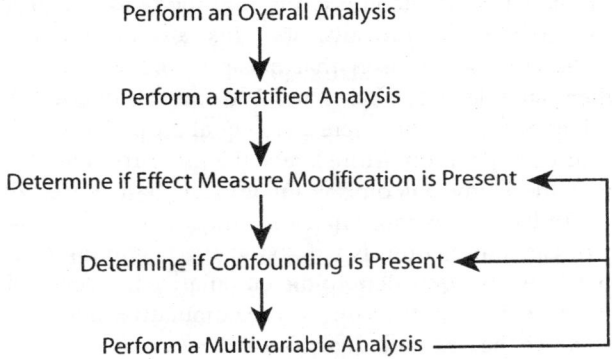

Unmatched case-control studies are those in which the controls are *not* individually matched with the cases during the selection process. The results from unmatched case-control studies are analyzed differently from matched studies as illustrated below. It is important to remember that a matched analysis is *only* appropriate when individual matching has been used in a study. If frequency matching (chapter 8) has been employed, an unmatched analysis should be performed. This is because the cases and controls have not been joined together as new units of analysis. With this short background, you are now ready to learn about the analysis and interpretation of both unmatched and matched case-control studies. We will first discuss unmatched analysis, which is the more common of the two procedures.

Unmatched Analysis

If we use dichotomous measures of exposure and outcome, an *unmatched case-control study* can be analyzed by placing the results in a 2 × 2 contingency table as follows:

	Outcome Status	
Exposure Status	Cases	Controls
Exposed	a	b
Unexposed	c	d

It is important to note that incidence measures for the exposed and unexposed groups, and hence risk or rate ratios, *cannot* be derived from the above contingency table. This is because the cases and controls have been selected separately on the basis of outcome status, and the ratio of controls (b + d) to cases (a + c) is fixed by the investigators. This ratio is rarely the same as the ratio of eligible controls to cases that exists in the source population. For instance, when one selects 100 cases and 100 controls (a control to case ratio of 1:1), this does not mean that there is an equal proportion of cases and controls in the source population. More likely, the proportion in the source population without the study outcome is far greater than those with it (a ratio between 10:1 and 1000:1 is more likely for most chronic disorders). Because the number of cases and controls is fixed at the beginning of a case-control study, a / (a + b) is not equivalent to the cumulative incidence in the exposed group, and c / (c + d) is not the same as the cumulative incidence in the unexposed group. Since the risk ratio depends on these measures (i.e., RR = [a / (a + b)] / [c / (c + d)]), it cannot be calculated in a standard case-control study.

The usual measure of association in case-control studies is the **exposure odds ratio**, which is the ratio of the odds of exposure among the cases (a / c) to the odds of exposure among the controls (b / d) (see formula 10.2). It is typically referred to as just the *odds ratio* (OR) or sometimes as the *relative odds* or **cross-product ratio**,[1] since it can be calculated from the above contingency table by ad / bc. This latter expression is also used to calculate the *disease odds ratio* (chapter 6), and as expected, provides an identical result. As with the exposure odds ratio, the disease odds ratio is generally known simply as the odds ratio. It may also be called the relative odds or the cross-product ratio like the exposure odds ratio. The difference between the exposure odds ratio and the disease odds ratio is largely one of interpretation since they can both be calculated in the same manner (i.e., as cross-product ratios) with the same numerical result.

(10.2)

$$OR = \frac{a/c}{b/d} = \frac{ad}{bc}$$

When OR = 1.0 there is no association between a **given** study exposure and outcome. When OR > 1.0 there is a positive association, and when OR < 1.0 there is an inverse association (i.e., the exposure is protective). The magnitude of the OR can be evaluated using the guidelines presented in chapter 6, specifically in table 6-3. Problem 10-1, which appears later in this chapter, provides additional details.

To illustrate the interpretation of the *exposure odds ratio* consider an association between a history of cigarette smoking and the incidence of bladder cancer where OR = 2.2. One could say that the odds of a history of cigarette smoking (the exposure) are 2.2 times greater among those who develop bladder cancer (the outcome) than those who do not. These odds, by the way, represent incidence odds as opposed to prevalence odds (see chapter 5). Alternatively, one could express the *disease odds ratio* by saying the odds of contracting bladder cancer are 2.2 times greater among those with a history of cigarette smoking than those without such a history. Since the derived formula for the OR (i.e., ad / bc) is the same whether the exposure odds or disease odds are used, either interpretation is acceptable.

Some authors refer to the OR as the relative risk (RR), specifically meaning the risk or the rate ratio. This is technically incorrect. While it is true that the OR approximates the risk or rate ratio when incident cases are used, subject selection is unbiased, and the study outcome is rare,[1] this practice should be discouraged. For one thing, the assumptions, especially the so-called **rare disease assumption**,* are not always met, and for another, the OR is a legitimate measure of association in its own right that does not need to be approximated by another measure. Nevertheless, there are situations where it

---

*Suggested estimates of what constitutes a "rare disease" vary in the literature. In general, these estimates typically range from two to 20 percent with figures like five or 10 percent being most commonly recommended.

meaningful to use the OR to estimate other measures of association. For example, calculating *attributable fractions* (chapter 6) from case-control studies is greatly simplified if the OR can be used to estimate the risk ratio (see formulas 6.17 and 6.19).

Technically, the meaning of the odds ratio and what it estimates depend on how the controls are sampled. Therefore, this should be specified in every study.[16] **Incidence density sampling** (also called **density sampling** or **density-based sampling**) is the method ordinarily used in nested case-control studies where controls are selected from the person-time experience that produced the cases. Typically, the controls are randomly selected from those who are at risk at the time each case develops. These at-risk subjects are referred to as the **risk set**. In this situation the odds ratio is an unbiased estimate of the *rate ratio* (i.e., the incidence density ratio or incidence rate ratio; defined in chapter 6) provided that incident cases are identified and subject selection is unbiased.[1] Importantly, there is *no* need for the rare disease assumption. This sampling method is also used in case-control studies based on disease registries. Cases are generally selected from the registry over a brief time period, and controls are sampled from the registry's source population during the same time period.[17] **Case-base sampling** is the method ordinarily used in case-cohort studies (chapter 4) where controls are randomly selected from the subjects in the source population free of the study outcome at the *beginning* of the study period. In this scenario the odds ratio is an unbiased estimate of the *risk ratio* (i.e., cumulative incidence ratio) given the same provisions as above. Again, there is no requirement for the rare disease assumption. Finally, **cumulative incidence sampling** normally entails selection of controls from subjects in the source population who are free of the study outcome at the *end* of the study period.[17] The odds ratio calculated in this situation approximates the risk ratio *only if* the study outcome is rare, and the other provisions referred to earlier are also met. In conventional case-control studies, before modern conceptions, cumulative incidence sampling was assumed to be the norm. In this type of sampling, the "study period" can be conceived as having already occurred by the time the controls are selected. An implication of these sampling methods is that the study outcome does not always have to be rare for the odds ratio to be a reliable estimate of the risk or rate ratio as just described.

An approximate 95 percent confidence interval for the OR can be calculated using a method described many years ago by Barnet Woolf (formula 10.3).[18] The letters a, b, c, and d refer to the frequencies in the contingency table shown at the beginning of this section. This formula is analogous to formula 9.6 and is calculated in the same manner.

(10.3)
$$95\% \ CI = \exp\left\{\ln\left(OR\right)\pm1.96\sqrt{\left(1/a\right)+\left(1/b\right)+\left(1/c\right)+\left(1/d\right)}\right\}$$

If desired, the statistical significance of the OR can be calculated using a chi-square test (χ^2) for independence.[19] The appropriate equation appears in formula 9.7, which is repeated here for convenience. A guide to interpreting the results of the chi-square can be found in table 9-3. A problem demonstrating the analysis of an unmatched case-control study appears later in problem 10-1.

(Repeated 9.7)

$$\chi^2 = \frac{n(ad - bc)^2}{(a+b)(c+d)(a+c)(b+d)}$$

Matched Analysis

Assuming dichotomous measures of exposure and outcome and a case to control ratio of 1:1, a *pair-matched* case-control study can be analyzed by placing the results in a 2 × 2 table like the one shown below. This table differs in important respects from that used to analyze unmatched studies. For one thing the frequencies (w, x, y, and z) represent *case-control pairs* and *not* individual cases or controls. The number of case-control pairs in which both cases and controls are exposed is represented by w, while the number of case-control pairs in which only the cases are exposed is x, and so on. The sum of the case-control pairs in the sample (w + x + y + z) is *one-half* of the total number of subjects in the study. If more than one control is matched to a case, the analysis will be more complicated. For a discussion of this situation one should consult an intermediate or advanced text on epidemiology or biostatistics.

Controls

Cases	Exposed	Unexposed
Exposed	w	x
Unexposed	y	z

The odds ratio calculated from a pair-matched case-control study may be referred to as the **matched pairs odds ratio** (OR-MP).[20] The OR-MP is calculated by taking the ratio of the **discordant pairs**, that is, those case-control pairs where exposure status differs between cases and controls. The **concordant pairs**, where exposure status is the same between cases and controls, are ignored in the analysis since they do not contribute information as to whether or not the exposure is related to the outcome. This is because the exposure status is the same in the cases and controls. Thus, the odds ratio for a matched pairs analysis is calculated as follows:

(10.4)   OR-MP = x / y

An approximate 95 percent confidence interval for the OR-MP can be calculated using formula 10.5.[3] The values of x and y should be relatively large, say at least 30 each, for this formula to provide a reasonable estimate of the exact confidence interval. An alternative method of estimating the 95 percent confidence interval depends on the usual test of significance for matched pairs analysis, which is known as **McNemar's chi-square test** (χ^2). The equations for this test statistic and the 95 percent confidence interval based on it are shown in formulas 10.6 and 10.7, respectively.

(10.5)
$$95\% \ CI = \exp\left\{\ln(x/y) \pm 1.96\sqrt{(1/x) + (1/y)}\right\}$$

(10.6)
$$\text{McNemar's } \chi^2 = (x - y)^2 / (x + y)$$

(10.7)
$$95\% \ CI = \exp\left\{\ln(x/y)\left(1 \pm 1.96\sqrt{\chi^2}\right)\right\}$$

The χ^2 depicted in formula 10.7 is McNemar's chi-square with one degree of freedom. The OR-MP, McNemar's χ^2, and the 95 percent CIs described in this section are interpreted in the same manner as their counterparts derived from unmatched studies. The basic analysis of a matched case-control study is illustrated later in problem 10-2.

CONTROLLING CONFOUNDING

In general, there are three main methods that can be used to control potential confounding in case-control studies. These are restriction, matching, and statistical adjustment in the analysis phase. Restriction (chapter 8) can be used in either unmatched or matched case-control studies alone or in combination with statistical adjustment in the analysis. As discussed in chapter 8, restriction can limit the generalizability of the findings, but it will not affect internal validity. Statistical adjustment in the analysis phase can also be used in unmatched or matched case-control studies alone or in combination with restriction. Matching in case-control studies is intended to control potential confounding, but it can have untoward consequences as discussed below.

Problems with Matching

In cohort studies, individual matching readily controls confounders, but in case-control studies things are not so simple. To begin to understand why it is helpful to recall that the control group for a case-control study should have an exposure distribution that is representative of that in the source population. Matching on extraneous variables, however, can influence the exposure distribution of the control group without affecting that of the case group. The reason is cases are selected first, and controls are then matched to the cases. The result can be a selection bias leading to a spurious association between exposure and outcome. This can occur when matched variables are associated with the exposure, which is true of all confounders by definition and some nonconfounders as well. The effect of matching in these circumstances is to make the control group more like the case group in terms of exposure status, thereby biasing the measure of association toward the null value (i.e., OR = 1.0).

In practical terms, this selection bias produces results typical of confounding.[21] Thus, it can be said that matching can create confounding in a case-control study even when it never existed in the source population.[22] While this confounding can be controlled statistically with the correct procedures, it is a generally underappreciated consequence of matching in case-control studies and can be a problem when matched studies are analyzed using methods designed for unmatched studies. Why then is matching even considered? The reason is there are some advantages to matching, which are summarized in table 10-2, along with the disadvantages. For one thing, matching can increase the **statistical efficiency*** (see chapter 8) of case-con-

Table 10-2   Major Advantages and Disadvantages of Matching in Case-Control Studies

Advantages	Disadvantages
1. It assures comparability between cases and controls on the selected variables.	1. Matched variables associated with the exposure may confound the measure of association and thus need to be controlled in the analysis.
2. It may increase the statistical efficiency of subgroup analyses based on the matched variables when the number of controls would otherwise be very small in one or more of the subgroups.	2. It may be difficult or costly to find a sufficient number of controls that meet the criteria for matching, especially if many variables are being matched.
3. It can be a convenient way to sample controls when random selection from the source population is not feasible (e.g., hospital controls matched to hospital cases based on time of admission).	3. It eliminates the possibility of examining the effects of the matched variables on the outcome.
	4. It can increase the difficulty or complexity of controlling for confounding by the remaining unmatched variables.
4. It can help control for unmeasured confounders that are difficult to quantify (e.g., matching by neighborhood as a proxy for certain aspects of socioeconomic status).	5. It may lead to overmatching with a consequent reduction in study efficiency.
	6. It can result in a greater loss of data since all the matched subjects in a unit have to be eliminated even if only one of them is lost or non-responsive.

*Statistical efficiency is a measure of the relative degree of precision in an analysis; that is, a measure of the extent to which random error is reduced. A statistically efficient analysis will have greater power, which is the ability to detect an association if it exists, for the same sample size than a statistically inefficient analysis.

trol analyses. Paradoxically, while matching alone does not prevent confounding in a case-control study, it can improve the statistical efficiency of controlling confounding in the analysis stage,[22] especially if the confounding is strong.[21] This is achieved in stratification, for example, by assuring a constant ratio of controls to cases in each stratum.[21] This in turn provides more precise estimates of the odds ratios and their associated confidence intervals.[22] On the downside, the matching process can be costly and time-consuming, while still producing findings that need to be adjusted for confounding. There can also be a loss of information since, for example, the effects of matched variables on the study outcome cannot be examined. Also, loss of a case in a pair-matched study automatically results in the loss of a control, and vice versa, since the cases and controls are paired as units of analysis. Finally, **overmatching**, which can be thought of as *inappropriate* or *unnecessary matching* (e.g., matching on a factor that is only associated with the exposure and not the outcome) may significantly *reduce* statistical efficiency, which is normally cited as one of the potential benefits of matching in case-control studies. In addition, one should be aware that overmatching in the design stage cannot be corrected in the analysis stage.[23]

As you can see from the foregoing discussion, a decision of whether or not to perform matching in a case-control study with the goal of controlling confounding is a complicated matter. On the whole, matching is most advantageous when the distribution of a particular confounder in the control group differs substantially from that in the case group. In this situation, matching adjusts for the discrepancy.[24] It may also be valuable in small studies where there are several nominal (categorical) confounders like occupation or neighborhood that have many subcategories.[22] Here, enhanced statistical efficiency should be important. Other factors, however, can reduce this efficiency (e.g., overmatching) or increase the costs of matching (e.g., difficulty in finding eligible controls). Generally speaking, the disadvantages of matching in case-control studies appear to outweigh the advantages, and, therefore, frequency matching (chapter 8) with statistical adjustment for confounding in the analysis phase might be a viable alternative.[3]

The basic methods for analyzing matched case-control studies to ensure adequate control of confounding, including that introduced by the matching process, include special forms of *stratification* or *multivariable analysis*. When pair matching is used, the analysis is relatively simple and has already been described in the previous section on matched analysis. Here it can be demonstrated that the OR-MP is equivalent to the *Mantel-Haenszel odds ratio* used in stratification[25] where each case and control pair makes up a single stratum.[26] Stratification and the Mantel-Haenszel odds ratio are discussed in the following section. The procedures are similar but somewhat more involved when multiple controls are matched to each case. These are not discussed here.

In summary, we can say that matching followed by a matched analysis is one way of controlling confounding in a case-control study. Multivariable approaches in the analysis phase are also available for controlling confounding in matched case-control studies. A commonly used method (i.e., conditional logistic regression) is described briefly in the next section since it relates to a frequently used method in unmatched studies (i.e., multiple logistic regression).

Confounding in Unmatched Studies

Confounding can be detected and controlled in the analysis phase of unmatched case-control studies using *stratification* or *multivariable analysis*. **Stratification** involves separating a sample into two or more subgroups according to specified levels or categories of a third variable (e.g., the confounding variable).[1] For example, to control for potential confounding by drinking status in a study of the effect of cigarette smoking on automobile injuries, one might examine the effect separately among drinkers and nondrinkers by calculating an odds ratio for each subgroup. These two subgroups represent two levels of stratification by drinking status, and their odds ratios represent the **stratum-specific odds ratios**. Since the stratum-specific odds ratios cannot be confounded by drinking status (i.e., everyone in a subgroup has the same drinking status), they should be alike except for random error.* If confounding by drinking status is present in the original relationship, we would expect the stratum-specific odds ratios to be similar but different from the **crude odds ratio** (OR$_c$), that is, the overall odds ratio prior to stratification. If there is no confounding, the stratum-specific and crude odds ratios should be similar except for random error.[†] This is will be illustrated shortly.

The number of stratification levels may vary depending on the level of precision desired. The goal is to produce subgroups whose subjects are similar with regard to the confounding factor. In the previous example, stratification on drinking status could have included several levels according to the number of drinks consumed per day if one thought that the degree of confounding varied depending on the amount of drinking. For example, drinking status might have been stratified by five levels (e.g., 0, 1–2, 3–4, 5–6, and more than 6 drinks per day). If stratification also included sex differences, then 10 categories would have been created (five categories for males plus five categories for females). If five age groups were also considered, then the number of stratification subgroups would rise to 50 (10 × 5 = 50), producing 50 separate odds ratios to compare. It is easy to see that stratification has its limits. As the number of subgroups increases, the analysis becomes more

---

*Random error can account for seemingly large differences in the stratum-specific odds ratios, which under ideal conditions would be the same if confounding were the only issue. Effect measure modification (described later) can also account for differences. Also, using only two strata to characterize drinking status may result in incomplete control of confounding (i.e., residual confounding) due to differences in risk by amount of drinking.

[†]Unfortunately, this is not always the case with odds ratios. It is possible for the odds ratios to be alike in the strata but different from the crude odds ratio when confounding is absent. This possibility emphasizes the need to consider the three requirements for confounding enumerated in chapter 8 in addition to examining differences in crude and stratum-specific odds ratios. More is said about this later and in chapter 11 in reference to stratification in *closed cohort studies*.

unwieldy, and the number of subjects in each subgroup decreases, which in turn reduces the power of the subgroup analyses resulting in decreased precision of the findings.

The decreased precision can be minimized by calculating a popular epidemiologic measure of association known as the **Mantel-Haenszel odds ratio** (OR_{MH}). This is an overall combined measure of the stratum-specific odds ratios. In essence, it is a summary odds ratio *adjusted for* the stratification factor(s) and represents a weighted average of the stratum-specific odds ratios where the weights depend on the number of observations in each stratum.[27] For dichotomous levels of exposure and outcome, the OR_{MH} is calculated using formula 10.8 first described by Nathan Mantel and William Haenszel in 1959.[28] The symbol Σ refers to "the sum of," and i represents each stratum.

(10. 8)

$$OR_{MH} = \frac{\Sigma\left(a_i d_i / n_i\right)}{\Sigma\left(b_i c_i / n_i\right)}$$

To illustrate the use of this formula briefly, imagine two levels of stratification on a factor. For each level (stratum) of the factor, a 2×2 contingency table is developed (see figure 10-3). The values in the cells of the first table are represented by a_1 through d_1 with a sum of n_1. The values in the cells of the second contingency table are represented by a_2 through d_2 with a sum of n_2. Therefore,

$$OR_{MH} = \frac{\left(a_1 d_1 / n_1\right) + \left(a_2 d_2 / n_2\right)}{\left(b_1 c_1 / n_1\right) + \left(b_2 c_2 / n_2\right)}$$

The OR_{MH} is produced by *pooling* the stratum-specific odds ratios as noted above. **Pooling** is a way of aggregating the data over the strata so as to summarize the effect of a given exposure on the outcome. It is based on the assumption that the effect is constant across the strata, so that each stratum-specific odds ratio provides a separate point estimate of the overall effect.[6] Importantly, the OR_{MH} represents an **adjusted odds ratio**, that is, the odds ratio after controlling for the confounding factor(s). Thus, it is unconfounded by the factor(s). There may still be some residual confounding (chapter 8), however, depending on whether confounding still exists *within* the strata chosen. For example, stratifying by broad age groups (e.g., 50 years or less, more than 50 years) for a study of the relationship between hypertension and congestive heart disease may not remove all confounding by age because within each age stratum those with hypertension probably tend to be older than those without it. Constructing additional age strata using smaller age intervals could reduce any residual confounding if it is considered significant.[26]

If it turns out that a potentially confounding factor is not a confounder, the OR_{MH} should be the same as the crude odds ratio except for random error (see previous footnote, however). If the factor is a confounder, it will differ from the crude odds ratio to an extent depending on the degree and direc-

Figure 10-3   Stratification in a Case-Control Study

Exposure status	Cases	Controls		Exposure status	Cases	Controls
Exposed	a_1	b_1		Exposed	a_2	b_2
Unexposed	c_1	d_1		Unexposed	c_2	d_2

n_1 $\qquad\qquad\qquad\qquad\qquad$ n_2

Stratum One $\qquad\qquad\qquad\qquad$ Stratum Two
(Level One) $\qquad\qquad\qquad\qquad\quad$ (Level Two)

$$OR_1 = a_1 d_1 / b_1 c_1 \qquad\qquad OR_2 = a_2 d_2 / b_2 c_2$$

$$OR_{MH} = \frac{(a_1 d_1 / n_1) + (a_2 d_2 / n_2)}{(b_1 c_1 / n_1) + (b_2 c_2 / n_2)}$$

$$OR_C = \frac{(a_1 + a_2)(d_1 + d_2)}{(b_1 + b_2)(c_1 + c_2)}$$

tion of confounding exhibited in the original relationship. Comparing the crude and adjusted odds ratios can be a convenient way to determine if confounding is likely and to what extent, although other factors should also be considered before concluding confounding is present. Ideally, one should be able to answer affirmatively to the following questions: (a) Is the potential confounder an independent risk factor for the outcome?, (b) Is the potential confounder associated with the exposure of interest in the source population?, and (c) Is the potential confounder not an intermediate step in the causal sequence between the exposure and outcome? You should recognize these as the three essential conditions for confounding outlined in chapter 8. Unfortunately, one cannot always answer all of these questions, although the first one should be a prerequisite for even considering a factor a potential confounder. Granting the foregoing, an alternative to comparing the crude and adjusted odds ratios is to compare the stratum-specific odds ratios to the crude odds ratio. This method tends to work best if there are only a few strata. It can be more difficult to reach a conclusion, however, if there are many strata and substantial random error due, for instance, to small sample sizes in the strata.

The Mantel-Haenszel odds ratio should *not* be used to adjust for confounding when the stratum-specific odds ratios depart substantially from uniformity, that is, when the differences in the stratum-specific odds ratios are not likely to be due only to random error. In these cases, a phenomenon known as *effect measure modification* may be occurring. This phenomenon should be described rather than controlled as will be discussed in the next section. Another common method of summarizing stratum-specific odds ratios that does not depend on the odds ratios being uniform across the strata is *standardization*, which was discussed in the chapter 6 in the context of age adjustment. This method produces standardized odds ratios and is described further in chapter 11.

Procedures for calculating an approximate 95 percent confidence interval and a statistical test of significance for the OR_{MH} are shown in formulas 10.9 and 10.10, respectively.[3]

(10.9)

$$95\% \ CI = \exp\left\{\ln\left(OR_{MH}\right)\left[1\pm\left(1.96\sqrt{\chi^2_{MH}}\right)\right]\right\}$$

Note that formula 10.9 relies in part on the **Mantel-Haenszel chi-square test** (χ^2_{MH}), which is the appropriate test statistic for the OR_{MH}. It has one degree of freedom, and is calculated from formula 10.10. The frequencies in formula 10.10 are those derived from the 2×2 tables produced when stratification is used to control for confounding (see figure 10-3). The entry $\Sigma \ a_i$, for example, based on figure 10-3, is equivalent to $a_1 + a_2$.

(10.10)

$$\chi^2_{MH} = \frac{\left\{\Sigma a_i - \Sigma\left[\left(a_i + c_i\right)\left(a_i + b_i\right)/n_i\right]\right\}^2}{\Sigma\left[\left(a_i + c_i\right)\left(b_i + d_i\right)\left(a_i + b_i\right)\left(c_i + d_i\right)/n_i^2\left(n_i - 1\right)\right]}$$

Multivariable methods* are statistically efficient alternatives to stratification that can also be used to detect and control confounding in unmatched (and matched) case-control studies. These methods use specific mathematical models to analyze effects of exposure status (an independent variable) on outcome status (the dependent variable) while controlling simultaneously for potentially confounding factors. The most common type of multivariable analysis used in unmatched case-control studies is **multiple logistic regression**, which is a type of multiple regression where the outcome variable is dichotomous (i.e., present or absent). It is often referred to, though not entirely correctly, as simply **logistic regression**, which technically is a form of the statistical method where there is only one dependent and one independent variable. Multiple logistic regression, on the other hand, by definition has one dependent variable but two or more independent variables in the model. It is an extension of logistic regression just as multiple linear regression is an extension of simple linear regression (see chapter 9). Aside from its efficiency and convenience, this multivariable method is popular in analyzing data from case-control studies because regression coefficients based on dichotomous independent variables can be easily transformed into estimates of the odds ratios by calculating their exponentials. For example, if a logistic

---

*Some authors use the term *multivariate* methods. In a strict sense, multivariable methods refer to those methods where there is only one outcome variable and two or more independent variables, whereas multivariate methods are those in which there are two or more outcome variables. Most of the advanced statistical methods used in epidemiology are in the strict sense multivariable methods.

regression coefficient is 0.724, the corresponding odds ratio would be 2.06 (i.e., exp (0.724) = 2.06). This is the odds ratio *adjusted* simultaneously for all the other independent variables (potential confounders) in the model. Most output from relevant computer application programs that provide multiple logistic regression contains the multiple logistic regression coefficients along with the adjusted odds ratios and their 95 percent confidence intervals. An overview of multiple logistic regression is presented in exhibit 10-2. Detailed discussion of multivariable analysis is beyond the scope of this text. There are, however, many intermediate to advanced epidemiology texts and biostatistics books that discuss multivariable methods in depth.

When a matched analysis has been conducted, **conditional logistic regression** (technically, conditional *multiple* logistic regression) may be used. Multiple logistic regression when applied to matched studies requires that the original matching be preserved in the analysis. This has the unfortunate consequence of forcing many additional parameters into the model resulting in a situation where there are more parameters in the model than there are cases. Conditional logistic regression, however, removes these additional "nuisance" parameters, while still maintaining the original matching. Thus, it is the standard multiple logistic regression procedure applied when analyzing matched case-control studies.[29] Conditional logistic regression can also be used when analyzing the findings of nested case-control studies. Since the controls are selected among cohort members at risk at the time each case occurs (i.e., among the risk set), these studies can be considered "matched case-control studies" where the matched factor is the length of the follow-up period.[30]

Stratification versus Multivariable Analysis

While multivariable analysis, particularly multiple logistic regression, is frequently employed in case-control studies to detect and control confounding in the analysis, stratification may be a better choice. Kenneth J. Rothman[6] lists three major advantages of stratification over multivariable analysis. First, stratified analysis allows the investigator to visualize the distributions of the subjects by exposure, outcome, and potential confounders. This way one can see patterns or oddities in the data that are not observable in a multivariable analysis. Second, those who read the published research can also see these distributions when appropriate tables are presented. If desired, they can verify the results or conduct their own stratified analysis from the data presented. Finally, there is a lesser chance of bias in stratified analyses due to fewer methodological assumptions.

The major disadvantage of stratified analysis is that it may not be practical when there are many potential confounders to control, especially if each has several categories. This can significantly decrease the number of subjects in the various strata resulting in statistical inefficiency and hence imprecision in the results. In this situation multivariable analysis may be preferred. It provides a more statistically efficient way to measure the effect of a given exposure on the outcome while simultaneously controlling for several potential

Exhibit 10-2
What Is Multiple Logistic Regression?

Multiple logistic regression, a popular mathematical model frequently used in analyzing data from case-control studies, is a multivariable method that may be used when the outcome or dependent variable is dichotomous (outcome present, outcome absent), and there are two or more independent variables that may be continuous or categorical. The basic multiple logistic regression equation can be expressed in a manner similar to that used in multiple linear regression in that there is an intercept (α), which is a constant, and two or more independent variables (Xs) multiplied by regression coefficients (βs). The dependent variable, however, is expressed as a transformed value that is equivalent to the natural logarithm (ln) of the odds of the outcome occurring. This is known as a *logit transformation*, and it has the effect of making the dependent dichotomous variable behave like a continuous variable that can take on values theoretically ranging from negative to positive infinity. This basic equation can be represented as follows:

$$\ln (\text{odds}) = \alpha + \beta_1 X_1 + \beta_2 X_2 + \beta_3 X_3 \ldots + \beta_k X_k$$

When an independent variable, say X_1, is dichotomous with possible values of 0 or 1, then $\exp(\beta_1)$ is the odds that the outcome will occur in those where X_1 is present ($X_1 = 1$) compared to the odds it will occur in those where X_1 is absent ($X_1 = 0$), controlling for all other factors in the model. This odds ratio (OR) represents an *adjusted OR* since all other factors (X_2 through X_k) are held constant. When X_1 is a continuous variable, $\exp(\beta_1)$ represents the OR associated with a unit increase in X_1, controlling for all other factors. Thus, $\exp(\beta_1)$ is the *adjusted OR* associated with a one unit increase in X_1, and $\exp(5 \times \beta_1)$ is the adjusted OR associated with a five unit increase and so on.

For example, imagine that stroke (SKE) is hypothesized to be related to systolic blood pressure (SBP), sex (SEX), and age (AGE) as follows:

$$\ln (\text{odds SKE}) = \alpha + \beta_1(\text{SBP}) + \beta_2(\text{SEX}) + \beta_3(\text{AGE})$$

If for the variable SEX, male = 1 and female = 0, then $\exp(\beta_2)$ equals the OR for stroke for males compared to females, controlling for differences in systolic blood pressure and age. If the variable SBP is continuous, then $\exp(\beta_1)$ equals the OR for stroke for subjects whose systolic blood pressure is one millimeter greater than the referents, controlling for sex and age differences. Thus, for subjects with a systolic blood pressure of 150, $\exp(\beta_1)$ would represent the OR for stroke where the referents are those with a systolic blood pressure of 149, controlling for sex and age differences. Likewise, $\exp(5 \times \beta_1)$ would represent the adjusted OR for stroke in those with a systolic blood pressure of 150 compared to those with a systolic blood pressure of 145.

In most computer application programs that calculate multiple logistic regression the equations are based on *maximum likelihood estimates* (i.e., the values of alpha and beta that have the greatest probability of having produced the observed data). The multiple logistic regression model is considered a *multiplicative model* since it is based on the assumption that a variable in the model multiplies the odds of the outcome by the same amount irrespective of the values of the other variables.

References: Cambell, M. J., and Machin, D. (1999). *Medical Statistics: A Common Sense Approach*, 3rd ed. Chichester: John Wiley & Sons Ltd.; Kelsey, J. L., Thompson, W. D., and Evans, A. S. (1986). *Methods in Observational Epidemiology*. New York: Oxford University Press.

confounders. Nevertheless, Rothman argues that a stratified analysis for the primary potential confounders should still be conducted before the multivariable analysis. In other words, multivariable analysis should be viewed as a supplement to a stratified analysis. [6]

EFFECT MEASURE MODIFICATION

Background

Even though assessment of confounding was discussed prior to *effect measure modification*, the latter should be assessed before the former in a study. **Effect measure modification** occurs when the magnitude of the effect of a study exposure on an outcome varies at different levels of a third factor (the first two factors being the exposure and the outcome), and this variation is not due to random or systematic error. This phenomenon, also referred to as **heterogeneity of effect**, is perhaps most clearly seen in a stratified analysis. For example, assume the crude odds ratio (OR_c) for the relationship between exposure A and outcome B is 3.0 in an unmatched case-control study. When this relationship is stratified by sex, assume the stratum-specific odds ratios are 1.0 for females and 5.0 for males. This suggests that sex is an **effect modifier**; that is, sex appears to modify the effect of A on B differently depending on the level of stratification. Among females, the odds of exposure to A is the same in cases and controls, but among males, the odds of exposure to A is five times greater in cases than controls. This implies that A is *not* associated with B among females but is strongly associated with B among males. If true, the implications for public health policy could be important depending on such factors as the seriousness of outcome B, the prevalence of exposure A, the proportion of males in the population, and, believe it or not, the type of measure of association that is used.

Unfortunately, many concepts in epidemiology are not always as simple as they first appear. Effect measure modification is no exception. It turns out that effect measure modification is *dependent* on the measure of association used. In fact, this concept was previously referred to as simply *effect modification*, but that terminology is now recognized by some as being too ambiguous because effect modification identified using a ratio measure of association may not exist if a difference measure of association is used, and vice versa. [6] Hence, the addition of the term "measure" represents an attempt to anchor effect modification to the type of measure of association being used. In general, we cannot make statements about effect measure modification without communicating the measure of association used since, as stated above, effect measure modification depends on the type of measure of association. Therefore, it is recommended that findings of effect measure modification be stated as specifically as possible. For example, it would be proper to say, "no heterogeneity of the odds ratio was found" or "effect measure modification was present using the odds ratio." The latter statement, in fact, would apply to the example cited in the previous paragraph. When statistical modeling is used (i.e., in multivariable analysis) one should refer to the nature of the statistical model since effect measure modification is dependent on the model chosen (i.e., additive or multiplicative; defined below). In statistical modeling, effect measure modification is often referred to as **statistical interaction**, or simply **interaction**, which are terms commonly used in the field of statistics, but frequently adopted by epidemiologists as well. In summary, effect measure modification (or statistical interaction) in a particular instance depends on the type of measure of association or the statistical model used in an analysis.[6] Therefore, these should be stated when reporting effect measure modification or statistical interaction.

Effect measure modification is distinct from confounding. Confounding can be viewed as an annoyance that needs to be identified and controlled so that we can get a valid look at the relationship between a given study exposure and outcome. Effect measure modification, on the other hand, is an effect that may help clarify the relationship between an exposure and outcome in the presence of other factors. Therefore, it should be described in a study. Although effect measure modification and confounding can occur together, effect measure modification should always take priority in the general sequence of analysis.

Assessing Effect Measure Modification (and Confounding)

A common method of identifying effect measure modification in case-control studies involves stratification. Often the procedure entails little more than viewing the stratum-specific odds ratios to see if they appear heterogeneous, taking into consideration that the differences could be due to random or systematic errors. If the differences appear real, effect measure modification (i.e., heterogeneity of effect) is suspected. In practice, stratification is often used to ascertain *both* effect measure modification and confounding as illustrated in table 10-3.

Table 10-3 provides some hypothetical results from case-control studies employing stratification on just two levels of a third factor. Comparison of the crude odds ratio with the unconfounded stratum-specific odds ratios provides an indication of whether effect measure modification or confounding is likely to be present. For example, in the second row of the table, the crude odds ratio appears to be confounded because it is larger than the unconfounded stratum-specific odds ratios. Effect measure modification is unlikely, however, because the unconfounded stratum-specific odds ratios are nearly identical, which we would expect if confounding is the only issue. In this example the confounding is considered *positive* (chapter 8) because the crude odds ratio is overestimated when compared to the unconfounded stratum-specific odds ratios. It would be appropriate in this example to calculate a Mantel-Haenszel odds ratio based on the stratum-specific odds ratios if one chooses to do so. It would represent a weighted average of the pooled stratum-specific odds ratios adjusted for the potential confounder. In row four of the table, effect measure modification appears to be present because the unconfounded stratum-specific odds ratios are very different (i.e., heterogeneous). Confounding is unlikely or insignificant because the unconfounded stratum-specific odds ratios are not both greater or less than the crude odds ratio, which we would expect if confounding were also an issue. Since the stratum-specific odds ratios are heterogeneous, it would not be appropriate to calculate a Mantel-Haenszel odds ratio based on these data. Such a summary measure would mask the apparent heterogeneity, which could represent an important public health finding. *Standardization* (chapter 11), however, could be used to summarize the odds ratios since it does not depend on the stratum-specific odds ratios being homogeneous. Finally, in the eighth row, the data appear to indicate both confounding and effect measure modification. The heterogeneity of the stratum-specific odds ratios implies effect measure

Table 10-3   Examples of Possible Confounding and Effect Measure Modification Using the Odds Ratio in Case-Control Studies

Row	Crude OR (OR_C)	Stratum-Specific ORs		Confounding	Effect Measure Modification
-----	------	OR_1	OR_2	------	------
(1)	4.00	4.00	4.02	None	Absent
(2)	3.50	1.05	1.01	Positive	Absent
(3)	1.00	2.50	2.48	Negative	Absent
(4)	2.75	1.20	6.35	None	Present
(5)	4.25	0.96	0.15	Positive	Present
(6)	2.00	1.00	1.10	Positive	Absent
(7)	3.75	0.75	2.85	Positive	Present
(8)	0.85	2.10	7.10	Negative	Present
(9)	2.35	0.50	4.12	None	Present

Summary

Confounding is likely to be present alone when:

$$OR_C \neq OR_1 = OR_2 \text{ or } OR_C \neq OR_{MH}$$

(Small differences in OR_1 and OR_2 are assumed to be due to random error.)

- If $OR_C > OR_1 = OR_2$, the confounding is considered *positive*.
- If $OR_C < OR_1 = OR_2$, the confounding is considered *negative*.

Effect measure modification for odds ratios is likely to be present when:

$$OR_1 \neq OR_2$$

(The difference should be more than that due to random error; differences in direction are most significant.)

Confounding and effect measure modification are likely to be present when:

$$OR_C < OR_1 \text{ and } OR_2, \text{ and } OR_1 \neq OR_2 \text{ or } OR_C > OR_1 \text{ and } OR_2, \text{ and } OR_1 \neq OR_2$$

Reference: Kleinbaum, D. G., Kupper, L. L., and Morgenstern, H. (1982). *Epidemiologic Research: Principles and Quantitative Methods.* Belmont, CA: Lifetime Learning Publications.

modification, while the fact that both stratum-specific odds ratios are larger than the crude odds ratio intimates that the crude odds ratio is underestimated due to *negative* confounding. The equations in table 10-3 can also be used to indicate whether confounding, effect measure modification, or both is more likely based on the observed odds ratios. An important *caution*, however, is necessary here. As indicated in the previous section on confounding, one should not rely on "the numbers" alone. Confounding requires, among other things, that the confounder be an independent risk factor for the study outcome, and this should be determined prior to selecting control variables (i.e., potential confounders) to analyze.[31] If there is no evidence to support that a factor may be a confounder, then despite what "the numbers" may appear to reveal, one should be hesitant to conclude that confounding is an issue. This concern is appropriately underscored in the following statement from a classic text in epidemiology:

> Prerequisite to any evaluation of confounding in the data is the consideration of causal relationships that the investigator believes to be operating in the target population. This latter point has not been fully appreciated by many investigators, and, if it is ignored the result may be unwarranted control of nonconfounders. Such unnecessary adjustment can lower precision and may even introduce bias into the estimate of effect.[31(p255)]

The above point is particularly *crucial* with regard to the odds ratio, which can sometimes exhibit apparent confounding in a stratified analysis even when it is absent. This may occur because the variable, although a risk factor for the outcome, is *not* associated with the study exposure. Because of this potential problem, it has been recommended that when neither confounding nor effect measure modification are suspected, *both* the crude and Mantel-Haenszel odds ratios be reported in characterizing the effect of the study exposure on the outcome.[32] The same recommendation, however, is *not* made for other common measures of association used in cross-sectional or cohort studies (e.g., prevalence or risk ratios). Also, it is possible that effect measure modification identified using odds ratios based on cumulative incidence sampling does not exist when the odds ratios are based on case-base or incidence density sampling (described earlier).[33] These are peculiarities of the odds ratio and reasons for identifying the measure of association *and* the sampling method used when reporting effect measure modification, or for that matter, confounding in case-control studies.

Another Approach to Assessing Effect Measure Modification

Another way of determining if effect measure modification is present involves comparing the *observed* and *expected* joint effect of the exposure and suspected effect modifier on the study outcome.[30] This approach is commonly applied in multivariable analysis, and like stratification, can be extended to more than just two independent variables. However, to keep the discussion simple, we will focus on situations where there is just one exposure variable and one potential effect modifier. In either case the concept remains the same. It is important to note that this approach has more flexibility than stratification when it comes to evaluating effect measure modification in unmatched case-control studies. This is because stratification using odds ratios only allows for the assessment of effect measure modification using a *multiplicative model*. A **multiplicative model** is one where the combined effect of two or more variables on an outcome is the *product* of their separate effects.[1] Since ratio measures of association, and hence the odds ratio, always indicate a multiplicative model, only **multiplicative effects** (those based on a multiplicative model) can be measured using the odds ratio. **Additive effects**, those based on an *additive model*, cannot be measured using the odds ratio. An **additive model** is one where the combined effect of two or more variables on an outcome is the *sum* of their separate effects.[1] Additive models are based on difference measures of association (e.g., risk differences), which generally cannot be derived from case-control studies. Thus, stratification in case-control studies using odds ratios only helps us identify effect measure modification based on a multiplicative model. Comparing observed and expected joint effects, however, allows for both types of comparison (multiplicative and additive) with just a little mathematical sleight of hand, as shall be demonstrated shortly. To recapitulate briefly, if a *ratio measure of association* is used, then any observed heterogeneity of effect will reflect a deviation from a multiplicative model, and if a *difference measure of association* is used, any observed heterogeneity of effect will represent a deviation from an additive model.

To get specific, using the odds ratio, the *observed joint effect* of the exposure and potential effect modifier on the study outcome will equal the *expected joint effect* of the two variables when there is *no* effect measure modification present. Thus, when effect measure modification is present, the observed and expected joint effects will differ. Since the use of the odds ratio assumes a multiplicative model, any observed effect measure modification (statistical interaction) can be referred to as **multiplicative interaction**; that is, statistical interaction based on a multiplicative model. Formula 10.11 summarizes the relationship when there is *no* multiplicative interaction.[30]

(10.11)

$$\text{Observed OR}_{E, M} = \text{Expected O}_{E, M} = \text{Observed OR}_E \times \text{Observed OR}_M$$

The subscripts E and M in formula 10.11 represent the exposure and potential effect modifier, respectively. This equation says that there is no multiplicative interaction present if the observed joint effect of the exposure and potential effect modifier ($\text{OR}_{E, M}$) equals the expected joint effect, which is the product of the separate observed effects of the exposure (OR_E) and the potential effect modifier (OR_M), respectively. If Observed $\text{OR}_{E, M}$ is *greater* than Expected $\text{OR}_{E, M}$, we have **positive interaction**, the extent to which depends on the magnitude of the difference. On the other hand, if Observed $\text{OR}_{E, M}$ is *less* than Expected $\text{O}_{E, M}$, we have **negative interaction**.[30] Thus, positive interaction means the observed joint effect of the variables is greater than the expected joint effect, and negative interaction means the observed joint effect is less than the expected joint effect, all other factors being equal. Of course, small differences may be inconsequential.

When there is no statistical interaction with *difference measures of association*, the observed joint effect of the exposure and potential effect modifier on the study outcome will equal the sum of the expected joint effect of the two variables. This latter sum is determined by adding their separate effects together (see formula 10.12). One cannot normally calculate a risk or rate difference in a case-control study (i.e., the difference in the absolute risk or rate between the exposed and unexposed subjects) due to the nature of the study design. Nevertheless, it is still possible to assess statistical interaction under an additive model (i.e., **additive interaction**) by evaluating the observed and expected joint effect of the exposure and potential effect modifier on the study outcome using **excess odds ratios** (i.e., those where the measures are OR – 1.0). These are a type of *relative effect* as suggested in chapter 6. The basic formula when there is *no* additive interaction is:[30]

(10.12)
Observed $OR_{E, M}$ = Expected $OR_{E, M}$ = Observed OR_E + Observed OR_M – 1.0

To use this formula, the OR_E and OR_M must each be at least one. One is subtracted from the sum of these values since $OR_{E, M}$, OR_E, and OR_M all represent *excess odds ratios*, and not odds ratios per se. Actually, the equation is: Observed $OR_{E, M}$ – 1.0 = Expected $OR_{E, M}$ – 1.0 = (Observed OR_E – 1.0) + (Observed OR_M – 1.0). Mathematically, this is equivalent to formula 10.12. When OR_E and OR_M are both less than one, the appropriate formula is:[30]

(10.13)   Observed $OR_{E, M}$ = Expected $OR_{E, M}$ =
1.0 / {[(1.0 / Observed OR_E) + (1.0 / Observed OR_M)] – 1.0}

Positive interaction exists when Observed $OR_{E, M}$ represents a stronger measure of association than Expected $OR_{E, M}$. Negative interaction exists when the association is weaker. Small differences, however, may not be of any practical significance, which is also true regarding formula 10.11. These formulas (10.11–10.13) are not applicable when one of the variables (E or M) is matched as in matched case-control studies. A stratified analysis assessing effect measure modification based on a multiplicative model, however, can be easily applied to matched studies.[30]

Table 10-4 illustrates how both multiplicative and additive interaction can be assessed by comparing the observed and expected joint effects of a study exposure (E) and a potential effect modifier (M) on a study outcome. In the example cited, the various odds ratios were calculated by determining the odds of the outcome in each category in which cases and controls were exposed to E or M and dividing these odds by the odds of the outcome in the referent group (chapter 6), which represents no exposure to either E or M. Please be aware that the numbers and calculations leading to the reported

Table 10-4   Assessment of Multiplicative and Additive Interaction in Case-Control Studies Using the Odds Ratio

Results of a hypothetical study of the relationship between E and M and a given outcome

Exposed?

E	M	OR	What's Measured
No	No	1.0	Referent
Yes	No	1.5	Independent effect of E
No	Yes	6.0	Independent effect of M
Yes	Yes	9.0	Observed joint effect

Key

E = the study exposure
M = the potential effect modifier
OR = observed odds ratio

Assessment of multiplicative interaction:

Observed $OR_{E, M}$ = Expected $OR_{E, M}$ = Observed OR_E x Observed OR_M

Since 9.0 = 1.5 x 6.0, there is *no* evidence of multiplicative interaction using the odds ratio.

Assessment of additive interaction:

Observed $OR_{E, M}$ = Expected $OR_{E, M}$ = Observed OR_E + Observed OR_M − 1.0

Since 9.0 > 1.5 + 6.0 − 1.0 = 6.5, there is evidence of additive interaction, and it is positive, using the odds ratio.

Reference: Szklo, M., and Nieto, F. J. (2000). *Epidemiology: Beyond the Basics.* Gaithersburg, MD: Aspen.

odds ratios are not shown in this table. The odds ratio for the referent group of no exposure to either factor is arbitrarily set at 1.0, which is common practice. In the example there is no evidence of multiplicative interaction because the observed joint effect (9.0) equals the expected joint effect (9.0), but there is evidence of additive interaction, which is positive, since the observed joint effect (9.0) exceeds the expected joint effect (6.5).

Summary and Conclusions

Effect measure modification based on a multiplicative model can be assessed in case-control studies using a stratified analysis. Basically, one looks for variations in the stratum-specific odds ratios that are unlikely due to random or systematic errors. The following steps should be considered:

- Observe the stratum-specific odds ratios to see if they differ materially in magnitude or direction, keeping in mind that odds ratios based on small sample sizes are more likely to vary due to random error.
- If necessary, perform a **test of heterogeneity** (also referred to as a **test of homogeneity**) to examine the probability that the stratum-specific odds

ratios represent nonrandom differences. Basically, these tests determine whether the stratum-specific odds ratios are significantly different from each other (see J. J. Schlesselman[3] for examples).

• Consider whether effect measure modification makes sense based on other studies or if there may be systematic errors that could produce similar results. Where possible, control for the systematic errors.

One should be cautious in using tests of heterogeneity (or homogeneity). When the sample sizes are large, even small differences in measures of association may be statistically significant. Also, even though statistical significance may not be reached in a particular analysis, it does not necessarily exclude the possibility of effect measure modification, especially when the differences in the measures of association are fairly large. It could be a problem of insufficient power.[30] Therefore, tests of heterogeneity should not be the sole reason for concluding that effect measure modification is either present or absent in a study. Reasons that may explain apparent differences in measures of association across strata other than random error include selective or residual confounding, bias, or differential intensity of the exposure.[30]

If the overall evidence points to effect measure modification, the stratum-specific odds ratios and their 95 percent confidence intervals should be reported and discussed in the study. Based on guidelines offered by Stephen C. Newman,[32] if in addition there is *no* evidence of confounding, the crude odds ratio should also be reported. However, if there is evidence of confounding, a standardized odds ratio (chapter 11) would be more informative since the crude odds ratio will be biased. Because of the peculiarities of the odds ratio, when effect modification is *absent*, the following measures should be reported:[32]

• No confounding present: Crude and Mantel-Haenszel odds ratios

• Confounding present: Standardized and Mantel-Haenszel odds ratios

In addition to using stratification, effect measure modification based on a multiplicative model may be examined by comparing the odds ratios derived from the observed and expected joint effects of the exposure and potential effect modifier on the study outcome. This can be done in the context of multivariable methods, such as multiple logistic regression. The observed and expected excess odds ratios may also be compared to evaluate whether effect measure modification is present based on an additive model. In both of these applications, effect measure modification is often referred to as statistical interaction or interaction, where the effect represents a departure from the underlying statistical model (i.e., multiplicity or additivity). For example, if the model is based on additivity of effects, a meaningful departure from additivity would indicate statistical interaction. However, even if there is no statistical interaction based on an additive model there may be some based on a multiplicative model, and vice versa. Thus, statistical interaction depends on the mathematical model, or as mentioned earlier, the measure of association used.[6]

It is also worth mentioning that epidemiologists often differentiate between two general types of effect measure modification (or statistical interaction). These are usually termed **quantitative interaction** and **qualitative interaction**, respectively. Briefly, the former represents effects of exposure on the outcome that differ from stratum to stratum but are in the same direction; that is, all odds ratios are greater than one, or all odds ratios are less than one (see, for example, row 4 in table 10-3). The latter represents interactions that differ in direction across the strata; that is, some odds ratios are equal to or greater than one, and some odds ratios are less than one (see, for example, row 9 in table 10-3). Qualitative interaction includes those situations where there is an effect in one of the strata but not the other (e.g., $OR_1 = 4.2$, $OR_2 = 1.0$).[30] An apparent example of qualitative interaction was reported by Korean investigators who found that the relationship between *H. pylori* seropositivity and gastric cancer appeared to be modified by the amount of daily vitamin C intake. Specifically, the authors found an OR of 4.68 between *H. pylori* seropositivity and gastric cancer in the low vitamin C intake group (less than or equal to 93.3 mg. per day) and an OR of 0.72 in the high vitamin C intake group (more than 93.3 mg. per day).[34] The example at the beginning of this section also illustrates qualitative interaction since one of the strata (females) showed no effect, while the other (males) did.

Finally, it should be emphasized that statistical interaction does not imply **biological interaction**, which represents the combined involvement of two or more factors in causing a given disease in a population. Biological interaction is not affected by the measure of association or the mathematical model used in a study,[6] since it represents a real effect. Technically, it correspond to *synergism* or *antagonism*. **Synergism** occurs when two or more factors acting together in a population result in a greater frequency of outcomes than would be expected if the factors operated independently (e.g., cigarette smoking and radon exposure together multiply the risk of lung cancer). **Antagonism** occurs when the combined factors result in a smaller frequency of outcomes than would be expected if the factors operated independently (e.g., nitrites and vitamin C together reduce the risk of stomach cancer). In essence, synergism implies that $1 + 1 > 2$, which antagonism implies that $1 + 1 < 2$. Both phenomena are based on the assumption that the relationships are causal. Although synergism and antagonism can be applied to multiplicative models, by strict definition they represent departures from additivity. Thus, in biological interaction deviations from additivity are the primary focus of interest.

From the preceding discussion, one can see that effect measure modification or statistical interaction is a relatively involved topic. For some this will all seem overly complicated, but, unfortunately, that is the nature of the beast so to speak. Perhaps this is why epidemiologists are paid the big bucks (not really, of course). A more complete discussion of the details of interaction may be found in intermediate-level texts, such as the one by Kenneth J. Rothman and Sander Greenland.[35] Effect measure modification (and confounding) are also referred to in subsequent chapters dealing with other epidemiologic study designs.

Problem 10-1 below illustrates the basic analysis of an unmatched case-control study, including the use of stratification. Problem 10-2, which follows, illustrates the basic analysis of a pair-matched case-control study. These problems are followed by a discussion of the major advantages and disadvantages of case-control studies and a brief description of the *case-crossover study*, a relatively new variation in case-control design.

Problem 10-1: Analysis of an Unmatched Case-Control Study

An epidemiologist wanted to test the hypothesis that cigarette smoking is a risk factor for fatalities from automobile crashes. To test her hypothesis, she selected as cases all licensed drivers in Hendricks County, 18–59 years of age, who were involved in fatal automobile crashes in the county while driving any time during the past two years. Controls were selected randomly from a state list of licensed drivers in the same age group and residing in Hendricks County. A total of 100 cases and 200 controls meeting the eligibility criteria were enrolled in the study. Cases and controls were frequency matched with regard to age group, sex, and race. Interviews with spouses, friends, and co-workers of the cases and with the controls indicated that 68 of the cases and 104 of the controls were cigarette smokers for at least five years prior to the dates of the crashes. Based on this information, determine if the findings support the investigator's hypothesis by calculating the crude odds ratio and its 95 percent confidence interval.

During the study, additional data were collected on the subjects' drinking habits. Among the 68 cases that smoked cigarettes, 58 were drinkers, and 10 were nondrinkers. Among the 32 cases that did not smoke cigarettes, 22 were drinkers, and 10 were nondrinkers. Similarly, among the 104 controls that smoked cigarettes, 70 were drinkers, and 34 were nondrinkers, and among the 96 controls that did not smoke cigarettes, 42 were drinkers, and 54 were nondrinkers. Based on this additional information, determine if drinking status is a confounder or an effect modifier for the hypothesized relationship.

Solution:
Step 1: Place the frequencies provided in the study description in the appropriate cells of a 2 × 2 contingency table. Where there are missing values, calculate them from the data provided. For example, since there were 100 cases, and 68 of these were cigarette smokers, the number of cases that did not smoke is $100 - 68 = 32$. Likewise, since 104 of the 200 controls were cigarette smokers those that did not smoke is $200 - 104 = 96$.

	Outcome Status	
Exposure Status	Cases	Controls
Smokers	68	104
Nonsmokers	32	96
	100	200

Step 2: Calculate the crude odds ratio from the contingency table using formula 10.2.

$$OR_c = ad / bc = (68 \times 96) / (104 \times 32) = 6{,}528 / 3{,}328 = 1.96$$

Step 3: Calculate the 95 percent confidence interval for the OR_c using formula 10.3.

$$95\% \ CI = exp\left\{\ln(OR_c) \pm 1.96\sqrt{(1/a)+(1/b)+(1/c)+(1/d)}\right\} =$$
$$exp\left\{\ln(1.96) \pm 1.96\sqrt{(1/68)+(1/104)+(1/32)+(1/96)}\right\} =$$
$$exp\left\{0.673 \pm 1.96(0.257)\right\} = exp(0.673 \pm 0.503) =$$
$$exp(0.170), \ exp(1.18) = 1.19, \ 3.25$$
$$95\% \ CI = 1.19 \ to \ 3.25$$

The crude odds ratio and its 95 percent confidence interval can be stated as OR_c = 1.96 (95% CI = 1.19 to 3.25). This finding appears to support the investigator's hypothesis that cigarette smoking is a risk factor for fatal automobile crashes.

Step 4: To determine if drinking status is a confounder or an effect modifier for the observed effect, one can stratify the analysis by drinking status. This can be done by creating contingency tables for each stratum as shown below. The values in the cells of the contingency tables are taken from the data provided in the study description.

Exposure Status	Cases	Controls		Cases	Controls
Smokers	58	70		10	34
Nonsmokers	22	42		10	54

Stratum 1: Drinkers   *Stratum 2: Nondrinkers*

Step 5: Calculate the stratum-specific odds ratios using formula 10.2.

$$Drinkers: OR_1 = (58 \times 42) / (70 \times 22) = 2{,}436 / 1{,}540 = 1.58$$
$$Nondrinkers: OR_2 = (10 \times 54) / (34 \times 10) = 540 / 340 = 1.59$$

Since the stratum-specific odds ratios are nearly identical (1.58 and 1.59), but different from the crude odds ratio (1.96), confounding by drinking appears to be present (see table 10-3). This is an apparent example of positive confounding, since the crude odds ratio appears inflated because of a failure to account for confounding by drinking status. Effect measure modification using the odds ratio does not appear to be present because the stratum-specific odds ratios do not display any material heterogeneity.

Step 6: Since effect measure modification is not apparent, a Mantel-Haenszel odds ratio (OR_{MH}) can be calculated using formula 10.8. The OR_{MH} is a weighted average of the stratum-specific odds ratios based on the strata sample sizes.

$$OR_{MH} = \Sigma \ (a_i \, d_i \, / \, n_i) \, / \, \Sigma \ (b_i \, c_i \, / \, n_i) =$$
$$\{[(58 \times 42) / 192] + [(10 \times 54) / 108]\} \, / \, \{[(70 \times 22) / 192] + [(34 \times 10) / 108]\} =$$
$$[(2{,}436 / 192) + (540 / 108)] \, / \, [(1{,}540 / 192) + (340 / 108)] =$$
$$(12.69 + 5.00) / (8.02 + 3.15) =$$
$$17.69 / 11.17 = 1.58$$

Since there are more drinkers than nondrinkers in this problem, it is not surprising that the OR_{MH} is weighted toward the odds ratio among the drinkers (i.e., 1.58). The Mantel-Haenszel odds ratio is most useful when there are multiple strata and more random variation among the stratum-specific odds ratios than observed here.

Answer: Based on the initial data, it appears that the hypothesis is supported by the study conducted in Hendricks County. That is, overall, cigarette smoking appears to be a risk factor for fatal automobile crashes (OR_C = 1.96; 95% CI = 1.19 to 3.25). Further analysis, however, reveals that the effect appears to be positively confounded by drinking status. That is, the crude OR appears inflated due to a failure to adjust for drinking status. The adjusted odds ratio (OR_{MH}) of 1.58 thus provides a better estimate of the true effect of cigarette smoking on fatal automobile crashes, assuming drinking status is the only important confounder and that there are no significant sources of bias in the study. Effect measure modification by drinking status using odds ratios is not apparent from the data.

Comments:

1. An unmatched analysis is appropriate in this problem because individual or pair matching was not employed in the study. Frequency matching was used, but it does not require a matched analysis. In fact, studies using frequency matching should always be analyzed using an unmatched analysis.

2. Since the outcome measure is death, we can be assured that the cases represent incident cases, which are desirable in a case-control study. Also, the exposure occurred prior to the outcome, which is the temporal sequence necessary to make statements about risk or causation.

3. This is a population-based case-control study. Both cases and controls were selected directly from a defined population in the county. Specifically, all cases, as defined in the study, were included, and controls were randomly selected from the source population. Therefore, it is reasonable to believe that the subjects are representative of licensed drivers in the county between 18 and 59 years of age. References to the population at large (i.e., licensed and unlicensed drivers) is not warranted, however, since the study was restricted, in addition to age, to licensed drivers in the county. This could limit the external validity of the study since unlicensed drivers may be more likely to be involved in fatal automobile crashes and may be more likely to smoke.

4. The crude odds ratio was 1.96. This represents an estimate of the overall odds ratio for the effect of cigarette smoking on fatal automobile crashes in the study population. Like any crude measure of association, a crude odds ratio may conceal confounding by other factors as it apparently did in this study.

5. The stratum-specific odds ratios are calculated in the same manner as the crude odds ratio. The only difference is that they represent odds ratios only for specific subgroups of the study population. Specifically, they represent odds ratios based on drinking status in this population

6. Using stratification as a means of detecting confounding is not as reliable when the measure of association is the odds ratio as opposed to other ratio measures of association. Specifically, it is possible for the stratum-specific odds ratios to be to be similar but different from the crude odds ratio even when confounding is *not* present. Because of this possibility, it is especially important to consider the evidence that confounding exists beyond what is revealed by the odds ratios. In this

study, drinking status is very likely a real confounder in that it meets the three conditions for confounding: (a) Drinking is a well recognized independent risk factor for automobile crashes; (b) It is known to be associated with cigarette smoking; and (c) It is not likely to represent an intermediate step in a causal sequence between cigarette smoking and automobile crashes.

7. Because there was apparent confounding by drinking status, the OR_{MH} of 1.58 is an appropriate measure of association to report when referring to the effect of cigarette smoking on fatal automobile crashes in this population. This means that the odds of cigarette smoking are 1.58 times greater in drivers involved in fatal automobile crashes than those not involved in fatal automobile crashes *after adjusting for drinking status*. This is the exposure odds ratio. Alternatively, we could say, the odds of being involved in a fatal automobile crash is 1.58 times greater among cigarette smokers than non-cigarette smokers after adjusting for drinking status. This is the disease odds ratio. Thus, the OR_{MH} is an adjusted odds ratio, and in this case it is the odds ratio adjusted for drinking status. Since the OR_{MH} is greater than one, it implies that there is still a moderate, positive effect (see table 6-3) of cigarette smoking on fatal automobile crashes after accounting for drinking status, although it is not as strong as the OR_C seemed to indicate. In other words, the apparent confounding by drinking status was only partial. If the overall effect were entirely due to confounding by drinking status, the OR_{MH} would be 1.0, implying no effect of cigarette smoking on fatal automobile crashes after adjustment for drinking status.

8. Though not done in this problem, one would normally calculate a 95 percent confidence interval for the Mantel-Haenszel odds ratio (OR_{MH}) in order to assess its relative precision. Formula 10.9 will do this, but since it also requires that formula 10.10 be calculated, it can be tedious to do by hand. It is easier to use a computer-assisted application. In any case, the approximate 95 percent confidence interval for the OR_{MH} is 0.94 to 2.68. This indicates a somewhat imprecise odds ratio, which probably reflects low power. In fact, based on the overall study size to detect a significant odds ratio as low as 1.96, the power is about 75 percent, and the power to detect an odds ratio as low as 1.58 is less than 50 percent. To get this to at least 80 percent, a commonly suggested minimum, would require about 225 cases and twice as many controls in the study. One criticism of the study represented in this problem is that power was apparently not examined before conducting the study. A more comprehensive look at the potential power of the study may have been helpful in increasing the statistical efficiency of the stratified analysis.

9. No evidence of effect measure modification was found in this study using the odds ratio. It is important to indicate that this finding is based on the odds ratio since the presence of effect measure modification is dependent on the measure of association used in a study. Since confounding appears to be present in this study, but effect measure modification appears to be absent, it is recommended that both the Mantel-Haenszel odds ratio and the standardized odds ratio be reported in the findings. Although we have not discussed the calculation of standardized odds ratios (it is discussed briefly in chapter 11), it turns out that the value of the standardized odds ratio, using the exposed group as the standard, is identical to the value of the Mantel-Haenszel odds ratio (1.58). This confirms that heterogeneity of effect (i.e., effect measure modification) is very unlikely in this study.

Problem 10-2: Analysis of a Matched Case-Control Study

An epidemiologist was interested in testing the hypothesis that antibiotic therapy during infancy is related to the development of asthma in later childhood. To test his hypothesis the epidemiologist identified 500 cases with newly diagnosed childhood asthma from the five medical facilities serving a large city in North Carolina. Five hundred controls were also selected from outpatients with diagnoses unrelated to asthma visiting the same facilities during the same time period as the cases. The cases and controls were pair matched on age (+/− 2 years), sex, and parental smoking status. The overall results of the study are summarized in the following table. Based on these data, calculate the appropriate measure of association and its 95 percent confidence interval. Also, interpret your findings.

Note: In the table below "exposed" refers to use of antibiotics during infancy (0–2 years), and "unexposed" refers to no use of antibiotics during the same period.

	Controls	
Cases	Exposed	Unexposed
Exposed	170	145
Unexposed	80	105

Step 1: Based on the data in the above table, calculate the matched pairs odds ratio (OR-MP) using formula 10.4.

$$OR\text{-}MP = x / y = 145 / 80 = 1.81$$

The matched pairs odds ratio (OR-MP) is interpreted in the same manner as an odds ratio based on an unmatched study. Therefore, it may be interpreted as follows: The odds of an infant developing later childhood asthma are 1.81 times greater (81 percent higher) in those infants who have had antibiotic therapy in infancy than those who have not, all other factors being equal. This interpretation represents the disease odds ratio. Based on table 6-3, the overall association is moderately strong.

Step 2: Calculate the 95 percent confidence interval for the OR-MP using formula 10.5.

$$95\% \ CI = \exp\left\{\ln(x/y) \pm 1.96\sqrt{(1/x)+(1/y)}\right\} =$$
$$\exp\left\{\ln(1.81) \pm 1.96\sqrt{(1/145)+(1/80)}\right\} =$$
$$\exp\left\{0.593 \pm 1.96(0.14)\right\} = \exp(0.593 \pm 0.273) =$$
$$\exp(0.320), \ \exp(0.866) = 1.38, \ 2.38$$
$$95\% \ CI = 1.38 \ to \ 2.38$$

This says that we are 95 percent confident that the true matched pairs odds ratio lies between 1.38 and 2.38. This relatively narrow confidence interval indicates that the estimate of the odds ratio (1.81) is fairly precise.

Answer: Based on data in the problem, the overall odds ratio is 1.81 (95% CI = 1.38 to 2.38). This means that infants who have had antibiotic therapy have nearly twice the odds of developing asthma in later childhood as those who have not, all other factors being equal. The 95 percent confidence interval indicates that the odds ratio is relatively precise.

Comments:
1. A matched analysis is appropriate in this problem because pair matching was used in the design of the study. Specifically, the cases and controls were matched on age, sex, and parental smoking status.

2. Matching in the design of the study followed by a matched analysis controls for confounding by the matched variables, assuming they were confounding factors in the study. Therefore, age, sex, and parental smoking status should not confound the overall odds ratio calculated in this study. The matched analysis for dichotomous measures of exposure and outcome using pair matching is relatively simple. It is more complicated, however, when there is more than one control per case.

3. The controls for the study were selected from the same facilities as the cases under the assumption that they came from the same source population, which may or may not be true. For example, the cases might tend to represent subjects from a wider geographic area and higher socioeconomic level than the controls if any of the facilities used in the study are referral hospitals for childhood asthma. This could create selection bias.

4. Controls with diagnoses known to be related to infant antibiotic use were excluded from the study since their inclusion could result in an overestimation or underestimation of the true effect of infant antibiotic use on later childhood asthma depending on whether the diagnoses are positively or negatively related to the antibiotic use.

ADVANTAGES AND DISADVANTAGES
OF CASE-CONTROL STUDIES

Case-control studies have a number of potential advantages and disadvantages. The major ones are summarized in table 10-5. In terms of advantages, case-control studies are usually quicker and less expensive than cohort studies, partly because sampling of controls is more efficient and the follow-up period has already occurred. Another advantage of case-control studies is that they are entirely appropriate when studying rare outcomes. Since subjects are selected on the basis of outcome status, it is generally possible to achieve a sufficient number of cases and controls with proper planning. In a cohort study the subjects are selected on the basis of exposure status, and, therefore, there is less control over how many cases actually develop during the follow-up period. If the disease is rare, the number of outcomes could be small, making a cohort study statistically less efficient than a comparable

---

Table 10-5   Major Advantages and Disadvantages of Case-Control Studies

Advantages	Disadvantages
1. They are relatively quick and inexpensive to conduct compared to cohort studies.	1. They may be more subject to selection and recall bias than cohort studies.
2. They are appropriate for studying rare outcomes.	2. Generally, incidence or prevalence measures cannot be calculated.
3. They usually require fewer subjects than cohort studies.	3. It may be difficult to determine the temporal relationship between a given exposure and outcome.
4. They allow multiple exposures to be examined in the same study.	4. They are not appropriate for studying rare exposures.
5. They are suitable for studying chronic diseases with long induction or latency periods.	5. They do not allow for the study of multiple effects from a single exposure.

---

case-control study. This latter point may suggest why case-control studies in general require fewer subjects than cohort studies. Case-control studies also allow investigators to examine multiple exposures in the same study whether or not *a priori* hypotheses have been developed (e.g., in exploratory studies). Since the exposures have to be defined at the outset of cohort studies, these studies do not provide the same flexibility. Finally, case-control studies may be more suitable for studying diseases with long induction or latency periods since cases are selected after the disease has already developed. Essentially, the cases have already passed through their induction and latency periods (e.g., when cumulative incidence sampling is used).

Case-control studies also share a number of potential disadvantages. First, case-control studies may be subject to selection bias because of difficulties in finding an appropriate control group that accurately represents the source population. Also, because the exposure data are usually selected retrospectively from among those with and without the study outcome, differential recall bias is more of a risk than in cohort studies. Those with the study outcome may be more likely to recall their prior exposures than those without the study outcome as discussed elsewhere in this text. Another disadvantage of case-control studies is the general inability to determine measures of incidence and prevalence due to the nature of the study design. While risk and rate ratios can be estimated under appropriate circumstances, case-control studies generally cannot provide information on risk or rate differences or the incidence or prevalence of the outcome among the exposed and unexposed groups. Because it is not clear in all case-control studies whether the outcomes represent prevalent or incident cases, it is sometimes difficult to determine the temporal sequence between exposure and outcome. This may limit speculation about cause and effect relationships. Case-control studies are also not appropriate for studying rare exposures since the investigators cannot determine ahead of time if a sufficient number of exposed subjects will be found in order to meet the minimum statistical requirements for an accurate analysis. Finally, case-control studies are not designed to examine multiple outcomes, which is possible in cohort studies. Despite these potential limitations, if properly and carefully designed and implemented, most case-control studies should be able to compare favorably with well-designed cohort studies in terms of the accuracy of the findings. Poorly designed and implemented studies are another story.

VARIATIONS IN THE CASE-CONTROL DESIGN

The evolution of the case-control study over the years has led to several variant designs. Two of these were discussed under the heading of hybrid studies in chapter 4 and referred to briefly in this chapter. These are the *nested case-control study* and the *case-cohort study*. Both are cost-efficient case-control studies embedded in existing cohorts; hence, their designation as hybrid studies. A more recent variant is the **case-crossover study.** This design uses only cases, but the cases also serve as their own controls; therefore, it is not simply a case series (chapter 4) but instead a type of case-control study. The case-crossover study is used in circumstances where the risk of the outcome is elevated for only a short time following exposure. This period is referred to as the **hazard period.** Typically, the frequency of the study exposure is examined during the hazard period (i.e., usually the time just before the occurrence of the outcome) and compared to its frequency during a designated control period.

Examples of published case-crossover studies should help in understanding the fundamentals of this design. Israeli investigators examined the association between seven potential trigger events during waking hours and the acute onset of ischemic stroke. Their study involved 200 new stroke patients who were interviewed one to four days after their strokes. According to the authors, "Reported exposure to potential triggers including negative and positive emotions, anger, sudden posture changes as response to a startling event, heavy physical exertion, heavy eating, and sudden temperature changes during a 2-hour hazard period prior to stroke onset were compared to the same period during the preceding day and to average exposures in the last year."[36(p2006)] The investigators found that 38 percent of the cases reported exposure to at least one of the seven trigger events during the hazard period. When all exposures were combined, the reported OR was 8.4 (95% CI = 4.5 to 18.1). This represents an estimated 740 percent increase in the odds of developing a stroke following exposure to one or more of the trigger events during the two-hour hazard period compared to the control periods.

Another case-crossover study was conducted in Italy. The cases for this study were 292 children with acute unintentional injuries presenting to a children's emergency center at an Italian university. Interviews were conducted with each eligible child or a parent. The purpose of the study was to determine if there was an association between sleep and wakefulness and unintentional childhood injury. The hazard period was the immediate 24 hours before the injury, and the control period was the 24 hours prior to the hazard period. Among the findings, the authors reported an association between injury risk and sleeping less than 10 hours among the boys in the study but not the girls (OR = 2.33, 95% CI = 1.07 to 5.09). They concluded that inadequate sleep "may increase the risk of injury among children."[37(p1)]

The main advantages of the case-crossover study stem from the fact that cases serve as their own controls. Thus, confounding by personal attributes like age, sex, or race and selection bias due to unrepresentative controls are not generally issues in these studies. Also, fewer subjects are required in case-crossover studies compared to conventional case-control studies due to the decreased variability among the subjects.[38] Decreased variability translates into increased statistical efficiency of a study. One potential disadvantage is recall bias since most studies rely on subject recall of prior events,[30] which may be more accurate during the hazard period than the control period. Another limitation is that only certain types of research questions can be answered using this design.[6] Specifically, the exposure must vary at different times for an individual. Therefore, a fixed exposure like the presence of a specific gene cannot be examined using a case-crossover design. Also, the effect of the exposure must be brief, and the study outcome must occur suddenly, as is the case with myocardial infarction, stroke, or unintentional injury.[6]

SUMMARY

- Case-control studies can be exploratory or analytic. Only analytic studies, however, test specified *a priori* hypotheses about possible causal associations between exposure and outcome.

- The contemporary analytic case-control study is considered an efficient sampling technique that shares elements in common with the cohort design. Ideally, a case-control study takes place within a source population or study base, which represents the group of persons or the person-time experience from which the cases are generated. Normally, the case group consists of all or a random sample of the cases occurring during a specified time period, and the control group is composed of a random sample of the entire source population that generated the cases.

- In terms of design, the starting point for an analytic case-control study is the development of a research hypothesis. This is followed by the identification and selection of appropriate cases and controls. Cases must be adequately defined. The goal is to strike a balance between an overly strict definition, which can result in exclusion of cases, and an overly general definition, which can result in inclusion of noncases. Proper control selection is extremely important. The control group should be representative of the source population in order to avoid selection bias. The main objective is to select a control group that reflects the actual proportion of exposed and unexposed individuals in the source population. Restricting a study to males only, for example, may affect the external validity of a study, but it will not affect its internal validity. Restrictions, however, must be applied equally to cases and controls as appropriate.

- When it is not feasible to conduct a population-based case-control study, cases and controls may be selected from hospitals or other sources. Hospital-based case-control studies are very common and can be appropriate as long as the controls can be considered representative of the source population. A good question to ask in this regard is whether the controls would have been cases at the study hospital had they developed the study outcome during the investigation. In general, some recommend that when hospital controls are used in a hospital-based study, they should come from a variety of diagnoses. Diagnoses that are known to be related to the study exposure should not be included, however.

- Exposure status in case-control studies needs to be assessed accurately to avoid potential information biases, especially interviewer and recall bias. Blinding interviewers to outcome status where possible and to the study hypothesis may help reduce interviewer bias, and blinding subjects to the study hypothesis and using objective means of confirming exposure status may help reduce recall bias.

- The analysis of case-control studies typically proceeds from an overall analysis to more specific analyses using stratification or multivariable methods in order to evaluate possible effect measure modification or confounding. The specific analytical procedures used will depend on whether cases and controls are individually matched or not. In both instances, however, the usual measure of association is an odds ratio.

- In general, confounding in a case-control study can be controlled by restriction, matching, or statistical adjustment in the analysis phase. In unmatched studies, confounding can be controlled alone or in combination with restriction using stratification or multivariable methods. In matched studies, confounding can be controlled using a special form of stratification or by multivariable analysis, which may or may not be used in combination with restriction.

- Effect measure modification, also known as heterogeneity of effect or statistical interaction, occurs in a case-control study when the magnitude of the measure of association varies at different levels of a third factor, and this variation is not due to random or systematic error. While confounding is considered an annoyance that needs to be controlled for valid findings, effect measure modification is a real effect that should be described in a study. The presence of effect measure modification is dependent on the measure of association used or the statistical model employed (additive or multiplicative). Therefore, the measure or model should be reported when discussing effect measure modification. Effect measure modification can be assessed by stratification or by comparing the observed and expected joint effects of the exposure and potential modifying factor on the study outcome. The latter method is used in the context of multivariable analysis.

- Case-control studies have a number of advantages and disadvantages compared to other epidemiologic study designs. Compared to cohort studies, for example, they are usually quicker and less expensive, more appropriate for studying rare outcomes, more statistically efficient, better adapted to studying diseases with long induction or latency periods, and suitable for examining multiple exposures for a single outcome. On the downside, they may be more subject to certain forms of bias. Also, they do not generally allow one to calculate incidence or prevalence measures or their derivative measures of association, although these can usually be estimated. In addition, they may not provide a clear temporal sequence between exposure and outcome, and they are not appropriate when the exposure is rare. Finally, they do not allow for the examination of the effects of multiple outcomes from a single exposure.

- In addition to nested case-control and case-cohort studies, a useful variant of the case-control study is the case-crossover study. In this design the cases serve as their own controls, thereby increasing statistical efficiency and eliminating some potential sources of bias and confounding. The design is used when the risk of the outcome is elevated for only a short period of time following the study exposure. This is known as the hazard period. Typically, the frequency of the exposure is examined during the hazard period and compared to that during a selected control period. Like the conventional case-control study, the usual measure of association is the odds ratio.

New Terms

- additive effects
- additive interaction
- additive model
- adjusted odds ratio
- antagonism
- biological interaction
- biomarker
- case-base sampling
- case-crossover study
- concordant pairs
- conditional logistic regression
- cross-product ratio
- crude odds ratio
- cumulative incidence sampling
- density sampling
- density-based sampling
- discordant pairs

- effect measure modification
- effect modifier
- excess odds ratio
- exploratory case-control study
- exposure odds ratio
- hazard period
- heterogeneity of effect
- hospital controls
- hospital-based case-control study
- incidence density sampling
- interaction
- logistic regression
- Mantel-Haenszel chi-square test
- Mantel-Haenszel odds ratio
- matched case-control study
- matched pairs odds ratio
- McNemar's chi-square test

- multiple logistic regression
- multiplicative effects
- multiplicative interaction
- multiplicative model
- multivariable method
- negative interaction
- overmatching
- pooling
- population controls
- population-based case-control study
- population-based disease registry
- positive interaction
- qualitative interaction
- quantitative interaction
- random digit dialing
- rare disease assumption
- risk set
- source population
- statistical efficiency
- statistical interaction
- stratification
- stratum-specific odds ratio
- study base
- synergism
- test of heterogeneity
- test of homogeneity
- unmatched case-control study

Study Questions and Exercises

1. Obtain a copy of the following article: MacMahon, B., Yen, S., Trichopoulos, D., Warren, K., and Nardi, G. (1981). Coffee and Cancer of the Pancreas. *New England Journal of Medicine* 304 (11): 630–633. Critique the study in terms of the validity of its design, conduct, and analysis.

2. A case-control study using two controls per case was designed to test the hypothesis that lack of regular exercise (the exposure) increases the risk of bone fractures (the outcome) in elderly women. Of the 600 women studied (200 cases and 400 controls), 128 were regular exercisers (26 cases and 102 controls). Based on this information, determine if a lack of regular exercise is a risk factor for bone fractures in this group. Report the crude odds ratio and its 95 percent confidence interval, the value of the test of significance, and its associated p-value. Also, interpret your results in words.

3. The investigators of the study described in the previous problem also collected data on the women's dietary habits, including average daily intake of calcium. Of those who did not exercise regularly, 50 of the cases and 112 of the controls had diets deficient in calcium. Of those who exercised regularly, seven of the cases and 49 of the controls had diets deficient in calcium. The remainder of the subjects had diets adequate in calcium. Based on this information, use stratification to determine if calcium intake is a likely confounder or effect modifier for the relationship between lack of regular exercise and bone fractures, and explain why or why not. Also, report the odds ratio for each stratum along with its 95 per cent confidence interval.

4. A case-control study was designed to see if body piercing by unlicensed merchants was associated with an increased risk of hepatitis B compared to those receiving piercing from licensed merchants. Cases with clinically diagnosed hepatitis B were pair matched to controls without hepatitis B by

age, sex, and number of previous body piercings. The results of the study appear in the contingency table below.

Controls

Cases	Exposed	Unexposed
Exposed	96	23
Unexposed	14	87
	110	110

Based on this information, calculate the applicable odds ratio, the 95 percent confidence interval, and the significance of the odds ratio based on the applicable chi-square test. Be sure to use a matched analysis. Also, interpret your findings in words.

References

1. Last, J. M., ed. (2001). *A Dictionary of Epidemiology*, 4th ed. New York: Oxford University Press.
2. Paneth, N., Susser, E., and Susser, M. (2002). Origins and Early Development of the Case-control Study: Part 2, The Case-control Study from Lane-Claypon to 1950. *Sozial- und Präventivmedizin* 47: 359–365.
3. Schlesselman, J. J. (1982). *Case-control Studies: Design, Conduct, Analysis*. New York: Oxford University Press.
4. Aschengrau, A., and Seage III, G. R. (2003). *Essentials of Epidemiology in Public Health*. Sudbury, MA: Jones and Bartlett Publishers.
5. Wacholder, S., McLaughlin, J. K., Silverman, D. T., and Mandel, J. S. (1992). Selection of Controls in Case-control Studies, I. Principles. *American Journal of Epidemiology* 135 (9): 1019–1028.
6. Rothman, K. J. (2002). *Epidemiology: An Introduction*. New York: Oxford University Press.
7. Mayne, S. T., Risch, H. A., Dubrow, R., Chow, W. H., Gammon, M. D., Vaughan, T. L., Borchardt, L., Schoenberg, J. B., Stanford, J. L., West, A. B., Rotterdam, H., Blot, W. J., and Fraumeni, J. F., Jr. (2006). Carbonated Soft Drink Consumption and Risk of Esophageal Adenocarcinoma. *Journal of the National Cancer Institute* 98 (1): 72–75.
8. Gill, J. S., Zezulka, A. V., Shipley, M. J., Gill, S. K., and Beevers, D. G. (1986). Stroke and Alcohol Consumption. *The New England Journal of Medicine* 315 (17): 1041–1046.
9. World Health Organization (1992). *International Statistical Classification of Diseases and Related Health Problems, Tenth Revision*. Geneva: World Health Organization.
10. Rosenthal, M. S. (1998). *The Gastrointestinal Sourcebook*. Los Angeles: Lowell House.
11. New York State Department of Health (1999). Chronic Disease Teaching Tools—Disease Registries. Available: http://www.health.state.ny.us/diseases/chronic/diseaser.htm (Access date: February 2, 2006).
12. National Cancer Institute (No date). Overview of the SEER Program. Available: http://seer.cancer.gov/about/ (Access date: February 2, 2006).

13. Edwards, C. G., Schwartzbaum, J. A., Lonn, S., Ahlbom, A., and Feychting, M. (2006). Exposure to Loud Noise and Risk of Acoustic Neuroma. *American Journal of Epidemiology* 163 (4): 327–333.

14. Baker, J. A., Beehler, G. P., Sawant, A. C., Jayaprakash, V., McCann, S. E., and Moysich, K. B. (2006). Consumption of Coffee, but Not Black Tea, Is Associated with Decreased Risk of Premenopausal Breast Cancer. *Journal of Nutrition* 136 (1): 166–171.

15. Wacholder, S., Silverman, D. T., McLaughlin, J. K., and Mandel, J. S. (1992). Selection of Controls in Case-control Studies, II. Types of Controls. *American Journal of Epidemiology* 135 (9): 1029–1041.

16. Pearce, N. (1993). What Does the Odds Ratio Estimate in a Case-control Study? *International Journal of Epidemiology* 22 (6): 1189–1192.

17. Checkoway, H., Pearce, N. E., and Crawford-Brown, D. J. (1989). *Research Methods in Occupational Epidemiology.* New York: Oxford University Press.

18. Woolf, B. (1955). On Estimating the Relation between Blood Group and Disease. *Annals of Human Genetics* 19: 251–253.

19. Ferguson, G. A. (1976). *Statistical Analysis in Psychology and Education*, 4th ed. New York: McGraw-Hill Book Company.

20. Rigby, A. S., and Robinson, M. B. (2000). Statistical Methods in Epidemiology. IV. Confounding and the Matched Pairs Odds Ratio. *Disability and Rehabilitation* 22 (6): 259–265.

21. Garey, K. W. (2004). The Role of Matching in Epidemiologic Studies. *American Journal of Pharmaceutical Education* 68 (3), Article 83. Available: http://www.ajpe.org/aj6803/aj680383.pdf (Access date: February 16, 2006).

22. Rothman, K. J. (1986). *Modern Epidemiology.* Boston: Little, Brown and Company.

23. Wacholder, S., Silverman, D. T., McLaughlin, J. K., and Mandel, J. S. (1992). Selection of Controls in Case-control Studies, III. Design Options. *American Journal of Epidemiology* 135 (9): 1042–1050.

24. Kelsey, J. L., Thompson, W. D., and Evans, A. S. (1986). *Methods in Observational Epidemiology.* New York: Oxford University Press.

25. Costanza, M. C. (1995). Theoretical Epidemiology: Matching. *Preventive Medicine* 24: 425–433.

26. Kahn, H. A., and Sempos, C. T. (1989). *Statistical Methods in Epidemiology.* New York: Oxford University Press.

27. Elwood, J. M. (1998). *Critical Appraisal of Epidemiological Studies and Clinical Trials*, 2nd ed. New York: Oxford University Press.

28. Mantel, N., and Haenszel, W. (1959). Statistical Aspects of the Analysis of Data from Retrospective Studies of Disease. *Journal of the National Cancer Institute* 22: 719–748.

29. MacMahon, B., and Trichopoulos, D. (1996). *Epidemiology: Principles and Methods*, 2nd ed. Boston: Little, Brown and Company.

30. Szklo, M., and Nieto, F. J. (2000). *Epidemiology: Beyond the Basics.* Gaithersburg, MD: Aspen.

31. Kleinbaum, D. G., Kupper, L. L., and Morgenstern, H. (1982). *Epidemiologic Research: Principles and Quantitative Methods.* Belmont, CA: Lifetime Learning Publications.

32. Newman, S. C. (2001). *Biostatistical Methods in Epidemiology.* New York: John Wiley & Sons, Inc.

33. Altman, D. G., and Matthews, J. N. S. (1996). Statistics Notes: Interaction 1: Heterogeneity of Effects. *British Medical Journal* 313: 486.

34. Kim, D-S., Lee, M-S., Kim, Y-S., Kin, D-H., Bae, J-M., Shin, M-H., and Ahn, Y-O. (2005). Effect Modification by Vitamin C on the Relation between Gastric Cancer and *Helicobacter pylori. European Journal of Epidemiology* 20: 67–71.

35. Rothman, K. J., and Greenland, S. (1998). *Modern Epidemiology*, 2nd ed. Philadelphia: Lippincott-Raven Publishers.

36. Koton, S., Tanne, D., Bornstein, N. M., and Green, M. S. (2004). Triggering Risk Factors for Ischemic Stroke: A Case-crossover Study. *Neurology* 63: 2006–2010.

37. Valent, F., Brusaferro, S., Barbone, F. (2001). A Case-crossover Study of Sleep and Childhood Injury. *Pediatrics* 107: 1–7. Available: http://www.pediatrics.org/cgi/content/full/107/2/e23 (Access date: February 28, 2006).

38. Maclure, M. (1991). The Case-crossover Design: A Method for Studying Transient Effects on the Risk of Acute Events. *American Journal of Epidemiology* 133 (2): 144–153.

CHAPTER ELEVEN

Cohort Studies

This chapter covers the basic design, analysis, and interpretation of cohort studies as well as their major advantages and disadvantages.

Learning Objectives

- Differentiate among prospective, retrospective, and mixed cohort studies.
- Differentiate between open and closed cohort studies.
- Discuss the key design features of cohort studies as they relate to selecting exposed and comparison groups.
- Discuss the key design features of cohort studies as they relate to determining exposure and outcome status in prospective and retrospective designs, including the common means of doing so.
- Discuss the common strategies for reducing losses to follow up in cohort studies.
- Discuss the key issues in assuring adequate power in a cohort study.
- Describe the approaches to the overall analysis of closed and open cohort studies, respectively.
- Calculate and interpret the appropriate measures of occurrence and association commonly used in the overall analysis of closed and open cohort studies, respectively, along with the appropriate 95 percent confidence intervals.
- Describe the advantages and disadvantages of restriction and matching, respectively, as methods of controlling confounding in cohort studies.
- Evaluate closed and open cohort studies for potential confounding and effect measure modification where stratification has been used.
- Calculate and interpret the appropriate pooled (Mantel-Haenszel) measure of association and its 95 percent confidence interval and the appropriate standardized measure of association based on the stratified analyses of closed and open cohort studies.
- Summarize the basic advantages and disadvantages of using multivariable analysis in cohort studies.
- Describe the major multivariable methods used in closed and open cohort studies, respectively, and their purposes.

- Explain the issue created by induction periods in cohort studies of chronic diseases and some possible solutions.
- List the major advantages and disadvantages of cohort studies.
- Define ambidirectional or ambispective cohort study, baseline data, cohort, concurrent cohort study, Cox proportional hazards model, descriptive cohort study, dynamic cohort study, external comparison group, fixed cohort study, general cohort, hazard ratio, historical cohort study, internal comparison group, nonconcurrent cohort study, person-time chi square test, Poisson regression, special exposure cohort, standardization, and 10 percent rule.

INTRODUCTION

Cohort studies were introduced in chapter 4 along with other common epidemiologic study designs. Cohort studies can be descriptive or analytic. Briefly, **descriptive cohort studies** have no *a priori* hypotheses and are often used to describe the incidence of one or more outcomes of interest. They may also suggest hypotheses for further study. An example of a descriptive cohort study is an investigation by researchers at the University of Medicine and Dentistry of New Jersey, New Jersey Medical School. This study was undertaken "To describe the clinical, immunologic, and psychosocial characteristics of children living with perinatally-acquired human immunodeficiency virus (HIV) infection beyond the age of 9 years."[1(p657)] Notice that the purpose of the study was descriptive. The researchers followed a group of 42 HIV-infected children for an average of 48 months from the time of diagnosis. They found that although approximately a quarter of the subjects remained asymptomatic, the rest had significant HIV-related symptoms, including considerable immunologic deterioration.[1] This can be considered a descriptive cohort study because it was descriptive and because it involved follow up of a specified *cohort* over time. A **cohort** is defined simply as a designated group of individuals who are followed over time.[2] It is also a descriptive study since no *a priori* hypotheses concerning exposure (HIV infection) and outcome (HIV complications) were examined. The remainder of this chapter focuses on the more familiar analytic cohort studies where one or more *a priori* hypotheses are investigated.

Of all the analytic study designs in epidemiology, cohort studies come closest to randomized controlled trials (chapter 12). Both designs involve cohorts, and in terms of directionality, both move from cause (exposure) to effect (outcome) over time. Both are thus follow-up or longitudinal studies, although exposure status is largely self-determined in cohort studies and randomly assigned in randomized controlled trials. In terms of classification, cohort studies are observational, while randomized controlled trials are experimental (see chapter 4).

TYPES OF COHORT STUDIES

As indicated in chapter 4, there are three basic types of cohort studies—*prospective cohort studies, retrospective cohort studies*, and *mixed cohort studies*. In each of these designs the unit of analysis is the individual, and the sequence of exposure-outcome assessment is the same. That is, exposure status is always determined prior to assessing outcome status. In *prospective cohort studies*, also known as **concurrent cohort studies**, or some less desirable names (see table 4-2), the exposure status of the subjects is determined at the beginning of the study before any study outcomes have occurred. The outcome status of each subject is then determined during a subsequent follow-up period that extends into the future. Generally, the length of the follow-up period is determined by the outcome's expected incubation or induction/latency period (chapter 3) depending on whether the outcome is an infectious or noninfectious condition, respectively. In *retrospective cohort studies*, also commonly referred to as **historical cohort studies** or **nonconcurrent cohort studies**, and less frequently to other names (table 4-2), the study exposure and outcome have already occurred. Therefore, the exposure status of each subject is determined for a time period that existed in the past, and outcome status is then determined during a subsequent time period that can stretch up to the present time (i.e., up to the time the study is initiated). This strategy maintains the same exposure-outcome assessment sequence as prospective cohort studies. **Mixed cohort studies**, sometimes referred to as **ambispective** (or **ambidirectional**) **cohort studies**, involve aspects of both prospective and retrospective cohort studies. Usually, past or historical exposure is assessed and follow up continues from that time up to the present and into the future.

The prospective cohort study provides a good illustration of what is meant by an *observational study* (chapter 4) because after selecting the subjects and identifying the exposed and unexposed groups, the investigators in essence allow nature to take its course while recording outcomes as they occur. No intervention is applied, nor is there any attempt to manipulate the conditions of the study as would be the case in experimental studies.

Open and Closed Cohort Studies

In addition to being classified by timing (prospective, retrospective, mixed), cohort studies may also be identified as open or closed. *Open cohorts studies* can be distinguished from *closed cohort studies* depending on whether or not new subjects can be added to the study once follow up begins. In **open cohort studies** (also known as **dynamic cohort studies**), eligible subjects may enter the study at any given time. In **closed cohort studies** (also known as **fixed cohort studies**), no one can be added once follow up begins.[3] The type of cohort study (open or closed) has implications for the type of analyses that should be performed. This aspect is discussed later in the chapter.

As well allowing new subjects to enter the cohort at different times, *open cohort studies* also allow subjects to leave the cohort at any given time. Thus, not all subjects are observed for the same length of time. Reasons that a subject may no longer be followed include: (a) development of the study outcome, (b) death due to competing risks (chapter 5), (c) voluntary withdrawal from the study, (d) a change in study eligibility requirements, (e) loss to follow up, or (f) termination of the study.* In general, none of these reasons affects the internal validity of the findings *except* when there are significant withdrawals or losses to follow up, *and* they are related to *both* exposure and outcome status. Withdrawals or losses related only to exposure or only to outcome will reduce the precision of the findings but not their validity.

Figure 11-1 presents a hypothetical open cohort study in which five subjects are followed during a six-year study period. Each line represents the length of follow up, and a solid black circle at the end of a line represents the occurrence of the study outcome. To illustrate, subject 1 began the study at the end of the first year and contracted the study outcome at the end of the fifth year. Thus, he was followed for a period of four years. Subject 2 began the study at the end of the second year and was followed until termination of the study. She therefore was also followed for four years. Subject 3 was followed for only two years. He entered the study at the start of the fourth year and exited at the end of the fifth year. Finally, subject 4 was followed for the maximum follow-up period of six years, and subject 5 was followed for four years from the beginning of the study until the end of the fourth year when she developed the study outcome. Overall, two cases developed over 20 person-years of follow up. Characteristic of open cohort studies, subjects may enter or leave the study at any given time. The observation time for each subject is taken into account in the analysis (discussed later). A somewhat offbeat but real life example of an investigation using an open cohort design is one that sought to determine if there was a link between occupational exposure to laboratory animals and the development of laboratory animal allergy (LAA). The setting was a pharmaceutical manufacturing plant where animals were used for laboratory testing. The subjects were workers with different levels of exposure to the laboratory animals. The findings were based on a total of 12 years of follow-up data collected from subjects who could enter or leave the study at different times. Overall, the investigators found that the incidence rate of LAA for the workers was 13.2 per 1,000 person-years (95% CI = 7.6 per 1,000 person-years to 18.7 per 1,000 person-years). They also reported that the rate ratios for LAA increased with greater work time exposure to laboratory animals.[4]

Conceptually, a *closed cohort study* is one in which the "subjects either develop the disease or not, and all those not developing it necessarily have the same length of follow-up, namely, the maximum observation time."[5(p34)] In practice, this ideal is only rarely achieved. An example is a retrospective cohort study of a foodborne outbreak where the disease is fairly common,

---

*It is interesting to note that all of these items *except* item a represent reasons for censoring observations in survival analysis (see chapter 5, exhibit 5-2). Voluntary withdrawals are often regarded as losses to follow up.

Figure 11-1   Illustration of Follow-up Times from an Open Cohort Study

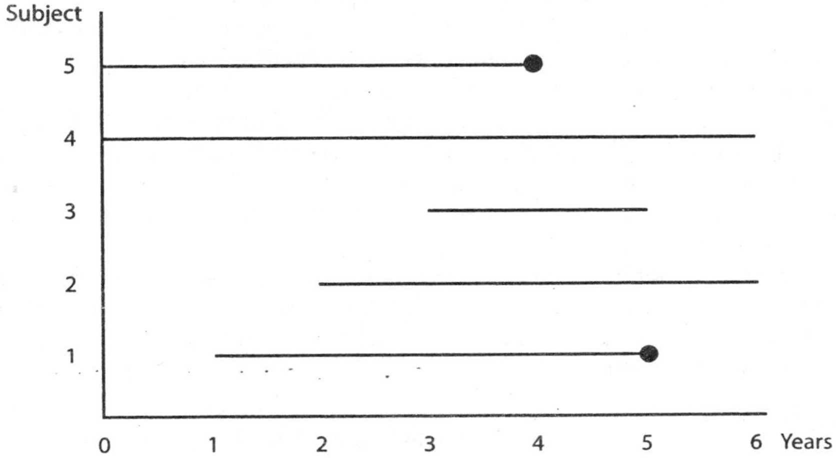

and the incubation period is short. In most studies of chronic diseases, deaths from competing risks, withdrawals, and losses to follow up complicate this idealized conception. In these instances investigators should attempt to trace losses of all types in order to determine their outcome status. This is because the members of a closed cohort represent a sort of "family" bound together because of a common experience. This experience might be a natural disaster, serving in the armed forces, drinking from a contaminated water supply, or some other event. The starting point for a closed cohort study is typically defined by the common experience, which does not change during the follow-up period. Because no one can be added to a closed cohort study once follow up begins, the number of subjects can be expected to decrease as the study progresses.[3] Also, the longer the follow-up period, the greater the risk of losses. These can have implications for the type of analysis to be performed as well as for the accuracy of the study findings.

Alexander Walker refers to the closed cohort study as "the nonrandomized cousin of a clinical trial."[6(p30)] This is because more than an open cohort study it resembles the design of a basic randomized controlled trial but without the randomization or the intervention. A classic example of a closed cohort are the survivors of the atomic bomb explosions at Hiroshima and Nagasaki, Japan. The survivors represent a closed cohort with a common experience of exposure to radiation from atomic bombs. This closed cohort, or subcohorts derived from it, have been followed and studied for decades. The findings of one prospective cohort study, for example, showed that median life expectancy decreased with increasing radiation dose.[7] Another example of a closed cohort study is one conducted in a district of Germany where the exposed group consisted of all blind subjects newly registered with the appropriate welfare administration during a specified time period. The comparison group was the general population of the German state in which the study took place. The subjects were followed for up to 48 months from the start of the study to determine if certain suspected risk factors, including diabetes, had an effect on mortality.[8] This investigation can be classified as a closed cohort study because no one could be added to the study during the follow-up period since the exposed group was fixed at the outset of the study (i.e., it included every eligible subject). The common experience shared by the cohort was blindness registration in the district during a defined time period. A more familiar example of a closed cohort study is the Framingham Heart Study referred to in chapter 1.

The remainder of this chapter discusses some key design issues as well as the basic approaches to analysis and interpretation of findings from cohort studies. It concludes with a summary of the major advantages and disadvantages of cohort studies.

KEY DESIGN ISSUES

Some of the more important issues in designing and conducting cohort studies have to do with the selection of the exposed and comparison groups, the types and quality of data collected, the efforts made to follow up the study participants, and assurance of adequate study power. This section addresses these and related issues. For convenience, both exposure and outcome are considered dichotomous measures unless otherwise indicated. In reality, exposure is often classified by level (e.g., low, medium, and high) with the lowest level typically serving as the referent (chapter 6). The basic concepts, however, are the same whether dichotomous or various levels of exposure are employed. In common with other analytic studies, one or more *a priori* study hypotheses should be evident.

Selecting Exposed and Comparison Groups

All cohort studies, prospective, retrospective, and mixed, have at least three essential features: (a) an exposed group, (b) a comparison group, and (c) a follow-up period. The exposed group is generally derived from a *general cohort* or composed of a *special exposure cohort*. A **general cohort** is usually a general population group defined by person, place, or time factors or another broadly based group, such as members of a health maintenance organization, trade union, or school. General cohorts may be selected based on several criteria, including how representative they are of the general population, expectations of high levels of participation, the quality or accessibility of relevant data, or simply convenience. Of course, findings from cohorts that are unrepresentative of the general population may have limited external validity. The initial cohort for the Framingham Heart Study (chapter 1) was a general cohort. It was defined as heart-healthy men and women between the ages of 30 and 62 living in Framingham, Massachusetts at the time of the study. General cohorts are usually used when a study exposure is expected to be fairly common. For example, cigarette smoking, hypertension, and high serum cholesterol were common enough exposures in the Framingham cohort to make it a suitable source for the exposed group. When a general cohort is used, the subjects in the cohort who are exposed to the study factor(s) serve as the exposed group. The unexposed subjects comprise the comparison group. In this scenario, the comparison group is referred to as an **internal comparison group** since it is part of the general cohort. A general cohort is illustrated in figure 11-2, item one, by the crosshatched oval. To reiterate, in a general cohort the exposed group is the subset of those cohort members who are exposed to the study factor(s), and the comparison group is the subset who are not exposed.

General cohorts may also be chosen from professional or other select groups (e.g., physicians, nurses, veterans, university alumni). These groups are often selected because they tend to be easier to maintain contact with during long follow-up periods, more willing to comply with the study protocol, or more likely to provide reliable information than general population groups. For example, physicians and nurses tend to report prior and current medical conditions more accurately and completely than members of the general population and are easier to trace because of their registration with licensing boards or memberships in well known organizations (e.g., American Medical Association, American Nurses' Association). This can result in more accurate and complete data collection and follow up. The Nurses' Health Study, for example, uses a general cohort made up of registered nurses

Figure 11-2   Possible Cohort Designs

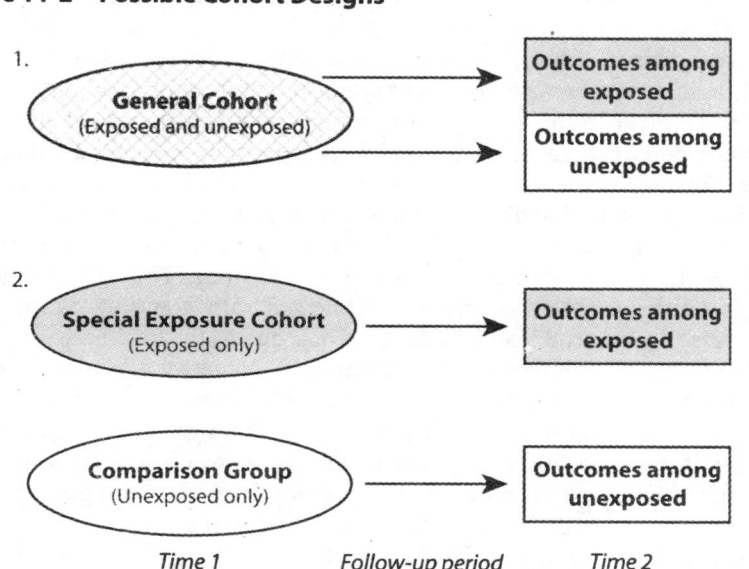

in several states throughout the United States. This prospective cohort study began in 1976 and has followed over 100,000 registered nurses continuously since that time. In 1989 the investigation was expanded to include an additional cohort of younger nurses, which is known as the Nurses' Health Study II. Participation rates in both studies have been reported to be high.[9]

Special exposure cohorts are typically used when the study exposure is uncommon or unique. These cohorts only represent the exposed group and may include certain occupational groups (e.g., radium dial painters), persons undergoing certain medical treatments (e.g., long-term users of Vioxx®), those with specific environmental exposures (e.g., New York residents in the vicinity of the former twin towers during 9/11), or members of organizations with unusual dietary habits or lifestyles (e.g., Seventh Day Adventists).[10] Studies of the link between benzene and aplastic anemia, for instance, have focused on occupational groups that work with the solvent since most individuals in the general population are not exposed to levels of benzene likely to be associated with this condition. Because of the relative infrequency or uniqueness of the exposures, special exposure cohorts provide a statistically efficient way of studying these factors, which would be rare or nonexistent in general cohorts. Special exposure cohorts, however, require a separate comparison group made up of unexposed individuals as illustrated in figure 11-2, item two. The comparison group for a special exposure cohort is usually referred to as an **external comparison group**, since it is not a part of the study cohort as is the case with general cohorts. To minimize the potential for selection bias and confounding, an external comparison group should be *as similar as possible* to the special exposure group except for the study exposure. In particular, the distribution of extraneous factors that may be related to the outcome should be comparable between the groups.[10] In some cases, more than one external comparison group may be used. If the results are similar using each comparison group, this may provide some reassurance that a finding is valid, assuming there are no other significant sources of systematic or nonsystematic error in the study. Many retrospective cohort studies use special exposure cohorts because of insufficient information on general cohorts that existed in the past.

Sometimes the incidence of the study outcome(s) in a special exposure cohort is compared to that in the general population, usually that segment with similar age, sex, or race/ethnicity distributions. This is frequently the case in occupational cohort studies. While generally convenient, this type of comparison group can lead to a negative bias due to the healthy worker effect or other types of membership bias (chapter 8). Negative bias may also result because the general population may include some exposed individuals, thereby minimizing any differences between the exposed and comparison groups. If the exposure is truly rare or unique, however, the consequence of this should be insignificant. Once again, multiple comparison groups may be used to account for differences that are due solely to the selection of a particular population as a comparison group. Generally speaking, an external comparison group based on the general population is probably a better choice than one based on a separate unexposed group because of the difficulty in finding groups that are really alike except for exposure status. For example, even though the groups appear to be similar with regard to demographic factors, they may differ with respect to unknown factors that are associated with the study outcome.

To summarize briefly, there are two major sources of exposed groups for cohort studies—general cohorts and special exposure cohorts. General cohorts make use of an internal comparison group consisting of those in the general cohort who are not exposed to the study factor(s). Special exposure cohorts generally require an external comparison group consisting of either a separate but similar cohort that is not exposed to the study factor(s) or the general population. In the latter case, the incidence of the outcome in the special exposure group is compared to that expected in the general population, usually within the same age, sex, or race/ethnicity categories. As a general rule of thumb, internal comparison groups provide better comparisons than external comparison groups, and general populations provide better external comparison groups than separate unexposed groups.

Determining Exposure Status

With general cohorts it is necessary to determine each subject's exposure status *before* follow up begins. Even with special exposure cohorts it is important to confirm exposure status (or determine the levels of exposure) before initiating follow up. It is also necessary to collect other relevant **baseline data**, that is, data collected at the beginning of a study.[2] These data include demographic factors that are used to characterize the subjects and data on potential confounders or effect modifiers that may need to be controlled or explained in the findings. Baseline data allow the investigators to perform appropriate subgroup analyses. To obtain this information, potential subjects may need to fill out questionnaires, respond to personal inquiries, or be tested. Because of some differences related to exposure assessment, prospective and retrospective cohort studies are discussed separately in this and the following segment.

Prospective cohort studies. Determining or confirming exposure status among the subjects of a prospective cohort study should be guided by considerations of accuracy, completeness, and practicality. Some of the more commonly used means of determining or confirming exposure status in prospective cohort studies are listed in table 11-1. Each method has its strengths and limitations, and no one method will be suitable in all cases. In general, because questionnaires and interviews rely on self-reported data, they may not always elicit complete or accurate responses, especially if the exposure relates to sensitive areas, such as illegal drug use or certain personal behaviors. On the other hand, questionnaires or interviews may be the only possible ways to collect information that is not recorded elsewhere or that

Table 11-1   Common Means of Determining Exposure and Outcome Status in Cohort Studies

Exposure Status	Outcome Status
• Medical records	• Medical records
• Employment records	• Disease registries
• Birth records	• Death certificates
• Questionnaires	• Questionnaires
• Interviews	• Interviews
• Physical examinations	• Physical examinations
• Specialized medical testing	• Diagnostic tests
• Biological specimens (blood, urine, tissue samples, etc.)	
• Environmental tests	

cannot be determined by testing. Also, questionnaires and interviews may provide a means of obtaining data on potential confounders that is not possible with other methods.

The use of other modes of obtaining exposure data, such as existing records, physical examinations, specialized medical testing (e.g., sonograms, cardiograms), biological specimens, or environmental testing, will depend on the specific circumstances of the study. Biological specimens, such as blood tests for elevated cholesterol levels, are highly objective means of determining exposure status but obviously cannot be used when the exposures of interest are variables like marital status, birth order, or seat belt use. Existing medical and other records may be convenient, but they may not always be complete for all members of the cohort, including the comparison group, especially when it comes to certain types of exposure data (e.g., smoking or drinking status). Tests for environmental exposures, such as tests for radon gas concentrations in homes, may be objective, but they may not give an accurate idea of the amount of toxicant actually absorbed by the individual. The amount of radon absorbed may vary, for example, due to the behaviors of the subjects, such as how much time is spent in the home and the extent to which windows are used for ventilation. In general, it is desirable to validate exposure status by using more than one data source whenever possible. Many studies of the effects of cigarette smoking, for instance, have queried subjects about smoking status using questionnaires or interviews, while taking blood measurements of cotinine, a *biomarker* (see chapter 10) for recent exposure to cigarette smoke.

Another issue relevant to exposure assessment in prospective cohort studies is change in exposure status during the follow-up period. In general, unless the exposure status is not subject to modification (e.g., blood type), it should be reassessed periodically to account for any changes. The frequency of reassessment will depend to some extent on the likelihood of change and the costs of reassessment. Where changes have occurred investigators can often take this into consideration in the analysis of the data. For example, investigators at the University of Massachusetts studied the possible relationship between alcohol consumption and cataracts in a cohort of female registered nurses (i.e., from the Nurses' Health Study).[11] Alcohol consumption status was reassessed via questionnaires every two years during the 12 years of follow up. Because person-years (see chapter 5) constituted the denominators of the calculated incidence rates in the exposed and unexposed groups, it was possible to account for changes in exposure status during the study period. For example, if a subject was classified as a drinker for the first six years of the study and then gave up drinking for the remaining six years, that subject would have contributed only six person-years of risk to the exposed group, assuming she had not developed a cataract within the first six years. By the way, the investigators in this study found no notable overall relationship between alcohol intake and the development of cataracts.

Retrospective cohort studies.   Determining or confirming exposure status in retrospective cohort studies presents some unique problems, and, therefore, not all of the means of exposure assessment listed in table 11-1 will be applicable in these studies. Questionnaires and interviews, for example, may have very limited use in retrospective cohort studies due to the historical nature of the cohort. In some instances, the subjects or close contacts who knew the subjects well may still be alive and can be questioned about exposure status. The quality of the data, however, may be compromised by faulty recall, inability to locate all the subjects or their proxies, etc. For many retrospective cohort studies past employment or company medical records will be the only available means by which to classify subjects on exposure status. These sources may not always be ideal because of incomplete or inaccurate data that can increase the probability of exposure misclassification, a consequence of information bias (chapter 8). In many cases, the investigators may have to rely on job titles or other uncertain means of deduction to classify subjects on exposure status. A classic example is a study of the relationship of asbestos to lung cancer, which assumed that shipbuilders were directly exposed to the asbestos that was used to line the interior of the ships' hulls. It is possible, however, that some of the shipbuilders actually had little or no direct contact with asbestos. The basic problem in retrospective cohort studies is that the available data sources on exposure status and other relevant factors are usually secondary sources that have been collected for other purposes. These sources may be less than ideal for testing specific research hypotheses because of missing or imprecise data. Changes in exposure status may also be difficult to ascertain.

In some retrospective, as well as prospective or mixed, cohort studies, birth records are used as a source of information about exposure status. For example, a retrospective cohort study conducted at Vanderbilt University in Nashville used birth certificates to classify the subjects on exposure status.[12] The study examined the relationship between certain maternal and child character-istics recorded on the birth certificates and mortality from community-acquired infections. The cohort for the study consisted of children who were less than five years old between 1985 and 1994. The authors found that chil-dren with three or more brothers and sisters and a birth weight of less than 1,500 grams had an approximate 20-fold increased risk of death from infection.

In some retrospective cohort studies it may be impossible to determine past exposure status due to a lack of valid and reliable information. In these instances the study simply cannot be completed. In those rare circumstances where accurate data on past exposures have been collected for some reason, there should be few impediments to proceeding with such a study.[13] One problem, however, that plagues many retrospective cohort studies is the unavailability of specific data on potential confounders or effect modifiers. This, of course, can lead to erroneous conclusions about suspected causal associations between exposures and outcomes.

Determining Outcome Status

With regard to determining outcome status, accuracy, completeness, and practicality are again the major considerations. In general, outcome status should be determined using valid and reliable methods; the methods should be applied equally to exposed and unexposed subjects; and, where applicable, the methods should be acceptable to those being studied. They should also be affordable. Even though cohort studies are often designed to examine more than one outcome, outcome status will be referred to in the singular in the dis-cussion that follows. This will avoid some potentially cumbersome phrases.

Prospective cohort studies.   Potential subjects for a prospective cohort study must be *at risk* of developing the study outcome. Since the usual purpose of a prospective cohort study is to determine if a given exposure increases or decreases the rate or risk of development of the study outcome, it is essential that the subjects are susceptible to the outcome at the time follow up begins. Therefore, those who have the outcome at the start of a study should be excluded from the study. An exception would be if the investigators are inter-ested in recurrences. Likewise, those who are not otherwise at risk of the out-come should be also excluded since they cannot contribute to the pool of new cases. It is quite obvious, for example, that women should not be included as subjects in a study of the effects of dietary factors on prostate cancer since women do not have a prostate gland and cannot possibly be at risk of the dis-ease. Likewise, women who have undergone a hysterectomy should not be included in a study of uterine cancer. Individuals who have had a particular disease in the past (e.g., stroke) may also be considered unsuitable if the inter-est is first occurrences of the study outcome as is usually the case. To ensure that all subjects are at risk of the study outcome, they may need to complete detailed questionnaires, respond to personal inquiries, or be tested for current *and* prior outcome status. Because large numbers of individuals may need to be examined, generally only the most efficient methods should be used. Determining if potential subjects are at risk of the study outcome may be fairly straightforward for infectious diseases where serum antibody levels can be measured.[13] It can be more problematic with noninfectious diseases since one may have to rely on individual recall or available medical records to determine disease history. Recall can be faulty, and though medical records are often a reliable source, sometimes they are incomplete or unavailable.

Once follow up is initiated, the investigators must monitor the subjects on a continuing basis to determine who develops the study outcome. Table 11-1 lists some of the more common means of outcome assessment used in prospective cohort studies. Medical records include reports from physicians, hospitals, and other health care facilities. When conclusive diagnostic tests are available, affordable, and safe these may be the best methods to use. Depending on the outcome of interest, other methods may be suitable. For example, if the outcome of interest is a particular disease, and a population-based disease registry (chapter 10) is available for that disease, it would be a good source to consider for outcome assessment. If the outcome is overall mortality, then death certificates may be an appropriate source since death reporting is nearly complete in the United States and many other countries. Death certificates or databases derived from death certificates (e.g., the National Death Index; see appendix B) are generally less reliable for determining *specific* causes of death, however, because of possible omissions or inaccuracies. If the outcome has a high case fatality, is rapidly fatal, and easily diagnosed, death certificates may be acceptable. Certain cancers fit these criteria (e.g., lung cancer), while many other chronic diseases (e.g., chronic bronchitis or diabetes) do not.[13] Thus, lung cancer is more likely to be reported on a death certificate as the *underlying cause of death* (see exhibit 2-1) than chronic bronchitis. Since lung cancer has a higher case fatality and is more rapidly fatal than chronic bronchitis, physicians are more likely to assign lung cancer as an underlying cause of death than they would chronic bronchitis. The latter is more likely to be assigned as an *antecedent cause of death* or *other significant condition* (exhibit 2-1). Where possible, it is a good idea to use several sources of data for cross-validation purposes. As with case-control studies (chapter 10), it is important to have adequate criteria for diagnosing outcomes that have been determined *before* the study is initiated. These criteria should be widely accepted and verifiable. They should be strict enough to exclude noncases, and not so strict as to exclude cases. Whenever possible, those determining outcome status should not be aware of exposure status in order to avoid any diagnostic suspicion bias (see chapter 8).

Retrospective cohort studies.   In retrospective cohort studies it may not be possible to determine which subjects were initially at risk of the study outcome because of a lack of available data. Determining outcome status during follow up can also be problematic. One problem is locating the subjects, many of whom may now be deceased or no longer living in the area or under the same name (e.g., women who have married and taken their spouse's surname). Of the methods listed in table 11-1, death certificates, disease registries, and medical records may be the most useful. As discussed earlier, death certificates are best used when overall mortality is the outcome of interest. With regard to specific diseases, they tend to be less reliable. Population-based disease registries can be an excellent source where applicable. Past medical records, if available, can be useful in identifying outcomes, but they may vary in quality, completeness, or comparability. Interviews, questionnaires, physical examinations, and diagnostic tests may also be used to assess outcome status if the survivors can be located and are able to participate. It will be necessary, however, to find equally reliable data on those who have died, cannot be located, or are unwilling to participate in the study.

In general, investigators have a more difficult task identifying suitable sources of outcome data in retrospective cohort studies compared to prospective cohort studies. They also typically face a greater challenge in locating all subjects. In both types of studies, however, it is incumbent upon the investigators to use the same or equally accurate methods of assessing outcome status for both the exposed and unexposed groups if the results are to be valid.

Following Up Study Participants

As a rule, cohort studies where chronic diseases or deaths are investigated tend to be relatively large and of long duration. In fact, some prospective cohort studies involve tens of thousands of participants who must be followed over the course of many years or even decades. A good example is the ongoing Nurses' Health Study, which began in 1976 with 122,000 registered nurses from 11 states.[9] Other cohort studies in their early stages, such as the Southern Community Cohort Study[14] and the National Children's Study,[15] anticipate more than 100,000 participants and follow-up periods spanning two or more decades. Maintaining close contact with the participants in these and other cohort studies while minimizing unnecessary losses can be a monumental and costly task. Nevertheless, it is a task that must be undertaken if the study results are to be useful. Significant losses due to nonparticipation, relocation, or other reasons can affect the accuracy of the study findings. Precision will decline because of decreased power due to smaller sample size, but more importantly, the findings may be biased if the losses are associated with *both* exposure and outcome status. That is, if those who are lost are more or less likely to have been exposed and develop the outcome than those who are retained in the study, a selection bias known as loss to follow-up bias may occur (see chapter 8). The best way to avoid this bias is to minimize losses to follow up.

Some of the common strategies aimed at reducing losses in prospective cohort studies are listed in table 11-2. Some may also apply to retrospective cohort studies. The most important are to obtain thorough and accurate contact information from each participant at the beginning of the study and to

Table 11-2   Strategies for Minimizing Losses in Cohort Studies

Initial Strategies

- Evaluate eligible participants for compliance potential
- Outline specific expectations and responsibilities of participants
- Require potential participants to complete typical tasks at baseline
- Train staff regarding good communication, enthusiasm, flexibility, and responsiveness
- Obtain complete contact information on participants

Ongoing Strategies

- Maintain up-to-date contact information on participants
- Maintain regular contact with participants
- Follow up all nonresponses, absences, etc. promptly
- Use contact information or other appropriate resources to follow up losses
- Offer incentives to participants

Reference: Hunt, J. R., and White, E. (1998). Retaining and Tracking Cohort Study Members. *Epidemiologic Reviews* 20 (1): 57–70.

update it periodically during the follow-up period. The study investigators should have basic contact information such as the participant's current full name, home and work addresses and phone numbers, e-mail address(es), and Social Security number. Date and place of birth and spouse or family member names can also be helpful. In addition, the name, address, and phone number of one or more friends or relatives not living with the participant but generally aware of his or her whereabouts should be obtained. Contact information for the participant's primary health care provider is also important. The above information can be invaluable when nonresponse occurs, and investigators need to locate a study subject.

The investigators or their staff should also maintain regular contact with the participants. This may take several forms, including periodic newsletters, letters or postcards, e-mails, and an up-to-date Web site featuring reports on the progress of the study, preliminary findings, frequently asked questions, statements about the significance of the study, and other relevant information, including how to contact the investigators. When nonresponses occur or individuals fail to show up for scheduled appointments, they need to be followed up promptly. Follow-up letters or postcards are standard, but phone calls or personal visits may be required if the mailings are unsuccessful. Research appears to indicate that certified mail may achieve a better response than other types of mail.[16] When losses to follow up occur and normal channels of communication are inadequate to ascertain a subject's whereabouts, other resources can be used. These might include postal services for changes of address, public records available through national, state, or local agencies (e.g., vital statistics registrars, departments of motor vehicles, taxing bodies, welfare and assistance programs), or other organizations such as credit bureaus, utilities, and election boards. Some of the major national organizations in the U.S. that might be contacted include the U.S. Postal Service, the Social Security Administration, the Centers for Medicare and Medicaid Services, and the Internal Revenue Service. The National Death Index maintained by the National Center for Health Statistics in Hyattsville, Maryland (see appendix B) is a useful source for identifying deceased persons.[17]

Regarding incentives, there appears to be some support for using modest financial or non-financial means to increase subject participation and retention in epidemiologic studies, although some have expressed concerns that such methods could lead to selection bias or other problems. The authors of a randomized controlled trial of financial incentives and delivery methods as a means of increasing responses to a questionnaire used in a prospective cohort study reported:

> Our randomized trial revealed that a small monetary incentive was effective in converting a number of reluctant responders. Cash yielded a significantly better response than did checks, and the response increased significantly with increasing incentive amounts ($0.00, $1.00, $2.00). The $2.00 bill, perhaps because of its novelty, achieved the best response. We found no advantage to using the more expensive Federal Express delivery method over first-class mail.[18(pp648-649)]

The topic of using incentives in a cohort study was discussed fairly comprehensively in a working paper related to planning the National Children's Study (NCS), which was referred to earlier in this section. This cohort study was expected to place a significant burden on the participants because of requirements for long interviews, detailed diaries, clinic and home visits, and biological and environmental sampling. Hence, the planners were concerned about issues related to recruitment and retention. The following comment in the report summarizes the view of the authors:

> Although the actual impact of offering an incentive to study participants is not altogether clear, prior research with other types of studies, and anecdotal evidence from recent studies that have imposed significant burden on respondents would suggest that some level of incentive be employed in the NCS. Because of the burden of the NCS, it may be necessary to consider incentives where the level of incentive increases with the length of participation and/or where an additional incentive is offered for the completion of the entire study.[19(pG-12)]

The Millennium Cohort Study being conducted in the United Kingdom is a national collaboration to study almost 19,000 babies born during 2000 and 2001. It has used some very modest non-financial incentives, including birthday cards and a "giraffe" wall chart for measuring growth, to give the participants a sense of connection with the study,[20] presumably in the hope of reducing losses to follow up. Other ideas that might be considered in cohort studies are annual drawings for cash or prizes, free or discount tickets for travel or entertainment, coffee mugs, hats, T-shirts, gift certificates, lottery tickets, etc. An obvious downside of this approach is the cost of the incentives, especially for large cohorts. Also, one has to wonder if incentives may bias subjective responses.

Assuring Adequate Power

As in other types of epidemiologic studies, it is important to have sufficient power in a cohort study so as to provide precise findings. As with case-control studies (chapter 10), sample size requirements for a given level of power can be estimated using various statistical software applications (see appendix A). The input required for determining the minimum sample size for cohort studies is similar to that for case-control studies (see chapter 10). One can also estimate the power of a cohort study based on desired sample size and other inputs using available software described in appendix A. Normally, one wants a sample size that provides at least 80 percent power. Because of the very real possibility of significant losses in cohort studies, however, the calculated sample size will probably be inadequate to maintain the desired level of power. Some recommend increasing the minimum estimated sample size by at least 25 percent to account for expected losses.[13] For example, based on one software application and assuming a general cohort with a desired sample size of 200 exposed and 4,000 unexposed subjects, an expected proportion with the outcome of 0.05 in the unexposed group, a 95 percent confidence level, and a desire to detect an association of at least RR = 2.00, the power of the study is estimated to be 80 percent. The total sample size of 4,200, however, is likely to be an underestimate of the actual number of subjects needed to maintain 80 percent power because of anticipated losses. Therefore, it would be better to select additional subjects, for example: (4,200 × 0.25) + 4,200 = 5,250. This represents an additional 1,050 subjects. Subgroup analyses may require separate sample size or power calculations in order to assure a reasonable level of precision.

OVERALL ANALYSIS OF COHORT STUDIES

The type of analysis performed in cohort studies depends to some degree on the type of cohort, the comparison group, and the objectives and preferences of the investigators. The major steps are similar to those outlined in figure 10-2 for case-control studies. Generally, the initial step is to perform an overall analysis without regard to potential confounding or effect measure modification, that is, to determine crude measures of occurrence and association and their 95 percent confidence intervals. This may be followed by stratification or multivariable analysis, both of which can help investigators identify and deal with confounding and effect measure modification.

Closed Cohort Studies

In closed cohort studies the standard measure of occurrence is cumulative incidence (CI; see chapter 5), and the applicable measure of association is the cumulative incidence ratio (CIR) or the cumulative incidence difference (CID). These measures were described in chapter 6. The odds ratio (OR) may also be used as the measure of association, and if the outcome is rare, it will approximate the CIR.* When a closed cohort study is subject to significant losses or competing risks, which is likely when the study has a long follow-up period, the findings may be analyzed in the same manner as *open cohort studies*, which is described in the next section.

For dichotomous measures of exposure and outcome, the results of a closed cohort study can be placed in a 2×2 contingency table as shown below. You will notice that this table is identical to that used in the analysis of cross-sectional studies (chapter 9).

	Outcome Status		
Exposure Status	Present	Absent	
Exposed	a	b	a + b
Unexposed	c	d	c + d
	a + c	b + d	n

Based on the frequencies a-d in the above table, the following measures can be readily calculated (see formulas 11-1 through 11-6).

(11.1) $$CI_c = [(a + c) / n] \times 10^n$$

CI_c is the crude or overall cumulative incidence of the study outcome for a given population base (10^n), and n is the total number of subjects in the cohort (i.e, a + b + c + d). The sum a + c represents the number of subjects who developed the study outcome.

(11.2) $$CI_e = [a / (a + b)] \times 10^n \text{ } and \text{ } CI_{ue} = [c / (c + d)] \times 10^n$$

CI_e is the cumulative incidence of the study outcome in the *exposed* group, and CI_{ue} is the cumulative incidence in the *unexposed* group. An approximate method for calculating a 95 percent confidence interval for cumulative incidence was described in chapter 5 (see formula 5.16). This can be applied to cumulative incidence calculated from either formula 11.1 or 11.2.

---

*The CIR may be referred to in studies as the risk ratio or relative risk. Technically, the CIR is a type of risk ratio, which is often referred to as relative risk. The CID is a type of risk difference or excess risk (see chapter 6).

(11.3) $CIR = [a / (a + b)] / [c / (c + d)]$

CIR in formula 11.3 is the cumulative incidence ratio, and the equation is equivalent to formula 6.4. It is often referred to generically as the risk ratio or relative risk (see chapter 6). An approximate 95 percent confidence interval for the CIR is given by formula 11.4.[21]

(11.4)
$$95\% \; CI = \exp\left\{\ln(CIR) \pm 1.96\sqrt{\left[(b/a)/(a+b)\right] + \left[(d/c)/(c+d)\right]}\right\}$$

Formula 11.4 is calculated in exactly the same manner as formula 9.5, which describes an approximate 95 percent confidence interval for the prevalence ratio. The expressions exp and ln were defined in chapter 9 and represent the exponential and natural logarithm, respectively.

(11.5) $CID = [a / (a + b)] \times 10^n - [c / (c + d)] \times 10^n$

CID or the cumulative incidence difference was described in chapter 6. The formula for its calculation (11.5) is equivalent to formula 6.9. The CID is often referred to generically as the risk difference or excess risk. An approximate 95 percent confidence interval for the CID can be calculated using formula 11.6.[22]

(11.6)
$$95\% \; CI = CID \pm 1.96\sqrt{\left[CI_e(1 - CI_e)/(a+b)\right] + \left[CI_{ue}(1 - CI_{ue})/(c+d)\right]}$$

In formula 11.6, CID is obtained using formula 11.5, and CI_e and CI_{ue} are calculated using formula 11.2. These measures should be *expressed as decimal fractions* when calculating the confidence interval. The resulting interval can then be restated using an appropriate population base. Problem 11-1 illustrates the basic overall analysis of a closed cohort study, including calculation of the above measures of association and their 95 percent confidence intervals.

If desired, though not necessarily recommended (see discussions of statistical significance testing in chapters 6 and 8), the statistical significance of the measures of association (CIR or CID) can be determined using a chi-square test for independence (χ^2) with one degree of freedom.[23] It is interpreted in the same manner as discussed in chapters 9 and 10 and delineated in table 9-3. It is repeated here for convenience.

(Repeated 9.7)
$$\chi^2 = \frac{n(ad - bc)^2}{(a+b)(c+d)(a+c)(b+d)}$$

Problem 11-1: Basic Overall Analysis of a Closed Cohort Study

A prospective cohort study was conducted among workers at a new pesticide manufacturing plant located in western Kentucky. All plant workers hired at the start of operations on March 15, 2006, comprised the cohort (n = 375). The workers were followed for one year from April 1, 2006, to March 31, 2007. The primary purpose of the study was to determine if routine exposure to airborne pesticide residues at the plant increased the risk of developing an acute respiratory infection (ARI). Airborne pesticide levels were monitored on a daily basis in two separate sections of the plant, one where raw materials and pesticides were stored and handled on a high volume basis (high exposure section) and one where non-pesticide operations (e.g., equipment maintenance, container manufacture) took place (low exposure section). Those workers assigned to the high exposure section were considered the exposed group, and those assigned to the low exposure section were considered the unexposed group. Before follow up began, the plant workers were given pre-employment physicals by a consulting physician and baseline data were collected on medical history, smoking status, and other factors. During follow up, monthly interviews were conducted by the director of occupational safety and health and her staff, which included a registered occupational health nurse and an industrial hygienist. Overall results of the study showed that at the end of follow up 57 members of the cohort had experienced at least one ARI, 48 among the exposed group (n = 254) and nine among the unexposed group (n = 121). Based on this information, calculate the crude cumulative incidence of ARI, the cumulative incidence in the exposed and unexposed groups, and the cumulative incidence ratio and difference along with their 95 percent confidence intervals. Interpret your results. Assume all subjects were followed up until development of an ARI or the conclusion of the study. Those subjects developing more than one ARI were only counted once (i.e., the interest was first ARI).

Solution:
Step 1: Place the results provided in the problem in the appropriate cells of a 2 × 2 contingency table as follows:

Outcome Status

Exposure Status	Present	Absent	
Exposed	48	206	254
Unexposed	9	112	121
	57	318	375

Step 2: Calculate the overall cumulative incidence of ARI using formula 11.1.
$$CI_c = 57 / 375 \times 10^n = 0.1520 \times 10^2 = 15.20 \text{ per } 100$$
Step 3: Calculate the cumulative incidence of ARI in the exposed and unexposed groups using formula 11.2.
$$CI_e = (48 / 254) \times 10^n = 0.1890 \times 10^2 = 18.90 \text{ per } 100$$
$$CI_{ue} = (9 / 121) \times 10^n = 0.0744 \times 10^2 = 7.44 \text{ per } 100$$
Step 4: Calculate the cumulative incidence ratio and cumulative incidence difference for ARI, along with their 95 percent confidence intervals, using formulas 11.3 to 11.6 as appropriate.

$$CIR = (48/254)/(9/121) = 0.1890/0.0744 = 2.54$$

$$95\% \text{ CI} = \exp\left\{\ln(2.54) \pm 1.96\sqrt{[(206/48)/254] + [(112/9)/121]}\right\} =$$

$$\exp\{0.9322 \pm 0.6782\} = 1.29 \text{ to } 5.00$$

$$CID = (48/254) \times 10^n - (9/121) \times 10^n = 0.1890 \times 10^2 - 0.0744 \times 10^2 = 0.1146 \times 10^2 =$$

$$11.46 \text{ per } 100$$

$$95\% \text{ CI} = 0.1146 \pm 1.96\sqrt{[0.1890(1-0.1890)/254] + [0.0744(1-0.0744)/121]} =$$

$$0.1146 \pm 0.0671 = 0.0475 \text{ to } 0.1817 = 4.75 \text{ per } 100 \text{ to } 18.17 \text{ per } 100$$

Answer: Based on the overall findings, the crude cumulative incidence of ARI is 15.20 cases per 100 workers for the period April 1, 2006, to March 31, 2007. This means that 15.20 cases of ARI developed for every 100 workers in the initial cohort during the course of follow up. This represents the overall risk of ARI in the cohort during the study period. The cumulative incidence of ARI in the exposed group is 18.90 cases per 100 workers and that in the unexposed group is 7.44 cases per 100 workers. Thus, the overall risk of ARI is higher in the exposed versus the unexposed group. Specifically, the cumulative incidence ratio (or risk ratio) is estimated to be 2.54 (95% CI = 1.29 to 5.00). This indicates that the exposed workers are an estimated 2.54 times more likely to develop an ARI than the unexposed workers in this cohort, all other factors being equal. We can be 95 percent certain that the true CIR lies between 1.29 and 5.00 based on the confidence interval. The cumulative incidence difference is 11.46 cases of ARI per 100 workers (95% CI = 4.75 per 100 to 18.75 per 100). This represents the estimated excess risk of ARI associated with the exposure during the study period. We can be 95 percent confident that the true excess risk of ARI lies between 4.75 and 18.75 cases per 100 workers based on the confidence interval.

Comments:
1. This was a *closed cohort study* since no one could be added to the study once follow up began. In other words, the cohort was closed or fixed at the outset; hence, the terminology closed or fixed cohorts. Furthermore, and characteristic of *pure* closed cohort studies, all subjects not developing the study outcome were followed for the entire observation period, which in this problem was one year. In practice, many closed cohort studies do not fully meet this criterion. This is especially true when the follow-up period is long. During long follow up subjects are more likely to die due to competing risks or be lost to follow up. This can be problematic if the objective is to estimate the risk of the outcome since risk measures like cumulative incidence are based on the assumption that the size of the population at risk remains constant. This is why closed cohort studies are often employed in the study of relatively high risk problems that occur in the short term (e.g., infectious diseases). Another problem with long-term cohort studies is aging of the sample. Since aging often increases the risk of an outcome, even in the unexposed group, the cumulative incidence ratio tends toward one over time, and the cumulative incidence difference tends toward zero. In these situations the measures commonly used in open cohort studies may be more appropriately applied.

2. The exposed group in this study was composed of only those plant workers hired on March 15, 2006, and working in the section of the plant where pesticides and

their ingredients were stored or handled. It was expected that airborne exposures to pesticide residues would be relatively high in this section. The referent group, representing an internal comparison group, was composed of those workers hired on the same day but working in another section of the plant where airborne exposures were expected to be relatively low. This was referred to as the unexposed group in that it was the group unexposed to high levels of the pesticide residues. Technically, however, it is the low exposed group. This should make it clear that the comparison group in a cohort study does not have to be a strictly non-exposed group, but it should be described by the investigators so the readers known to whom the exposed group is being compared.

3. Cumulative incidence is an estimate of the risk of a given outcome, specifically a group member's average risk (see chapter 5) for a given time period, which in this case was one year. In this problem, risk was estimated for the overall sample, the exposed group, and the unexposed group. The risk was unadjusted, however, and could be positively or negatively influenced by confounding due to factors such as age, health status, and cigarette smoking even if we assume there are no other sources of error in the study.

4. The cumulative incidence ratio represents the relative risk of ARI in the exposed versus the unexposed group during a one year time period. As discussed in chapter 6, it does not have any units but is a useful measure of association or effect between a given exposure and outcome. It expresses the number of times the outcome is more likely to occur in the exposed group compared to the unexposed group. The cumulative incidence difference represents the absolute difference in risk between the exposed and unexposed groups for a given time period (see chapter 6). It represents the excess risk associated with the outcome. In this problem the excess risk of ARI was estimated to be 11.46 cases per 100 workers for a one year period, April 1, 2006, to March 31, 2007. The 95 per cent confidence intervals indicate the relative precision of the measures of association. The measures of association do not appear overly precise. For example, the percent relative effect (defined in chapter 6) ranges from 29 percent to 400 percent. This is perhaps due to the unequal size of the exposed and unexposed groups, which does not affect the validity of the findings but does affect their precision. The overall power of the study assuming seven percent of the unexposed workers develop the outcome, a 95 percent confidence level, and an ability to detect a cumulative incidence ratio of at least 2.50 is about 81 percent, which is generally considered acceptable.

5. In step 4, calculation of the CIR and CID could have been simplified since the cumulative incidence in the exposed and unexposed groups had already been calculated in step 3.

Open Cohort Studies

The analysis of open cohort studies differs from that for closed cohort studies. This is due to the fact that, unlike closed cohort studies, not all subjects in open cohort studies are followed for the same length of time. For one thing, subjects in open cohort studies may enter or leave the study at various times. This can result in differences in follow-up time between the exposed and unexposed groups, and these differences must be accounted for in the analysis. One way to do this is to use measures of occurrence and association that are based on person-time units. As noted in chapter 5, person-time units represent a way of accounting for differences in follow-up time among the subjects. Thus, in open cohorts studies the standard measure of occurrence is incidence density, and the applicable measure of association is the incidence density ratio or the incidence density difference, each of which was described in chapter 6. These measures take into account the variable times at risk among the subjects, which is not true with cumulative incidence and its derivative measures of association used in closed cohort studies. The use of person-time units, however, is based on an assumption that the risk of the study outcome is *constant* during the follow-up period. This assumption becomes less tenable as the length of follow up increases. An alternative approach is to use *survival analysis* in which the study findings are analyzed over relatively short, successive periods of time where the risk of the study outcome is likely to be uniform. The fundamentals of survival analysis are summarized briefly in exhibit 5-2, and the topic is treated comprehensively in many biostatistical texts (see, for example, *Biostatistical Methods in Epidemiology* by Stephen C. Newman).[5] Survival analysis may also be used in the analysis of closed cohort studies, especially if there are significant losses to follow up. Our focus, however, will be on measures based on incidence density. Multivariable procedures frequently used in survival analysis will be treated briefly in the section dealing with confounding and effect measure modification in open cohort studies later in the chapter.

Given the foregoing, the overall findings from an open cohort study based on a general cohort or a special exposure cohort with a comparable unexposed group can be analyzed with the aid of the following tabular display. Notice that row totals cannot be calculated for this table. This is because the two columns represent different types of measurements that cannot be added together.

Exposure Status	Outcome	Person-time
Exposed	a	T_e
Unexposed	c	T_{ue}
	a + c	T

The values a and c are analogous to those in the contingency table used in analyzing closed cohort studies, and therefore the total number of outcomes is also a + c. The values T_e and T_{ue} represent the total person-time units (e.g., person-years) generated during follow up of the exposed and unexposed groups, respectively. The value T is the sum of T_e and T_{ue}, and it is the total number of person-time units generated in the study at the time of analysis.

Based on the above table, the following measures can be calculated (see formulas 11.7 through 11.13).

(11.7) $$ID_c = [(a + c) / T] \times 10^n$$

ID_c is the crude or overall incidence density (incidence rate) for a given population base measured in person-years or other person-time units (see chapter 5).

(11.8) $$ID_e = (a / T_e) \times 10^n \ and \ ID_{ue} = (c / T_{ue}) \times 10^n$$

ID_e is the incidence density in the *exposed* group, and ID_{ue} is the incidence density in the *unexposed* group. These are the rates of outcome development by exposure status. A method for calculating an approximate 95 percent confidence interval for incidence density was described in chapter 5 (see formula 5.17) and is not repeated here. It is applicable to ID_c, ID_e, and ID_{ue}.

(11.9) $$IDR = (a / T_e) / (c / T_{ue})$$

Formula 11.9, which defines the incidence density ratio, is equivalent to formula 6.6. It is often referred to generically as the rate ratio, and though not correctly, sometimes the relative risk (see chapter 6). An approximate 95 percent confidence interval for the IDR is given by formula 11.10.[22]

(11.10)

$$95\% \ CI = \exp\left\{\ln(IDR) \pm 1.96\sqrt{(1/a)+(1/c)}\right\}$$

The values a and c in this formula are the number of exposed and unexposed subjects with the study outcome, respectively (see above tabular display). As with formula 11.4, the expressions exp and ln represent the exponential and natural logarithm, respectively (see chapter 9).

(11.11) $$IDD = (a / T_e) \times 10^n - (c / T_{ue}) \times 10^n$$

Formula 11.11, which defines the incidence density difference, is equivalent to formula 6.11. It is a type of rate difference or excess rate (see chapter 6). An approximate 95 percent confidence interval for the IDD is given by formula 11.12.[22]

(11.12)

$$95\% \ CI = IDD \pm 1.96\sqrt{\left(a/T_e^2\right)+\left(c/T_{ue}^2\right)}$$

The IDD in formula 11.12 should be *stated as a decimal fraction* (e.g., 0.016 per person-year versus 1.6 per 100 person-years). The calculated confidence limits can then each be multiplied by a selected population base as desired. Note that this formula does *not* require natural logarithms or exponentials to calculate the confidence interval. Neither does formula 11.6.

If preferred, the statistical significance of the measures of association (IDR or IDD) can be determined using the **person-time chi-square test** (χ^2_{P-T}) with one degree of freedom.[24] It is interpreted similarly to the chi-square test for independence discussed in earlier chapters and shown in table 9-3. The formula is:

(11.13)

$$\chi^2_{P-T} = \frac{\left\{a - \left[T_e\left(a+c\right)\right]/T\right\}^2}{\left[\left(T_e\right)\left(T_{ue}\right)\left(a+c\right)\right]/T^2}$$

The symbols used in formula 11.13 are based on those in the generic tabular display shown above. Problem 11-2 illustrates an approach to the basic overall analysis of an open cohort study based on a general cohort.

Problem 11-2: Basic Overall Analysis of an Open Cohort Study

A prospective cohort study was designed to determine if there is an association between diabetes and Alzheimer's disease. The subjects included men and women, 50–59 years of age at entry into the study. New subjects could enter the study at various points during follow up after an assessment of their eligibility and disease status. Overall, the subjects were followed for an average of 12 years. Outcome assessments for Alzheimer's disease were made by a team of specialists knowledgeable of the condition. Of the 95 subjects with diabetes at entry into the study, 25 were diagnosed with Alzheimer's disease during follow up. Of the 780 subjects without diabetes, 120 were diagnosed with Alzheimer's disease. The exposed group (diabetics) contributed a total of 680 person-years of observation during the study, while the unexposed group (non-diabetics) contributed 6,500 person-years of observation. Based on these findings, calculate the crude incidence density, the incidence density in the exposed and unexposed groups, and the incidence density ratio and difference along with their 95 percent confidence intervals. Interpret your results.

Solution:
Step 1: Place the data provided in the problem in the appropriate cells of a tabular display as shown below. It is important to keep in mind that the values in the right-hand column of this display are person-time units. In this particular problem they represent person-years.

Exposure Status	Outcome	Person-time
Exposed	25	680 years
Unexposed	120	6,500 years
	145	7,180 years

Step 2: Calculate the crude incidence density for Alzheimer's disease using formula 11.7.

$$ID_c = (145 / 7{,}180) \times 10^n = 0.0202 \times 10^2 = 2.02 \text{ per 100 person-years}$$

Step 3: Calculate the incidence density for Alzheimer's disease in the exposed and unexposed groups using formula 11.8.

$$ID_e = (25 / 680) \times 10^n = 0.0368 \times 10^2 = 3.68 \text{ per 100 person-years}$$

$$ID_{ue} = (120 / 6{,}500) \times 10^n = 0.0185 \times 10^2 = 1.85 \text{ per 100 person-years}$$

Step 4: Calculate the incidence density ratio and incidence density difference for Alzheimer's disease along with their 95 percent confidence intervals using formulas 11.9 to 11.12 as appropriate.

$$IDR = (25/680)/(120/6{,}500) = 1.99$$

$$95\% \text{ CI} = \exp\left\{\ln(1.99) \pm 1.96\sqrt{(1/25)+(1/120)}\right\} =$$

$$\exp\{0.6881 \pm 0.4309\} = 1.29 \text{ to } 3.06$$

$$IDD = (25/680) \times 10^n - (120/6{,}500) \times 10^n = 0.0368 \times 10^2 - 0.0185 \times 10^2 =$$

$$0.0183 \times 10^2 = 1.83 \text{ per 100 person-years}$$

$$95\% \text{ CI} = 0.0183 \pm 1.96\sqrt{(25/680^2)+(120/6{,}500^2)} =$$

$$0.0183 \pm 0.0148 = 0.0035 \text{ to } 0.0331 =$$

$$0.35 \text{ per 100 person-years to } 3.31 \text{ per 100 person-years}$$

Answer: Based on the overall findings, the incidence density of Alzheimer's disease in this cohort is 2.02 cases per 100 person-years. This represents the overall rate of development of Alzheimer's disease in the cohort (i.e., 2.02 cases of Alzheimer's disease developed for every 100 person-years of observation). The incidence density of Alzheimer's disease in the exposed group is 3.68 cases per 100 person-years, and the incidence density in the unexposed group is 1.85 cases per 100 person-years. Thus, the overall rate of Alzheimer's is higher among diabetics than non-diabetics. In fact, the incidence density ratio is an estimated 1.99 (95% CI = 1.29 to 3.06). This indicates that the rate at which Alzheimer's disease developed in the cohort is almost two times greater among diabetics than non-diabetics, all other factors being equal. The confidence interval indicates that we can be 95 percent certain that the true IDR is between 1.29 and 3.06. The incidence density difference is 1.83 cases of Alzheimer's disease per 100 person-years (95% CI = 0.35 per 100 person-years to 3.31 per 100 person-years). This represents the excess rate of Alzheimer's disease in the cohort associated with diabetes. We can be 95 percent certain that the true difference is between 0.35 and 1.83 cases per 100 person-years based on the confidence interval.

Comments:

1. This was an *open cohort study* because new subjects could be added during the follow-up period. While it is not stated in the problem, it is presumed that subjects could also leave the cohort at any time, which is another characteristic of open cohort studies. The terminology, open cohort study, implies that the cohort is open to new members at any given time. A synonymous term, dynamic cohort study, perhaps better illustrates the potential for subjects to enter or leave the cohort during follow up.

2. Open cohort studies are analyzed in a way that accounts for only the time the subjects are observed to be at risk of the study outcome. In this study the average follow-up time was 12 years. If a subject died due to a competing risk after only two years of observation, he or she would only contribute two person-years to the denominator of the incidence density. On the other hand, if another subject was observed for 10 years until development of the study outcome, he or she would contribute 10 person-years to the denominator. In this way a subject's contribution to the denominator is proportional to his or her time at risk. This is not true in closed cohort studies using cumulative incidence as the measure of occurrence. Both subjects would contribute equally to denominator even though their risks of the outcome are different. Total person-time is not always calculated by summing the person-time units contributed by each individual in the cohort. In some cases it is estimated as described in chapter 5.

3. A concern in long-term open (and closed) cohort studies is aging of the cohort. Calculation of person-time is based on an assumption that the risk of the outcome is approximately equal during the period of observation.[25] This is necessary if, for example, 10 person-years are to be considered equivalent to five persons followed for two years or 10 persons followed for one year, which is presumed in calculating person-time units. In this study the subjects were defined as being 50–59 years of age at entry. Since some of these subjects may have been followed for more than 10 years (i.e., the average follow-up time was 12 years), some could have been in their sixties or seventies before conclusion of the study. From what we know about Alzheimer's disease (and most other chronic diseases) risk increases with age. Therefore, an overall incidence density and its derivative measures of association could be misleading in this study. Time in general is related to risk; therefore, it is standard practice in long-term cohort studies to determine incidence density for relatively narrow age groups or over smaller intervals of time in which the risk of the outcome is likely to be independent of time of observation. This is done in *survival analysis* (exhibit 5-2).

4. Conceptually, the reported incidence density represents the flow of Alzheimer's disease into the study population. It is the rate at which the disease occurred. The incidence density ratio is a measure of association between the exposure (diabetes) and the outcome (Alzheimer's disease). Unlike the cumulative incidence ratio, it does not measure the relative *risk* of developing Alzheimer's disease. Instead, it measures the relative *rate* at which Alzheimer's develops. When the risk of the outcome is small (e.g., less than 0.05 in the exposed and unexposed groups), however, the IDR approximates the CIR rather well.[13] The incidence density difference represents the absolute rate at which the disease occurred. It is often referred to as the excess rate associated with the exposure (see chapter 6). Like IDR, it is also a measure of association.

5. Overall, the ratio measure of association in this problem was more precise than the difference measure of association based on the widths of the 95 percent confidence intervals. The same was true for in the previous problem (10-1). This may be partly due to the different methods used to estimate these values.

EVALUATING CONFOUNDING AND
EFFECT MEASURE MODIFICATION

The discussion in the previous section concerned the overall analysis of closed and open cohort studies using appropriate measures of occurrence and association. The findings from such analyses may be considered preliminary since no attempt is made to control confounding or explain effect measure modification at this stage of analysis. Confounding can be controlled in the design stage of a cohort study by restriction or matching. *Restriction* is effective in controlling confounding by assuring the exposed and unexposed groups are the same or similar with regard to potential confounders like age, sex, or race/ethnicity. Furthermore, it does not affect the internal validity of the findings; in fact, it improves it by controlling systematic error due to confounding.[10] Nevertheless, restriction has some disadvantages. It may limit the external validity of a study; that is, the degree to which the findings may be generalized to other populations. It may also limit the pool of eligible subjects, thereby reducing sample size and hence a study's power. Also, it may leave residual confounding (chapter 8) if the restriction is based on broad categories. For example, restricting eligibility for a study of the effect of sunlight exposure on cataract development to those 25-65 years of age would undoubtedly result in some residual confounding by age since the frequency of both sunlight exposure and cataracts can be expected to vary significantly within this broad age group. Of course, restriction also limits any consideration of the restricted variables as potential risk factors for the study outcome.[10]

Unlike that in case-control studies (chapter 10), *individual matching* is relatively straightforward in cohort studies and can be a very effective means of controlling confounding in the design stage. Even so, it is rarely used. There are several reasons for this. First, multiple outcomes are often examined in cohort studies, and it is not always clear at the outset what factors are likely to be potential confounders for all of these outcomes. Second, obtaining information on potential confounders can be expensive and inefficient. It may require detailed interviews or testing among large numbers of people, perhaps in the hundreds of thousands. Third, there may be a loss of potential subjects who cannot be matched to the exposed subjects on the chosen variables.[13] A fourth problem has to do with the fact that matching involves individuals while the analysis often involves person-time units (e.g., in open cohort studies). Therefore, the distribution of person-time during follow up may not reflect the original distribution of matched subjects.[26] Unlike restriction, however, matching in cohort studies still allows one to evaluate the role of the matched variables on the study outcomes and to assess their role as possible effect modifiers. Also, a special matched analysis is not generally required when matching is used in cohort studies, although it will maximize study efficiency.[27]

The following two sections deal with some common methods for detecting and controlling confounding and identifying possible effect measure modification in the analysis phase of unmatched closed and open cohort studies. Restriction in the design stage, while useful, is unlikely to address all potential confounders in a study and does not address the issue of effect measure modification. As noted above, matching is rarely used in cohort studies, and where it is, it is likely to be limited to variables like age and sex, which are relatively easy to ascertain from subjects. For these reasons detecting and controlling confounders and identifying potential effect modifiers in the analysis phase are common objectives in cohort studies. The usual methods of achieving these objectives involve *stratification* or *multivariable analysis*. Though not necessarily discussed in this order, an evaluation of effect measure modification should normally precede that of confounding in the analysis phase of a study.

Stratification

Because the statistical procedures used in stratification differ somewhat in closed and open cohort studies, the following discussion is presented separately for each design. The basic principles, however, remain the same for all cohort studies.

   Closed cohort studies.   *Stratification*, along with pooling to produce a summary Mantel-Haenszel odds ratio (OR_{MH}), was described in chapter 10 in the context of case-control studies. The same procedures can be used to detect and control confounding in closed cohort studies when the odds ratio is the chosen measure of association. One can also use stratification in closed cohort studies to identify effect measure modification. When effect measure modification is evident one should *not* calculate the OR_{MH}, however, since it is based on the assumption that the stratum-specific odds ratios are constant across the strata.[3] In effect, the OR_{MH} could conceal the heterogeneity of the stratum-specific odds ratios. Instead, effect measure modification should be identified and described in the study.

   One must be *cautious* when using the odds ratio to estimate the risk ratio in closed cohort studies. This is because the results of stratification do not always correspond between these two measures of association even when the study outcome is rare. In some cases, effect measure modification detected using odds ratios may not exist when risk ratios are used.[28] This problem underscores a point made in chapter 10. Effect measure modification is dependent on the measure of association being used; therefore, the measure of association (e.g., OR, CIR, CID) should be reported when assessing effect measure modification. In fact, this is why it is referred to as effect *measure* modification. Also, as noted in chapter 10, when the stratification factor is not a true confounder (i.e., it is a risk factor for the outcome but not associated with the exposure), using the odds ratio can sometimes lead to a false conclusion of confounding that is not apparent with other ratio measures of association. Therefore, it is also a good idea to report the measure of association used when evaluating confounding in a closed cohort study.

Methods analogous to those described in chapter 10 with regard to the odds ratio can be used to generate Mantel-Haenszel estimates of the cumulative incidence ratio (risk ratio) and the cumulative incidence difference (risk difference). These measures are generally referred to in the literature as the **Mantel-Haenszel risk ratio** (RR_{MH}) and the **Mantel-Haenszel risk difference** (RD_{MH}).[3] When the frequency of the outcome is relatively high (e.g., in studies of disease outbreaks), the cumulative incidence difference is generally the preferred measure of association in closed cohort studies,[27] and, hence, in this circumstance the RD_{MH} will be the appropriate Mantel-Haenszel estimate.

Formulas for calculating the RR_{MH} and RD_{MH} are shown below along with their approximate 95 percent confidence intervals.[3] The symbol Σ refers to "the sum of," and i represents each stratum. The frequencies a_i–d_i and n_i are based on the standard 2×2 contingency table referred to on p. 332. Like the OR_{MH}, use of the RR_{MH} and the RD_{MH} are based on an assumption that the applicable measures of association are homogeneous across all strata (i.e., there is no effect measure modification).

(11.14)

$$RR_{MH} = \frac{\Sigma\left(a_i M_{ui} / n_i\right)}{\Sigma\left(c_i M_{ei} / n_i\right)}$$

where $M_{ei} = a_i + b_i$ and $M_{ui} = c_i + d_i$

(11.15)

$$95\% \text{ CI} = \exp\left\{\ln\left(RR_{MH}\right) \pm 1.96 \sqrt{\frac{\Sigma\left[\left(M_{pi} M_{ei} M_{ui} / n_i^2\right) - \left(a_i c_i / n_i\right)\right]}{\left[\Sigma\left(a_i M_{ui} / n_i\right)\right]\left[\Sigma\left(c_i M_{ei} / n_i\right)\right]}}\right\}$$

where $M_{pi} = a_i + c_i$, $M_{ei} = a_i + b_i$, and $M_{ui} = c_i + d_i$

(11.16)

$$RD_{MH} = \frac{\Sigma\left[\left(a_i M_{ui} - c_i M_{ei}\right)/ n_i\right]}{\Sigma\left(M_{ei} M_{ui} / n_i\right)}$$

where $M_{ei} = a_i + b_i$, and $M_{ui} = c_i + d_i$

(11.17)

$$95\% \text{ CI} = RD_{MH} \pm 1.96 \times \sqrt{\frac{\Sigma\left(M_{ei} M_{ui} / n_i\right)^2 \left\{\begin{matrix}\left[a_i d_i /\left(M_{ei}^2 \left(M_{ei}-1\right)\right)\right]+ \\ \left[b_i c_i /\left(M_{ui}^2 \left(M_{ui}-1\right)\right)\right]\end{matrix}\right\}}{\left[\Sigma\left(M_{ei} M_{ui} / n_i\right)\right]^2}}$$

where $M_{ei} = a_i + b_i$, and $M_{ui} = c_i + d_i$

Despite their complex appearances, these formulas are mathematically simple, though tedious to calculate by hand. Software applications are available from various sources that can be used to solve these equations with just a few keystrokes on a computer. Problem 11-3 illustrates stratification and pooling in a closed cohort study using two strata. The calculation of RR_{MH}, RD_{MH}, and their 95 percent confidence intervals are also demonstrated.

An alternative to producing Mantel-Haenszel estimates via pooling is **standardization**. Standardization was discussed in chapter 6 in the context of rate adjustment (also known as rate standardization) and in chapter 10 in terms of the odds ratio. The principles discussed there also apply here. Like pooling, standardization is used in the stratification process to produce a summary measure of association that is *adjusted* for confounding by one or more factors. Unlike pooling, however, standardization does *not* require that the stratum-specific measures of association be constant across the strata. Therefore, the technique is applicable even in the presence of effect measure modification. The standardized measure may not be very informative, however, if the stratum-specific measures of association vary widely, especially in direction. In this case it is a good idea to report the individual measures of association and their confidence intervals along with the standardized estimate.

In the context of cohort studies, standardization involves taking a weighted average of the stratum-specific measures of association where the weights are commonly based on the distribution of the potential confounder(s) in the exposed group, or alternatively, in the unexposed (comparison) group. The former practice is reminiscent of "indirect adjustment" (chapter 6) where the exposed group represents the study (non-reference) population, while the latter is characteristic of "direct adjustment" where the unexposed group represents the standard population.*

A major difference between standardization and pooling using the Mantel-Haenszel procedure is the weighting system. The Mantel-Haenszel estimate is a weighted average of the stratum-specific measures of association where the weights are based on the amount of data in each stratum. Those strata with more data are weighted more, and those with less data are weighted less. Standardization also utilizes a weighted average of the stratum-specific measures of association, but the weights are based on the proportions of the potential confounder(s) in the exposed or unexposed groups (i.e., the applicable standard population). For example, if we were to standardize the stratum-specific risk ratios by sex, and there were 40 percent males and 60 percent females in the applicable standard population, our weights would be 0.40 and 0.60, respectively. While the Mantel-Haenszel procedure tends to produce more precise estimates than standardization, standardization is based on clearly specified weights that enhance the comparability of study results from one analysis to another as long as the same standard population or weighting system is used.[3]

---

*Actually, in both cases the standard population is represented. You will recall from chapter 6 that the study (non-reference) population is actually the standard population in indirect adjustment. Therefore, we can say that standardization uses weights based on the distribution of potential confounder(s) in the standard population whether the standard population is represented by the exposed or unexposed group.

Standardized measures of association that may be employed in closed cohort studies include the **standardized risk ratio** (SRR), **standardized risk difference** (SRD), and the **standardized odds ratio** (SOR). For example, the SRR can be calculated using formula 11.18 when the weights are standardized to the potential confounder distribution in the exposed group. Similarly, the SOR can be calculated as shown in formula 11.19.[10]

(11.18)

$$SRR = \frac{\sum a_i}{\sum \left[c_i \left(a_i + b_i \right) / \left(c_i + d_i \right) \right]}$$

The symbols a_i through d_i are frequencies based on standard 2×2 contingency tables as illustrated earlier. Using the data in problem 11-3, which appears below, we have:

$$SRR = \frac{(28+40)}{\left[(46)(28+27)/(46+68) \right] + \left[(22)(40+101)/(22+98) \right]}$$

$$= 68 / 48.0430 = 1.42$$

This result is close to the RR_{MH} of 1.39 calculated in problem 11-3. In general, standardized and pooled measures of association will be fairly close when there is little heterogeneity among the stratum-specific measures of association,[29] as is the case in problem 11-3.

In the above example the SRR can be interpreted as the estimated risk ratio *adjusted* for cigarette smoking status. It indicates that the estimated overall risk of an acute respiratory infection is 1.42 times greater among those exposed to airborne pesticide residues than those not exposed *after controlling for* cigarette smoking status. The adjusted risk ratio was standardized to the exposed group. The result would not be expected to be the same, however, if the adjusted measure had been standardized to the unexposed group. This is because different standard populations usually have different distributions of the potential confounders that affect the magnitude of the estimate differently. For this reason it is always recommended that the standard population or the weights be specified when using standardization.

(11.19)

$$SOR = \frac{\sum a_i}{\sum \left[b_i c_i / d_i \right]}$$

In summary, both the Mantel-Haenszel and standardization procedures produce summary measures of association that control for confounding by the stratification factor(s). The former method tends to provide a more precise estimate of the adjusted measure of association, while the latter method tends to provide a more comparable estimate as long as the same standard population or weights are used. The Mantel-Haenszel estimates (RR_{MH}, RD_{MH}, or OR_{MH}) should not be used when there is effect measure modification, but it makes no difference when estimates are derived by standardization (SRR, SRD, or SOR). However, when effect measure modification is not present, analogous estimates (e.g., RR_{MH} and SRR) should be similar.

Problem 11-3: Basic Stratified Analysis in a Closed Cohort Study

The study referred to in problem 11-1 concerning routine exposure to airborne pesticide residues and the risk of acute respiratory infection was replicated at a pesticide manufacturing plant in West Virginia. As part of the analysis the investigators stratified the findings by cigarette smoking status. These results appear below.

Exposure Status	Outcome Status Present	Absent		Outcome Status Present	Absent
Exposed	28	27		40	101
Unexposed	46	68		22	98
			169		261
	Non-Cigarette Smokers			*Cigarette Smokers*	

Based on these results, calculate both the cumulative incidence ratio (CIR) and cumulative incidence difference (CID) overall and for each stratum of cigarette smoking status. Based on your findings does effect measure modification or confounding appear to be present? Why or why not? If appropriate, calculate the Mantel-Haenszel risk ratio (RR_{MH}) and risk difference (RD_{MH}) and their 95 percent confidence intervals using the proper formulas. Compare these measures to the crude measures. What do these comparisons suggest?

Solution:
Step 1: Calculate the overall CIR and CID using formulas 11.3 and 11.5, respectively. Note that the tables must be combined to get the overall measures.

$$CIR = [(28 + 40) / (28 + 27 + 40 + 101) \times 10^n] / [(46 + 22) / (46 + 68 + 22 + 98) \times 10^n] =$$
$$[(68 / 196) \times 10^n] / [(68 / 234) \times 10^n] =$$
$$34.69 \text{ per } 100 / 29.06 \text{ per } 100 = 1.19$$
$$CID = 34.69 \text{ per } 100 - 29.06 \text{ per } 100 = 5.63 \text{ per } 100$$

Step 2: Calculate the stratum-specific CIR and CID using formulas 11.3 and 11.5, respectively.

$$CIR \text{ (non-cigarette smokers)} = [28 / (28 + 27) \times 10^n] / [46 / (46 + 68) \times 10^n] =$$
$$50.91 \text{ per } 100 / 40.35 \text{ per } 100 = 1.26$$
$$CIR \text{ (cigarette smokers)} = [40 / (40 + 101) \times 10^n] / [22 / (22 + 98)] \times 10^n] =$$
$$28.37 \text{ per } 100 / 18.33 \text{ per } 100 = 1.55$$
$$CID \text{ (non-cigarette smokers)} = 50.91 \text{ per } 100 - 40.35 \text{ per } 100 = 10.56 \text{ per } 100$$
$$CID \text{ (cigarette smokers)} = 28.37 \text{ per } 100 - 18.33 \text{ per } 100 = 10.04 \text{ per } 100$$

Step 3: Determine whether effect measure modification or confounding appears to be present. Note that general guidelines appear in table 10-3. These guidelines may be applied to the CIR and CID as well as the odds ratio.

From Step 1:

Crude CIR = 1.19; Crude CID = 5.63 per 100

From Step 2:

CIR: 1.26 (non-cigarette smokers) vs. 1.55 (cigarette smokers)

CID: 10.56 per 100 (non-cigarette smokers) vs. 10.04 per 100 (cigarette smokers)

Based on the CID, and assuming no bias in the study, cigarette smoking appears to be a confounder for the association between exposure to airborne pesticide residues and acute respiratory infection. Using the guidelines in table 10-3, which can also be applied to measures of association other than the odds ratio, the stratum-specific CIDs are relatively homogeneous, and both are greater than the crude CID. Based on the CIR, there also appears to be some confounding and possibly some effect measure modification as well.

Step 4: Calculate RR_{MH} and it 95 percent confidence interval using formulas 11.14 and 11.15. Also, calculate RD_{MH} and its 95 percent confidence interval using formulas 11.16 and 11.17.

$$RR_{MH} = \frac{\left[(28)(114)/169\right]+\left[(40)(120)/261\right]}{\left[(46)(55)/169\right]+\left[(22)(141)/261\right]} = 1.39$$

$$95\%\ CI = \exp\left\{\ln(1.39)\pm1.96\sqrt{\frac{\begin{array}{c}\left\{\left[(74)(55)(114)/169^2\right]-\left[(28)(46)/169\right]\right\}+\\ \left\{\left[(62)(141)(120)/261^2\right]-\left[(40)(22)/261\right]\right\}\end{array}}{\begin{array}{c}\left\{\left[(28)(114)/169\right]+\left[(40)(120)/261\right]\right\}\times\\ \left\{\left[(46)(55)/169\right]+\left[(22)(141)/261\right]\right\}\end{array}}}\right\}$$

$$= \exp\left[0.3293\pm1.96\sqrt{20.6519/1{,}001.1284}\right]$$

$$= \exp\left[0.3293\pm0.2815\right] = 1.05\ \text{to}\ 1.84$$

$$RD_{MH} = \frac{\left\{\left[(28)(114)-(46)(55)\right]/169\right\}+\left\{\left[(40)(120)-(22)(141)\right]/261\right\}}{\left[(55)(114)/169\right]+\left[(141)(120)/261\right]}$$

$$= 10.4229/101.9282 = 0.1023\ \text{or}\ 10.23\ \text{per}\ 100$$

$$95\%\ CI = 0.1023\pm1.96\times$$

$$\sqrt{\frac{\begin{array}{c}\left[(55)(114)/169\right]^2\left\{\left[(28)(68)/55^2(55-1)\right]+\left[(27)(46)/114^2(114-1)\right]\right\}+\\ \left[(141)(120)/261\right]^2\left\{\left[(40)(98)/141^2(141-1)\right]+\left[(101)(22)/120^2(120-1)\right]\right\}\end{array}}{\left\{\left[(55)(114)/169\right]+\left[(141)(120)/261\right]\right\}^2}}$$

$$= 0.1023\pm1.96\sqrt{(28.5763/10{,}389.3535)}$$

$$= 0.1023\pm0.1028 = -0.0005\ \text{to}\ 0.2051\ \text{or}\ -0.05\ \text{per}\ 100\ \text{to}\ 20.51\ \text{per}\ 100$$

Answer: Based on the cumulative incidence difference (CID), there appears to be confounding due to cigarette smoking status. The stratum-specific CIDs (10.56 per 100 in non-cigarette smokers and 10.04 per 100 in cigarette smokers) are relatively homogeneous, and both are greater than the crude CID. Based on the cumulative incidence ratio (CIR), there also appears to be some confounding due to cigarette smoking and possibly some effect measure modification. This is due to the fact that the stratum-specific CIRs (1.26 in non-cigarette smokers and 1.55 in cigarette smokers) are both greater than the crude CIR but also somewhat different from each other. A comparison of the crude and adjusted measures of association also suggests confounding. The Mantel-Haenszel risk difference is 10.23 per 100 (95% CI = -0.05 per 100 to 20.51 per 100) versus a crude CID of 5.63 per 100. The Mantel-Haenszel risk ratio is 1.39 (95% CI = 1.05 to 1.84) versus a crude CIR of 1.19. These results suggest negative confounding since the crude measures are lower than the adjusted measures.

Comments:

1. Stratification is a useful procedure that allows one to assess whether or not effect measure modification or confounding is likely to be present in a study. Assuming there are no significant selection or information biases, if the stratum-specific measures of association are heterogeneous beyond what one might expect due to random error, effect measure modification is likely for that measure. In this problem, there may be some effect measure modification using the risk ratio (cumulative incidence ratio), although the apparent difference could be due simply to random error. A test of heterogeneity could be employed to test the likelihood that the difference between the stratum-specific risk ratios is statistically significant. While statistical testing alone does not confirm effect measure modification, given what we know about cigarette smoking and its interaction with other environmental pollutants, it is certainly a possibility. Stratifying the data on several levels of cigarette smoking (e.g., heavy, moderate, light, and none) may have made it easier to draw a conclusion in this regard. Effect measure modification does not appear to be present using risk differences (cumulative incidence differences), and if present using risk ratios, it does not appear to be very strong. One should always remember that effect measure modification is dependent on the measure of association used (see chapter 10), so these findings are not contradictory.

2. Evidence of confounding by cigarette smoking was found in this study for reasons outlined in the responses to the problem. A rule of thumb for assessing suspected confounding for ratio measures of association is referred to as the 10 percent rule. It was introduced in chapter 8 and is discussed later in this chapter. Basically, when the adjusted ratio measure of association is more than 10 percent higher or lower than the comparable crude measure of association, confounding is indicated. Use of the rule assumes that there is also non-numerical evidence to support confounding (i.e., it meets or appears to meet the criteria for confounding outlined in chapter 8). In this problem, the Mantel-Haenszel risk ratio was more than 10 percent higher than the crude cumulative incidence ratio, and cigarette smoking appears to meet the criteria for confounding (e.g., those working in pesticide plants are more likely to smoke cigarettes, and cigarette smoking is a risk factor for acute respiratory infections).

3. One may wonder why a Mantel-Haenszel risk ratio was calculated if effect measure modification was possible using the cumulative incidence ratio. The reason is that the evidence was inconclusive. Kenneth J. Rothman has suggested:

> The assumption [of homogeneity of effect] does not imply that the estimates of effect will be the same, or even nearly the same, in each stratum.

It allows for statistical variation over the strata. . . . Unless the data demonstrate some clear pattern of variation that undermines the assumption that the effect is uniform over the strata, it is usually reasonable to use a pooled approach, despite the fiction of the assumption.[3(pp150-151)]

4. Though not shown here, the estimated overall power of the study is less than 50 percent, probably due to the relatively small sample size for a cohort study. The negative lower confidence limit for the Mantel-Haenszel risk difference (i.e., -0.05 per 100) is not an anomaly. Risk differences can be less than or greater than zero, which is the null point indicating no difference (see problem 11-4, comment number 3).

Open cohort studies.   As with closed cohort studies, *stratification* can be used in open cohort studies to assess potential confounding or effect measure modification. The main difference is that the primary measures of association are typically based on incidence density rather than cumulative incidence. Nonetheless, the general principles are the same, and the strategies used in table 10-3, and explained in chapter 10, are still appropriate. Also, findings from closed cohort studies where there have been significant losses to follow up or deaths due to competing risks may be analyzed as open cohort studies in order to account for uneven follow-up times.

As in closed cohort studies, when there is no effect measure modification, confounding, if present, can be controlled by *pooling* the stratum-specific measures of association to produce an unconfounded estimate of the overall measure of association. When effect measure modification is present, *standardization* can be used to control confounding, but as in closed cohort studies, the resulting measure alone may conceal the actual degree of the heterogeneity across the strata. Therefore, it is a good idea to present the stratum-specific measures of association and their confidence intervals along with the standardized measure.

The basic formulas for pooling the incidence density ratio and the incidence density difference using Mantel-Haenszel procedures are shown below along with their 95 percent confidence intervals.[3] The **Mantel-Haenszel incidence density ratio** (IDR_{MH}) is also known as the **Mantel-Haenszel incidence rate ratio** (IRR_{MH}) and more commonly as the **Mantel-Haenszel rate ratio** (RR_{MH}). Similarly, the **Mantel-Haenszel incidence density difference** (IDD_{MH}) is also known as the **Mantel-Haenszel incidence rate difference** (IRD_{MH}) and more commonly as the **Mantel-Haenszel rate difference** (RD_{MH}). The symbols RR_{MH} and RD_{MH}, unfortunately, can be confused with the Mantel-Haenszel risk ratio and risk difference, respectively, since they use the same symbols. Therefore we will use IDR_{MH} and IDD_{MH} to avoid any confusion between the measures. An unfortunate aspect of epidemiology, which is true for other disciplines as well, is a lack of uniformity in the use of many key terms (see table 6-4, for example). This situation continues to improve with time, however.

The values in the formulas below are based on the tabular display shown earlier in the section dealing with the overall analysis of open cohort studies (see p. 337). As with closed cohort studies, the symbol Σ refers to "the sum of," and i represents each stratum.

(11.20)
$$IDR_{MH} = \frac{\Sigma(a_i T_{uei} / T_i)}{\Sigma(c_i T_{ei} / T_i)}$$

(11.21)
$$95\% \ CI = \exp\left\{ \ln(IDR_{MH}) \pm 1.96 \sqrt{\frac{\Sigma\left[(a_i + c_i)(T_{ei})(T_{uei})/T_i^2\right]}{\left[\Sigma(a_i T_{uei} / T_i)\right]\left[\Sigma(c_i T_{ei} / T_i)\right]}} \right\}$$

(11.22)
$$IDD_{MH} = \frac{\Sigma\left[(a_i T_{uei} - c_i T_{ei})/T_i\right]}{\Sigma(T_{ei} T_{uei} / T_i)}$$

(11.23)
$$95\% \ CI = IDD_{MH} \pm 1.96 \sqrt{\frac{\Sigma\left[(T_{ei} T_{uei} / T_i)^2\right]\left[(a_i / T_{ei}^2) + (c_i / T_{uei}^2)\right]}{\left[\Sigma(T_{ei} T_{uei} / T_i)\right]^2}}$$

Standardized measures of association employed in open cohort studies and based on incidence density include the *standardized mortality* (or *morbidity) ratio* (SMR), which was discussed in chapter 6, and the **standardized rate ratio** (SRR). Like their risk-based counterparts, these adjusted measures of association tend to be less precise than pooled estimates based on the Mantel-Haenszel procedure but are easier to compare from one analysis to another as long as the same standard population or weighting system is used.[3] There is also a *standardized rate difference*, which is less commonly used. It is not discussed here.

In the context of open cohort studies, the standardized morbidity ratio is sometimes referred to as the **standardized incidence ratio** (SIR) where morbidity is represented by incidence. It is calculated as shown in formula 11.24.[30] The symbols used on the right-hand side of the equation are the same as those used in the Mantel-Haenszel estimates above. In the context of open cohort studies, both the SIR and SRR are considered types of *standardized rate ratios*.

(11.24)
$$SIR = \frac{\Sigma a_i}{\Sigma\left[T_{ei}(c_i / T_{uei})\right]}$$

The SIR (or SMR) as calculated in formula 11.24 is based on weights derived from the distribution of potential confounders in the *exposed group*. It can be interpreted as the sum of the observed cases in the exposed group divided by the sum of the expected cases in the exposed group "where the expected numbers are based on rates in the reference population."[30(p123)] The reference population is defined in chapter 6 in the description of indirect adjustment. Formula 11.24 can be conceived as an adjusted form of the more familiar equation, SMR = OE / EE (formula 6.1).

The SRR as calculated in formula 11.25 is based on the weights derived from the distribution of potential confounders in the *unexposed group*. It can be interpreted as the sum of the expected cases in the unexposed group, where the expected numbers are based on rates in the non-reference population as defined in chapter 6, divided by the sum of the observed cases in the unexposed group.[30] It is calculated as follows:

(11.25)
$$SRR = \frac{\sum \left[T_{uei} \left(a_i / T_{ei} \right) \right]}{\sum c_i}$$

Since this measure has the same acronym as the standardized risk ratio, one must be careful to distinguish between the two in the literature. If they are not precisely specified, the context should help one determine which measure is being referred to.

Problem 11-4: Basic Stratified Analysis in a Open Cohort Study

The investigators of the study referred to in problem 11-2 concerning the possible relationship between diabetes and Alzheimer's disease in middle-aged men and women decided to stratify the results by subject status with regard to a history of stroke. The stratified data are presented in the tables which follow. Based on these results, report the overall incidence density ratio (IDR) and incidence density difference (IDD) along with their 95 percent confidence intervals. Also, report the stratum-specific IDR and IDD, respectively, based on stroke history along with their 95 percent confidence intervals. Based on your findings, does effect measure modification or confounding appear to be present? Why or why not? Calculate appropriate summary measures of association using the Mantel-Haenszel procedure or standardization as appropriate. If the Mantel-Haenszel procedure is used, also calculate the applicable 95 percent confidence interval. What do these findings suggest?

Exposure Status	Outcome	Person-time		Outcome	Person-time
Exposed	10	370 years		15	310 years
Unexposed	58	2,700 years		62	3,800 years
	No History of Stroke			*History of Stroke*	

Solution:
Step 1: The overall IDR and IDD were already calculated in problem 11-2. These results are represented below.

IDR = 1.99 (95% CI = 1.29 to 3.06)

IDD = 1.83 per 100 person-years

(95% CI = 0.35 per 100 person-years to 3.31 per 100 person-years)

Step 2: Calculate the stratum-specific IDR and IDD and their 95 percent confidence intervals using formulas 11.9 through 11.12, respectively.

$$\text{IDR (no stroke history)} = (10 / 370) / (58 / 2,700) = 0.02703 / 0.02148 =$$
$$1.26 \ (95\% \ CI = 0.64 \text{ to } 2.47)$$
$$\text{IDR (stroke history)} = (15 / 310) / (62 / 3,800) = 0.04839 / 0.01632 =$$
$$2.97 \ (95\% \ CI = 1.69 \text{ to } 5.22)$$
$$\text{IDD (no stroke history)} = (10 / 370) \times 10^n - (58 / 2,700) \times 10^n =$$

2.70 per 100 person-years – 2.15 per 100 person-years = 0.55 per 100 person-years
95% CI = –0.01214 to 0.02314 = -1.21 per 100 person-years to 2.31 per 100 person-years

$$\text{IDD (stroke history)} = (15 / 310) \times 10^n - (62 / 3,800) \times 10^n =$$

4.84 per 100 person-years – 1.63 per 100 person-years = 3.21 per 100 person-years
95% CI = 0.007278 to 0.05692 = 0.73 per 100 person-years to 5.69 per 100 person-years

Step 3: Determine if effect measure modification or confounding is likely to be present. Note that general guidelines appear in table 10-3. These guidelines may be applied to both the IDR and IDD.

Crude IDR = 1.99; Crude IDD = 1.83 per 100 person-years (from step 1)

IDR: 1.26 (no stroke history) vs. 2.97 (stroke history) (from step 2)

IDD: 0.55 per 100 person-years (no stroke history) vs.
3.21 per 100 person-years (stroke history) (from step 2)

Based on these results, it appears that stroke status is an *effect modifier* for the association between diabetes and Alzheimer's disease using both the IDR and the IDD. The stratum-specific IDRs appear heterogeneous as do the IDDs. Confounding by stroke status does not appear to be an issue since the crude measures are not less than or greater than both of the stratum-specific measures (see table 10-3). It is possible that the observed differences for both the stratum-specific IDRs and IDDs are due to random error given the relatively small number of events in the strata and the generally broad confidence intervals. To be more confident in concluding that effect measure modification is present one could employ a test of heterogeneity (see chapter 10) to determine if the differences are large enough to conclude that random error is an unlikely explanation for the findings.

Step 4: Calculate the standardized measures of association using formulas 11.24 and 11.25. Note that these measures only apply to the IDR and not the IDD.

$$SIR = \frac{(10 + 15)}{\left[(370)(58/2,700)\right] + \left[(310)(62/3,800)\right]}$$
$$= 25.00 / 13.0060 = 1.92$$

$$SRR = \frac{\left[2,700(10/370)\right] + \left[3,800(15/310)\right]}{(58 + 62)}$$
$$= 256.8439 / 120.00 = 2.14$$

Answer: The overall or crude incidence density ratio is 1.99 (95% CI = 1.29 to 3.06). The crude incidence density difference is 1.83 per 100 person-years (95% CI = 0.35

per 100 person-years to 3.31 per 100 person-years). The stratum-specific incidence density ratio for those without a history of stroke is 1.26 (95% CI = 0.64 to 2.47), and for those with a history of stroke it is 2.97 (95% CI = 1.69 to 5.22). The stratum-specific incidence density difference for those without a history of stroke is 0.55 per 100 person-years (95% CI = -1.21 per 100 person-years to 2.31 per 100 person-years). For those with a history of stroke it is 3.21 per 100 person-years (95% CI = 0.73 per 100 person-years to 5.69 per 100 person-years). These findings appear to suggest that there is effect measure modification using both the incidence density ratio and incidence density difference due to the heterogeneity of these measures across the strata. The incidence density ratio among the subjects with a history of stroke is over two times that of those without a history of stroke, and the incidence density difference among those with a history of stroke is over five times that of those without a history of stroke. Confounding by stroke status is unlikely since the crude incidence density ratio and difference are not both greater or less than the stratum-specific measures (see table 10-3). The standardized incidence ratio is 1.92, and the standardized rate ratio is 2.14. Both of these are close to the crude incidence density ratio suggesting that if confounding by stroke status is present in the study it is minimal.

Comments:

1. In open cohort studies the incidence density ratio tends to be favored over the incidence density difference even though both measures of association are reported in this problem. According to Alexander Walker, "this is the result of an empirical observation in chronic disease research, that incidence rate ratios tend to be more constant from study to study or from stratum to stratum of a single study than are rate differences."[6(p108)] This is one reason why standardized rate differences are not discussed in this chapter.

2. Because the stratum-specific measures of association are relatively heterogeneous, we concluded that effect measure modification appears to be present in the study for both the incidence density ratio and the incidence density difference. It is most pronounced using the difference measure, which represents additive effects (see chapter 10), but nevertheless also appears to be present using the ratio measure, which represents multiplicative effects (see chapter 10). This is not always the case. It is quite possible in a study that there could be effect measure modification on an additive scale but not on a multiplicative scale and vise versa. This is why when reporting effect measure modification one should always indicate the effect measure being used or the type of statistical model being employed (i.e., additive or multiplicative).

3. The lower 95 percent confidence limit for the incidence density difference in the stratum representing those subjects without a history of stroke is negative. This simply means that it is possible that the true incidence density is higher in those subjects without diabetes than in those with it. Since the incidence density difference is determined by subtracting the incidence density in the unexposed group (i.e., those without diabetes) from the incidence density in the exposed group (i.e., those with diabetes), a negative difference will result when the rate is higher in the unexposed versus the exposed group. The relatively broad confidence interval in this stratum (probably due to the small number of cases) simply means the range of likely incidence density differences include three possibilities: (a) the rate in the unexposed group exceeds that in the exposed group, (b) there is no difference between the rates in the exposed and unexposed groups (possible because zero is included in the confidence interval, and (c) the rate in the exposed group exceeds

that in the unexposed group. In traditional hypothesis testing we would refer to this result as not statistically significant (p > 0.05). The confidence interval for the stratum representing subjects with a history of stroke, on the other hand, did not include zero, and thus traditionally it would represent a statistically significant (p ≤ 0.05) result although the broadness of the interval still indicates a relatively imprecise finding.

4. Since there is evidence of effect measure modification in the study using both the incidence density ratio and difference, Mantel-Haenszel estimates of the measures of association were not calculated. Mantel-Haenszel estimates should only be used when effect measure modification is not suspected (e.g., observed variation appears to be due to random error) or at least is inconclusive as in problem 11-3. Adjusted summary measures of association, however, were calculated using standardization. Standardization is appropriate even when heterogeneity of effect (effect measure modification) is present. The standardized measures summarize the overall association between diabetes and Alzheimer's disease after adjusting for differences in stroke status. The two methods used produced somewhat different findings. This is not unexpected since different standard populations (weights) were used.

5. There is no evidence of significant confounding by stroke status in this study. The differences between the adjusted and crude incidence density ratios are relatively small indicating that confounding is either unlikely or minimal at most. As discussed in the next section, the adjusted and crude ratios were well within limits sometimes used to assess confounding. Once again, the main concern in this study appears to be effect measure modification, which should be described and discussed in light of suspected causal mechanisms. It makes biological sense, for example, that stroke *and* diabetes may increase the risk of Alzheimer's disease, a form of dementia.

Multivariable Analysis

While stratification has several advantages as a method of addressing confounding and effect measure modification, it has its limitations as well. As stated in chapter 10, a major disadvantage is that it may not be practical when there are many potential confounders to control, especially if each has multiple categories. This can greatly increase the number of strata resulting in statistical inefficiency and a loss of power due to small numbers in each stratum. There may even be empty strata. *Multivariable analysis*, however, is generally a more statistically efficient way to measure the effect of an exposure or combination of exposures on the study outcome while controlling simultaneously for several other factors. Multivariable analysis also allows investigators to examine continuous independent variables like height or weight, which would otherwise have to be reduced to meaningful categories in a stratified analysis. Nevertheless, as indicated in chapter 10, multivariable analysis is best conceived as a supplement to a stratified analysis since the latter procedure tends to provide a clearer picture of what the data actually reveal. Even when the number of variables makes stratification impractical, it should be carried out at least for the major study variables.[3] Together, these approaches can facilitate the analysis of the findings. Finally, it should be emphasized that selection of an appropriate multivariable model requires an adequate knowledge of the nature of the variables, the underlying assumptions about the relationship between the study exposures and outcomes, and the limitations of the various procedures.[10] Without this knowledge it is too easy to draw erroneous conclusions given the ease of use and wide availability of software application programs that perform multivariable analyses.

The most common type of multivariable analysis used in both closed and open cohort studies to address confounding and effect measure modification is multiple regression analysis.[31] Although *multiple linear regression* (chapter 9) is the standard when the outcome variable is continuous and certain other assumptions can be met, other types of multiple regression analysis tend to be more common in cohort studies. The following segments delineate briefly the most common methods of multiple regression analysis used in closed and open cohort studies, respectively. Each of these methods may be used to detect and control confounding or identify effect modifiers (i.e., interaction). The specific details of the methods can be found in several intermediate or advanced texts of epidemiologic methods or biostatistics and are not discussed here.

Closed cohort studies. When the outcome is dichotomous, as is often the case, multiple logistic regression is one of the most frequently used methods of regression analysis for assessing confounding or interactions in closed cohort studies. A concise overview of multiple logistic regression can be found in exhibit 10-2. You will recall that this method is also commonly used in case-control studies. As indicated in the exhibit, multiple logistic regression can provide odds ratios adjusted for confounding variables. It can also be used to examine possible interactions between selected variables by entering their product (e.g., X_1X_2) in the regression equation.

Open cohort studies. Confounding and effect measure modification can also be assessed in open cohort studies using multiple regression analysis.* Multiple logistic regression, which can achieve this objective in closed cohort studies, as well as in case-control and cross-sectional studies, is not, however, applicable to open cohort studies. This is because follow-up times may vary in these studies, and the procedure is not designed to deal with this. Therefore, other types of multivariable analysis must be used. One method that is frequently employed in open cohort studies is the **Cox proportional hazards model**, which is a multiple regression technique used in *survival analysis* (see exhibit 5-2). The method is appropriate when the study outcome represents *time-to-event* versus the *occurrence of an event*.[31] Specifically, the Cox model predicts the time to the study outcome for each subject in the study, while controlling for differences in time under observation and differences in subject characteristics.[32] Like multiple logistic regression, the method can be used to assess confounding and interaction. Exhibit 11-1 provides a concise overview of the technique. To illustrate its use in a nutshell, consider the following

*The procedures mentioned here also apply to closed cohort studies that are analyzed like open cohort studies due to significant losses to follow up or deaths due to competing risks.

Exhibit 11-1
What Is the Cox Proportional Hazards Model?

The Cox proportional hazards model is a popular multiple regression technique that is applicable to situations where there are unequal follow-up times, such as in the analysis of findings from open cohort studies. Its use is most closely associated with survival analysis (see exhibit 5-2). As with multiple logistic regression (see exhibit 10-2), the dependent variable in the Cox model is dichotomous (outcome present, outcome absent), and the independent variables are either continuous or categorical. The regression equation for the Cox model may be presented as follows:

$$\ln (\text{hazard rate}) = \alpha(t) + \beta_1 X_1 + \beta_2 X_2 + \beta_3 X_3 \ldots + \beta_k X_k$$

This equation is similar to that for multiple logistic regression. Both equations take the natural logarithm (ln) of a specific measure of the outcome variable, and both equations have intercepts and two or more independent variables (Xs) multiplied by regression coefficients (βs). The Cox model, however, has two distinctive features. First, the dependent variable is a transformed value that is equivalent to the natural logarithm of the *hazard rate* of the study outcome. The hazard rate is an instantaneous incidence density that can vary with time, specifically time since follow up began. Thus, it is a time-dependent measure. Second, the intercept $\alpha(t)$ represents the *baseline* hazard rate; that is, the hazard rate where all the Xs are zeros (e.g., the hazard rate in the unexposed group). An important assumption of the Cox model is known as the *proportional hazards assumption*. This assumption says that the ratio of the hazard rates (e.g., that in the exposed group to that in the unexposed group) is constant over time for each independent variable in the model. The ratio of hazard rates is referred to as the *hazard ratio*, which is a type of relative risk. Though hazard rates can vary with time, the hazard ratio will always be same in a study since the time functions cancel out when the ratio is calculated. A hazard ratio of 2.0 implies that those in the exposed group have twice the hazard as those in the unexposed group *at any given point in time* during the follow-up period, all other factors being equal. Likewise, a hazard ratio of 0.5 says that the hazard in the exposed group is only half that in the unexposed group at any given point in time. Many researchers interpret hazard ratios as risk ratios.

Similar to multiple logistic regression (exhibit 10-2), if an independent variable, say X_1, is dichotomous with possible values of 0 and 1, $\exp(\beta_1)$ will represent the hazard ratio, controlling for all other factors in the model. This corresponds to the adjusted hazard ratio. When X_1 is a continuous variable, $\exp(\beta_1)$ represents the hazard ratio associated with a unit increase in X_1, controlling for all other factors. Thus, $\exp(\beta_1)$ is the adjusted hazard ratio associated with a one unit increase in X_1, and $\exp(5 \times \beta_1)$ is the adjusted hazard ratio associated with a five unit increase and so on. The examples in exhibit 10-2 for multiple logistic regression are applicable to the Cox model as well. Like multiple logistic regression, the Cox model is a multiplicative model based on maximum likelihood estimates.

References: Friedman, G. D. (2004). *Primer of Epidemiology*, 5th ed. New York: McGraw-Hill; Kelsey, J. L., Thompson, W. D., and Evans, A. S. (1986). *Methods in Observational Epidemiology*. New York: Oxford University Press; McNeil, D. (1996). *Epidemiological Research Methods*. Chichester: John Wiley & Sons; Morton, R. F., Hebel, J. R., and McCarter, R. J. (2001). *A Study Guide to Epidemiology and Biostatistics*, 5th ed. Gaithersburg, MD: Aspen Publishers, Inc.

study. Investigators examined the effect of stroke on the subsequent occurrence of dementia using a cohort design. They examined the incidence of dementia from baseline assessments among incident stroke patients (the exposed group) and non-stroke patients (the unexposed group). Using the Cox proportional hazards model, they found the relative risk (RR) of incident dementia associated with stroke was 3.83 (95% CI = 2.14 to 6.84) after adjusting simultaneously for various demographic variables and baseline mental measurements. Before adjustment the RR was 6.12 (95% CI = 3.57 to 10.50), suggesting that as a whole these factors positively confounded the association between stroke and dementia.[33] The Cox proportional hazards model may also be used to identify interactions by adding a product term (e.g., age by sex) to the regression equation. While RR is often reported in open cohort studies using the Cox model to assess confounding or interaction, the actual measure of association is known the **hazard ratio**, which is defined in exhibit 11-1.

Another common type of multiple regression analysis that may be used in open cohort studies to address confounding and interaction is **Poisson regression**. It is a multiple regression technique that is appropriate when the study outcome is dichotomous, and the independent variables are categorical.[25] It is best suited to open cohort studies where the study population is large, the outcome is rare, and person-time units are measured. The appropriate measure of association is the incidence density ratio.[34] As a brief example, consider a prospective cohort study that evaluated the independent and joint effects of parental atopy (a history of maternal or paternal asthma or allergic rhinitis) and exposure to molds on the occurrence of childhood asthma. The investigators used a Poisson regression to adjust for a number of potential confounders (i.e., age, sex, duration of breast-feeding, parents' highest education, single parent or guardian, maternal smoking during pregnancy, exposure to environmental tobacco smoke, gas cooking, presence of furry or feathery pets at home, and type of child care) and to examine possible interactions. They found that, after controlling for the confounding variables, parental atopy (adjusted IDR = 1.52; 95% CI = 1.08 to 2.13) and the presence of mold odor in the home (adjusted IDR = 2.44; 95% CI = 1.07 to 5.60) were independent determinants of asthma incidence in childhood. They did not find any evidence of interaction between these determinants using an additive model described elsewhere.[35]

Concluding Remarks

Confounding. Confounding occurs in a cohort study because the confounding variables are *unevenly distributed* between the exposed and unexposed groups and because of their particular relationship to both the study exposure and outcome. Identification and control of confounding are important since confounding represents a source of systematic error that can affect the internal validity of the study findings. Confounding can be identified by comparing the stratum-specific measures of association to the crude measure of association during stratification or by multivariable analysis. Assuming confounding exists, it can be controlled by pooling or standardization. The degree of confounding in a study can be determined by comparing the adjusted and crude measures of association. The greater they depart from each other, the greater the degree of confounding. A handy rule of thumb referred to in chapter 8 is applicable to all ratio measures of association (e.g., odds ratios, risk ratios, rate ratios). This rule of thumb states that a difference of more than 10 percent between the adjusted and crude ratio measures of association is indicative of confounding.[36, 37] Anything less suggests that confounding is either negligible or nonexistent. We can refer to this rule informally as the **10 percent rule**. The percent difference is determined as follows:

(11.26)   % Difference = $| [(MA_a - MA_c) / MA_a] | \times 100$

where $| |$ refers to the absolute value, MA_a is the adjusted ratio measure of association, and MA_c is the crude ratio measure of association. Using findings from problem 11-4 (steps 1 and 4), the percent differences are:

For the SIR: $| (1.92 - 1.99) / 1.92 | \times 100 = 3.65\%$
For the SRR: $| (2.14 - 1.99) / 2.14 | \times 100 = 7.01\%$

These results are *not* indicative of significant confounding since the percentages are not greater than 10 percent. This, of course, assumes that the potentially confounding factor (in this example stroke history) meets the criteria for confounding outlined in chapter 8 (i.e., independent risk factor for the outcome, associated with the study exposure, not an intermediate step in the causal chain).

Effect measure modification.   Effect measure modification or interaction can be assessed in a stratified analysis by again comparing the stratum-specific measures of association to the crude measure of association or tested using an appropriate multiple regression technique. However, testing for potential interactions is best done when the interactions have been hypothesized on an *a priori* versus an *a posteriori* basis.[38] As was done in chapter 10, we can assess effect measure modification (interaction) by comparing the observed and expected joint effects of the exposure and suspected effect modifier on the study outcome.[25] This is typically done in the context of multiple regression. With regard to multiplicative effects, the same formula used in chapter 10 for this assessment (formula 10.11) can be used by simply substituting risk or rate ratios for the odds ratios as appropriate. To assess additive effects, however, we should substitute the *risk or rate differences* for the odds ratios in formula 10.12 and *not* subtract one.[25] Risk and rate differences were discussed in chapter 6. For example, there is *no* evidence of additive effects for a risk difference (RD) when: Observed $RD_{E, M}$ = Expected $RD_{E, M}$ = Observed RD_E + Observed RD_M. When these equations are *not* equal, however, there is evidence of interaction, the degree to which depends on the size of the disparity.

INDUCTION AND LATENCY PERIODS

So far in this chapter it has been assumed that follow up for subjects in open or closed cohort studies begins immediately after assessment of subject eligibility and determination of exposure status and other personal characteristics at baseline. For many chronic diseases like cancer, however, immediate follow up of the exposed group can result in nondifferential misclassification with consequent bias of the measure of association toward the null value.[39] This can happen because subjects in the exposed group are not technically "at risk" of manifesting the outcome due to the study exposure until a sufficient *induction period* (chapter 3) has transpired. For example, consider an occupational cohort study of the relationship between exposure to trichloroethylene (TCE; an industrial cleaning solvent) and the incidence of liver cancer. A case of liver cancer that is diagnosed just two months after exposure to TCE is extremely unlikely to be due to this exposure because of what we know about the occurrence liver cancer. Liver cancer normally takes years to develop, and, therefore, liver cancer that occurs after only two months of follow up is almost certainly due to other causes, which likely began several years ago. A simple analogy may be helpful. Suppose you develop a foodborne illness about an hour after eating dinner. The illness is confirmed by laboratory testing to be salmonellosis. It is highly doubtful that your salmonellosis was caused by anything you ate at dinner, however, because the disease has an incubation period of six to 48 hours (average 12 to 24 hours). Therefore, it is more likely that the disease was contracted at an earlier meal, perhaps at breakfast or a meal during the previous day.

Theoretically, the relevant follow-up period for exposed subjects should correspond to the expected *latency period* (chapter 3) for the study outcome, based on the study exposure, since the exposed subjects are not considered at risk of manifesting the outcome until after the induction period has occurred. Conceptually, the induction period is the time it takes for the causative agents to initiate the disease process, and the latency period is the time it takes from disease initiation to disease manifestation or diagnosis. Thus, until the induction period has occurred, the exposed subjects are not at risk of manifesting the study outcome due to the study exposure. In other words, sufficient exposure time has not yet occurred. Figure 11-3 illustrates the follow-up time for a subject in the exposed group of a hypothetical cohort study. The subject is followed until she develops the study outcome. Note, however, that the relevant follow-up time for measurement purposes is that equivalent to the latency period since theoretically the subject was not at risk of exhibiting the outcome, due to the study exposure, during the induction period.

Several suggestions have been made for dealing with this issue.[30] One option is to begin follow up of the exposed group after a specified interim period thought to be consistent with the induction period based on the study exposure. Another option is to assume several possible induction periods and analyze and report the findings based on each assumption. Because it is

Figure 11-3   Hypothetical Induction and Latency Periods for an Exposed Subject

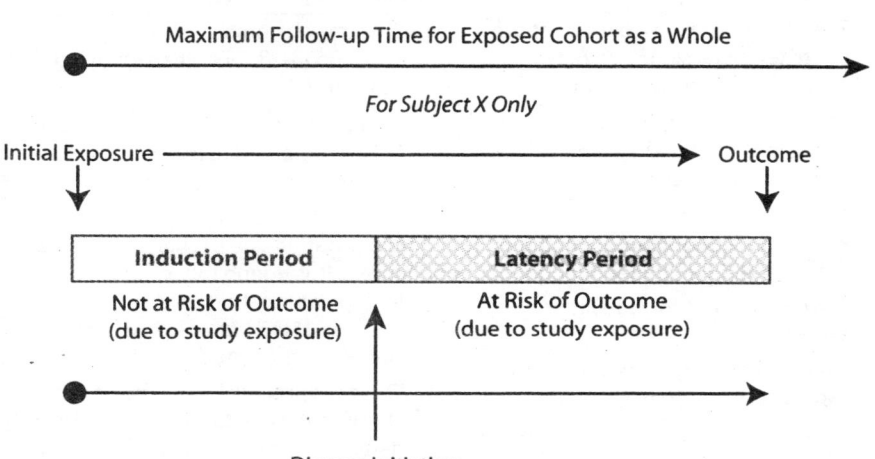

impossible to measure the induction period, the latter alternative may be a better option. It provides more information and may indicate which assumptions are the best since the measures of association should be larger the closer the assumptions are to reality.[26] That is, the more realistic the assumption, the less likely the measure of association is significantly biased toward the null value due to nondifferential misclassification.[39]

There is another wrinkle associated with this issue. What is to be done with the follow-up time (e.g., person-years) among the exposed subjects prior to the completion of the hypothesized induction period? Kenneth J. Rothman makes two suggestions: (a) ignore it, or (b) combine it with the follow-up time of the unexposed subjects.[3] Each option, of course, will lead to a different estimate of the measure of association. In the latter case, the theory is that this follow-up time represents unexposed time and therefore could be appropriately added to the follow-up time of the unexposed group.

ADVANTAGES AND DISADVANTAGES OF COHORT STUDIES

Table 11-3 summarizes the major advantages and disadvantages of cohort studies. While these advantages and disadvantages are meant to apply to cohort studies in general, some may be more applicable to prospective, and some to retrospective, cohort studies as indicated in the table. Mixed cohort studies will share the advantages and disadvantages of both types.

Table 11-3　Major Advantages and Disadvantages of Cohort Studies

Advantages	Disadvantages
1. They demonstrate a clear and appropriate temporal sequence between exposure and outcome status.	1. They may be time consuming, expensive, and inefficient when studying rare conditions.
2. They permit direct calculation of incidence measures and their derivative measures of association.	2. There is a greater potential for subject losses compared to other types of analytic studies.
3. They allow one to study multiple effects of a single exposure in the same study.	3. There is a potential for exposure misclassification due to changes in exposure status during follow up (prospective cohort studies) or or because of inadequate data (retrospective cohort studies).
4. They are suitable for studying rare exposures.	
5. They are not likely to be subject to exposure suspicion bias.	4. There is a potential for outcome misclassification due to advances in disease detection during the follow-up period.
6. They are helpful in establishing cause-effect relationships if properly conducted.	5. They may be subject to diagnostic suspicion bias.
	6. They may not be feasible when historical records are unavailable or unreliable (retrospective cohort studies).

Major Advantages

Well-designed cohort studies offer a number of advantages. First, they clearly demonstrate an appropriate temporal sequence between exposure and outcome status. Since exposure status is determined *first* and in a time period *preceding* assessment of outcome status, it is easier to ascribe the outcomes to exposure status than in study designs where the temporal sequence is more difficult to ascertain (e.g., cross-sectional studies). You will recall that it is essential for exposure to precede outcome in order to demonstrate causal associations (chapter 7). Of all the analytic studies discussed in this text, the cohort study best meets this criterion, all other factors being equal.

A second advantage of cohort studies is that they permit the direct calculation of incidence measures (i.e., cumulative incidence or incidence density) in both the exposed and unexposed groups. This makes it easy to derive risk or rate ratios (or differences) as appropriate. Third, cohort studies permit investigators to examine the multiple effects of a single exposure in the same study. Thus, one may look at the possible effects of hypertension, for example, on heart disease, stroke, and kidney disease in the same investigation. Fourth, they are suitable for studying rare exposures. Because exposure status is determined first, cohort studies can be designed to assure that there are an adequate number of exposed and unexposed subjects at the study outset even if a special exposure cohort must be used. This is not possible in case-control studies because exposure status is assessed after the subjects (cases and controls) have already been selected. Fifth, prospective cohort studies are unlikely to be subject to exposure suspicion bias, which can occur when knowledge of outcome status influences the assessment of exposure status (see chapter 8). This is not likely since exposure status is always assessed *before* outcome status. The same advantage exists in retrospective cohort studies provided they are conducted appropriately; that is, exposure status is determined before examining outcome status. Finally, well designed and executed cohort studies come closest to experimental studies in establishing cause-effect relationships. One reason is because in practice they tend to be less subject to bias than other analytic studies. Nevertheless, as pointed out in chapter 10, a well designed case-control study can produce results that are about as convincing as a well designed cohort study.

Major Disadvantages

One of the potential disadvantages of cohort studies is the time and expense that may be involved in following up large numbers of subjects over long periods of time. In prospective cohort studies of chronic diseases, for example, thousands or tens of thousands of people may need to be enrolled and followed for years or even decades to produce a sufficient number of outcomes for valid statistical comparisons. The Nurses' Health Study, for instance, established a cohort in 1976 consisting of 121,700 female registered nurses from 11 states. Periodic follow-up to assess current exposure and outcome status has been conducted every two years since that time.[40] When the outcome is particularly rare, such a study may be impractical in terms of the number of subjects and resources needed.

Another potential disadvantage of cohort studies is losses to follow up. Significant subject losses can reduce the precision of study findings, and if they are systematically different from the original cohort with respect to exposure *and* outcome status, they can introduce study bias (i.e., loss to follow-up bias). Loss to follow-up bias, a type of selection bias, was discussed in chapter 8. Losses can be a particular problem in prospective cohort studies when the follow-up time extends over many years. A similar issue arises in retrospective and mixed cohort studies when subjects cannot be found because of the long time between initial exposure and outcome. An additional disadvantage of cohort studies is potential exposure misclassification. This may occur, for example, in prospective cohort studies when subjects change their exposure status during the follow-up period. If the investigators do not take the changes into account, the study results could be inaccurate due to information bias (chapter 8). Therefore, periodic reassessments of those study exposures that can be modified by participants (e.g., cigarette smoking, dietary habits) are important in prospective cohort studies. Exposure misclassification can also be an issue in retrospective cohort studies since exposure is often determined from historical records that may be incomplete or inaccurate.

A further disadvantage of cohort studies is possible outcome misclassification. Advances in the ability to detect a particular disease during the course of follow up may bring prior classifications of outcome status into question and lead to inaccurate study results. Also, diagnostic suspicion bias (chapter 8) is possible in cohort studies to the extent that knowledge of a subject's exposure status influences the accuracy with which outcome status is determined. If the investigators are more likely to classify exposed subjects as having the study outcome than unexposed subjects, perhaps simply because they believe the exposure is related to the outcome, diagnostic suspicion bias will result.[41]

Finally, there is a disadvantage to the cohort design in that retrospective cohort studies cannot be conducted when historical data on exposure status (or, less likely, outcome status) is unavailable. This, unfortunately, is not an uncommon problem. In these instances, a prospective cohort study or some other study design may be feasible. Also, when the historical data are known to be unreliable it does not make much sense to proceed with a retrospective cohort study.

SUMMARY

- Cohort studies can be descriptive or analytic. Analytic cohort studies are of three basic types—prospective, retrospective, and mixed. In each type exposure status is assessed first, and outcome status is assessed later. Only the time periods in which the assessments take place differ.

- Cohort studies may be classified as open or closed. In open cohort studies subjects may enter or leave the cohort at any given time. In closed cohort studies new subjects cannot be entered once follow up begins. Conceptually, all subjects not developing the study outcome are observed for the entire follow-up period. This ideal is rarely achieved in practice, however, due to unavoidable losses.

- Cohort studies have at least three essential features—an exposed group, a comparison group, and a follow-up period. The exposed group is typically from a general cohort or a special exposure cohort. A general cohort is usually a general population or other broadly based group expected to have a relatively high frequency of exposed individuals, who serve as the exposed group. Those in the general cohort who are not exposed serve as the internal comparison group. Special exposure cohorts are exposed groups. They are used when the study exposure is uncommon. Special exposure cohorts require an external comparison group of unexposed but similar individuals. As a general rule, internal comparison groups provide better comparisons than external groups.

- Before follow up begins in a cohort study exposure status must be ascertained, and relevant baseline data must be collected. In addition, it should be determined that the subjects are actually at risk of the study outcome. Common means of collecting these data include questionnaires, interviews, existing medical or employment records, and examinations. Changes in exposure status during follow up also need to be addressed. In general, obtaining adequate information is easier in prospective versus retrospective cohort studies.

- The methods used to determine outcome status in cohort studies should be valid and reliable and applied equally to exposed and unexposed subjects. Common means of assessing outcome status include medical records, disease registries, death certificates, and diagnostic tests. In general, the task is more difficult in retrospective versus prospective cohort studies.

- Minimizing losses in cohort studies is very important. Studies with significant losses will be imprecise at best and possibly invalid if losses are related to exposure and outcome status. Strategies for minimizing losses include initial screening to evaluate compliance potential, maintaining current contact information, training staff, maintaining contact with participants, and offering modest incentives for initial and continuing participation.

- In general, the analysis of cohort studies begins with an overall or crude analysis. The standard measure of occurrence in closed cohort studies is cumulative incidence, and the applicable measure of association is the cumulative incidence ratio or difference. The odds ratio may also be used as a measure of association. The standard measure of association in open cohort studies is incidence density, and the applicable measure of association is the incidence density ratio or difference.

- The overall analysis should be followed by stratification, which can be used to evaluate confounding and effect measure modification. In closed cohort studies, adjusted measures of association commonly include the Mantel-Haenszel risk ratio or risk difference when effect measure modification is absent and the standardized risk ratio, risk difference, or odds ratio when effect measure modification is present. In open cohort studies, some analogous measures are the Mantel-Haenszel incidence density ratio or difference and the standardized incidence ratio (or standardized mortality ratio) and the standardized rate ratio, respectively.

- Multivariable analysis can also be used to assess confounding and interaction and is generally more efficient than stratification. Nevertheless, it is best conceived as a supplement to a stratified analysis, which tends to provide a clearer picture of the data. In closed cohort studies multiple logistic regression is the most frequently used method of multivariable analysis. In open cohort studies the Cox proportional hazards method or other methods associated with survival analysis are more common procedures.

- In general, if confounding is present, its magnitude can be determined by comparing the adjusted and crude measures of association. The greater they depart from each other, the greater the confounding. A 10 percent difference is often used as a threshold. Testing for effect measure modification is best done when the interactions have been hypothesized on an *a priori* basis.

- In following up subjects in a cohort study involving a chronic disorder consideration should be given to the induction and latency periods. With diseases like cancer subjects may not technically be at risk of manifesting the outcome until the induction period is completed. Therefore, the appropriate follow-up period for the exposed group is the length of the latency period. Several suggestions have been made to deal with this issue.

- Cohort studies have several advantages and disadvantages. Some of the advantages include a clear temporal sequence between exposure and outcome status, an opportunity to calculate incidence-based measures, suitability for studying rare exposures, and support for establishing cause-effect relationships. Disadvantages include the substantial time commitments and expenses to study certain outcomes, the potential for significant losses to follow up, and the possibility of exposure misclassification and diagnostic suspicion bias.

New Terms

- ambidirectional cohort study
- ambispective cohort study
- baseline data
- closed cohort study
- cohort
- concurrent cohort study
- Cox proportional hazards model
- descriptive cohort study
- dynamic cohort study
- external comparison group
- fixed cohort study
- general cohort
- hazard ratio
- historical cohort study
- internal comparison group
- Mantel-Haenszel incidence density difference
- Mantel-Haenszel incidence density ratio
- Mantel-Haenszel incidence rate difference

- Mantel-Haenszel incidence rate ratio
- Mantel-Haenszel rate difference
- Mantel-Haenszel rate ratio
- Mantel-Haenszel risk difference
- Mantel-Haenszel risk ratio
- mixed cohort study
- nonconcurrent cohort study
- open cohort study
- person-time chi-square test
- Poisson regression
- special exposure cohort
- standardization
- standardized incidence ratio
- standardized odds ratio
- standardized rate ratio
- standardized risk difference
- standardized risk ratio
- 10 percent rule

Study Questions and Exercises

1. Describe how you would design a valid prospective cohort study to test the hypothesis that cigarette smoking during pregnancy increases the risk of Sudden Infant Death Syndrome (SIDS). Include in your description how you would select the cohort, how you would assess exposure and outcome status, and how you would analyze the data. Also indicate how you would evaluate potential confounding and effect measure modification in the study.

2. In January 2007, epidemiologists with the Frantrac Research Institute in Copenhagen were contracted by the Denmark Chemical Manufacturers Association to study the possible relationship between XG-47, an industrial solvent, and liver cancer. The epidemiologists collected the work records of all those who had been employed from 1975 to 1985 at the only plant using XG-47 to establish exposure levels and demographic profiles of the workers. Next, the epidemiologists conducted an extensive search to see what happened to the identified employees. This included an examination of the national cancer registry in Denmark to determine which workers had contracted liver cancer. There were a total of 345 workers, 145 of whom were exposed to XG-47. There were 12 cases of liver cancer among the exposed group, and 19 cases of liver cancer altogether. Based on this information, answer the following questions: (a) what type of study is represented here and why, (b) what is the applicable overall measure of association, and (c) what is the value of the applicable measure of association and its 95 percent confidence interval? Based on your findings, what would you conclude about the relationship between XG-47 and liver cancer, assuming no significant sources of bias or confounding in the study?

3. A prospective cohort study of the effect of alcohol consumption on gall bladder disease was designed to follow a group of 400 healthy men over a five-year period. The men were tested for the presence of gall bladder disease at the end of each year during the follow-up period. Only new cases of gall bladder disease were recorded at each annual assessment. The results of the study were as follows:

Among the 200 drinkers:
10 subjects were positive for gall bladder disease in year three.
15 subjects were positive for gall bladder disease in year five.

Among the 200 nondrinkers:
6 subjects were positive for gall bladder disease in year two.
4 subjects were positive for gall bladder disease in year three.

Based on these data, calculate the crude incidence density ratio for gall bladder disease in this group and its 95 percent confidence interval. Interpret your results.

4. Indicate whether each of the following statements is true or false (T or F). For each false statement, indicate why it is false.

___ a. If the results of a well conducted closed cohort study showed a crude cumulative incidence ratio of 3.5 and an RR_{MH} of 6.3, one would be correct in concluding that effect measure modification is present.

___ b. Exposure suspicion bias is common in prospective cohort studies.

___ c. Death certificates tend to be relatively unreliable sources for determining specific causes of death in retrospective cohort studies.

___ d. External comparison groups are always preferable to internal comparison groups in cohort studies.

___ e. A potential source of error in closed cohort studies is loss to follow-up bias.

___ f. By design, subjects not developing the study outcome in a closed cohort study should be followed for the entire length of the follow-up period.

___ g. In terms of external comparison groups in cohort studies, general populations tend to be a better choice than separate unexposed groups.

___ h. Compared to pooling, standardization is a more precise method of adjusting for confounding in a cohort study.

___ i. Multivariable analysis is preferred over stratification as a method of assessing confounding and effect measure modification in an open cohort study.

___ j. Matching is rarely used in cohort studies; however, when used, it still allows one to evaluate the role of the matched variables on the study outcome and to assess their role as possible effect modifiers.

References

1. Grubman, S., Gross, E., Lerner-Weiss, N., Hernandez, M., McSherry, G. D., Hoyt, L. G., Boland, M., and Oleske, J. M. (1995). Older Children and Adolescents Living with Perinatally Acquired Human Immunodeficiency Virus Infection. *Pediatrics* 95 (5): 657–663.

2. Last, J. M., ed. (2001). *A Dictionary of Epidemiology*, 4th ed. New York: Oxford University Press.

3. Rothman, K. J. (2002). *Epidemiology: An Introduction*. New York: Oxford University Press.

4. Elliot, L., Heederik, D., Marshall, S., Peden, D., and Lewis, D. (2005). Incidence of Allergy and Allergy Symptoms Among Workers Exposed to Laboratory Animals. *Occupational and Environmental Medicine* 62 (11): 766–771.

5. Newman, S. C. (2001). *Biostatistical Methods in Epidemiology*. New York: John Wiley & Sons, Inc.

6. Walker, A. M. (1991). *Observation and Inference: An Introduction to the Methods of Epidemiology*. Chestnut Hill, MA.: Epidemiology Resources Inc.

7. Cologne, J. B., and Preston, D. L. (2000). Longevity of Atomic Bomb Survivors. *The Lancet* 356 (9226): 303–307.

8. Trautner, C., Icks, A., Haastert, B., Plum, F., Berger, M., and Giani, G. (1996). Diabetes as a Predictor of Mortality in a Cohort of Blind Subjects. *International Journal of Epidemiology* 25 (5): 1038–1043.

9. The Nurses' Health Study: History (No date). Available: http://www.channing.harvard.edu/nhs/history/index.shtml (Access date: March 28, 2006).

10. Hennekens, C. H., and Buring, J. E. (1987). *Epidemiology in Medicine*. Boston: Little, Brown and Company.
11. Chasan-Taber, L., Willett, W. C., Seddon, J. M., Stampfer, M. J., Rosner, B., Colditz, G. A., Speizer, F. E., and Hankinson, S. E. (2000). A Prospective Study of Alcohol Consumption and Cataract Extraction Among U.S. Women. *Annals of Epidemiology* 10 (6): 347–353.
12. Cooper, W. O., Hickson, G. B., Mitchel, E. F., Jr., Edwards, K. M., Thapa, P. B., and Ray, W. A. (1999). Early Childhood Mortality from Community-acquired Infections. *American Journal of Epidemiology* 150 (5): 517–527.
13. Kelsey, J. L., Thompson, W. D., and Evans, A. S. (1986). *Methods in Observational Epidemiology*. New York: Oxford University Press.
14. Southern Community Cohort Study: An Introduction to the Southern Community Cohort Study (No date). Available: http://www.southerncommunitystudy.org/about.html (Access date: March 22, 2006).
15. The National Children's Study: What is the National Children's Study? (2005). Available: http://www.nationalchildrensstudy.gov/about/mission/overview.cfm (Access date: March 22, 2006).
16. Rimm, E. B., Stampfer, M. J., Colditz, G. A., Giovannucci, E., and Willett, W. C. (1990). Effectiveness of Various Mailing Strategies Among Nonrespondents in a Prospective Cohort Study. *American Journal of Epidemiology* 131 (6): 1068–1071.
17. Hunt, J. R., and White, E. (1998). Retaining and Tracking Cohort Study Members. *Epidemiologic Reviews* 20 (1): 57–70.
18. Doody, M. M., Sigurdson, A. S., Kampa, D., Chimes, K., Alexander, B. H., Ron, E., Tarone, R. E., and Linet, M. S. (2003). Randomized Trial of Financial Incentives and Delivery Methods for Improving Response to a Mailed Questionnaire. *American Journal of Epidemiology* 157 (7): 643–651.
19. Pierce, B., and Hartford, P. (2004). White Paper on Recruitment and Retention for the National Children's Study. Available: http://nationalchildrensstudy.gov/events/advisory_committee/AppendixG.pdf (Access date: April 6, 2006).
20. Institute of Child Health (2004). Children of the New Century. Available: http://www.ich.ucl.ac.uk/publications/research_review03/48population1.html (Access date: April 6, 2006).
21. Katz, D., Baptista, J., Azen, S. P., and Pike, M. C. (1978). Obtaining Confidence Intervals for the Risk Ratio in Cohort Studies. *Biometrics* 34: 469–474.
22. Ahlbom, A. (1993). *Biostatistics for Epidemiologists*. Boca Raton: Lewis Publishers.
23. Ferguson, G. A. (1976). *Statistical Analysis in Psychology and Education*, 4th ed. New York: McGraw-Hill Book Company.
24. Elwood, M. (1998). *Critical Appraisal of Epidemiological Studies and Clinical Trials*, 2nd ed. Oxford: Oxford University Press.
25. Szklo, M., and Nieto, F. J. (2000). *Epidemiology: Beyond the Basics*. Gaithersburg, MD: Aspen.
26. Rothman, K. J. (1986). *Modern Epidemiology*. Boston: Little, Brown and Company.
27. MacMahon, B., and Trichopoulos, D. (1996). *Epidemiology: Principles and Methods*, 2nd ed. Boston: Little, Brown and Company.
28. Campbell, U. B., Gatto, N. M., and Schwartz, S. (2005). Distributional Interaction: Interpretational Problems When Using Incidence Odds Ratios to Assess Interaction. *Epidemiologic Perspectives & Innovations* 2. Available: http://www.epi-perspectives.com/content/2/1/1 (Access date: February 28, 2006).
29. Kleinbaum, D. G., Kupper, L. L., and Morgenstern, H. (1982). *Epidemiologic Research: Principles and Quantitative Methods*. Belmont, CA: Lifetime Learning Publications.
30. Checkoway, H., Pearce, N., and Crawford-Brown, D. J. (1989). *Research Methods in Occupational Epidemiology*. New York: Oxford University Press.
31. Normand, S-L. T., Sykora, K., Li, P., Mamdani, M., Rochon, P. A., and Anderson, G. M. (2005). Readers Guide to Critical Appraisal of Cohort Studies: 3. Analytical Strategies to Reduce Confounding. *British Medical Journal* 330: 1021–1023.
32. Morton, R. F., Hebel, J. R., and McCarter, R. J. (2001). *A Study Guide to Epidemiology and Biostatistics*, 5th ed. Gaithersburg, MD: Aspen Publishers, Inc.

33. Desmond, D. W., Moroney, J. T., Sano, M., and Stern, Y. (2002). Incidence of Dementia After Ischemic Stroke: Results of a Longitudinal Study. *Stroke* 33: 2254–2260.
34. McNeil, D. (1996). *Epidemiological Research Methods*. New York: John Wiley & Sons.
35. Jaakkola, J. J. K., Hwang, B-F., Jaakkola, N. (2005). Home Dampness and Molds, Parental Atopy, and Asthma in Childhood: A Six-Year Population-Based Cohort Study. *Environmental Health Perspectives* 113 (3): 357–361.
36. Sonis, J. (1998). A Closer Look at Confounding. *Family Medicine* 30 (8): 584–588.
37. Maldonado, G., and Greenland, S. (1993). Simulation Study of Confounder-selection Strategies. *American Journal of Epidemiology* 138: 923–936.
38. Altman, D. G., and Matthews, J. N. S. (1996). Statistics Notes: Interaction 1: Heterogeneity of Effects. *British Medical Journal* 313: 486.
39. Rothman, K. J. (1981). Induction and Latent Periods. *American Journal of Epidemiology* 114 (2): 253–259.
40. Rim, E. B., Manson, J. E., Stampfer, M. J., Colditz, G. A., Willett, W. C., Rosner, B., Hennekens, C. H., and Speizer, F. E. (1993). Cigarette Smoking and the Risk of Diabetes in Women. *American Journal of Public Health* 83 (2): 211–214.
41. Sackett, D. L. (1979). Bias in Analytic Research. *Journal of Chronic Diseases* 32: 51–63.

CHAPTER TWELVE

Experimental and Quasi-Experimental Studies

*This chapter covers important aspects of the design, analysis,
and interpretation of randomized controlled trials,
group randomized trials, and quasi-experimental studies.*

Learning Objectives

- Describe the essential differences among randomized controlled trials, group randomized trials, quasi-experimental studies (quasi-experiments), and natural experiments, respectively.
- Compare and contrast efficacy trials and effectiveness trials.
- Summarize the major steps in designing and conducting a randomized controlled trial, including the purpose of each step.
- Calculate the minimum sample size required for a randomized controlled trial based on the expected difference between the proportions of outcomes in the experimental and control groups for specified parameters.
- Explain the significance of randomization and describe the major methods of randomization used in randomized controlled trials along with the objectives of each method.
- Identify the specific types of blinding (masking) and respective benefits in randomized controlled trials.
- Compare the various design options commonly used in randomized controlled trials, including their advantages and disadvantages.
- List some common reasons for noncompliance (nonadherence) in randomized controlled trials as well as some practical ways of increasing and assessing compliance (adherence) in a trial.
- Compare and contrast intention-to-treat and per protocol analysis, including the advantages and disadvantages of each method.
- Analyze and interpret the findings of randomized controlled trials using incidence density as the measure of effect.
- Assess the strengths and weaknesses of subgroup analyses in randomized controlled trials.

371

- Discuss the purpose, use, and strengths and weaknesses of meta-analysis.
- Describe the basic statistical approaches to meta-analysis and the common methods for assessing and dealing with statistical heterogeneity.
- Explain the major advantages and disadvantages of randomized controlled trials.
- Describe three common reasons for conducting group randomized trials.
- Summarize the major methodological issues in the conduct of group randomized trials, including the clustering effect.
- Calculate and interpret the effective sample size of a given group randomized trial.
- Describe the basic approaches to analyzing the findings of group randomized trials, including the types of models commonly used.
- Distinguish among the major design variations in group randomized trials.
- Compare the ethical principles applicable to randomized controlled trials with those applicable to group randomized trials.
- Describe the most common before and after and time-series designs used in quasi-experimental studies, including their respective strengths and weaknesses.
- Define active treatment, arm, carryover effects, clinical heterogeneity or diversity, Cochrane Collaboration, community trial, contamination, covariate, crossovers, cumulative meta-analysis, data and safety monitoring board or committee, Declaration of Helsinki, design effect, effect size, efficacy analysis, eligibility criteria, endpoints, equipoise, exclusion criteria, forest plot, futility, Hawthorne effect, hierarchical modeling, homogenous, I^2, inactive treatment, inclusion criteria, informed consent, institutional review board, intervention study, intraclass (or intracluster) correlation coefficient, Mantel-Haenszel method, maturation, methodological heterogeneity or diversity, multilevel modeling, narrative review, overview, Peto method, placebo, placebo effect, placebo-controlled trial, primary prevention trial, prognostic factor, prospective meta-analysis, publication bias, qualitative systematic review, quantitative systematic review, recruitment, recruitment period, regression to the mean, research ethics committee, restricted randomization, rho, run-in period, secondary prevention trial, sensitivity analysis, sham procedure, stopping rules, study protocol, systematic review, variance inflation factor, washout period.

INTRODUCTION

Unlike descriptive and analytic studies, *experimental studies* are those in which the conditions of the study are controlled directly by the investigators.[1] Most importantly, the investigators control the exposure status of the subjects. In fact, experimental studies in epidemiology are often referred to as **intervention studies** since the investigators "intervene" into the lives of their subjects by manipulating their exposure status. In observational studies, no such intervention occurs. Investigators simply observe and record subject status regarding inherent or acquired exposures of interest.

As discussed in chapter 4, there are two major types of experimental studies in epidemiology. These are *randomized controlled trials* and *group randomized trials*. Synonyms for these terms appear in table 4-2. A major difference between these two types has to do with who is randomized. In randomized controlled trials *individuals* are randomly allocated to experimental and control groups, while in group randomized trials *groups of individuals* are randomly assigned. In randomized controlled trials there may be one or more experimental groups and one or more control groups in any given study. In the simplest design, a single experimental group is given a potentially promising but unproven intervention (i.e., a novel treatment, procedure, program, or service), while a single control group is subject to an alternative strategy (e.g., the standard treatment, procedure, program, or service) or no intervention at all. In group randomized trials multiple groups are typically assigned to intervention or control conditions.

In addition to experimental studies, there are related studies in epidemiology known as *quasi-experimental studies*. These were discussed briefly in chapter 4 and consist of studies in which the investigators do not have full control over the over the assignment or timing of the intervention but where the studies are still conducted as if they were experiments.[1] They are nonrandomized trials and are discussed later in the chapter. Another related type of study is the *natural experiment*, which was referred to in chapter 4. A natural experiment is an *unplanned* situation in nature where the levels of exposure to an assumed causal factor differ among subgroups in a population in a way that is relatively unaffected by extraneous factors so that the situation resembles a planned experiment.[1] This was the case in John Snow's 19th-century investigation of cholera deaths. A natural experiment existed due to the almost random fashion in which drinking water was supplied to area homes by two rival water companies (see chapter 2). Another example has to do with the conditions produced by the Chernobyl nuclear power plant disaster in the former Soviet Union. This created an unplanned opportunity to study the health effects of radiation exposure on populations according to the distance from the disaster site. Natural experiments are not true experiments because there is no planned intervention nor any randomization of subjects. In fact, they are observational studies masquerading as experimental studies (see chapter 4). Because they are relatively rare, natural experiments are not discussed further.

This chapter focuses on key design features of experimental and quasi-experimental studies in epidemiology. Basic approaches to the analysis and interpretation of findings from experimental studies are also described.

RANDOMIZED CONTROLLED TRIALS

A randomized controlled trial (RCT) is a planned epidemiologic experiment where individual subjects are randomly assigned to one or more experimental or control groups to assess the effects of a preventive or therapeutic treatment, procedure, or other type of intervention.[1] Randomized controlled trials are frequently referred to as the *gold standard* (defined in chapter 1) of epidemiologic studies.[2] This is because when they are well designed and conducted they provide the strongest possible evidence of causation that epidemiologic studies can deliver. This is due to the tightly controlled conditions of the experiment and the randomization of the subjects, which tend to preclude other possible explanations for the findings. When properly executed, RCTs can be replicated by other investigators who use the same **study protocol** (i.e., detailed written plan and procedures for the trial).

One of the early forerunners of the RCT was a study by Johannes Fibiger in a Copenhagen hospital in 1898.[2] In this study, diphtheria patients were assigned to two groups based on day of admission. The purpose was to test the *efficacy* (defined in chapter 1; also see exhibit 12-1) of serum injection compared to traditional treatment for the disease. While the assignment to experimental and control groups was not truly random, the design represents a *clinical trial* (chapter 4) that has many of the hallmarks of an RCT. It was not until the middle of the 20th century, however, that RCTs became established in the United States. A classic example is the large-scale polio vaccine field trials conducted in 1954. These studies demonstrated that the polio vaccine was highly effective in preventing poliomyelitis.[3] A more recent example is a study of the effect of pravastatin (a cholesterol-lowering drug) in reducing the risk of stroke.[4] As part of the findings, the authors reported that among heart patients pravastatin therapy reduced the risk of nonhemorrhagic stroke by 23 percent when compared to controls who were given a **placebo**, a similar appearing but pharmacologically inactive substance (i.e., in common parlance, a "sugar pill," though it may or may not contain any sugar).

As described in chapter 4, RCTs can be grouped into two basic categories—*preventive* (or *prevention*) *trials* and *therapeutic trials*. Preventive trials can be further classified as **primary prevention trials** or **secondary prevention trials**. The former focus on individuals in the stage of susceptibility, whereas the latter

---

Exhibit 12-1
Efficacy and Effectiveness in Randomized Controlled Trials

In the language of randomized controlled trials (RCTs), the terms *efficacy* and *effectiveness* have different meanings. *Efficacy* is a measure of the extent to which an intervention is beneficial under ideal conditions. *Effectiveness*, on the other hand, is a measure of the degree to which an intervention is beneficial under ordinary, real life situations. *Efficacy trials* (those that focus on measuring efficacy) seek to answer the question: Does the intervention work among those who accept it? In contrast, *effectiveness trials* (those that focus on measuring effectiveness) deal with the question: Does the intervention work among those to whom it is offered? It is helpful to think of efficacy and effectiveness trials as representing opposite ends of a spectrum of RCTs. The trials lying between these ends have more or less of the characteristics of an efficacy or effectiveness trial depending on where they are situated on the spectrum.

Efficacy Trial ◄─────────────────────────────► *Effectiveness Trial*

Differences in efficacy and effectiveness trials are reflected in their design, conduct, and analysis. Efficacy trials tend to be more tightly controlled than effectiveness trials. For example, they tend to have more restrictive eligibility requirements. The objective is to avoid, to the extent possible, enrolling subjects who could compromise the internal validity of the findings, for instance, due to the presence of "co-interventions" or noncompliance with the study protocol. Thus, investigators of efficacy trials are willing to sacrifice some of the external validity of the study in order to preserve its internal validity. In addition, the analysis of efficacy trials focuses on subjects who have been compliant with the study protocol, although the goal is to achieve high enough levels of compliance where this is not an issue. Effectiveness trials, on the other hand, place less emphasis on these matters since the main objective is to determine if the intervention is likely to work in real world situations where some members of a more diverse group will, for example, not comply with recommended practices or choose to use other "interventions." A finding of effectiveness should mean that the intervention is expected to be successful when applied in non-experimental settings. Generally speaking, maintaining external validity is more important to investigators involved with effectiveness trials than with efficacy trials. In terms of analysis, effectiveness trials generally use an *intention-to-treat analysis* (defined in the chapter), which does not take into consideration the extent of compliance with the intervention. Essentially, everyone gets counted.

Although it is not essential, it is generally recommended that the efficacy of an intervention be established before conducting studies of its effectiveness. If the findings from an effectiveness trial indicate that the intervention is not effective, it may be because it is not efficacious, it is not acceptable to the participants, or a combination of the two. It therefore makes logical sense to establish efficacy before attempting to determine effectiveness. It should also be kept in mind that an intervention that is efficacious in an epidemiologic experiment may not be effective in the real world. For example, an efficacy trial may show that selected heart patients who follow a strict low-fat and cholesterol diet and perform vigorous daily exercise are less likely to suffer a second myocardial infarction (MI) compared to a control group. Life-long adherence to this regimen, however, by a more diverse group of heart patients may prove much more difficult outside the experimental setting, leading to less desirable outcomes than expected. In other words, an efficacious intervention may not be very effective in ordinary circumstances.

There is another sense in which it is helpful to differentiate between efficacy and effectiveness. This has to do with the extent of compliance in an RCT. As in real life, complex, rigorous, or long-term regimens may be difficult to follow even in the context of an experiment. Therefore, many investigators who intend to measure the efficacy of an experimental intervention may in fact end up measuring its effectiveness because of high levels of noncompliance or significant withdrawals from the study. The present chapter focuses primarily on design and analysis issues that are most appropriate for efficacy trials.

References: Fletcher, R. H., Fletcher, S. W., and Wagner, E. H. (1988). *Clinical Epidemiology: The Essentials*, 2nd ed. Baltimore: Williams & Wilkins; Jadad, A. R. (1998). *Randomised Controlled Trials: A User's Guide*. London: BMJ Books; Pittler, M. H., and White, A. R. (1999). Efficacy and Effectiveness. *Focus on Alternative and Complementary Therapies* 4 (3): 109–110; Streiner, D. L. (2002). The 2 "Es" of Research: Efficacy and Effectiveness Trials. *Canadian Journal of Psychiatry* 47: 552–556.

focus on those in the stage of presymptomatic disease (see chapter 3). Primary prevention trials seek to test modes of preventing study outcomes *before* they develop (e.g., trials of the effect of vitamin supplementation on disease prevention in healthy volunteers). Secondary prevention trials typically seek to test methods that might impede the development of the study outcome in *high risk* individuals (e.g., trials of the effect of behavioral modification in reducing the risk of type 2 diabetes among pre-diabetic individuals). The polio vaccine field trials referred to in the previous paragraph represent primary prevention trials, while the study of pravastatin in heart patients represents a secondary prevention trial. Its focus is on prevention of stroke in high risk individuals (e.g., heart patients). Therapeutic trials seek to test ways of reducing suffering, recurrences, or death in patients with the *existing* study disease (e.g., trials of the effect of specific therapies on the survival of cancer patients). Therapeutic trials are often referred to as clinical trials, although not all clinical trials involve randomization (see chapter 4). Another example of a therapeutic trial is a study of the effect of an investigational drug in relieving joint pain in patients with rheumatoid arthritis. The focus of therapeutic trials is *tertiary prevention* (chapter 3).

While each type of RCT has a specific aim (primary, secondary, or tertiary prevention), the basic study design is the same. One of the first steps in planning an RCT is to develop the *primary research hypothesis*, which is the major question the investigators seek to answer. There may also be secondary hypotheses. This is followed by such steps as selecting the study population, determining sample size requirements, collecting baseline data on the subjects, randomly allocating the subjects into experimental and control groups, applying the intervention, and assessing the study outcomes during a follow-up period. These and other considerations, such as ethical policies, should be part of the study protocol, which was referred to earlier.

In terms of ethics, in the United States, all federally funded research on human subjects must first be approved by the appropriate **institutional review board** (IRB). Many institutions, such as universities and medical centers, also require non-federally funded research on human subjects to go through the same process. The IRB is a standing committee within the sponsoring institution that reviews research protocols using ethical guidelines designed to protect the safety and well-being of the study participants.[1] Although the intensity of review differs based on the nature of the research, the IRB rules apply to all research on human subjects whether it is experimental, quasi-experimental, or observational. In other countries, the equivalent review bodies are often referred to as **research ethics committees** or similar names.[1, 5]

Selecting the Study Population

As indicated in chapter 4, selecting the study population for an RCT begins with the selection of a source population from which volunteers meeting the study eligibility requirements are recruited. The source population for a study of the efficacy of a new treatment for cervical cancer, for example, will be restricted at a minimum to women with cervical cancer, since men cannot contract the disease. Other restrictions, such as age, race, geographical location, and stage of cancer, may also be applied especially if they are believed to be important factors that may affect the outcome of the trial. The most important consideration in identifying the source population, however, is its ability to produce valid results for the hypothesis being tested. Therefore, it must be large enough to be likely to produce enough **endpoints** (study outcomes) so as to permit accurate statistical comparisons between the experimental and control groups.[6]

The study population will be more restrictive than the source population to enhance compliance with the study protocol and improve the accuracy of the data collected. Generating the study population involves enrolling members of the source population into the study. These must be individuals who are fully informed and willing to participate in the trial and who meet other predetermined qualifications. This enrollment process is known as **recruitment**, and the time during which it takes place is the **recruitment period**. By fully informed and willing participants we mean those who have given **informed consent**, that is, those who have agreed voluntarily to take part in the trial after receiving an adequate explanation of its purpose, methods and procedures, and the potential risks and benefits of participation.[7] In RCTs informed consent is typically sought in writing, and the method must be approved by the IRB or equivalent oversight body.

The predetermined qualifications for entry into an RCT are termed **eligibility criteria**. These are based on the study objectives and should guide the identification of the source population as well as the selection of the study population. The eligibility criteria define who is to be included in the study (**inclusion criteria**) as well as who is to be excluded from the study (**exclusion criteria**). The purpose of the eligibility criteria is to optimize the conditions for successful testing of the effects of the intervention. The inclusion criteria are usually based on demographic, geographic, medical, or temporal characteristics with the goal of optimizing the testing of the primary research hypothesis.[8] The exclusion criteria have to do with subject characteristics that may affect the validity of the study findings and with ethical issues related to questionable benefits or potential risks to individuals if they were included in the study. For example, a therapeutic drug trial may exclude severely ill patients who are unlikely to complete the study due to their illness and whose inclusion would therefore threaten the study's internal validity. Similarly, such a trial may exclude those currently taking medications known to interfere with the effectiveness of study drug, thereby decreasing any potential benefits to participation in the study.

In general, the eligibility criteria for an RCT should involve due regard for the study objectives, the possible effects on the internal and external validity of the study, the potential benefits or risks to the subjects, and factors related to practicality and efficiency. To illustrate the application of eligibility criteria, consider an RCT that was conducted at a hospital in Philadelphia.[9] The study was designed to evaluate the efficacy of lithium in treating aggressive behavior in children and adolescents. This study employed the following *inclusion criteria*: male and female patients, 10–17 years of age, residing in an acute-care child and adolescent psychiatric inpatient ward of a teaching hospital with a history of severe aggressive behavior and a diagnosis of conduct disorder. The *exclusion criteria* included mental retardation, pervasive developmental disorder, recent substance dependence, and a number of other psychiatric disorders, in addition to pregnancy, certain major medical problems, recent prescriptions for psychoactive drugs, and previous inclusion in a lithium trial. As you can see from this example, the eligibility criteria were very restrictive due to a number of considerations, including the study objective (e.g., includes only 10–17 year olds), convenience (e.g., includes only patients in a given hospital), threats to internal validity (e.g., excludes groups that may present compliance problems), and risks to the subjects (e.g., excludes pregnant adolescents and those with certain medical conditions). Table 12-1 summarizes some of the more common eligibility criteria that may be employed

---

Table 12-1   Eligibility Criteria Commonly Used in Randomized Controlled Trials

Reasons for Inclusion	Reasons for Exclusion
• **Certain age, sex, or racial/ethnic characteristics** (e.g., African-American men, 60–79 years, for a study with an outcome of stroke—provides a high risk group likely to produce sufficient endpoints for analysis)	• **Potential harm to participants** (e.g., patients with a previous history of hemorrhagic stroke for a study of a blood-thinning medication on memory improvement—may initiate another stroke)
• **Absence of certain diseases or conditions** (e.g., persons free of heart disease in a study of the efficacy of dietary management in preventing coronary heart disease—prevents erroneous results)	• **Intervention unlikely to be effective** (e.g., persons with a previous episode of mumps for a preventive trial of a new vaccine for mumps—mumps confers lifelong immunity)
• **Not currently receiving the proposed intervention** (e.g., persons not currently taking vitamin C in a study of vitamin C and colds—prevents possible inflation of the magnitude of the effect)	• **Potential for poor compliance with the study protocol** (e.g., persons with drug or alcohol addiction—less likely to comply with the intervention in a study of the efficacy of meditation in treating anxiety)
• **Located in certain communities, hospitals, or clinics** (e.g., patients at ABC Community Hospital—convenient for investigators)	• **Practical difficulties with participation** (e.g., persons with certain mental disabilities—might result in inaccurate responses to study questions)
• **Meets eligibility criteria during certain time periods** (e.g., meets eligibility criteria between June 1 and December 31 of a given year—the period of initial recruitment)	• **Do not meet the inclusion criteria** (i.e., all who do not meet the inclusion criteria for a study are automatically excluded from the study)

Reference: Hulley, S. B., Cummings, S. R., Browner, W. S., Grady, D., Hearst, N., and Newman, T. B. (2001). *Designing Clinical Research*, 2nd ed. Philadelphia: Lippincott Williams & Wilkins.

in RCTs. In general, the eligibility criteria become more specific as one moves from the source to the study population. This may affect the external validity of a trial, but it will not affect its internal validity as long as the restrictions are applied equally to the experimental and control groups.

Determining Sample Size Requirements

Since many in the source population of an RCT may be ineligible or unwilling to participate in the study, the size of the study population is often substantially smaller than that of the source population. Small sample size can present serious concerns in RCTs because of low power. As a consequence, small but clinically significant differences may go undetected. The solution to this problem is to determine the minimum sample size required to detect what is considered a clinically significant value for the desired measure of association *before* an RCT is initiated. In fact, this is critical. There have been too many trials where this advice has been ignored, resulting in inconclusive findings. Curtis L. Meinert, for example, states that some of these studies may be considered "unethical in that they require patients to accept the risks of treatment, however small, without any chance of benefit to them or future patients."[7(p74)] If an RCT has such low power that investigators are unlikely to detect clinically significant differences between the experimental and control groups when they exist, it has little chance of influencing medical or public health policies for the better.

There are several ways to determine the minimum sample size required to detect a predetermined effect. In general, sample size determination is based on addressing the primary research hypothesis. Formula 12.1 provides one method of estimating the minimum sample size requirements for RCTs when the study results are measured as the difference between the proportions of outcomes (e.g., disease, death, recovery) in the experimental and control groups.[10] This formula applies, however, *only* if the following conditions are met: (a) there are only two groups to be compared (i.e., an experimental and control group), and (b) the two groups are designed to be equal in size. In addition, it is assumed that the following parameters apply: p-value = 0.05, beta = 0.10, and power = 90%.[10]

(12.1)
$$n = \frac{P_C(1 - P_C) + P_E(1 - P_E)}{(P_E - P_C)^2} \times 10.5$$

The n in formula 12.1 refers to the number of subjects required in *each* group (experimental and control). P_C is the proportion of outcomes *expected* in the control group, and P_E is the proportion of outcomes *expected* in the experimental group. The difference $P_E - P_C$ is known as the **effect size**, which can be defined as the size of the difference one would like to be able to detect if it exists.[10] Ideally, the effect size should be based on practical or clinical significance (chapter 6).

To illustrate the use of formula 12.1, consider the following example. Suppose that one expected those receiving an investigational drug (the experimental group) to experience a simple survival rate (formula 5.13) of 35 percent after one year of follow up and those *not* receiving the drug (the control group) to experience a one-year simple survival rate of 25 percent. This represents an effect size of 10 percent. Given the parameters stated above, the minimum sample size required for *each* group would be calculated as follows:

$$\{[(0.25 \times 0.75) + (0.35 \times 0.65)] / (0.35 - 0.25)^2\} \times 10.5 =$$
$$(0.415 / 0.01) \times 10.5 = 436$$

Thus, a total of 872 subjects (436 in each group) would be the minimum number of subjects required for the study. If the expected simple survival rates were 30 percent and 25 percent, respectively, the minimum sample size required in each group would be 1,670 or 3,340 total. Here, the effect size would be five percent. As this example illustrates, the smaller the effect size, the greater the sample size required, all other factors being equal. This is because, in general, it takes more power to detect a small difference than it does to detect a large difference. Normally, investigators would have some idea of the expected outcome for the control group (P_C) based on a literature review as well as a sense of a meaningful effect size. This information would allow the investigator to determine the expected outcome for the experimental group (P_E) for use in formula 12.1 since P_E is mathematically equal to the sum of the effect size and P_C (i.e., $P_E = [P_E - P_C] + P_C$) based on the above definitions of these terms.

Determining the required sample size at the beginning of a study is only part of the solution to maintaining adequate power in RCTs. Because of potential losses during the course of an investigation, the **effective sample size** (i.e., the sample size remaining after losses) may be significantly below the original requirements. Therefore, it is a good idea to include more than the minimum number of subjects in a study whenever possible. As with cohort studies (chapter 11), one can increase the required sample size by say 25 percent or more in order to account for potential losses during follow up. In some cases, however, it may be necessary to relax the eligibility requirements in order to recruit enough subjects. The advisability of doing so will depend on the specific study and its research objectives. Another possibility is to make contingency plans for obtaining additional subjects if needed.[8] Other strategies include targeting high risk groups and extending the follow-up period where possible. Targeting groups at high risk of the study outcome has the effect of increasing the number of predicted endpoints and decreasing the sample size requirements for the groups being compared. For example, since stroke incidence increases with age, one might restrict a trial designed to test whether a particular intervention reduces the incidence of stroke to adults 65 years of age and older. This age group, being at a higher risk of stroke than younger age groups, is more be likely to produce the number of endpoints needed for an accurate comparison in a shorter time period than a younger group. A downside of this approach is that it may limit the generalizability of the study findings. Extending the follow-up period of an RCT can have a similar effect.[6] In many cases, RCTs are *multicenter studies* that pool resources to ensure there are adequate numbers of subjects and endpoints for accurate statistical comparisons. Finally, the basic strategies for minimizing losses in cohort studies can be applied to RCTs as well (see table 11-2).

While low participation in an RCT, whether due to strict eligibility requirements or a general lack of interest among potential participants, will not affect the internal validity of a trial, losses to follow up can *if* they are associated with *both* the exposure (intervention) and the outcome. If not, like low participation, losses will still affect the precision of the findings and hence the power of the trial. Another related issue is noncompliance with the study protocol. This is discussed later in the chapter.

Randomly Allocating Subjects into Experimental and Control Groups

Allocating subjects into experimental and control groups in RCTs involves *randomization* (chapter 4) by definition. Randomization, or random allocation, means that the assignment of subjects into experimental and control groups is strictly by random means. This assures that the subjects have the *same* probability of being assigned to either the experimental or control group. Trials that do not involve random allocation are not RCTs, and do not carry the same status in epidemiology as their randomized counterparts. Randomization, properly executed, eliminates selection bias in subject assignments and increases the probability that the experimental and control groups will be comparable in terms of baseline factors other than the intervention being applied. Where these factors are predictive of the study outcome, it is essential that they be equally balanced between the study groups in order to control confounding and thus obtain a fair and accurate evaluation of the efficacy of the intervention. A key benefit of randomization, therefore, is its potential to assure that **prognostic factors**, that is, factors that are predictive of the study outcome,[5] are distributed similarly in the experimental and control groups. Randomization is more likely to achieve this objective when the sample size is large.

To comprehend this better, it is helpful to understand that prognostic factors, such as age, sex, or health status, cannot confound the effect of an intervention on a study outcome when they are equally balanced between the study groups. When they are unequally balanced, however, confounding will occur. This is because prognostic factors that are not evenly distributed between the study groups are not only risk factors for the study outcome, they are associated with the exposure (i.e., the intervention) as well.[11] Therefore, as long as they do not represent intermediate steps in the causal sequence that leads to the effect, they meet the three conditions for being confounders (see chapter 8). Imbalance between study groups indicates that they are associated with the intervention. This is because they are more or less likely to be in the experimental or control group and thus are positively or inversely associated with the intervention. Only if their distribution is the same in the study groups can they be considered unassociated with the intervention.[11]   .

The magic of randomization is that when properly performed it not only eliminates selection bias in subject assignments, but it also tends to produce study groups that are similar with regard to the distribution of anticipated, and even *unanticipated*, prognostic factors. Thus, it can be an efficient and effective method of controlling confounding in RCTs. Barring measurement errors, any differences in baseline factors between the study groups, other than the intervention to be applied, should only be due to chance. Furthermore, this chance decreases with the size of the study population. Because randomization is capable of controlling unknown confounders, as well as expected ones, it is considered more effective in controlling confounding than restriction, matching, or stratification, which can only control anticipated confounders.

There are several methods of randomization that can be used in RCTs. **Simple randomization**, which can be thought of as randomization without modifications, works best at producing comparable groups when the study population is large. When the study population is small (say, less than 100 subjects per group),[12] chance differences between the groups are more likely to occur. It is important to remember that randomization is based on probability; therefore, randomization alone cannot guarantee that experimental and control groups will always be comparable despite a large sample size. Nevertheless, the larger the sample, the greater the probability the study groups will be similar. In general, RCTs with study populations over a thousand tend to produce experimental and control groups that are relatively balanced with respect to baseline factors.[8]

When the study population in an RCT is small it may be helpful to employ a modified randomization technique that increases the probability that important prognostic factors will be equally distributed between the experimental and control groups. One such technique is **stratified randomization** (see figure 12-1). This technique has the effect of reducing random error. First, the subjects are deliberately separated into different strata of the factor(s) for which the technique is being employed (e.g., into groups of males and females). Next, the subjects are randomly allocated from each stratum into experimental and control groups, which are then combined into the final experimental and control groups. The use of this technique should result in study groups that are nearly identical with regard to the stratification variables. Stratified randomization is best suited to studies based on relatively small sample sizes, while simple randomization is best used in larger studies. Stratified randomization can also be used to detect effect measure modification in a trial.[7] The method becomes inefficient, however, when more than a few factors are stratified, so it should only be used with regard to the most important prognostic variables (e.g., disease severity).

Another potential issue that can arise with simple randomization is unequal numbers of subjects in the study groups. If the disparity is large, it can reduce the statistical efficiency of a trial, resulting in decreased power. This is more likely to be a problem when the sample size is small. A random-

Figure 12-1   Example of Stratified Randomization in a Randomized Controlled Trial

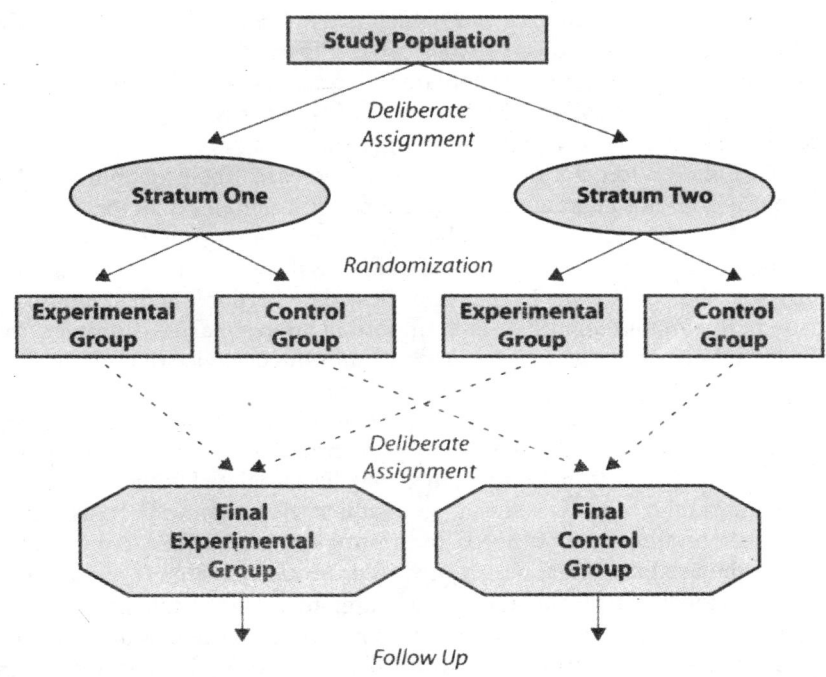

Reference: Fletcher, R. H., Fletcher, S. W., and Wagner, E. H. (1988). *Clinical Epidemiology: The Essentials,* 2nd ed. Baltimore: Williams and Wilkins.

ization technique that is commonly used to prevent this problem is **block randomization**. During the recruitment period, subjects are divided into small blocks or groupings of equal size as they enter the trial. Within each block the subjects are then randomly assigned to the experimental or control groups in such a way that equal numbers are assigned to each group.[13] For example, with blocks of four subjects every time four subjects are recruited, two are assigned to the experimental group and two to the control group. Thus, block randomization assures perfect balance in the number of subjects in each study group as long as complete blocks of subjects are assigned. If the recruitment is terminated prior to completing a block, the difference in size between study groups should still be small depending on the block size. A disadvantage of block randomization is that assignments at the end of a block may be discerned by investigators who have observed the previous assignments. Therefore, it may be helpful to vary the size of the blocks in a random fashion. Block randomization can also present problems when used in multicenter studies, but these difficulties can be overcome in some fairly straightforward ways. Other methods of modified randomization have also been developed to deal with balance issues related to size and the distribution of prognostic factors. These are described in more advanced textbooks under the label **restricted randomization**, which is the technical term for modified randomization (e.g., stratified or block randomization).

It is always a good idea to compare the experimental and control groups on baseline factors following the randomization process. The main reason is to see if the resulting distributions of important factors are similar in each group. Simple randomization, for example, increases the probability of balance, but it does not guarantee it since chance still remains a factor. If important variables are not balanced between the study groups, appropriate adjustments may need to made in the analysis phase of the trial using techniques described in chapter 11 (i.e., stratification with pooling or standardization or multivariable analysis). It is important to emphasize, however, that while imbalance on prognostic factors indicates the presence of confounding, it does not tell us the extent of the confounding. Even widely disparate values of a factor between the experimental and control groups may not signal significant confounding if the factor is a weak predictor of the study outcome. Then again, a relatively small imbalance may be associated with considerable confounding if the factor is a strong predictor of the outcome.[11] To assess the degree of confounding, one needs to control for it and then compare the results to the crude estimate as outlined in previous chapters. It is *not* appropriate to perform statistical significance testing to evaluate imbalances. First, the amount of confounding is not necessarily related to the amount of imbalance as just described. Second, the results of statistical significance testing are influenced by sample size, while confounding is not (see chapter 8), and third, statistical significance testing is illogical in this application. Rejecting the null hypothesis says that chance is an unlikely explanation for the observed difference, and yet we know that the difference is due to chance given that randomization has been used.[11]

Table 12-2 presents data on baseline factors for an RCT following simple randomization. In this example, the distributions of the data are quite similar between the experimental and control groups indicating that randomization was successful in producing study groups that are balanced on the selected factors, and presumably on unmeasured factors as well. Thus, we would feel fairly confident that confounding is not a significant issue in this study.

Applying the Intervention and Assessing Outcomes During Follow Up

In a typical RCT the members of the *experimental group* receive a potentially promising but unproven intervention, and the results are compared to the experience of the members of the *control group* after a suitable follow-up period. The follow-up period may be short or long depending on the nature of the outcome (e.g., lifestyle changes, symptom relief, pain control, acute or chronic disease reduction, survival). The members of the control group usually receive the standard regimen, a placebo, a *sham procedure*, or nothing at

Table 12-2   Distribution on Baseline Factors Following Randomization for a Hypothetical Randomized Controlled Trial of the Effect of Meditation on Stress Reduction in Young Adults

Baseline factor	Experimental Group (n = 2,500) %	Control Group (n = 2,500) %
Male	58	57
Age (years)		
18–22	26	24
23–27	44	46
28–32	30	30
White	78	78
Fitness level		
High	32	32
Medium	59	60
Low	9	8

all. A **sham procedure** is one designed to appear like a real procedure but without any anticipated effects. It is analogous to the use of a placebo in a drug trial. For example, RCTs of the efficacy of acupuncture for various medical conditions often employ a sham procedure in the control **arm** of the experiment.* The participants in the experimental arm receive the customary acupuncture, while those in the control arm receive simulated acupuncture where the needles do not penetrate the skin.[14] Placebos, sham procedures, or nothing at all may be referred to as **inactive treatments**. In contrast, standard regimens are known as **active treatments**. Thus, the control group in an RCT may receive an active treatment, an inactive treatment, or some combination of the two.

The reporting of outcomes during follow up in an RCT may be subject to bias, especially if the outcomes are subjective like pain control or symptom relief. One way this bias can occur is when the study participants know their group assignments. This knowledge can lead to differential misclassification on outcome status. It can also have a differential effect on compliance with the study protocol. To illustrate, consider an RCT to assess the efficacy of a new medication in the treatment of migraine headaches where the experimental group receives the new medication, and the control group receives a placebo. If the subjects know to which study group they have been assigned (i.e., the experimental or control group), those in the experimental group may be more likely to report a reduction in the severity and duration of their symptoms compared to those in the control group even if the medication is

*_Arm_ is a term commonly used in experimental trials and is synonymous with group.[5] Therefore, the control arm is the control group, and the experimental arm is the experimental group in a two-arm RCT.

not beneficial. Essentially, there is a tendency for those receiving a new treatment to report positive benefits due to their own expectations for the treatment. The members of the control group would not be expected to report positive benefits knowing that they are receiving an inactive treatment. They may also be less likely to comply with the study protocol or withdraw from the trial than those in the experimental group for the same reason. Either way, this could lead to bias in reporting the outcomes of the trial. If the subjects in the example did not know their group assignments, however, this bias would be unlikely since expectations between the groups would probably be similar. Also, greater noncompliance with the study protocol or increased withdrawals among members of the control group should be less likely since the subjects could not be sure they are not in the group receiving the new medication (i.e., the experimental group).

One way of minimizing these problems is *blinding* or *masking** the subjects to their study group assignments. **Blinding** or **masking** refers to concealing certain information so as to avoid bias.[5] This is facilitated by the use of a placebo or sham procedure in the control arm of an experiment. This makes it more difficult for the subjects to know which group they are in. In the language of epidemiology, this is known as a **single-blinded study** (or *single-masked study*). This is a study in which the subjects are kept unaware of their group assignment, although the investigators are still aware. While a single-blinded study can minimize bias introduced by the subjects, it has no effect on bias on the part of the investigators (specifically, those assessing outcome status). For example, by knowing the subjects' group assignments, the investigators (assessors) may tend to record more positive outcomes in the experimental group than in the control group if they believe the intervention is likely to be beneficial. This is most likely to occur when the study outcome is relatively subjective, such as severity of symptoms. In a **double-blinded study** (or *double-masked study*) *neither* the subjects nor the investigators (assessors) are aware of the subjects' group assignments. This design helps to overcome bias on the part of both the subjects and the investigators. A double-blinded study is generally accomplished by using a sealed code for the group assignments that is only broken at the conclusion of the study. Double-blinded studies have been the standard for RCTs for decades. A **triple-blinded study** (or *triple-masked study*) also keeps those who are analyzing the data, if different from those assessing the outcomes, unaware of the subjects' group assignments. This minimizes any data manipulation that might be attempted, consciously or unconsciously, to support the study hypotheses.

Blinding is also helpful in reducing confounding that occurs *during* the follow-up period. Confounding during follow up can arise when the investi-

*The terms blinding and masking and their derivatives (e.g., blinded and masked) are used interchangeably in epidemiology. Some prefer the use of masking over blinding, since the latter may be subject to confusion, especially when the outcome of interest is blindness (i.e., loss of vision).[7] The use of the term *blinding*, however, has a longer tradition than that of masking and may be more familiar to most people.

gators pay more attention to the subjects in the experimental group than to those in the control group, perhaps by suggesting, consciously or unconsciously, other ways that subjects in the experimental group can improve their condition. This can increase the probability that the intervention appears successful when in fact it is due to confounding by these other means. Confounding can also occur among the subjects when, for example, those in the control group of a therapeutic trial seek other treatments more frequently than those in the experimental group because they learn they are taking a placebo. These so-called "cointerventions," which were not part of the original design, can confound the study results during the follow-up period.[8]

While double or triple blinding can help minimize information bias in ascertaining the study outcomes or confounding during the follow-up period, it is not always feasible. Some studies, for example, cannot be blinded. A therapeutic trial to determine if back surgery is more efficacious than prescribed exercises in reducing chronic lower back pain cannot be double blinded since it would be obvious to patients and investigators alike who is receiving which treatment. In other cases, blinding may be difficult because of the problem of producing a suitable placebo, especially where the intervention is likely to produce soon-to-be-discovered side effects like dry mouth, gastrointestinal upset, or fatigue that are not experienced by those taking the placebo. As implied earlier, blinding is most important when the outcomes being assessed are subjective. When the outcome is truly objective (e.g., overall mortality), blinding is less important since the outcomes are unlikely to be influenced by knowledge of treatment status. When double or triple blinding is not feasible, extra efforts should be made to reduce potential information bias. Some recommendations include: (a) using as objective criteria as possible in assessing outcomes, (b) following up the experimental and control groups with the same level of intensity, and (c) using independent assessors who do not know the group assignments or study hypotheses.[6]

In general, a well-designed **placebo-controlled trial** (a trial in which the control group receives a placebo or sham procedure) with randomization and double-blinding (or triple-blinding if necessary) represents the ideal RCT from a scientific perspective, although not necessarily from an ethical perspective (see below). A double-blinded, placebo-controlled randomized trial requires that the intervention demonstrate a level of superiority that exceeds any *placebo effect* found in the control group. The **placebo effect** is the effect due, presumably, to subject expectations that a treatment is beneficial. Since this effect may be operating in both the experimental and control arms of a double-blinded RCT, the beneficial effects of the intervention would have to exceed the placebo effect in the control group in order to be considered efficacious.

Ideally, the intervention in an RCT should be shown to be superior to the experience of the control group in order to warrant its acceptance. Superior, however, may mean better outcomes or similar outcomes but with fewer risks. For example, some of the newer anti-depressant medications produce fewer adverse side effects than older varieties without necessarily being more effective at reducing clinical depression. Thus, their demonstrated superiority relates to their potential applicability to a wider group of patients. In practice, new medications may be approved if they demonstrate they are no worse than current treatments or superior to placebos and hence the placebo effect.

Beyond Informed Consent: Some Ethical Considerations

A generally accepted prerequisite to the conduct of RCTs, particularly those involving patients, is the principle of **equipoise**. This refers to "a state of genuine uncertainty about the benefits or harms that may result from each of two more regimens."[1] Genuine uncertainty about whether or not an intervention is better or worse than the standard regimen or an inactive treatment (i.e., when an effective regimen does not exist), is important so that subjects are not intentionally denied the more effective regimen. In fact, RCTs are performed specifically to reduce this uncertainty. The reasoning is that if there is consensus as to which is the more effective regimen, it would be unethical *not* to offer it to all subjects. In general, there should be enough confidence in the *potential* benefits of an intervention to expose some individuals to it, especially if it may involve serious risks, but not so much confidence that it would be unethical not to offer it to others who might benefit from it.[6] In short, according to the principle of equipoise, an RCT is only possible when there are honest doubts about the efficacy of a proposed intervention. If an intervention is known to be superior to conventional regimens or no active treatment, then it would be unethical to proceed with an RCT. Generally speaking, the research objective should be to determine if an intervention is beneficial when compared to a control group.

Equipoise has implications for the use of placebos or sham procedures in the control arm of an RCT. If an effective active treatment exists, it would appear to be unethical to assign an inactive treatment (i.e., placebo, sham procedure, or no treatment) to the control group in an RCT. To do so would deny these participants of the more effective regimen. This appears to be the intent of the **Declaration of Helsinki**,[15] a highly regarded and widely adopted policy statement of the World Medical Association (WMA). The Declaration enumerates principles for the ethical practice of medical research involving human subjects. Specifically, paragraph 29 states:

> The benefits, risks, burdens and effectiveness of a new method should be tested against those of the best current prophylactic, diagnostic, and therapeutic methods. This does not exclude the use of placebo, or no treatment, in studies where no proven prophylactic, diagnostic or therapeutic method exists.[15]

Notice that this principle allows inactive treatments in the control arm but *only if* effective active treatments do not exist. This particular paragraph of the Declaration has been controversial.[16-18] Shortly after adopting the above language in 2000, a note of clarification was appended to paragraph 29, effectively expanding the role of placebo-controlled trials. The note stated:

The WMA hereby reaffirms its position that extreme care must be taken in making use of a placebo-controlled trial and that in general this methodology should only be used in the absence of existing proven therapy. *However, a placebo-controlled trial may be ethically acceptable, even if proven therapy is available* (emphasis added), under the following circumstances:

- Where for compelling and scientifically sound methodological reasons its use is necessary to determine the efficacy or safety of a prophylactic, diagnostic or therapeutic method; or
- Where a prophylactic, diagnostic or therapeutic method is being investigated for a minor condition and the patients who receive placebo will not be subject to any additional risk of serious or irreversible harm.[15]

This change was apparently in response to criticisms aimed at the perceived restrictive nature of paragraph 29[17] and was a setback to those who favored the more restrictive language. Advocates on both sides appear to have strong beliefs on the issue (see figure 12-2 and table 12-3). Compliance with the Declaration of Helsinki is voluntary, and while some ethics committees have adopted it outright, agencies such as the U.S. Food and Drug Administration continue to promote placebo-controlled trials in drug testing even when an effective treatment exists.[19]

Another issue with ethical implications has to do with whether or not investigators should consider stopping an RCT before the planned termination date. This issue is discussed further in the next section. In general, there are at least three reasons to consider stopping an RCT based on preliminary findings. These are: (a) discovery of significant harm to subjects that out-

Figure 12-2   Placebo Cartoon

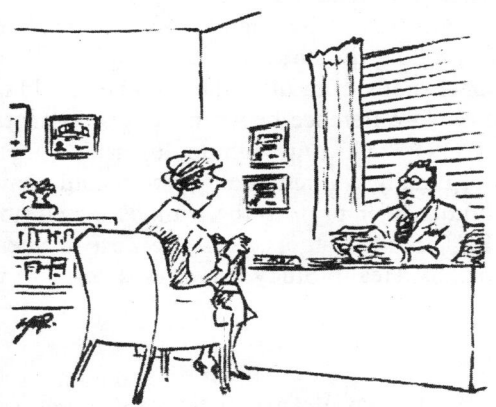

Pepper . . . and Salt
THE WALL STREET JOURNAL

"No one likes placebos, but someone has to take them."

From *The Wall Street Journal*—permission, Cartoon Features Syndicate.

Table 12-3   The Ethics of Using Placebos when Effective Treatment Exists: Two Points of View

For Placebo Use	Against Placebo Use
"Investigators have a duty to avoid exploiting research participants, not a therapeutic duty to provide optimal medical care. Accordingly, enrolling patient volunteers in placebo-controlled trials that withhold proven effective treatment is not fundamentally unethical as long as patients are not being exploited." Source: Miller, F. G., and Brody, H. (2002). What Makes Placebo-Controlled Trials Unethical? *American Journal of Bioethics* 2 (2): 5.	"[I]t is unethical to use a placebo in any trial if there is already an accepted treatment for the condition. . . . Instead, an investigator must treat a new therapy against the existing standard. . . . [N]o researcher should deny a patient the best available treatment solely for the purpose of learning whether a new treatment is better than a placebo." Source: Rothman, K. J. (2002). *Epidemiology: An Introduction.* New York: Oxford University Press, p. 212.

weighs any possible benefits of the trial, (b) clear evidence that the intervention is more or less effective than the control regimen, and (c) strong indications that the research question cannot be adequately answered.[7, 8] A decision to stop an RCT early should not be made lightly based on preliminary information. Investigators should be sure the findings are not a transitory phenomenon and therefore likely to change as additional data are collected and analyzed. Though of lesser importance, at least when it comes to safety issues, it should be remembered that to varying degrees the participants, investigators, and sponsors of the trial have made commitments of time, effort, and expense to answer what was originally considered an important research question. Therefore, stopping a trial on a hunch might be considered unethical or at least unwise. With regard to item c, there are several reasons it may no longer be possible to answer the original research question. One could be substantial losses to follow up that leave the sample size too small to draw any meaningful conclusions from the data. Another could be interim findings indicating little or no difference between the experimental and control groups after several years of follow up with no discernible possibility of a change in the situation. Finally, the research question could have been answered definitively by another RCT prior to the planned conclusion of the study.[8] An example of an RCT that was stopped early because of a beneficial finding was the first Physicians' Health Study, which is referred to in the next section.

Variations in Design

The most common design for RCTs is the **parallel group design**, also referred to as a **parallel treatment design** or **noncrossover design**.[7] In this design all of the subjects are assigned independently to one of the study groups, and no subjects receive more than one of the study regimens.[5] In the simplest parallel group design each subject is allocated to either the experimental or control group (see figure 4-7). The parallel group design is the type of RCT we have been discussing so far. An alternative to this design is the *crossover design*.

The **crossover design** is a variation of the parallel group design in which the intervention is applied at different times to each subject. In the most basic application of this design, the study population is randomized into an experimental and control group as in a parallel group design. After a specified period of time, however, the subjects in the original experimental group become the control group, and the subjects in the original control group become the experimental group as illustrated in figure 12-3. Only one primary hypothesis is being tested here, but the investigators can examine the effect of the intervention both within and between the two groups being compared. The major advantages of the crossover design are reduced sample size requirements and decreased potential for confounding due to the fact that the subjects serve as

Figure 12-3   Example of a Randomized Controlled Trial Using a Crossover Design

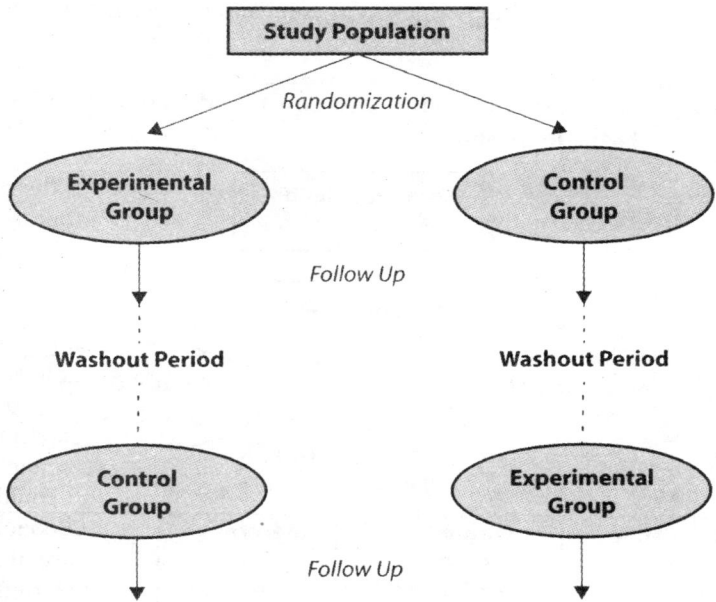

After the washout period, a time during which the subjects do not receive any intervention, those in the original experimental group become the control group, and those in the original control group become the experimental group. In a placebo-controlled trial, those receiving the intervention "crossover" to receive the placebo after a washout period, and those receiving the placebo "crossover" to receive the intervention after the same washout period.

their own controls.[8, 20] Comparing the same subjects in the experimental and control groups produces less statistical variance in the results, which in turn increases the power of the study, thereby reducing sample size requirements.[8] One of the disadvantages of this design is the longer time it takes to complete the study due to the need to follow the subjects twice (once with the intervention and once without the intervention). This can also increase the withdrawal rate due to subject fatigue. Another disadvantage is **carryover effects**, which are residual effects of the intervention during the period after it has ended. A common way to deal with carryover effects is to introduce a **washout period**, a stage during which the effects of the intervention are believed to wear off. The assignment of the subjects in the experimental group to the control group and vice versa begins only after the washout period has ended (see figure 12-3). Other disadvantages of the crossover design include its application only to interventions that provide temporary relief and the complexity of the analysis compared to that of the traditional parallel group design.[20]

Another variation in the design of an RCT is the **factorial design**, which is intended to answer more than one research question. This design can provide significant cost savings over separate trials. The simplest factorial design is the 2 × 2 design, which is illustrated in figure 12-4. In this design the study population is randomized into an experimental and control group to test one

Figure 12-4   Example of a Randomized Controlled Trial Using a 2 × 2 Factorial Design

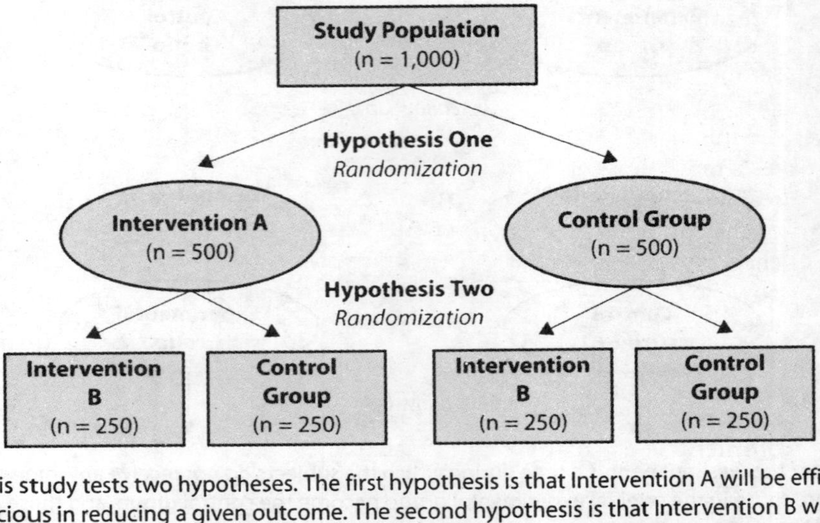

This study tests two hypotheses. The first hypothesis is that Intervention A will be efficacious in reducing a given outcome. The second hypothesis is that Intervention B will be efficacious in reducing another outcome. Note that the number of subjects being tested under Hypothesis One (n = 1,000) is the same as the number of subjects being tested under Hypothesis Two (n = 4 × 250 = 1,000). Therefore, the 2 × 2 factorial design is equivalent to two separate parallel group randomized controlled trials.

hypothesis, and the subjects in each of these groups are then randomized into an additional experimental and control group to test a second hypothesis. A potential limitation of this design is possible interactions between the interventions that can affect the magnitude of the outcomes. Therefore, unless one intends to test the effects of the interactions between the interventions, the design is best suited to interventions that operate independently of each other.[8] More complex designs are 2 × 2 × 2, 3 × 3, etc.

A good example of a 2 × 2 factorial design is the first Physicians' Health Study that involved over 22,000 male physicians, 40–84 years of age.[21] This was a preventive trial using a factorial design. It was planned to test two major research hypotheses: (a) that aspirin reduces total cardiovascular mortality, and (b) that beta-carotene reduces cancer incidence. The first randomization produced an experimental group consisting of physicians who took a standard aspirin every other day and a control group that took a placebo. The subjects in the experimental group were further randomized into experimental and control groups that took beta-carotene or a placebo, respectively. The subjects in the original control group were similarly divided into experimental and control groups that took beta-carotene or a placebo. Thus, the second hypothesis was tested among both the aspirin users and nonusers for a total sample size equivalent to that of the original study population. In effect, two equally sized RCTs were conducted at the same time. As a point of information, the aspirin trial of the Physicians' Health Study was stopped prematurely after only 4.8 years of the planned eight-year follow-up period due in part to a significant reduction in nonfatal myocardial infarctions among those taking the aspirin regimen compared to the controls (RR = 0.56).[8] The beta carotene trial was continued, however, because of no compelling reasons to stop the trial.

Another way that the design of RCTs can vary can be related to how sample size is determined. In a **fixed sample size design** (or *fixed sample design*, for short), the sample size is normally *fixed* before the trial begins,[7] and the findings are not generally analyzed until the conclusion of the trial.[22] Subjects may be enrolled all at once or over time until the specified sample size is reached. The predetermined sample size should be based on a consideration of the minimum number of subjects required to detect an important difference in the primary outcome between the study groups at a desired level of power. Other considerations such as cost and subject availability may also be taken into account. The fixed sample size design is the type of RCT we have been describing up to this point.

An alternative to the fixed sample size design is a *sequential design*. In a **sequential design** sample size is *not fixed* but varies depending on the results of interim analyses of the accumulating data. Basically, before a new subject (or pair of subjects) is enrolled in a sequential trial, the data generated up to that point are analyzed to determine whether or not the study should continue. Inherent in a sequential design is consecutive enrollment of subjects during the recruitment period and repeated analyses of the data in order to reach a decision about the efficacy or safety of the intervention as soon as possible. The main motivation for reaching an early decision should be ethics, although other factors may also be considered (see table 12-4). If, for example, the data clearly indicate that the intervention is superior or inferior to the control regimen, then it is generally considered unethical to allow the trial to continue since some of the subjects would be known to be receiving an inferior treatment, which violates the principle of equipoise.

Table 12-4   Major Reasons for Conducting Interim Analyses in Randomized Controlled Trials

Ethical	Administrative	Economic
Assure subjects not exposed to unsafe, inferior, or ineffective regimens	Assure trial is being conducted as planned (i.e., in accordance with the study protocol)	Potentially reduce sample size requirements, follow-up time, and hence the cost of the trial

Reference: CTriSoft International (2004). Tutorials: Group Sequential Trial Design; Overview of Group Sequential Trial Design. Available: http://www.ctrisoft.net/tutorials/seqdes.html (Access date: July 6, 2006).

Sequential designs require well thought-out **stopping rules**, which are rules for deciding when to terminate a trial.[5] Stopping rules may not be specified in fixed sample size designs since interim analyses are not usually planned.[22] In sequential trials, stopping rules should be stated in the study protocol and invoked as soon as the applicable criteria are satisfied. Table 12-5 lists common reasons for stopping sequential trials. The second one is often referred to in the epidemiologic literature as **futility** (defined later).

Table 12-5   Common Reasons for Stopping Sequential Trials

- The intervention is clearly superior or inferior to the control regimen.
- There is no clear difference between the experimental and control regimens.
- Serious adverse effects are associated with the experimental or control regimen.
- The quality of the data is poor.
- Subject recruitment is too slow.
- There is convincing evidence from other sources that the trial is unnecessary or unethical.
- The research question is no longer relevant.
- Compliance with the study protocol is unacceptably low.
- The resources needed to complete the trial are no longer adequate.
- The integrity of the trial has been significantly compromised.

Reference: Piantadosi, S. (1997). *Clinical Trials: A Methodologic Perspective*. New York: John Wiley and Sons.

Increasingly, **data monitoring committees** (also known as **data and safety monitoring boards** or **committees**)[23] are charged with making the these decisions. They consist of various outside experts who regularly review the accumulated data in a sequential trial in order to determine if the trial should be stopped or modified in some way based on interim findings.[5] Exhibit 12-2 lists the U.S. Food and Drug Administration's recommendations for when a data monitoring committee should be used in clinical trials. According to the FDA, data monitoring committees are not needed in most other instances, such as short-term studies investigating the relief of mild to moderate symptoms of disease.[23]

A popular variation of the sequential design is the **group sequential design**. In this type of sequential trial, analysis of the accumulated findings is conducted at predetermined intervals following enrollment of a specified number or block of subjects. Generally, only two or three interim analyses are planned in a group sequential design,[5] rather than the continuing analyses that are characteristic of conventional sequential designs. In most other respects, the designs are similar. A group sequential trial sponsored by the National Heart, Lung, and Blood Institute ARDS Clinical Trials Network was conducted to compare the effects of higher and lower positive end-expiratory pressure (PEEP) levels among patients receiving mechanical ventilation

---

Exhibit 12-2
U.S. Food and Drug Administration Recommendations for Data Monitoring Committees

According to the U.S. Food and Drug Administration, a Data Monitoring Committee should be considered when:

- The study endpoint is such that a highly favorable or unfavorable result, or even a finding of futility, at an interim analysis might ethically require termination of the study before its planned completion;

- There are *a priori* reasons for a particular safety concern, as, for example, if the procedure for administering the treatment is particularly invasive;

- There is prior information suggesting the possibility of serious toxicity with the study treatment;

- The study is being performed in a potentially fragile population such as children, pregnant women or the very elderly, or other vulnerable populations, such as those who are terminally ill or of diminished mental capacity;

- The study is being performed in a population at elevated risk of death or other serious outcomes, even when the study objective addresses a lesser endpoint;

- The study is large, of long duration, and multi-center.

Source: U.S. Food and Drug Administration, Center for Biologics Evaluation and Research (2006). *Guidance for Clinical Trial Sponsors: Establishment and Operation of Clinical Trial Data Monitoring Committees.* Available: http://www.fda.gov/cber/gdlns/clintrialdmc.htm (Access date: July 6, 2006).

and suffering from acute lung injury and acute respiratory disease syndrome (ARDS). Interestingly, the trial was stopped for *futility*. The authors stated:

> The data and safety monitoring board stopped the trial at the second interim analysis, after 549 patients had been enrolled, on the basis of the specified futility stopping rule. At this time it was calculated that if the study had continued to the planned maximal enrollment of 750 patients, the probability of demonstrating the superiority of the higher-PEEP strategy was less than 1 percent under the alternative hypothesis based on the unadjusted mortality difference.[24(p331)]

Sequential designs are most applicable when the study outcomes are likely to occur in a relatively short period of time. If the outcomes have long induction or latency periods, sequential designs will not be practical.[7] The main advantage of sequential designs is the ability they provide to minimize the time that subjects are exposed to an ineffective or harmful intervention or an inferior control regimen. In a traditional fixed sample size design such exposure would ostensibly continue until the end of the planned study period even though interim analyses, had they been performed, might have revealed that one of the study arms was clearly beneficial or harmful to participants. Thus, sequential designs have a potential ethical advantage over fixed sample size designs, while also being potentially more economic due to their generally smaller sample sizes and shorter follow-up periods. A disadvantage may be difficulty in planning for the actual size and length of the trial since they are unknown at the outset of the study. As with the trial sponsored by the National Heart, Lung, and Blood Institute ARDS Clinical Trials Network, some sequential trials set a maximum sample size so that the trial can be stopped if the outcomes are nearly equal in both study-arms when the sample size is reached.[7] Another disadvantage of sequential trials is the number of analyses to be performed, particularly in conventional sequential trials where analyses are frequent. Also, investigators need to adjust standard analytical methods in sequential trials to take into account the repeated nature of the analyses, which could otherwise diminish the precision of the findings.

Reducing Noncompliance

An important issue that needs to be considered in the design stage of an RCT is the likelihood of **noncompliance** (or **nonadherence**) with the study protocol, particularly as it relates to the experimental and control regimens. Failure of subjects to follow the study protocol can affect the accuracy of the study findings. In particular, noncompliance tends to reduce the power of a trial and hence the probability of detecting a true difference between the study outcomes in the experimental and control groups. High levels of noncompliance make the findings of a study suspect. Some of the reasons for noncompliance include confusion about specific requirements, unpleasant side effects from a study regimen, forgetfulness, desire for alternative treatments, and declining interest in the study. In general, the longer subjects are expected to be compliant and the more difficult or complex the protocol, the greater the degree of noncompliance.[6] Noncompliance tends to be less of an issue when the intervention is administered directly by the investigators or other health professionals under their direction than when it relies on the subjects to administer it to themselves. Also, trials that only require one administration of the intervention produce less noncompliance than trials that require repeated administrations over time.[25] For example, a six-month trial of the efficacy of a surgical technique to relieve symptoms of Parkinson's disease is likely to result in greater **compliance** (or **adherence**) than a comparable three-year trial using a new medication that must be taken by the subjects four times a day.

Strategies for increasing compliance are similar to those for reducing losses to follow up and have already been discussed in the context of cohort studies (see chapter 11 and table 11-2 in particular). In an RCT it is especially important to select interested individuals who have a strong motivation to participate in the trial and persevere to its completion. One way to facilitate this is to utilize a **run-in period**, which is a pre-trial phase during which eligible subjects are given the control (or sometimes the experimental) regimen for a specified period of time, usually for several weeks or a few months. The primary purpose is to increase compliance in the trial by screening out those who are noncompliant during the run-in period (see figure 12-5). The first Physicians' Health Study (referred to earlier) and the second Physicians'

Figure 12-5   The Use of a Run-In Period in a Randomized Controlled Trial

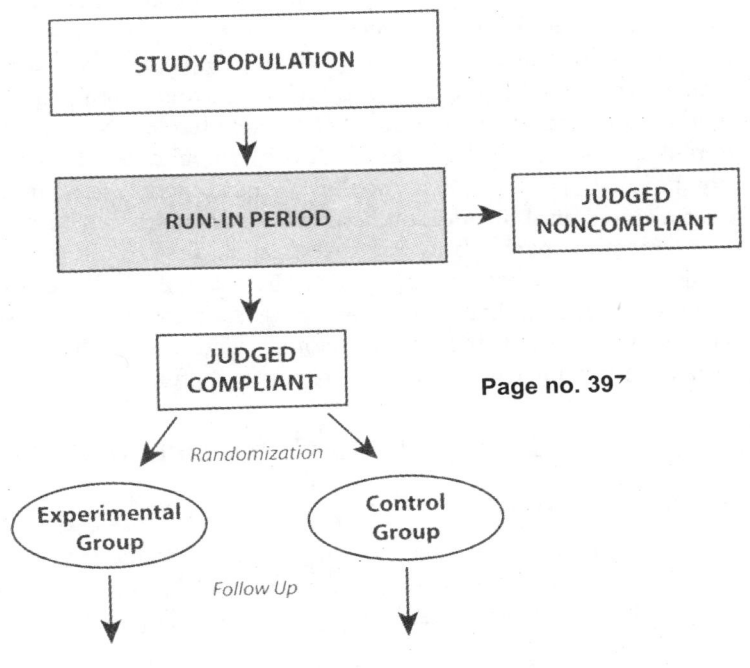

Health Study, which examined the roles of vitamins C and E, beta-carotene, and multivitamins in the prevention of cardiovascular disease, total cancer, and prostate cancer, are examples of RCTs using a run-in period to increase compliance with the study protocol. In the first Physicians' Health Study, for instance, nearly one-third of the potential participants were screened out as a result of the run-in period.[26] The use of physicians in these studies also reflects the investigators' beliefs that this group would be more likely to comply with the study protocol. In fact, the study authors give five reasons for selecting physicians as the study population: (a) ability to give true informed consent, (b) knowledge of possible side effects, (c) accuracy and completeness of information, (d) ease of follow up, and (e) opportunity to conduct the trials by mail.[26]

Even with the best efforts to maintain compliance in RCTs not all subjects will adhere to the study regimens. Therefore, compliance must be assessed during the conduct of the trial. Unfortunately, there is no foolproof way to do this. Surveys or interviews based on self-reports represent one method of assessing compliance, but as you can imagine, they are not always reliable. In studies of drug efficacy, dispensing more medication than required and counting the number of unused pills at designated intervals is another strategy. For example, investigators may instruct subjects to bring any unused medications to follow-up visits or at other specified times so they can determine the actual quantity consumed. This method can also be unreliable since it does not prove that the missing medications were actually used as prescribed. Perhaps the most reliable method of assessing compliance is to measure specific biomarkers (chapter 10) whenever possible. For example, if the experimental drug or one of its metabolites used in a placebo-controlled drug trial can be measured in a blood or urine sample, this would provide objective confirmation that the drug was taken. The aim here is the same as that for certain job applicants or athletes competing in the Olympics, namely to determine if a particular drug was used. Most biomarkers, however, have relatively short half-lives in the body so they are not generally good indicators of long-term compliance. In addition, testing for biomarkers can be expensive and inconvenient for participants and investigators alike. In addition, there may be false positives or false negatives (see chapter 13). Finally, it is important to emphasize that investigators should always attempt to follow up noncompliant subjects using the same methods and thoroughness as for compliant subjects if the trial results are to be meaningful.[6]

ANALYSIS OF RANDOMIZED CONTROLLED TRIALS

Planning the Analysis

Before beginning the analysis phase of an RCT one should examine if the experimental and control groups are similar with regard to important prognostic factors. While simple randomization, especially with large samples, should equalize the distribution of these and other factors between the experimental and control groups, chance can still play a role. Therefore, it is important to see if the randomized groups appear to be comparable. If there are notable differences for any given factors, then these factors can be controlled in the analysis using methods such as stratification with pooling or standardization or multivariable analysis in order to reduce confounding (see chapter 11).

In general, the preferred approach to analyzing the findings of RCTs is known as **intention-to-treat analysis**. This means that the trial results are analyzed based on the *original* subject assignments to the experimental and control groups as determined by randomization. Intention-to-treat analysis does *not* take into consideration whether or not all of the subjects complied with the study protocol. If there are a significant number of *crossovers* (defined below), an intention-to-treat analysis will tend to *underestimate* the effect of the intervention on the study outcome. Nevertheless, this is still preferable to focusing the analysis only on compliant subjects, which nullifies the benefits of randomization and can therefore invalidate the study results.[1, 8] **Crossovers** (not to be confused with planned crossovers in a crossover design) occur when subjects in the experimental group do not complete the assigned intervention, or subjects in the control group seek the intervention or other active treatments.[8] They are referred to as "crossovers" because in a sense they crossover from the experimental arm to the control arm of the trial, or vice versa, as a result of their noncompliance with the assigned regimen. Intention-to-treat analysis is the analytical approach used in *effectiveness trials*, although it is also recommended for *efficacy trials* for reasons stated above. See exhibit 12-1 for definitions and descriptions of effectiveness and efficacy trials. When there is a high level of compliance in both arms of a trial, intention-to-treat analysis should produce results similar to those of *per protocol analysis*, which is defined in the next paragraph.

An alternative to intention-to-treat analysis is known as **per protocol analysis**. It has also been referred to as **efficacy analysis** since it focuses on the efficacy of the intervention, while intention-to-treat analysis focuses on its effectiveness (see exhibit 12-1 for an explanation). In this approach, data on subjects who did not adequately comply with the study protocol are excluded from the analysis.[5] Thus, only data on compliant subjects are used. This approach may sound good in theory, but it has a number of drawbacks. For one thing, it removes the benefits of randomization. As discussed earlier in the chapter, randomization is effective in eliminating selection bias in subject assignments and minimizing confounding due to anticipated and unanticipated differences between the experimental and control groups. Compliant subjects, however, are a select group that is unlikely to be representative of the study groups to which they were originally and randomly assigned. Therefore, those in the experimental and control groups probably differ from each other with regard to the distribution of certain prognostic variables, thereby introducing confounding in the data. If the degree of compliance differs between the study groups and is also related to the probability of the outcome, then a selection bias analogous to loss to follow-up bias (see chapter 8) could result.[6] In short, restricting the analysis to compliant subjects can cause systematic errors than can invalidate the findings of an RCT. Removing those who did not comply with the study protocol may also limit one's ability to apply the findings to medical or public health practice, since it does not make sense to recommend interventions that are likely to result in high levels of noncompliance.[27] Finally, focusing only on compliant subjects reduces the effective sample size of a trial with a subsequent loss of power. For these reasons, per protocol analysis is not recommended as the sole method for analyzing the results of an RCT. Sometimes investigators will analyze the results of a trial in terms of compliance in order to compare the findings with an intention-to-treat analysis. If the findings are similar, this increases confidence in the study results. If there are differences, however, the intention-to-treat analysis should prevail.[8]

Overall Analysis

A number of techniques can be used to analyze the overall findings of RCTs depending on the interests and objectives of the investigators and the specific design of the trial. These techniques range from the relatively simple to the more complex. In a parallel group and fixed sample size design where there are two study groups and the primary outcome variable is dichotomous, the overall results can be analyzed using procedures similar to those that have already been described in relation to cohort studies (see chapter 11). For example, one can calculate the incidence density of the outcomes in the experimental and control groups, respectively, and determine the incidence density ratio (formula 11.9) and its 95 percent confidence interval (formula 11.10). Often investigators of RCTs seek to determine if the intervention decreases the occurrence of unfavorable outcomes. Thus, the amount of reduction in the *percent relative effect* (chapter 6) may be of interest (see formula 6.5, partially repeated here for convenience). An approximate 95 percent confidence interval for the decreased percent relative effect can be calculated using formula 12.2.

(Repeated 6.5)   % Decreased Change = (1 – Ratio) × 100

The ratio referred to in the above example is the incidence density ratio (IDR) or rate ratio, which can be calculated using formula 11.9.

(12.2)
95% CI = (1 – 95% UCL for IDR) × 100 to (1 – 95% LCL for IDR) × 100

The CI in formula 12.2 refers to the confidence interval, UCL and LCL refer the upper confidence limit and lower confidence limit, respectively, and IDR refers to the incidence density ratio (or rate ratio). The confidence limits are those calculated for the IDR using formula 11.10. *However, the upper confidence limit for the IDR is used to calculate the lower confidence limit for the decreased relative effect, and the lower confidence limit for the IDR is used to calculate the upper confidence limit for the decreased relative effect.* This is shown in formula 12.2 and illustrated in problem 12-1.

One could also analyze the overall findings of a parallel group and fixed sample size design if the outcome measure is expected to increase when the intervention is successful (e.g., increased expiratory volume, increased survival). In this case, an increase in the percent relative effect may be of interest. Other common measures that might be used in analyzing parallel group designs are proportions or cumulative incidence. If the outcome data are continuous (e.g., weekly blood pressure measurements over the course of a study), one might want to compare means between the experimental and control groups using t-tests. Though in practice most investigators using RCTs test for statistically significant differences between the outcome measures in the experimental and control groups, significance testing is not recommended as discussed in previous chapters. Therefore, problem 12-1 employs a confidence interval.

Problem 12-1: Overall Analysis of a Randomized Controlled Trial

A double-blinded randomized controlled trial was initiated to determine if saw palmetto berry extract (an herbal remedy) is efficacious in reducing initial emergency urinary retention due to benign prostatic hyperplasia (BPH) in men. Initial emergency urinary retention was defined as the first episode during the study period of an inability to urinate due to BPH that required emergency medical attention. The study population included a select group of adult men, 60–69 years of age, with diagnosed BPH, who were members of a large health maintenance organization (HMO). One thousand men who met the study eligibility criteria were randomized into two equally sized experimental and control groups. Those in the experimental group were instructed to take a standardized dose of 320 milligrams of saw palmetto berry extract each evening during dinner. The extract was provided in capsule form and free of charge by the HMO. Those in the control group were given the same instructions but were supplied with a placebo instead. The participants were given free prostate examinations by trained staff urologists every six months for the planned two-year study and were instructed to seek medical assistance if needed using a designated 24-hour telephone hotline that directed the subjects to a nearby treatment center. The endpoint of interest was initial emergency urinary retention, as defined in the study. This typically requires immediate urinary catheterization.

At the conclusion of the study, the following data were reported:

- *Experimental group*: 40 incidents of initial emergency urinary retention during 960 person-years of follow-up
- *Control group*: 65 incidents of initial emergency urinary retention during 935 person-years of follow-up

Assuming the study was properly designed and conducted, and based on the above data, determine if the treatment was efficacious.

Solution:
Step 1: Place the data provided in the appropriate cells of a tabular display as follows:

Exposure Status	Outcome	Person-time
Exposed	40	960 years
Unexposed	65	935 years
	105	1,895 years

It is important to keep in mind that the values in the right-hand column of the display are person-years, and those in the left-hand column are frequencies. Using symbols defined in chapter 11, $a = 40$, $c = 65$, $T_e = 960$, $T_{ue} = 935$, and $T = 1895$.

Step 2: Calculate the incidence density of initial emergency urinary retention in the experimental (exposed) and control (unexposed) groups and the incidence density ratio (rate ratio) using formulas 11.8 and 11.9, respectively.

$ID_e = (a \ / \ T_e) \times 10^n = (40 \ / \ 960) \times 10^n = 0.042 \times 10^2 = 4.2$ per 100 person-years

$ID_{ue} = (c \ / \ T_{ue}) \times 10^n = (65 \ / \ 935) \times 10^n = 0.070 \times 10^2 = 7.0$ per 100 person-years

$IDR = ID_e \ / \ ID_{ue} = (4.2$ per 100 person-years$) \ / \ (7.0$ per 100 person-years$) = 0.60$

Step 3: Calculate the 95 percent confidence interval (95% CI) using formula 11.10.

$$95\% \ CI = \exp\left\{\ln(IDR) \pm 1.96\sqrt{(1/a) + (1/c)}\right\}$$
$$\exp\left\{\ln(0.60) \pm 1.96\sqrt{(1/40) + (1/65)}\right\} =$$
$$\exp\left(-0.51 \pm 1.96\sqrt{0.025 + 0.015}\right) =$$
$$\exp(-0.51 \pm 0.39)$$

The 95 percent *lower* confidence limit (LCL) is: $\exp(-0.51 - 0.39) = \exp(-0.90) = 0.40$
The 95 percent *upper* confidence limit (UCL) is: $\exp(-0.51 + 0.39) = \exp(-0.12) = 0.90$
Therefore, the 95 percent confidence interval is 0.40 to 0.90.

Step 4: Calculate the decreased percent relative effect using formula 6.5 and its 95 percent confidence interval. The 95 percent confidence interval can be calculated using formula 12.2 along with the 95 percent upper confidence limit and the 95 percent lower confidence limit already calculated for the IDR in step 3.

% Decreased Change $= (1 - Ratio) \times 100 = (1 - 0.60) \times 100 = 0.40 \times 100 = 40.0\%$

95% CI $= (1 - 95\% \ UCL \ for \ IDR) \times 100$ to $(1 - 95\% \ LCL \ for \ IDR) \times 100 =$

$(1 - 0.90) \times 100$ to $(1 - 0.40) \times 100 = 10.0\%$ to 60.0%

Thus, the 95 percent confidence interval for the percent relative effect is 10.0% to 60.0%.

Answer: Based on the data in this problem, the treatment with saw palmetto berry extract is efficacious. Those in the experimental group had a 40.0% (95% CI = 10.0% to 60.0%) reduction in initial episodes of emergency urinary retention due to BHP compared to those in the control group.

Comments:

1. This problem assumes that the investigators intended to use person-time units (i.e., person-years) in their analysis. Person-years were provided in the problem, but normally they would need to be calculated or estimated as described in chapter 5. Although not required, the tabular display provides a convenient way of exhibiting the data needed to calculate the incidence density ratio and its 95 percent confidence interval.

2. The incidence density ratio is a measure of association or effect between the exposure (treatment with the standardized saw palmetto berry extract) and the primary outcome (initial emergency urinary retention due to BHP). Since this RCT was designed to see if the intervention decreased the occurrence of the outcome, one would expect the incidence density ratio to be *less than one* if the intervention is efficacious. In this problem the ratio was 0.60. Those in the experimental group developed initial emergency urinary retention at a rate only 0.60 times as great as those in the control group (i.e., there was a 40 reduction in the primary outcome in the experimental group compared to the control group).

3. An incidence density ratio of 0.60 indicates a moderate association between the exposure and outcome (see table 6-3). Based on the 95 percent confidence interval for the incidence density ratio, we can say that we are 95 percent sure that the true ratio lies between 0.40 and 0.90, all other factors being equal. Since this interval does not contain one, we can also say that the incidence density ratio in this problem is statistically significant at $p \leq 0.05$. Statistical significance could also have been tested using the person-time chi-square test as described in chapter 11 (formula 11.13). Note that significance testing, though widely practiced, is not recommended for reasons discussed in earlier chapters. Based on the information provided in the problem, we conclude that the findings of this study support the hypothesis that saw palmetto berry extract is efficacious in reducing initial emergency urinary retention due to BHP in the study population. One could speculate whether this finding is likely to apply to other groups. Details related to compliance rates might be examined in considering whether the use of the treatment is likely to be effective (see exhibit 12-1). One could also speculate, or seek to demonstrate with additional clinical testing, if it reduces the size of enlarged prostate glands thereby improving urinary flow or acts by other mechanisms.

4. The *percent relative effect* as described in this problem is a convenient and simple way to communicate the efficacy of an experimental intervention. The percent relative effect ranges from zero to 100 percent, and the closer it is to 100 percent, the more efficacious the intervention. In this problem the percent relative effect was 40.0 percent. This indicates a 40.0 percent reduction in the outcome is due to the intervention, all other factors being equal. Since the incidence density ratio was statistically significant, and since the percent relative effect in this problem is based on the incidence density ratio, we can conclude that the percent relative effect is also statistically significant. It is more informative, however, to provide a 95 percent confidence interval for the percent relative effect. As illustrated in the solution to this problem, this can be derived from the confidence interval for the incidence density ratio. The 95 percent confidence interval for the percent relative effect also indicates statistical significance as long as it does not contain zero. Based on the calculated 95 percent confidence interval for the percent relative effect, we can be 95 percent sure that the true percent relative effect is between 10.0 percent and 60.0 percent in the study population, all other factors being equal.

A more complex way of analyzing the data from RCTs involves *survival analysis* (see exhibit 5-2). This method can be useful when follow-up periods vary widely for subjects or when the subjects enter a trial at different times.[10] Basically, in survival analysis one plots the time for each subject from application of the intervention to a nonrecurrent event, such as death, disease, or another predetermined endpoint, on a *survival curve*. Survival curves can provide data on the percent survival (time until outcome) for any given time period, median survival time for a group as a whole, and other useful information.[28] The Cox Proportional Hazards model (see exhibit 11-1) is an efficient method of multivariable survival analysis that allows one to control for several confounding factors simultaneously.[10] A more detailed discussion of survival analysis is beyond the scope of this text. Those who are interested in the topic should consult more advanced books. As indicated in chapter 11, survival analysis is also frequently used in the analysis of the results of cohort studies, particularly open cohort studies.

Subgroup Analyses

In addition to an overall analysis of the data in RCTs, many investigators perform **subgroup analyses**. These are typically performed in observational studies as well. They refer to analyses that are performed on subcategories of the study population usually based on potential risk factors for the primary outcome, such as age, sex, race/ethnicity, body mass index, exercise frequency, or prior medical conditions. The purpose of subgroup analyses is to detect effect measure modification (defined in chapter 10). Specifically, in the context of RCTs, subgroup analyses are performed to determine if certain characteristics of the study subjects "modify the effect of the intervention under study."[29(p79)] Subgroup analyses in RCTs are controversial because the findings can be misleading. Andrew Oxman and Gordon Guyatt,[29] for instance, cite an RCT where a subgroup analysis suggested that aspirin was beneficial in preventing stroke in men with cerebrovascular disease (CVD) but not in women. As a result, many women with CVD were not given aspirin therapy by their physicians until later studies discounted the original negative finding among women.

Subgroup analyses can be problematic for a number of reasons. The most serious concerns are associated with *a posteriori* comparisons (chapter 6), that is, comparisons that were not planned prior to initiation of the trial. These analyses have been referred to disparagingly as exploratory analyses, fishing expeditions, data dredging exercises, and the like. Even subgroup analyses based on *a priori* hypotheses are not immune to criticism, however. In general, subgroup analyses can increase the probability of chance findings due to smaller sample sizes, increased variance, and multiple comparisons.[30] Small sample size and increased variance decrease the power of a study to detect clinically significant differences, and multiple comparisons increase the probability of type I errors. The values of randomization may also be lost in improperly planned subgroup analyses, resulting in biased or confounded findings. This is the same problem that can occur when the findings of RCTs are based on a per protocol analysis. As a matter of fact, per protocol analysis is a type of subgroup analysis where the subgroup is defined by compliance. According to Douglas Altman and John Matthews,

> Results of tests for interactions are likely to be convincing only if they were specified at the start of the study. In any study that presents subgroup analyses it is important to specify when and why the subgroups were chosen. Studies which present analyses without such justification can be difficult to interpret.[31(p486)]

The number of subgroup analyses should also be reported, along with the reasons for deciding which findings to report.[29]

Ideally, subgroup analyses should be restricted to those that were planned prior to the start of a trial and described in the study protocol. They should be also be limited to an examination of baseline factors measured prior to the trial so as to preserve the values of randomization.[8] In addition, there should be some scientifically plausible reasons for selecting the factors.[32] *A posteriori* comparisons, if conducted, should be limited to generating hypotheses for additional study.[6] Even with these qualifications, the findings of subgroup analyses should be interpreted cautiously so as not to mislead medical or public health practice. Oxman and Guyatt[29] offer seven guidelines for evaluating the likelihood that apparent differences found in subgroup analyses are real. These are reproduced in table 12-6. While subgroup analyses are performed in all types of epidemiologic studies, they are usually of more concern in RCTs since the results are more likely to impact clinical or community practice with the potential for detrimental effects if the findings are incorrect.

Table 12-6   Guidelines for Deciding Whether Apparent Differences in Subgroup Response Are Real

1. Is the magnitude of the difference clinically important?
2. Was the difference statistically significant?
3. Did the hypothesis precede rather than follow the analysis?
4. Was the subgroup analysis one of a small number of hypotheses tested?
5. Was the difference suggested by comparisons within rather than between studies?
6. Was the difference consistent across studies?
7. Is there indirect evidence that supports the hypothesized difference?

Source: Oxman, A. D., and Guyatt, G. H. (1992). A Consumer's Guide to Subgroup Analyses. *Annals of Internal Medicine* 116: 78-84. Permission granted by the American College of Physicians.

Meta-Analysis

Besides overall and subgroup analyses of *individual* RCTs, *multiple* RCTs addressing the same research question can often be integrated in a orderly way so as to provide an overall statistical summary of the results. This process is known as **meta-analysis**. It is especially useful when individual studies tend to be inconclusive due to insufficient sample size. A properly conducted meta-analysis can provide a statistically efficient, and hence, precise estimate of the effect of a given intervention by combining the results of relevant studies in a systematic manner. Meta-analyses may also offer several other advantages, including: (a) hypotheses for future trials, (b) answers to questions not considered in the original trials, (c) consensus about the effectiveness of an intervention, and (d) explanations for differences in individual trial results. Accordingly, meta-analysis is considered an important area of epidemiologic research. This is underscored by a commonly held view that the results of any single study are unlikely to represent the final word on the effectiveness of an intervention.[33] Meta-analysis also has its limitations, however, which are discussed later in this section.

Background.   Ostensibly, meta-analysis was first defined in 1976 by Gene Glass, a researcher in the field of education. He described it in the following manner:

> Meta-analysis refers to the analysis of analyses. I use it to refer to the statistical analysis of a large collection of analysis results from individual studies for the purpose of integrating the findings. It connotes a rigorous alternative to the casual, narrative discussions of research studies which typify our attempts to make sense of the rapidly expanding research literature.[34(p3)]

As indicated in the above definition, a meta-analysis differs from a **narrative review**, such as that found in a traditional research review article. Narrative reviews tend to be subjective in that there are no established rules for the authors to follow with regard to which studies to include or exclude from the review. Moreover, it is not uncommon for authors to select studies that tend to support their own points of view.[35] Meta-analysis, on the other hand, is a type of *systematic review.* A **systematic review** (also called an **overview**) denotes a comprehensive, rigorous, and standardized approach to selecting, assessing, and synthesizing all relevant studies on a given topic.[1] Systematic reviews are designed specifically to minimize subjectivity and hence improve the accuracy of the inferences. Systematic reviews that summarize studies without combining the results statistically may be referred to as **qualitative systematic reviews**. Those that also combine study results statistically to produce an overall summary effect may be designated **quantitative systematic reviews**. Quantitative systematic reviews are therefore equivalent to meta-analyses.[36]

Meta-analyses involve more than just applying statistical techniques to combine study results. Mark Elwood[12] has summarized eight steps included in standard meta-analysis. These steps should be part of a comprehensive study protocol and may be restated as: (a) defining the research question, (b) defining the criteria for study selection, (c) finding all eligible studies, (d) reviewing the methods and results of each study critically, (e) summarizing the results of each study using a standardized format, (f) using proper statistical methods to produce a summary result when appropriate, (g) assessing variation (heterogeneity) between the studies, and (h) reviewing, interpreting, and reporting the findings.[12] As these steps indicate, standard meta-analysis is designed to be a carefully planned retrospective observational study of studies with a statistical goal of producing a summary estimate of the effect of a given exposure (e.g., treatment, procedure) on a given outcome. Some basic questions to ask when reviewing a meta-analysis are provided in table 12-7. For the most part, these are based on Elwood's summary of the steps involved meta-analysis.

As a practical example, consider a meta-analysis that was conducted to assess the effectiveness of pharyngeal anesthesia in improving patient tolerance and the ease of upper endoscopy during sedation. The authors of this study searched relevant databases for reports of RCTs in the English language that compared the efficacy of pharyngeal anesthesia to either a placebo or no treatment. Data on patient tolerance and physician assessment of the ease of the endoscopy were analyzed. Five out of a possible 53 RCTs provided interpretable data. Based on the integrated findings, the authors reported greater patient tolerance of upper endoscopy during sedation among those receiving pharyngeal anesthesia compared to those not receiving it or receiving a placebo (OR = 1.88, 95% CI = 1.13 to 3.12). They also found that physicians performing sedated upper endoscopy were more likely to rate it as "not difficult" when patients received pharyngeal anesthesia compared to when they

---

Table 12-7   Some Basic Questions to Ask When Reading a Meta-Analysis

- Was the primary research question clearly stated and appropriate?
- Were the criteria used to select studies reasonable?
- Were the selected studies comparable in terms of objectives and methods?
- Did the authors made a comprehensive search for all eligible studies?
- Were sound reasons provided for excluding studies from consideration?
- Were the studies critically and objectively reviewed?
- Were appropriate statistical methods used and adequately explained?
- Was the format for summarizing the findings appropriate and clearly presented?
- Were the findings adequately interpreted and discussed?
- Were differences in study designs taken into consideration?
- Were differences among study findings considered and explained where possible?
- Were the methods used in the meta-analysis reproducible?
- Did the authors reveal possible conflicts of interest?

did not or when they received a placebo (OR 2.60, 95% CI 1.63 to 4.17). The authors reported heterogeneity in the patient-tolerance portion of the meta-analysis due to a lack of standardized outcome measures and sedation procedures but concluded that pharyngeal anesthesia improves upper endoscopy and patient tolerance.[37] One potential weakness of this meta-analysis was restricting the universe of trials to those published in the English language.

Meta-analysis can be applied to experimental, quasi-experimental, or observational studies, although up until recently it has been most frequently employed with regard to RCTs. Use with observational studies in particular introduces more opportunities for bias and confounding because of the lack of subject randomization in these studies and less control over the study conditions. There can also be problems when findings from various types of observational designs are integrated into the same meta-analysis. Nevertheless, the popularity of meta-analysis almost assures that its use with observational studies will continue to increase.[38] Furthermore, there are many important health-related questions that RCTs cannot address due to ethical concerns. When one considers the escalating amount of research on any given health-related issue, it seems both logical and appealing to have a systematic way of summarizing the findings of multiple studies so as to provide practical guidance to medical and public health practitioners. In addition to providing an overall effect estimate where feasible, meta-analysis examines commonalities, differences, and trends in the findings of the component studies.

In one sense, meta-analysis can be thought of as a sort of "bottom line" based on a planned statistical review of the findings of multiple relevant studies. Nonetheless, a meta-analysis is *not always* the definitive word when it comes to a research question. In fact, the findings of some meta-analyses have contradicted large well-designed RCTs evaluating the same research hypothesis.[39] Like any epidemiologic study, a meta-analysis can be poorly designed, executed, and interpreted leading to erroneous conclusions. For example, meta-analyses may be influenced by the accuracy, thoroughness, objectivity, or knowledge of the researchers. They may also be limited by the quality or representativeness of the component studies. Biased studies or those with dissimilar subjects, interventions, or results may affect the accuracy of the findings from meta-analyses. Also, meta-analyses that exclude relevant studies may produce misleading findings. One potential problem in this regard is **publication bias**. This can result when the search for relevant investigations is restricted to published studies. In general, published studies tend to report positive findings more often than unpublished studies. They also tend to be unrepresentative in other ways. For example, they are usually larger studies and more likely to be studies sponsored by public or nonprofit organizations.[27] Publication bias can occur any time investigators rely too heavily on published works, and the findings from these works are not representative of all eligible studies. Preventing publication bias requires a concerted effort to identify and include unpublished reports in the meta-analysis. This may involve contacting experts in the field, reviewing registries of clinical trials, and contacting private companies dealing with the issue. Even with published research it is important to conduct a thorough search of relevant databases and registries as well as sources for identifying relevant dissertations, conference proceedings, and the like. It is also important to ensure that less well known, smaller circulation, or Internet-only journals are not overlooked. The same recommendations apply to qualitative systematic reviews. One helpful resource of information for both qualitative and quantitative systematic reviews is the **Cochrane Collaboration**, which is "an international, non-profit, independent organization, established to ensure that up to date, accurate information about the effects of healthcare interventions is readily available worldwide."[40] Formed in 1993 by epidemiologist and physician Archie Cochrane, the Cochrane Collaboration consists of Collaborative Review Groups that prepare, maintain, and update qualitative and quantitative systematic reviews that are contained in the Cochrane Library along with the Cochrane Controlled Trials Register, a database of RCTs, and other important and useful resources.[40] A detailed summary of the resources of the Cochrane Collaboration may be found by visiting their main Web site at http://www.cochrane.org.

In an effort to enhance the value of the information that can be gained from meta-analyses, modifications have been introduced over the years. **Cumulative meta-analysis**, for example, involves repeating a meta-analysis each time a new study meeting the eligibility criteria has been conducted.[35] It can be thought of as being analogous to a sequential trial in that interim analyses are performed each time new data become available. Rather than being static, this type of meta-analysis is ongoing and therefore always current. Also, while the standard meta-analysis is retrospective in nature (i.e., the investigators review studies that have already been conducted), a relatively new variety of meta-analysis takes a prospective approach. This type of meta-analysis is known as a **prospective meta-analysis**. It is one in which the studies "are identified, evaluated and determined to be eligible before the results of any of the studies become known."[41] In contrast to retrospective designs, prospective meta-analyses allow the research questions, the study selection criteria, and the proposed analyses, including any subgroup analyses, to be planned *before* the results of the component studies are available.[41] This reduces the potential for bias that this foreknowledge might introduce into a meta-analysis.

Perhaps a good conclusion to this short introduction to meta-analysis is that expressed by Janice Pogue and Salim Yusuf of McMaster University in Hamilton, Ontario. In a persuasive article on improving meta-analysis they wrote:

> For a meta-analysis to give definitive information, it should meet at least the minimum standards that would be expected of a well-designed, adequately powered, and carefully conducted randomised controlled trial. These minimum standards include both qualitative characteristics—a prospective protocol, comparable definitions of key outcomes, quality control of data, and inclusion of all patients from all trials in the final

analysis—and quantitative standards—an assessment of whether the total sample is large enough to provide reliable results and the use of appropriate statistical monitoring guidelines to indicate when the results of the accumulating data of a meta-analysis are conclusive. We believe that rigorous meta-analyses undertaken according to these principles will lead to more reliable evidence about the efficacy and safety of interventions than either retrospective meta-analysis or individual trials.[42(p47)]

Statistical procedures. A detailed discussion of the statistical procedures involved in meta-analysis is beyond the scope of this chapter. However, it should be helpful to highlight briefly some of the more common approaches used to create statistical summaries. More comprehensive information on this topic can be found in many advanced or specialized texts on the topic.

Broadly speaking, there are two major approaches to integrating ("pooling") the findings of individual studies in a meta-analysis. One is based on what has been referred to as an **equal effects model**.[43] This model is based on the assumption that the underlying effect is *equal* in all studies included in the meta-analysis. Therefore, it is assumed that the reported effects for each component study differ only because of random error. In practice, this model is more commonly called a **fixed effects model**.* Therefore, you should be aware of this terminology. The second approach is based on what is commonly referred to as a **random effects model**. It is based on the assumption that the underlying effect *varies* in each component study due to actual differences in effect as well as random error.[44] In general, when the findings of the component studies are similar, both models produce about the same summary estimate, although the associated confidence interval tends to be wider with the random effects model.[44] When the findings of the component studies vary appreciably, the models can be expected to produce divergent results. Because of the assumption inherent in the random effects model, it is important to look not only at the summary estimate of effect when using this model but the distribution of effects as well.[45]

Given the foregoing, what model should be used in a particular instance? Since the models are based on unverifiable assumptions, there is no easy answer to this question. Generally speaking, it is sometimes recommended that a test of heterogeneity (see chapter 10) be performed to see if different results among the component studies of a meta-analysis are more or less likely to be due to chance alone. If the test results indicate that the different findings are *unlikely* to be due to chance alone, then the random effects model

---

*Technically, a fixed effects model is based on the assumption that the effects in the component studies are fixed but unknown quantities.[43] Use of the model further "assumes that the differences between the studies are so important that pooling is not indicated and that individual effect sizes should be retained."[43(p131)] An equal effects model is also based on the assumption that the effects of the component studies are fixed but unknown quantities but that they are *random* estimates of one effect. Therefore, pooling is indicated. Thus, the term "fixed effects model" can be ambiguous when used without explanation. Equal effects model, however, is a more precise term that avoids this confusion.

would be more appropriate; if not, the equal effects model would be satisfactory.[27] Others suggest using both models. If the summary effects are similar then either model is acceptable; if they differ, however, the one showing the more conservative result is recommended.[45] One problem with tests of heterogeneity is that they tend to have low power when the number of studies in a meta-analysis is small and "excessive" power when the number of studies is large.[46] A proposed alternative to a standard test of heterogeneity is I^2. According to its developers, I^2 is a new measure that quantifies the "degree of inconsistency" among the results of studies comprising a meta-analysis. The measure ranges from zero to 100 percent with zero indicating no heterogeneity and 100 percent indicating maximal heterogeneity. Tentative guidelines assign I^2 values of 25 percent, 50 percent, and 75 percent as markers of low, moderate, and high inconsistency, respectively. In addition to quantifying the extent of apparent heterogeneity in study results, I^2 has the advantages of allowing comparisons among meta-analyses that have different numbers of component studies, studies of different designs, and studies using different effect measures.[46] An *uncertainty interval*, which is analogous to a confidence interval, can be calculated for I^2 to assess the precision of the measure. More is said about heterogeneity in meta-analysis near the end of this section on meta-analysis.

Where the results of a meta-analysis are expressed dichotomously, the odds ratio (OR) is a common and convenient measure of effect to use.[44] Common alternatives include the risk ratio and risk difference, although other familiar and less familiar measures may also be used. When the data are continuous, the *mean difference* or *standardized mean difference* is often employed. Our discussion, however, will focus on dichotomous measures.

Two frequently used techniques for producing summary estimates of effect based on an *equal effects model* are the **Mantel-Haenszel method** and the **Peto method**. You should already be familiar with the Mantel-Haenszel method, which is often used with stratification in case-control studies (chapter 10), and sometimes in cohort studies as well (chapter 11), to produce a summary measure of association. It is used in the same way in meta-analysis but where the individual studies comprise the strata. Basically, a weighted average of the study-specific measures of effect are used to produce a Mantel-Haenszel estimate of effect. Appropriate confidence intervals or tests of significance are then applied to this estimate. In the Peto method, an overall summary odds ratio (OR_S) can be calculated by first producing 2 × 2 tables for each component study and then determining the number of observed (O_i) and expected (E_i) events in the experimental groups. The differences between the observed and expected events for each study are then summed and divided by the sum of the variances of the expected number of events (V_i) in each component study. The exponential (exp; defined in chapter 9) of this equation produces the OR_S as follows:[12]

(12.3) $$OR_S = \exp\left(\Sigma\,(O_i - E_i)\,/\,\Sigma\,V_i\right)$$

The subscript i in formula 12.3 represents each individual study estimate so that if there are five studies in the meta-analysis, we will have O_1 through O_5, E_1 through E_5, and so on. The calculation of the expected events and variances is not discussed here, but concise examples can be found in Elwood's text.[12] Other methods of calculating summary estimates based on an equal effects model are also commonly used. The methods used to estimate summary effects based on a *random effects model* tend to be more complicated and are not discussed here.

There are several available computer application programs that will perform the statistical procedures involved in a meta-analysis. These programs typically generate descriptive diagrams known as **forest plots**, which are usually reproduced in published meta-analyses. These provide readers with a visual representation of the effect estimates and applicable confidence intervals for each component study as well as the "pooled" estimate and its confidence interval.[44, 47]

Figure 12-6 shows an example of a forest plot from a published meta-analysis of observational studies testing the hypothesis that abuse during pregnancy is a risk factor for low birth weight. The analysis is based on an equal effects (fixed effects) model using the odds ratio as the measure of effect.[48] As is typical of forest plots, the squares represent point estimates of the effects measured in each component study with the relative size of the squares weighted according to the influence they are to have on the overall estimate. Commonly used weights include study sample size, proportion of study outcomes, inverse of the study variance, indexes of study quality, and other factors.[49] Different summary measures have different weighting systems. For example, the weights for the Mantel-Haenszel estimate of the odds ratio depend on the number of observations in each stratum (i.e., study).[12] The horizontal lines running through the squares represent the applicable confidence intervals (usually 95 percent), and the solid vertical line indicates no effect (e.g., OR = 1.0). At the bottom of the forest plot there is usually a diamond-shaped object that corresponds to the overall summary estimate of effect with its confidence limits equal to the outer horizontal tips of the diamond.[47] In figure 12-6, the pooled estimate of effect based on the meta-analysis is an OR of 1.36 (95% CI = 1.06 to 1.75). The study-specific ORs range from 0.84 to 1.75 with the smallest estimate coming from a study assigned a relatively small weight based on the inverse of the variance in the study. This small weight is reflected by the small size of the square. The relatively high variance in this study is also indicated by the wide 95 percent confidence interval (noted by the length of the horizontal line through the square).

Overall, the results of the meta-analysis in this example suggest that abuse during pregnancy increases the odds of low birth weight offspring by 36 percent. Before any firm conclusions are drawn, however, one needs to consider the soundness of the meta-analysis as a whole. For example, are the studies represented in the meta-analysis sufficiently inclusive of all relevant studies on the topic and sufficiently exclusive of irrelevant studies? Some

Figure 12-6   Example of a Forest Plot Based on a Meta-Analysis of Eight Studies Assessing the Relationship between Abuse during Pregnancy and Low Birth Weight (LBW) Outcomes

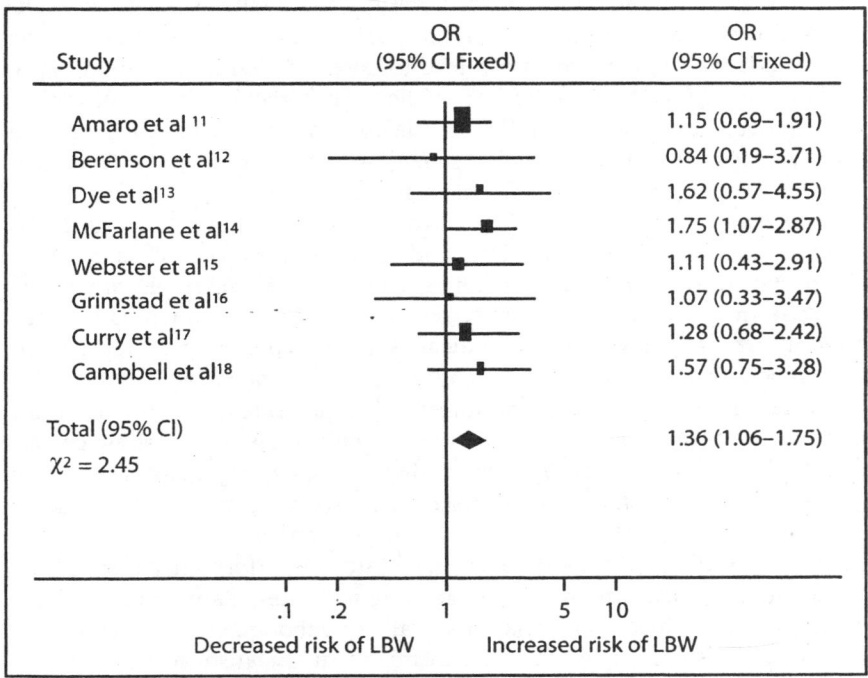

Study	OR (95% CI Fixed)	OR (95% CI Fixed)
Amaro et al [11]		1.15 (0.69–1.91)
Berenson et al[12]		0.84 (0.19–3.71)
Dye et al[13]		1.62 (0.57–4.55)
McFarlane et al[14]		1.75 (1.07–2.87)
Webster et al[15]		1.11 (0.43–2.91)
Grimstad et al[16]		1.07 (0.33–3.47)
Curry et al[17]		1.28 (0.68–2.42)
Campbell et al[18]		1.57 (0.75–3.28)
Total (95% CI) $\chi^2 = 2.45$		1.36 (1.06–1.75)

.1   .2   1   5   10

Decreased risk of LBW   Increased risk of LBW

Source: Murphy, C. C., Schei, B., Myhr, T. L., and DuMont, J. (2001). Abuse: A Risk Factor for Low Birth Weight? A Systematic Review and Meta-analysis. Reprinted from *Canadian Medical Association Journal* 29 May 2001; 164 (11), pp. 1567–1572 by permission of the publisher. © Canadian Medical Association.

other important questions to ask are listed in Table 12-7. One should be able to obtain answers to these questions from the qualitative portion of the meta-analysis. The main point is that one needs to look deeper than just the statistical summary of effect when reviewing the results of a meta-analysis. The next segment deals with the sometimes challenging issue of *heterogeneity.*

Assessing heterogeneity.   An important consideration in meta-analysis is an assessment of **heterogeneity,** which, broadly defined, refers to differences among the component studies of a meta-analysis. These differences may be due to variations in the study interventions, outcomes, or subjects (sometimes called **clinical heterogeneity** or **clinical diversity**) or to differences in trial design or quality (sometimes called **methodological heterogeneity** or **methodological diversity**). Heterogeneity is most often reflected in differences in the effect estimates among the component studies of a meta-analysis (sometimes referred to as **statistical heterogeneity**).[50] Since statistical heterogeneity may represent nonrandom differences, it should be examined in a meta-analysis, especially if it is substantial. Ideally, the studies included in a meta-analysis using an *equal effects model* should be **homogenous**, that is, similar in terms of study interventions, outcomes, subjects, design, and quality, so that the results are consistent except for random variation. If not, the underlying assumption of the model is violated, which can lead to false conclusions and inappropriate recommendations for medical or public health practice. Apparent statistical heterogeneity, however, could be due to chance in which instance an overly zealous examination of heterogeneity would be misguided.[51] Thus, statistical heterogeneity presents a dilemma for epidemiologists. Is it real, or is it a just a result of random error? The answer to this question has implications for the model used in meta-analysis and for other decisions. As a practical matter, statistical heterogeneity is of most concern when the results are widely divergent. In a forest plot this may be seen when there are numerous *non-overlapping* horizontal lines, which, as indicated earlier, represent confidence intervals. When the horizontal lines tend to overlap, statistical heterogeneity should be of less concern. In the forest plot represented in figure 12-6, for example, the confidence intervals all overlap indicating at least some consistency in the results of the component studies. Thus, heterogeneity is less likely to be a major issue in the study represented by this forest plot, and the choice of an equal effects (fixed effects) model seems reasonable.

Notwithstanding the above remarks, researchers performing a meta-analysis need to take great care in the selection and inclusion of appropriate studies so as not to introduce unnecessary clinical or methodological heterogeneity. They should also anticipate factors that might cause statistical heterogeneity and make provisions for an examination of these factors in the study protocol.

On a practical level, there are several strategies that can be used to deal with apparent heterogeneity in a meta-analysis.[50]

- *Do not perform a meta-analysis.* Sometimes serious concerns about clinical or methodological diversity are best handled by limiting the analysis to a qualitative systematic review. When a meta-analysis shows substantial statistical heterogeneity, especially when the effects differ widely in direction and the confidence intervals do not overlap, a single summary estimate of effect is unlikely to be meaningful.

- *Conduct a subgroup analysis.* Subgroup analyses may be helpful in identifying factors causing the heterogeneity. One needs to be very cautious, however, in performing subgroup analyses for the same reasons discussed earlier in this chapter with regard to individual RCTs. Unless the subgroup analyses have been pre-specified in the study protocol, along with a logical rationale, they should be considered exploratory at best (i.e., hypothesis generating for future studies).

- *Perform a meta-analysis based on a random effects model.* This option was mentioned earlier in this section. While it is one way of dealing with heterogeneous results, it should only be used only when the heterogeneity cannot be readily explained by other factors. In other words, it is not a substitute for examining potential sources of clinical and methodological heterogeneity in a meta-analysis.

- *Change the effect measure used in the meta-analysis.* In some circumstances, certain effect measures may introduce an artificial heterogeneity in a meta-analysis. Using a different effect measure may help to detect this.
- *Perform a sensitivity analysis.* **Sensitivity analyses** are "secondary analyses carried out by varying the assumptions that are made about the data and models used. . . . The purpose of such analyses is to see if the results and conclusions from a study are robust."[5(p177)] An example would be excluding studies of poor quality in a meta-analysis to see if their exclusion makes any difference in the overall measure of effect. The idea is to calculate the summary effect before and after certain changes in the analysis so as to identify possible explanations for the statistical heterogeneity. Subgroup analyses can also be performed as sensitivity analyses.

   Concluding remarks.   It should be helpful at this point to refer to some of the terms and issues described in this section in the context of an actual meta-analysis. Two medical researchers, one from the University of British Columbia and the other from the University of Alberta, teamed up to "reconduct" a meta-analysis of RCTs assessing the efficacy of β-blockers in the treatment of hypertension.[52] The motivation for the review was a recent and widely publicized meta-analysis on the topic concluding that β-blockers should no longer be a first choice in the treatment of hypertension.

   In discussing the findings of the previous meta-analysis, the researchers pointed out several potential flaws: (a) not all relevant trials were included in the meta-analysis, (b) the study outcome was inconsistent with that used in most trials on the topic and even with most outcomes examined in the meta-analysis, and (c) the data used in the study were clinically and statistically heterogeneous. To overcome these problems, the researchers sought to include all relevant trials, to define the study outcome in accordance with those most frequently reported in clinical trials, and to explore and explain heterogeneity as it relates to age differences (i.e., patients less than 60 years of age and patients 60 years of age and older). The subgroup analysis based on age groups was apparently decided upon *a priori*, and the grouping selected was based prior research findings. To locate appropriate trials for possible inclusion in their meta-analysis, the authors searched major databases (i.e., MEDLINE and the Cochrane Library) and contacted experts in the field. A total of 21 trials were included in the review involving over 145,000 subjects. Because of suspected heterogeneity, the analysis was based on a random effects model. Forest plots were produced for those studies that included a placebo in the trial (see figure 12-7) as well as for the other studies. The effect measure was the risk ratio, and 95 percent confidence intervals were calculated. Sensitivity analyses were performed based on study intervention differ-

Figure 12-7   Example of Forest Plots Based on a Meta-Analysis Assessing the Efficacy of Beta Blockers on Hypertension in Randomized Controlled Trials Employing Placebos

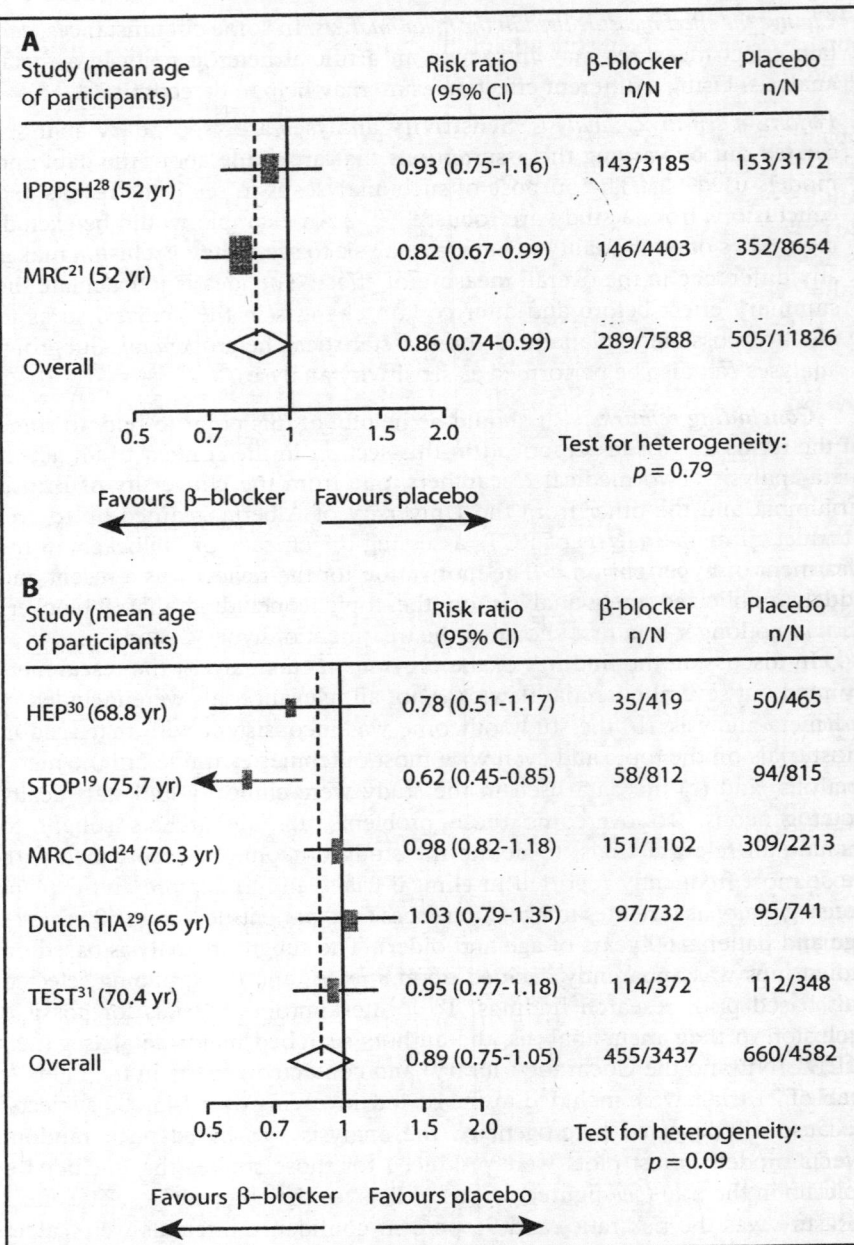

Source: Khan, N., and McAlister, F. A. (2006). Re-examining the Efficacy of B-blockers for the Treatment of Hypertension: A Meta-analysis. Reprinted from *Canadian Medical Association Journal* 06 June 2006; 174 (12), pp. 1737–1742 by permission of the publisher. © Canadian Medical Association.

ences and other factors, and the results remained robust. Although the researchers reached essentially the same conclusion as those conducting the previous meta-analysis (i.e., that β-blockers should not be the first line of defense against hypertension unless there were other indications for its use) in the older patients, they reached a *different* conclusion with regard to the younger group of patients (i.e., that β-blockers should remain an option). The implications for medical practice are significant.

As this study illustrates, conducting a meta-analysis requires a great deal of planning and anticipation concerning potential issues such as heterogeneity. Because the results of a meta-analysis can affect medical and public health policy, it is critical that the authors do a thorough, careful, and accurate job that is subject to adequate peer review. Poorly conducted meta-analyses do not serve to advance knowledge and practice in medicine and public health. In fact, they are more likely to undermine them.

MAJOR ADVANTAGES AND DISADVANTAGES OF RANDOMIZED CONTROLLED TRIALS

The major advantages and disadvantages of RCTs are summarized in table 12-8. The most significant advantage of RCTs is their ability to demonstrate causal relationships when well designed and conducted. As indicated earlier in this chapter, RCTs have certain design features that enhance their internal validity. Randomization, in particular, tends to assure that the experimental and control groups in RCTs are similar with regard to anticipated and even unanticipated prognostic factors. This effectively controls confounding. It also eliminates selection bias in subject assignments. In addition, it is generally easier to blind (mask) subjects and investigators in RCTs than in analytic studies. Double blinding, when possible, helps to prevent certain forms of information bias (e.g., diagnostic suspicion bias) and tends to reduce certain types of post-randomization confounding that can occur during the follow-up period of a trial. Another significant advantage of RCTs is that the investigators have direct control over the exposure. This permits them to establish precise doses or detailed procedures most appropriate to the trial. Such levels of precision or detail can rarely be achieved in analytic studies. Because of these strengths RCTs are widely accepted as the gold standard of epidemiologic studies. They are also the basis for many established medical and public health practices, such as the use of statin drugs in the prevention and management of heart disease, the use of streptokinase as a "clot buster" in cases of acute myocardial infarction, and vaccination for measles and other communicable diseases.

Despite their significant advantages, RCTs have a number of potential disadvantages. One of the chief weaknesses of RCTs has to do with their limited applicability. As suggested earlier in this chapter, ethical concerns limit the use of RCTs to circumstances of uncertainty. There must be enough confidence in the potential benefits of a medical intervention, for example, to expose some

Table 12-8   Major Advantages and Disadvantages of Randomized Controlled Trials

Advantages	Disadvantages
1. They can provide convincing evidence of causal relationships if well designed and conducted.	1. They have limited applicability due to ethical considerations and possibly the artificial setting of the experiment.
2. They allow investigators to control exposure levels so as to achieve the desired level of precision.	2. They may have limited external validity due to a reliance on volunteers and use of generally strict eligibility requirements.
	3. They can be expensive and time consuming to organize and conduct.
	4. They may be subject to bias due to differential rates of compliance, withdrawals, or losses to follow up among the experimental and control groups.
	5. It may be difficult to achieve adequate sample size due to a reliance on volunteers and strict eligibility criteria.
	6. They may require large sample size to detect small but clinically significant differences.

individuals to it but not so much confidence that it would be unethical not to offer it to others as well. Ethical considerations would also preclude, for example, an RCT to examine the effects of ionizing radiation exposure on the development of cataracts because it would be unethical to expose individuals to a known biological hazard without any expected benefits. This is why RCTs generally focus on interventions that have the potential to *reduce* rather than increase the risks of morbidity or mortality. In some cases, RCTs may need to be concluded early on ethical grounds because of cumulating evidence that the intervention is either highly beneficial or harmful to participants. Randomized controlled trials are also limited in their applicability by the fact that they tend to address narrowly focused questions in relatively artificial settings. The relevance of the findings to the real world is not always clear. That is to say, what seems to work well in an experimental situation may not work as well in real life. For example, having subjects following a strict low-fat vegan diet to reduce the progression of atherosclerosis may prove to be efficacious in an experimental setting but may not be very effective in actual life situations.

Another disadvantage of RCTs relates to their reliance on volunteers and the use of generally strict eligibility criteria. Volunteers are necessary in RCTs partly because of the potential health risks associated with many experimental treatments. Generally strict eligibility criteria are also necessary in order to protect the integrity of the experiment and the safety of the participants as well as to help ensure the successful completion of the trial. Unfortunately, the resulting study population is often quite different from the original source population or any other identifiable population for that matter. This will limit the generalizability of the findings and hence the external validity of the study. Neither the use of volunteers nor strict eligibility criteria, however, will have a negative impact on the internal validity of a trial. In fact, they should enhance it.

A further disadvantage of RCTs is the amount of time and money that are generally required to organize and carry out a reasonably sized trial, especially one that may require many years of follow up due to the nature and frequency of the defined study outcome. Prevention trials concerned with the prevention of chronic diseases, for example, may take years to complete at relatively high costs due to the long induction and latency periods and the relatively low incidence of the outcomes. One way to partially short circuit these problems is to focus on indicators of the outcomes (e.g., reduction in certain risk factors) rather than on the diseases per se.

Randomized controlled trials also have the potential disadvantage of the bias that can be introduced when there are differential rates of compliance, withdrawal, or losses to follow up between the experimental and control groups. If any of these factors are significant, they can alter the magnitude or direction of the effect measure. To minimize bias resulting from these sources, it is often helpful to: (a) exclude individuals who are likely to deviate from the study protocol at the outset of the study, (b) make the intervention as simple to comply with as possible, (c) maintain close contact with the subjects throughout the trial, (d) encourage participation by emphasizing the scientific importance of the study, and (e) follow up withdrawals or other losses or their family or friends to determine subject outcomes wherever possible.[6] Getting information on compliance, withdrawals, and losses to follow up is very important since it can be used to substantiate or refute the findings of a study. Sometimes where losses cannot be traced it is advisable to assume that none and all received the intervention and none and all had the study outcome so as to determine the potential range of the study results. In general, noncompliance, withdrawals and losses to follow up, even if equally distributed among the experimental and control groups, will diminish the power of a study. The RCTs most likely to experience problems with noncompliance, withdrawals, or losses to follow up are those that involve long, complex protocols; interventions with disagreeable side effects; or patients with severe or fatal diseases who fail to respond to the intervention. Some of the latter may seek other interventions during the course of the study, possibly introducing systematic errors.

Reliance on volunteers and use of strict eligibility requirements can not only affect the external validity of a trial as indicated above, but they can also make it difficult to recruit a sufficient number of subjects to answer the research questions reliably. In some cases there may be barely enough volunteers for a study, and the eligibility requirements may limit that number even further. If there are also significant withdrawals or losses to follow up, the effective sample size may be too small to detect modest but clinically significant differences between the experimental and control groups. Finally, because most RCTs are designed to detect relatively small effects, the number of subjects required for a study can be substantial. It is not uncommon for investigators of RCTs to look for benefits that represent a modest 10 to 20 percent reduction in the frequency of adverse outcomes.[6] Detecting a difference as little as 10 percent with 95 percent confidence where the expected incidence of the study outcome in the control group is 10 percent would require about 20,000 subjects in *both* the experimental and control arms of an RCT employing a parallel group design.

GROUP RANDOMIZED TRIALS

Group randomized trials (GRTs), also frequently referred to as *cluster randomized trials* and sometimes **community trials*** or similar names (see table 4-2), were introduced briefly in chapter 4. In a nutshell, they are planned epidemiologic experiments in which *groups of people* (i.e., clusters of people) are randomly allocated to experimental (intervention) or control conditions in order to evaluate the effectiveness of one or more interventions. A distinctive feature of GRTs is that the units of assignment are intact groups of people versus individual persons. These groups may be defined geographically (e.g., neighborhoods, census tracts, communities), socially (e.g., religious congregations, social organizations), or structurally (e.g., worksites, schools, hospitals).[53] In the medical field they often represent physician practices. Like RCTs, GRTs should be guided by a detailed study protocol that includes study objectives and hypotheses, research methods, proposed statistical analyses, ethical considerations, and other pertinent matters related to their design and implementation.

This part of the chapter focuses on the rationale for GRTs, some important methodological issues, basic approaches to analysis, and common design variations. Ethical issues are also addressed. In general, the methods for GRTs are more complex than those for RCTs. When properly conceived and conducted, however, GRTs are considered the gold standard for evaluating interventions applied to groups.[54]

Reasons for Conducting Group Randomized Trials

There are three commonly cited reasons for undertaking a GRT as opposed to an RCT when assessing an intervention.

- The intervention may be more appropriate at the group level.
- The intervention group may be "contaminated" by members of the control group.
- The intervention may be more convenient at the group level.

---

*The term community trial encompasses both randomized and nonrandomized designs. It is also frequently assumed to apply only to studies involving entire communities, although this is not the case. Group (or cluster) randomized trials is a more precise term in that it denotes randomization and implies a broader applicability.[53]

With regard to the first reason, consider a GRT "that implemented and evaluated a community-organizing effort to change community policies and practices to reduce youth access to alcohol."[55(p209)] The study intervention was implemented in seven communities with eight other communities serving as controls.[55] It is difficult to conceive how this intervention could be tested in an RCT since the intervention involved changing community-wide policies and practices. Therefore, communities were the appropriate units to randomize to the intervention and control conditions. In general, interventions that are applicable to groups versus individuals are most appropriately tested among groups. Hence, interventions like health education programs, mass media safety campaigns, or policy changes in physician practices are more appropriately applied to groups of people than to individual subjects.

The second common reason for conducting a GRT instead of an RCT is to avoid what is generally termed *contamination*. **Contamination,** in this context, effectively represents *crossovers* (defined earlier) from the control group to the experimental group. Consider, for example, an RCT conducted at a well-baby clinic at a large county health department. The purpose of the trial is to determine if one ten-minute self-hypnosis session a week effectively relieves maternal stress. If the mothers in the experimental group tell mothers in the control group about the technique, the mothers in the control may decide to try it on their own. This "contamination" would tend to bias the findings of the trial toward the null value (i.e., no effect). A suitably conducted GRT could significantly reduce or eliminate this contamination if the intervention was offered to all mothers at the clinic, and the control groups comprised mothers attending well-baby clinics in other counties where contact with the mothers in the intervention group would be unlikely. The same problem could occur in a medical practice experiment. For example, say an RCT is designed to determine if offering patients with moderately elevated cholesterol levels a free information packet on recommended dietary and lifestyle modifications, along with coupons for free or discounted items and services, will result in lower cholesterol levels after 12 and 24 weeks, respectively. Eligible patients are randomly assigned to receive from their physician either the intervention or the standard verbal recommendation to follow a prudent diet and exercise program. Contamination could occur in this setting in more than one way. The patients in the experimental group might share the information packets and coupons with friends or acquaintances who happen to be in the control group, and the participating physicians might provide them to selected control subjects. This contamination can occur with good intentions. Perhaps some patients in the experimental group are excited about the information and coupons and are not aware that their contacts are in the control group. Also, it could be that the participating physicians feel obligated to provide the packets and coupons to anyone requesting them or to those patients they believe would be most likely to benefit from them regardless of their study group assignment. A better approach would be to randomly assign the physicians to the intervention or control conditions. In this case, the physicians represent groups, that is, their collective patients. A physician in the intervention group would supply the information packet and coupons to all his or her patients with moderately elevated cholesterol levels, and a physician in the control group would provide his or her patients with the standard verbal recommendation. This would tend to avoid contamination as long as the participating physicians are not in such close contact with each that they introduce the contamination. Finally, it should be interesting to note that a sort of "contamination," broadly defined, within an intervention group *of a GRT* can be considered beneficial. It is a way of dispersing the intervention among the members of the group.[56]

Group randomized trials may also be employed for reasons of convenience or practicality. Sometimes it is less expensive or problematic to randomize intact groups in a trial than it is to assemble, screen, and assign individuals. This may be true, for example, in a large school. Assigning entire classes to the intervention and control conditions may be more convenient and cost efficient than assigning individual students to newly created experimental and control groups.

Major Methodological Issues

There are several methodological issues that need to be considered in conducting GRTs. Failure to address these adequately can affect the validity or precision of a study, possibly leading to spurious findings. A thorough discussion of these issues is beyond the scope of this textbook. Those wanting a detailed discussion are referred to classic texts, such as that by David M. Murray,[53] or other more recent works dealing with the design and analysis of GRTs.

We will focus on three important and overlapping methodological issues facing those who conduct GRTs. One of these has to do with the *number of groups or clusters* in the experiment. When the number is small, it is less likely that randomization will achieve its goal of reducing selection bias and confounding.[53, 54] Using a small number of groups also decreases the power of a GRT, resulting in a loss of precision. Another significant issue that must be dealt with is the *expectation that individuals within groups may be more alike in their responses than individuals between groups.*[57] Since standard statistical procedures do not take this into account when individuals outcomes are of interest, appropriate changes must be made in the design and analysis of GRTs compared to RCTs. Failure to deal with this issue can result in an overestimation of the precision of the findings as evidenced by artificially narrow confidence intervals or small p-values associated with statistical tests of significance. A third interrelated issue concerns the *units of inference,* that is, the units on whom the data are collected *and* to whom the results are to be applied. These units can affect the design, analysis, and interpretation of GRTs.[58] These three related methodological issues and their repercussions are described briefly in the following segments.

Number of groups.   Ideally, selection bias and confounding can be controlled in GRTs by randomization because it increases the probability that potential sources of these errors will be evenly distributed among the study conditions. In this regard, group randomization works best when the number of groups or clusters is large. When the number of groups is small, the probability of assignment to intervention or control conditions will still be the same with randomization, but the sources of systematic errors may not be because they may not have been evenly distributed among the groups prior to randomization. Consider, for example, a GRT with just two groups, one of which is comprised of a significantly older population than the other. Randomization will assure that each group has the same probability of being assigned to intervention or control conditions, but it will not change the different age distributions of these groups. One of the study groups will still be older than the other after randomization since entire groups and not individuals are being assigned. If age is a confounder, that confounder will not be controlled by randomization. Now consider a GRT where there are 50 groups to be randomly allocated to intervention or control conditions. Say that 10 of these groups differ significantly with regard to age. It is much more likely that randomization of the 50 groups will result in a balance where there are approximately the same number of older and younger groups assigned to both the intervention and control conditions. Thus, the more groups the better the chances that randomization will achieve its goal of reducing selection bias and confounding in GRTs. Studies in which there are only two groups (one per condition) are unable to distinguish the effects of the intervention from the natural variability between the groups. Therefore, they are not recommended for GRTs.[56] A small number of groups also affects the precision of a GRT by reducing its power. The power of a GRT is partly dependent on the number of groups, much more so than the number of individuals within the groups. This problem is addressed in the following segment. In general, GRTs should employ as many groups as possible, and generally no less than four groups in each study arm.[56] In fact, some authors believe that "it is unusual for a GRT to have adequate power with fewer than 8 to 10 groups per condition."[54(p424)] An adequate number of groups is especially important when the intervention effect is expected to be small.[56]

Within group similarity.   While entire groups are randomized to intervention and control conditions in GRTs, the units of observation are usually individuals, as they are in RCTs. In RCTs, however, individual outcomes are assumed to be independent of each other. This assumption is *not* tenable in GRTs. The reason is that individuals in the same group tend to be more alike than individuals in different groups, and, therefore, they are more likely to have similar outcomes. This is usually explained by one or more of following reasons: (a) common influences in their surroundings; (b) shared ideas, experiences, or values; or (c) self selection into groups.[57] Members of the same household, for example, are more likely to respond to a dietary intervention in the same way than members of different households, probably because of qualities they share in common. This tendency to be similar within groups is sometimes referred to as the **clustering effect**.[59] It is an important phenomenon in GRTs and is reflected in a measure known as the **intraclass** (or **intra-**

cluster) correlation coefficient, which represents the correlation between individual outcomes in the same group.[60] It is important to note, however, that the clustering effect depends on *both* the intraclass correlation coefficient *and* the size of the groups in a GRT.[61] This relationship is demonstrated following a short description of the intraclass correlation coefficient.

The formula for the intraclass correlation coefficient in the above context is:

(12.4)
$$ICC = \frac{SD_B^2}{SD_B^2 + SD_W^2}$$

The term SD_B^2 is the variance in the outcome between groups, and SD_W^2 is the variance in the outcome within groups. Note that the variances are equivalent to the squares of the standard deviations (SDs). The ICC, often designated as **rho** (ρ), is the intraclass (or intracluster) correlation coefficient. In practice, ρ ranges from zero to one. The greater the clustering effect, the greater the ICC. Conversely, the smaller the clustering effect, the smaller the ICC. In general, ICCs tend to be relatively small, typically less than 0.05. Although the ICC is an indication of the degree of correlation between individual outcomes within the same group, it is more precisely defined as the proportion of the total variation in the outcome that is due to the variation between the groups.[56]

The ICC is important because it takes into account the two sources of variation in individual outcomes from GRTs—that within groups and that between groups. Standard statistical methods, such as those used with RCTs, do not account for the variation between groups. Hence, if used to measure individual outcomes from GRTs, they can significantly underestimate the total variance, which can lead to an inflated assessment of the precision of the findings as evidenced by artificially narrow confidence intervals or small p-values compared to those of similarly sized RCTs. Also, standard sample size calculations used in the design of a GRT will tend to underestimate the actual sample size needed to achieve the same level of power as a similarly sized RCT.[56, 62] This underestimation can sometimes be dramatic.[62, 63]

To illustrate this latter problem, we can calculate the *effective sample size* for a GRT using formula 12.5 below. In this context, effective sample size corresponds to the sample size of a GRT after *adjusting* for the clustering effect.[64] This is a slightly different definition than that used for effective sample size earlier in this chapter, though the concept is similar.

(12.5)
$$ESS = \frac{mk}{1 + \rho(m+1)}$$

In this formula, m = the average number of subjects per group in the trial;* k = the number of groups, and ρ = the intraclass correlation coefficient. Estimates of ρ for sample size calculations are often obtained from pre-

---

*If the groups in the trial vary significantly in size, a weighted average should be used instead.[62]

viously published studies with similar objectives using similar populations or from pilot studies conducted on the population of interest. In addition, several investigators have compiled these for use with specific populations. The denominator of the ESS is commonly known as the **design effect** or the **variance inflation factor**. The design effect expresses the ratio of the number of subjects needed in a GRT to the number of subjects needed in a comparable RCT in order to achieve the same level of statistical efficiency or power, all other factors being equal.[65] It can be thought of as a *correction factor* for the clustering effect. As noted earlier, the clustering effect depends on the ICC (ρ) *as well as* the sample size in each group (m), which the formula for the design effect takes into account.

Assume a GRT is being planned throughout a large school district including 10 elementary schools with the objective of determining if frequent safety messages and demonstrations at school reduce playground injuries. Five fourth-grade classes in five different schools are to receive the intervention, and five fourth-grade classes in five other schools are to serve as controls. The average class size will be 40 students, and the estimated ICC based on a similar study is 0.03. The ESS is calculated as follows:

$$\text{ESS} = [40 \times 10] / [1 + 0.03 (40 - 1)] = 400 / 2.17 = 184$$

Although the researchers plan to enroll 400 students (mk = $40 \times 10 = 400$) in the trial, the *effective sample size* is only 184. Since power is related to sample size, this indicates that the power of the study will be substantially less than the planned enrollment size might have suggested based on standard sample size calculations. In other words, the power of the study should be based on a sample of 184 students versus a sample size of 400. The *design effect* or *variance inflation factor* in this example is a rather large 2.17. This tells us that we would need 2.17 times the required sample size for an individually randomized trial to achieve the same level of power. If a comparable RCT with a sample size of 400 students had 85 percent power, we would need $2.17 \times 400 = 868$ students in a GRT just to achieve that same level of power, all other factors being equal.

It is important to keep in mind that the design effect depends on both the ICC *and* the average group sample size of a GRT. Thus, even if ρ is very small, but still greater than zero, the design effect could still be fairly large if the average group sample size is large.[64] In the previous example, if $\rho = 0.001$, and there were 500 students per group, the design effect would be: $1 + 0.001 (500 - 1) = 1.499$. This means that the total required sample size would need to be about 50 percent higher than that for a comparable RCT in order to achieve the same level of power. Since the sample size in a GRT is equivalent to mk, that is, the average number of subjects per group times the number of groups (see the numerator in formula 12.5), this larger sample size could be achieved by either increasing the average number of subjects per group (m) or by increasing the number of groups (k). Generally speaking, it is better to increase k than m.[56, 66] The reasoning is: (a) it is statistically more efficient; (b) it tends to increase the generalizability of the findings; and (c) it increases the precision of estimates of the intraclass correlation coefficient.[56] Because of the latter point, it is best to only use estimates of ICCs that come from studies employing a large number of clusters per study condition (i.e., at least eight).[54]

In summary, because of the clustering effect, which is responsible for additional variance in GRTs compared to similar sized RCTs, standard analytical methods or sample size calculations designed for data at the individual level cannot be applied to GRTs without appropriate statistical adjustment. If this adjustment is not made, the results using these procedures will tend to *overstate* the significance of the findings or the power of the study to detect significant findings. In some cases the overestimation can be substantial. The design effect or variance inflation factor, which depends on the intraclass correlation coefficient and average group size in a GRT, can be used to adjust for the clustering effect, thereby assuring the precision of the findings when standard statistical procedures are used. Unfortunately, this need for adjustment has not always been considered by researchers employing GRTs, sometimes resulting in spurious findings.

Units of inference. As should be clear from the above discussion, the units of assignment in GRTs (i.e., groups) are not always the same as the units of inference. In fact, the problem caused by the clustering effect can only occur when investigators of GRTs apply their findings to individuals instead of groups. A simple example of a GRT where the units of inference are individuals is an experimental trial to determine if medical practice changes result in improved patient outcomes. The interest here is in the effect of the group intervention on individual patient responses. Now consider a GRT to determine if large families receiving a new technique of family therapy have more favorable outcomes (e.g., less family quarrelling, more social activities as a family) than those receiving standard family therapy. Eligible families are randomly assigned to receive either the new treatment (the intervention condition) or the standard treatment (the control condition). The units of assignment and the units of inference in this example are both groups of individuals, that is, families. Individual responses to the intervention are not measured. Therefore, the findings from this study would not be subject to the clustering effect, and there would be no need to modify standard analytical methods nor standard techniques for estimating sample size as there would be if the units of inference were individuals.[58] An *ecological fallacy* (see chapter 4), however, would be committed if the results of this study were applied to individuals within the families.[56] For example, it would be inappropriate to conclude that increased family harmony implies increased contentment among individual family members. Some family members may go along with family wishes but resent them at the same time. To gauge individual responses to the therapy accurately individuals would need to be the units of inference.

Basic Approaches to Analysis

There are two basic approaches to analyzing the results of GRTs. These are: (a) analysis at the group level, and (b) analysis at the individual level that takes into account the clustering effect. Both of these approaches may involve elementary or more advanced statistical methods. Only the more advanced statistical methods, however, allow investigators to adjust for individual or group level **covariates,**[67] that is, variables that are potentially predictive of the study outcome (e.g., potential confounders).[1]

The first approach is conceptually the simplest. A summary measure of effect is calculated for each group in the trial. For continuous measures this is often based on group means. For dichotomous measures it may be group proportions or log odds. Since only one measure is calculated for each group in the trial, the outcomes can be considered independent, and therefore standard parametric or non-parametric statistical methods, such as those used in RCTs, can be employed.[56, 67] In this approach, the group outcomes are treated as if they were individual outcomes generated from an individually randomized trial. For example, some investigators have compared the overall mean effect for the intervention condition with the overall mean effect for the control condition using a standard t-test. However, when the size of the groups is highly variable, a weighted t-test, using the size of the groups as weights, is recommended.[67, 68] Other simple or more complex analyses can be performed at the group level. For example, multiple regression analysis can be used to adjust directly for group level covariates (e.g., group size, geographic area, community governance). Individual level covariates can then be incorporated in the model using a two-stage process.[67, 69] While analysis at the group level does not require adjustment for the clustering effect,* generally speaking, it is not a highly efficient approach to the analysis of GRTs except under certain specific conditions.[67] The second approach involves analysis of outcomes at the individual level using elementary or advanced statistical procedures. These procedures must take into account the clustering effect in order to produce precise results. For elementary statistical tests, this is accomplished by incorporating the design effect or variance inflation factor into the calculation of the standard error.[56] With a t-test or z-test, for example, one can divide the value of the test statistic by the square root of the design effect (i.e., the denominator in formula 12.5), and for a chi-square test one can divide it by the design effect.[67] Advanced statistical procedures, such as *multilevel analysis* (also called **multilevel modeling** or **hierarchical modeling**), which was first defined in chapter 9, can account for the clustering effect in the modeling procedure while simultaneously adjusting for both group and individual level covariates.[61, 67] *Multilevel analysis* can be described concisely as:

> An analytical approach that is appropriate for data with nested sources of variability—that is, involving units at a lower level or micro units (for

---

*It should be noted that some epidemiologists refer to the analysis of GRTs at the group level as a method of accounting for the clustering effect. Strictly speaking, however, there is no consideration of clustering in this approach other than perhaps choosing this approach to avoid dealing with the clustering effect.

example, individuals) nested within units at a higher level or macro units (for example, groups such as schools or neighborhoods). Multilevel analysis allows the simultaneous examination of the effects of group level and individual level variables on individual level outcomes while accounting for the non-independence of observations within groups.[70(p591)]

The "non-independence of observations within groups" mentioned in the above description is the clustering effect that we have been referring to. Multilevel analysis, which is an extension of multiple regression analysis, has some significant advantages as summarized by Amanda Woods.[71]

• The "ability to partition the variance between individual and group level characteristics and also explore the interaction between them." (p. 560)

• An "opportunity to look at the different levels of hierarchy in the population and then to see where the effects are occurring. It allows for better estimates of simple questions and also allows for more complex questions to be answered." (p. 560)

Increasingly sophisticated statistical software for conducting multilevel modeling and other advanced statistical techniques for analyzing the findings of GRTs at the individual level is available to epidemiologists and other researchers. While these programs are very useful, they involve complex procedures that rely on a number of assumptions and decisions. Therefore, they should not be used without an adequate understanding of their strengths and limitations. For many researchers this will mean seeking expert guidance from knowledgeable biostatisticians *before* a GRT is initiated.

Design Variations

As with RCTs, a number of corresponding designs have been used in GRTs. Consequently, parallel group, crossover, factorial, and sequential designs have all been employed in GRTs. For example, in a *crossover design* each group is subjected to both the intervention and control conditions in sequence during separate time periods.[72] A *factorial design* is exemplified by the National Workplace Health Project, Australia's largest workplace intervention trial.[73] This GRT used a 2×2 factorial design to examine socio-behavioral and environmental interventions focusing on a number of key health behavior outcomes. Twenty worksites were randomly allocated to either the social-behavioral treatment or its control condition and then separately to the environmental treatment or its control condition creating four combinations each composed of five worksites.

Like RCTs, GRTs may also be based on *completely randomized*, stratified, or matched-pair designs. A **completely randomized design** is one in which the units of assignment are made without any pre-stratification or matching.[74] It is the design assumed in the preceding section on basic approaches to analysis. Its counterpart in RCTs is what we defined as *simple randomization*. In the context of GRTs, a completely randomized design is most appropriate when the number of groups for randomization is large. This tends to assure that groups randomly assigned to the intervention and control conditions are balanced with respect to baseline factors.[60] A *stratified design* involves dividing groups into strata according to suspected prognostic factors and then randomly assigning the groups to intervention or control conditions. The goal is the same as that of a completely randomized design, namely to provide groups that are balanced with regard to baseline factors, specifically those for which stratification is performed.[60] Common group stratification factors include geographic area, overall indicators of socioeconomic status, and group size.[74] A *matched-pair design* is a specific form of stratification where each stratum consists of only two groups. One group is randomly assigned to the intervention condition and the other to the control condition.[74] When the total number of groups is relatively small in a GRT, stratification or a matched-pair design may be more statistically efficient than a completely randomized design.[60] A matched-pair design, in particular, can produce "very tight and explicit balancing of important base-line risk factors."[74(p97)] This could potentially reduce bias and increase the power of a given trial, especially when the number of groups is limited.[53, 75] This design has its weaknesses, however, including consequences from overmatching (defined in chapter 10), difficulty in estimating the intraclass correlation coefficient, and a significant loss of information when a group withdraws since its matched pair must also be eliminated from the analysis.[58, 60]

The design of GRTs can also vary depending on when or how often the study outcomes are measured. A **posttest-only design**, for example, involves measuring study outcomes in the intervention and control groups only at the conclusion of the trial. A **pretest-posttest design**, on the other hand, entails measuring the outcomes before and after the intervention. Finally, a **multiple pretest-posttest design** requires that outcome measurements be made at several different points before and after the intervention. This design option allows investigators to examine patterns in the data, which can help to explain observed differences. It can also be extended to include continuous surveillance.[53] When the number of randomized groups is relatively large, each of these design variations tends to produce results that are internally valid since selection bias and confounding tend to be eliminated. When the number of randomized groups is small, however, the results of these designs could still be affected by sources of systematic error. This will make it difficult to attribute observed differences in outcomes exclusively to the intervention. While it is impossible to enumerate a "sufficient number" of groups that applies in all cases, some authors have suggested that eight groups (four per study condition in a two-arm trial) might represent a lower limit.[56]

Finally, GRTs involving follow up may be designed based on whether the primary objective is to measure the effects of the intervention on the study population as a whole or on the individuals within the population.[56] Basically, these are sampling strategies. In the former case, a *repeated cross-sectional design* (for GRTs) is more appropriate, and in the latter case, a *cohort design* (for GRTs) is more appropriate. A **repeated cross-sectional design** (for

GRTs) is one in which a *new sample* of individuals is selected from each group each time outcome measurements are to be made during follow up. A **cohort design** (for GRTs) is one in which the *same individuals* are sampled each time outcome measurements are to be made. Each design has its own advantages and disadvantages.[53] Both designs, however, can be used in GRTs to sample individuals within groups.[56] Generally speaking, in those situations where either design would be appropriate, the repeated cross-sectional design is less susceptible to bias than the cohort design. When bias is absent, however, the cohort design will usually have greater power than the repeated cross-sectional design.[56] These designs and the previous ones referred to in this section are not all mutually exclusive. For example, a repeated cross-sectional design of a GRT could be based on a parallel group design that is completely randomized using a multiple pretest-posttest design.

Loss to Follow Up

Group or cluster randomized trials may be subject to losses to follow up, which can affect the precision as well as the validity of the findings (i.e., cause loss to follow-up bias; see chapter 8). While losses to follow up can be a problem in RCTs, they can have a greater impact in GRTs since entire groups, often containing numerous individuals, can withdraw from a study.[74] This is specifically a problem in GRTs using a cohort design (see above) and is more likely to occur when the follow-up period is long.[56] A GRT using a repeated cross-sectional design should not experience this problem since different samples are selected at different times. Nonresponse from individual subjects, however, can be a problem in both types of designs.[56, 74]

Ethical Issues

Overall, ethical practices with regard to the conduct of RCTs are well established. Those with regard to GRTs, on the other hand, are less well established and are sometimes more controversial.[58] One problem, for example, concerns informed consent. A natural question is, who needs to be informed and when? While it is clear, for instance, that key community leaders must be consulted before initiating a GRT involving entire communities, it is less clear whether the individuals living in the communities also need to be given informed consent prior to data collection, particularly if the risks of participation appear to be minimal, such as in a health education campaign to reduce sunlight exposure. Related questions might include: Which community leaders need to be informed? and If residents of the communities need to be notified, are general announcements in the media sufficient? A host of other ethical questions concerning GRTs can be raised as well as logistical problems in implementing ethical guidelines.

In comparing ethical issues of RCTs with GRTs, J. L. Hutton concluded:

> [C]luster randomised controlled trials raise new issues on the nature and practice of informed consent, because of the levels at which consent can be

sought, and for which it can be sought. In addition, careful consideration of the principles relating to the quality of the scientific design and analysis, balance of risk and benefit, liberty to leave a trial, early stopping of a trial and the power to exclude people from potential benefits is required.[76(p473)]

Many pertinent issues still need to be resolved before ethical guidelines for GRTs can approach the level of consensus that now exists for the conduct of RCTs.

QUASI-EXPERIMENTAL STUDIES

Quasi-experimental studies, also known as **quasi-experiments**, were introduced in chapter 4. To reiterate, they are studies in which the investigators do not have full control over the assignment or timing of the intervention but where the studies are still conducted as if they were experiments.[1] Fundamentally, the defining characteristics of quasi-experimental studies in epidemiology are an identifiable intervention and the absence of random allocation. In addition, some quasi-experimental studies do not have separate control groups. Quasi-experimental studies may be conducted for a variety of reasons, including political, ethical, or practical limitations.[77] For example, some of the groups for a proposed GRT may not consent to the intervention making random allocation of groups impossible.

There are a large variety of potential quasi-experimental designs, and the units of assignment may be individuals or groups. Many of these designs have features analogous to RCTs or GRTs, although some are unique. To keep our discussion concise, we will only focus on the most common quasi-experimental designs. These fall into two broad categories: (a) *before and after studies*, and (b) *time-series studies*.[77] Other design options, as well as appropriate analytical methods for quasi-experimental studies, are discussed in more specialized texts.

Before and After Studies

As indicated by their name, **before and after studies** involve measurements and comparisons of the study outcomes before and after the intervention. The **one-group pretest-posttest design**[78] is the simplest before and after design. It is considered an *uncontrolled* before and after study.[77] Unfortunately, this design is weak from the standpoint of internal validity and therefore has been classified by some as a "pre-experimental design,"[78] implying that it lacks sufficient rigor to produce convincing results. Controlled designs offer better protection against bias and confounding than this strategy. The design may be represented diagrammatically as follows:

$$O_1 \times O_2$$

The Os represent the outcome measures before (O_1) and after (O_2) the intervention, and the $\times$ represents the intervention. One must be very circumspect in attributing any change from O_1 to O_2 exclusively to the intervention.

The reason is that several alternate explanations are usually possible. For example, external influences affecting O_2 may have occurred during the time lapse between measurements of study outcomes. Consider a trial in which the units of assignment are entire communities. Say, specific risk factors for heart disease are measured on individuals in the study community prior to an intervention involving mass education on heart disease prevention and implementation of a low cost community-wide screening program to detect major risk factors for heart disease. Post-intervention measurements are made one year following the intervention. During the year following the intervention, it is possible that other unrelated events occurred in the community and had an effect on the magnitude of O_2. This could be other prevention-oriented programs instituted by other groups; increased community awareness of risk factors, perhaps due to deaths from heart disease of well-known, prominent persons in the community; and so on. In addition to external influences, other common explanations for the findings of one-group pretest-posttest designs include **maturation** (i.e., factors associated with the passage of time, such as aging of the subjects), secular trends (chapter 1) in the outcomes, and the **Hawthorne effect**,* which is the tendency of research subjects to change their behaviors due purely to the fact that they are being studied.[79]

Another type of before and after design is the **nonequivalent control group design**.[78] In contrast to the one-group pretest-posttest design, this strategy has a separate control group. Thus, it is considered a *controlled* before and after study.[77] It may be diagrammed as follows:

$$O_1 \quad \times \quad O_2$$
$$O_1 \qquad\quad O_2$$

The fact that the control group (represented by the bottom row) does not include an "×" indicates that typically it does not receive any intervention. The control group is called "nonequivalent" because randomization has not been used in assigning the subjects to the study groups. Therefore, we cannot be sure the groups are equivalent (i.e., comparable) on pertinent factors. The addition of a separate control group, however, strengthens the internal validity of this design compared to the one-group pretest-posttest design, all other factors being equal. The design can be strengthened even further to the degree to which the experimental and control groups can be shown to be alike, that is, where pertinent pre-intervention measurements are similar.[78] Nonetheless, the findings of even a well-designed nonequivalent control group study can be affected by the interaction of selective differences between the study groups and other factors, particularly maturation, or by a phenomenon known as *regression to the mean*.[78] In this context, **regression to the mean** represents the tendency for extreme values on a pretest to be closer to the mean value on a posttest regardless of the intervention. Hence, an initial difference between O_1 in the experimental and control groups when O_2 in each

*The name of this source of bias comes from classical studies conducted on workers at the Hawthorne Western Electric Plant in Cicero, Illinois, beginning in the 1920s.

group is similar might be explained by regression to the mean in the experimental group. To illustrate, say that O_1 was uncharacteristically high in the experimental group and thus different from that in the control group where it represented a more typical value. Now if there was no change from O_1 to O_2 in the control group but a sizeable decrease in the experimental group, this could be due solely to regression to the mean. Students often experience this phenomenon in new classes when they score very high or very low on the first exam and then closer to the average score on the second exam.

Time-Series Studies

There are two common variations of **time-series studies**. The first, has been referred to as an **interrupted time-series design**.[56] In this quasi-experimental design, multiple measurements of the study outcome are made prior to and following the intervention without the use of a separate control group. The design may be represented as follows:[78]

$$O_1 \quad O_2 \quad O_3 \quad O_4 \quad \times \quad O_5 \quad O_6 \quad O_7 \quad O_8$$

In general, this design permits the effect of the intervention to be estimated while taking into account secular trends or cyclic patterns (chapter 1) affecting the study outcomes.[77] It is relatively effective in controlling threats to internal validity due to maturation, regression to the mean, and selection bias as well as that due to the Hawthorne effect, but the findings are still susceptible to external influences on the outcome, such as competing prevention programs.[56, 77, 78] Generally speaking, interrupted time series designs should have *at least* four measurements before and after the intervention to provide convincing results.[56] An extension of this design is known as the **multiple time-series design**. The difference is that the latter design employs a separate control group (see below):

$$
\begin{array}{ccccccccc}
O_1 & O_2 & O_3 & O_4 & \times & O_5 & O_6 & O_7 & O_8 \\
O_1 & O_2 & O_3 & O_4 & & O_5 & O_6 & O_7 & O_8
\end{array}
$$

The addition of a separate control group allows investigators to account better for external influences on the outcome.[56] However, it is possible that interactions between selective differences in the study groups and external influences may affect the results.[78] According to Donald T. Campbell and Julian C. Stanley, "In general, this is an excellent quasi-experimental design, perhaps the best of the more feasible designs."[78(p57)]

While well-designed quasi-experimental studies are likely to produce results that are more convincing than observational studies, all other factors being equal, they are still generally inferior to true experimental studies in terms of scientific rigor. Randomization, a key element of experimental epidemiologic studies, helps to eliminate selection bias and prevent confounding with regard to known and unknown prognostic factors by creating similar groups prior to the intervention. This same level of equivalency between study groups is more difficult to achieve in quasi-experimental studies due to the lack of random allocation. Hence, selection bias and confounding can still be significant factors in these studies.

Like other epidemiologic study designs, quasi-experimental studies need to be carefully planned, executed, analyzed, and interpreted in light of their particular strengths and weaknesses. As just mentioned, the chief limitation of quasi-experimental studies is the absence of randomization, which makes these studies more vulnerable than their randomized counterparts to certain types of systematic errors. These threats to internal validity increase the probability that there may be alternate explanations for the findings.[77] To minimize this possibility it is important to use control groups in quasi-experimental studies whenever feasible. It is also advantageous to select experimental and controls groups that are as similar as possible at the start of the study and that are likely to remain so throughout the trial period except for any effects that may result from the intervention. This requires that investigators attempt to anticipate changes due to external influences, differential levels of maturation, regression to the mean, and so forth. It also requires that they attempt to account for them during the design and analysis phases. Strategies like matching on important prognostic factors and statistically adjusting for unmatched confounders in the analyses may help to minimize some of these problems. In some cases, quasi-experimental studies may exhibit greater external validity their randomized counterparts since they often represent more "real-world" conditions.[80]

Methods of data collection for quasi-experimental studies are varied but similar to those used in experimental studies. They may include surveys, interviews, subject testing, and other common techniques. Analytical procedures can be quite complex, and advanced statistical procedures are required to account for the lack of random allocation.[81] For details one should consult specialized texts on the topic.

SUMMARY

- Experimental studies are those in which study conditions are controlled directly by the investigators. The two major types in epidemiology are randomized controlled trials (RCTs) and group randomized trials (GRTs). The major difference is that in RCTs individuals are randomly assigned to study groups while in GRTs groups of individuals are randomly assigned. Quasi-experimental studies are those in which the investigators do not have full control over the assignment or timing of the intervention but where the studies are still conducted as if they were experiments. Natural experiments are unplanned situations in nature where the levels of exposure to presumed causes differ among subgroups such that the situations resemble planned experiments. They are, however, observational studies.

- Randomized controlled trials, the gold standard of epidemiologic studies, provide the strongest possible evidence of causation in epidemiology when well-designed and conducted. They can be categorized as preventive or therapeutic trials. Preventive trials can be further classified as primary or secondary prevention trials depending on their specific focus. Therapeutic trials focus on tertiary prevention.

- Typical steps in an RCT include development of a primary research hypothesis, selection of a study population, determination of sample size requirements, collection of baseline data, random allocation of subjects into experimental and control groups, application of an intervention, and assessment of outcomes during a follow-up period. The plans for these and other considerations, such as the adoption of ethical policies, should be part of the study protocol.

- Selection of the study population begins with the selection of a source population from which volunteers meeting the eligibility requirements are recruited. The eligibility requirements and informed consent help to protect the study integrity and the safety of the participants. Since many may be ineligible or unwilling to participate, the size of the study population is often substantially smaller than the source population. This can result in a study with low power. The solution is to determine the minimum sample size required to detect clinically important differences before an RCT is initiated.

- Randomization means that the assignment of subjects to experimental and control groups is strictly by random means. Properly executed, randomization eliminates selection bias in subject assignments and increases the probability that study groups will be comparable thereby controlling confounding. Randomization is most likely to achieve these objectives when sample size is large. Because randomization controls both known and unknown confounders, it is considered more effective than restriction, matching, or stratification in achieving comparable groups. Common randomization procedures include simple, stratified, and blocked. Simple randomization works best when sample size is large; the others are best used when sample size is small.

- In a typical RCT the members of the experimental group receive a promising but unproven intervention, and the results are compared to the experience of the members of the control group after an appropriate follow-up period. The members of the control group usually receive the standard treatment, a placebo, a sham procedure, or no treatment at all.

- Blinding (masking) is a method of controlling bias that may result from a knowledge of subject assignments. Single-blinded studies are those in which subjects are kept unaware of their group assignments. Double-blinded studies are those in which both the subjects and the investigators (specifically, those assessing outcome status) are unaware of subject assignments. These have been the traditional standard for RCTs. Triple-blinded studies also keep those who analyze the data unaware of subject assignments. Blinding can also reduce confounding that occurs during the follow-up period. Blinding may not always be feasible, however, due to practical or ethical considerations. It is most valuable when study outcomes are subjective. When double-blinding cannot be used extra efforts should be made to use objective criteria in assessing outcomes, to follow up study groups equally, and to use independent assessors not knowledgeable of group assignments or study hypotheses.

- A widely accepted ethical prerequisite to RCTs is the principle of equipoise, which refers to a genuine uncertainty about the benefits or risks of an intervention. An RCT is ethically feasible only when there are potential benefits but honest doubts about the efficacy of a given intervention. According to the principle, subjects should not be intentionally subject to harm or denied known benefits of an intervention. Randomized controlled trials normally must be pre-approved by an appropriate institutional review board or research ethics committee.

- There are several possible design variations in RCTs. These include parallel group, crossover, factorial, fixed sample size, and sequential, including group sequential, designs. Not all of these variations are mutually exclusive. Sequential and group sequential designs require stopping rules, which are rules for deciding when to terminate a trial. Common reasons include early demonstrated superiority or inferiority of the intervention and futility, a statistical judgment that no difference is likely to be found between the study groups even with continued follow up.

- An important issue that must be considered in RCTs is the likelihood of noncompliance with the study protocol. This can affect the accuracy of the findings. Noncompliance tends to be greatest when a study is long or the protocol is complex. A run-in period is one way of helping assure that only committed subjects are included in an RCT. The preferred approach to the analysis of RCTs is known as intention-to-treat analysis. This means that trial results are analyzed based on original subject assignments as determined by randomization regardless of subsequent compliance with the study protocol. Focusing only on compliant subjects (i.e., per protocol analysis) nullifies the benefits of randomization, which can invalidate study results. A variety of statistical methods can be used to analyze findings from RCTs, including survival analysis.

- In addition to an overall analysis, the findings of an RCT may undergo subgroup analyses. Their purpose is to detect interactions. Subgroup analyses can be problematic for a number of reasons. For example, they may nullify the values of randomization or result in inconclusive findings due to small sample sizes. Ideally, if performed at all, they should be planned before the start of a trial and limited to baseline factors measured prior to the trial.

- Meta-analysis is an orderly way of integrating the findings of similar studies so as to provide an overall statistical summary of the results. Traditionally, it has been used mostly with RCTs, but it is applicable to other epidemiologic study designs as well. Meta-analysis represents a quantitative systematic review and requires careful planning. The statistical approach to integrating the findings of individual studies may be based on equal effects (fixed effects) or random effects models. Forest plots provide a visual representation of the effect estimates and confidence intervals for each component study as well as a "pooled" estimate and its confidence interval. An important consideration in meta-analysis is the assessment of heterogeneity. This has implications for the model used in performing the meta-analysis. Because the results of meta-analysis can affect policy, it is critical that authors do a thorough and accurate job that is subject to adequate peer review.

- Randomized controlled trials have a number of advantages and disadvantages. Advantages include the ability to provide convincing evidence of causal relationships due largely to effective control of selection bias and confounding by randomization, the relative ease of blinding subjects and investigators to exposure status when feasible, and direct control of the exposure level. Potential weaknesses include limited applicability due to ethical concerns and reliance on volunteers. Also, the normally strict eligibility criteria may limit external validity. In addition, RCTs can be expensive and time consuming due to large sample size requirements. Finally, they tend to be prone to losses to follow up and noncompliance, which can affect the accuracy of the results.

- Group randomized trials, like RCTs, should be guided by a detailed study protocol. When properly conducted, they are considered the gold standard for evaluating interventions applied to groups of people. They are usually undertaken when: (a) the intervention is more appropriate at the group level, (b) the members in the intervention group are likely to be contaminated by members in the control group, or (c) when an intervention at the group level is more convenient.

- There are several methodological issues that need to be addressed in GRTs. These include having an adequate number of groups in the study to assure that randomization achieves its objective of minimizing selection bias and confounding and to assure the study has adequate power, accounting for the clustering effect when the units of inference are individuals, and avoiding interpretation problems based on the units of inference (e.g., an ecological fallacy). These concerns are not entirely independent of each other. The clustering effect is usually dealt with by taking the design effect into account in sample size estimation and in the analysis. The design effect depends on the intraclass correlation coefficient and the size of the study groups. Failure to consider the clustering effect can result in an overestimation of the power of a study and the precision of its findings.

- There are two basic approaches to analyzing results from GRTs—analysis at the group level or analysis at the individual level. The latter must take into account the clustering effect. Both approaches may employ elementary or more advanced statistical procedures. Only the more advanced procedures, however, allow investigators to adjust for individual or group covariates. Multi-level analysis is one such approach.

- As with RCTs, there are a number of design variations possible with GRTs, not all of which are mutually exclusive. These include parallel group, crossover, factorial, and sequential designs; completely randomized, stratified, or matched-pair designs; repeated cross-sectional and cohort designs; and other options (e.g., posttest-only, pretest-posttest designs).

- Group randomized trials may be subject to losses to follow up, which can affect study precision and validity. The impact of losses can be greater than in RCTs because entire groups of individuals can be lost. Ethical policies regarding GRTs are not as well established as those for RCTs but are still evolving.

- Quasi-experimental studies use an intervention but do not involve randomization to study groups. In addition, some quasi-experiments do not have separate control groups. In some cases quasi-experimental studies parallel RCTs or GRTs but without random allocation. Broadly speaking, the most common quasi-experimental designs in epidemiology include before and after studies (e.g., the nonequivalent control group design) and time-series studies (e.g., the interrupted time-series design). While well-designed quasi-experimental studies are likely to produce results that are more convincing than comparable observational studies, they are generally considered inferior to experimental studies in terms of scientific rigor. A major reason is that they are more vulnerable to systematic errors.

New Terms

- active treatment
- adherence
- arm
- before and after studies
- blinding
- block randomization
- carryover effects
- clinical diversity
- clinical heterogeneity
- clustering effect
- Cochrane Collaboration
- cohort design (for GRTs)
- community trial
- completely randomized design
- compliance
- contamination
- covariate
- crossover design
- crossovers
- cumulative meta-analysis

- data and safety monitoring board
- data and safety monitoring committee
- data monitoring committee
- Declaration of Helsinki
- design effect
- double-blinded study
- effect size
- effective sample size
- efficacy analysis
- eligibility criteria
- endpoints
- equal effects model
- equipoise
- exclusion criteria
- factorial design
- fixed effects model
- fixed sample size design
- forest plot
- futility

- group sequential design
- Hawthorne effect
- heterogeneity
- hierarchical modeling
- homogenous
- I^2
- inactive treatment
- inclusion criteria
- informed consent
- institutional review board
- intention-to-treat analysis
- interrupted time-series design
- intervention study
- intraclass correlation coefficient
- intracluster correlation coefficient
- Mantel-Haenszel method
- masking
- maturation
- meta-analysis
- methodological diversity
- methodological heterogeneity
- multilevel modeling
- multiple pretest-posttest design
- multiple time-series design
- narrative review
- nonadherence
- noncompliance
- noncrossover design
- nonequivalent control group design
- one-group pretest-posttest design
- overview
- parallel group design
- parallel treatment design
- per protocol analysis
- Peto method
- placebo
- placebo effect
- placebo-controlled trial
- posttest-only design
- pretest-posttest design
- primary prevention trial
- prognostic factor
- prospective meta-analysis
- publication bias
- qualitative systematic review
- quantitative systematic review
- quasi-experiment
- random effects model
- recruitment
- recruitment period
- regression to the mean
- repeated cross-sectional design (for GRTs)
- research ethics committee
- restricted randomization
- rho
- run-in period
- secondary prevention trial
- sensitivity analysis
- sequential design
- sham procedure
- simple randomization
- single-blinded study
- statistical heterogeneity
- stopping rules
- stratified randomization
- study protocol
- subgroup analyses
- systematic review
- time-series studies
- triple-blinded study
- variance inflation factor
- washout period

Study Questions and Exercises

. Describe how you would design a valid randomized controlled trial to test the hypothesis that Low-Chol, a new oral medication to lower serum cholesterol, decreases the risk of death from coronary heart disease (CHD) in healthy men, 40–54 years of age, at high risk for the disease. Include in your description how you would select the study population, determine the subject eligibility criteria, ascertain the appropriate sample size, allocate the subjects into experimental and control groups, apply the intervention, and assess the outcomes during follow up.

2. Assume the randomized controlled trial you designed in item 1 was implemented with the following results:

Exposure Status	CHD deaths	Person-years
Low-Chol	29	16,500
No Low-Chol	62	19,350
	91	35,850

Assuming that the study was designed to minimize bias and confounding, determine if Low-Chol is efficacious in reducing deaths due to CHD based on the study findings. To support your conclusion provide the percent relative effect and its 95% confidence interval. Interpret these measures.

3. Why was the technique used by Johannes Fibiger (see p. 374) for assigning subjects to experimental and control groups not considered a method of random allocation? Be specific.

4. Describe how you would design a valid group randomized trial to test the hypothesis that aggressive traffic control measures to reduce air pollution in large cities is associated with fewer hospital emergency room visits due to acute asthmatic attacks in children. Include in your description how you would select the units of assignment, allocate them to study conditions, apply the intervention, and evaluate the effectiveness of the intervention. Also, indicate how you would account for the clustering effect in your analysis.

5. What is the effective sample size of a two-arm group randomized trial where there are 12 groups to be assigned to each arm of the study, and the average group consists of 125 individuals? Assume the intraclass correlation coefficient, estimated from a study on a similar population, is 0.008 and that the intended units of inference are individuals. Also, based on your results, (a) what can you conclude about the power of this study, and (b) how might the power of the study be increased?

6. Indicate whether each of the following statements is true or false (T or F). For each *false* statement, indicate why it is false.

_____ a. There are three major types of unplanned experimental epidemiologic studies—randomized controlled trials, group randomized trials, and natural experiments.

_____ b. Prognostic factors cannot confound the effect of an intervention on a study outcome when they are equally balanced between the study groups in a randomized controlled trial.

_____ c. In general, matching tends to be more effective than randomization in controlling confounding.

_____ d. Blinding tends to reduce confounding during the follow-up period in a randomized controlled trial.

_____ e. The internal validity of a randomized controlled trial is not affected by a study population that is unrepresentative of the general population.

_____ f. According to the principle of equipoise, it is only legitimate to design a randomized controlled trial when there is strong evidence that the planned intervention will be beneficial to the participants.

_____ g. In a factorial design of a randomized controlled trial each subject is assigned to the experimental group at one time or another.

_____ h. The sample size for a randomized controlled trial using a group sequential design is normally determined at the beginning of the study.

_____ i. Intention-to-treat analysis tends to underestimate the magnitude of the association between a study intervention and outcome in a randomized controlled trial when the number of crossovers is large.

_____ j. Subgroup analyses in a randomized controlled trial can increase the probability that the study findings are due to chance alone.

_____ k. If heterogeneity appears to be present in a meta-analysis of randomized controlled trials, it is always best to use a fixed effects model to characterize the findings so as to maximize the precision of the analysis.

_____ l. Overly strict eligibility requirements for a randomized controlled trial may have the effect of invalidating the study findings.

_____ m. Group randomized trials tend to reduce the potential for contamination due to crossovers from control to intervention groups.

_____ n. Failure to account for the clustering effect in a group randomized trial where individuals are the units of inference can result in an underestimation of the significance of the findings.

_____ o. Where both the intraclass correlation coefficient and the average group sample size are very small, a group randomized trial will have a very large design effect.

____ p. A matched-pair design of a group randomized trial is simply a special type of stratified design.

____ q. Group randomized trials that focus on the effects of an intervention on the study population as a whole are best analyzed using a repeated cross-sectional versus a cohort design.

____ r. Quasi-experimental study designs do not employ separate control groups.

____ s. The weakest quasi-experimental design commonly used in epidemiology is the multiple time-series design.

____ t. The tendency for extreme measurements on a pretest in a quasi-experimental study to be closer to the mean value on a posttest regardless of the effect of the intervention is known as the Hawthorne effect.

References

1. Last, J. M., ed. (2001). *A Dictionary of Epidemiology*, 4th ed. New York: Oxford University Press.
2. Meldrum, M. L. (2000). A Brief History of the Randomized Controlled Trial: From Oranges to the Gold Standard. *Hematology/Oncology Clinics of North America* 14 (4): 745–760.
3. Francis, T., Jr., Napier, J. A., Voight, R. B., Hemphill, F. M., Wenner, H. A., Korns, R. F., Boisen, M., Tolchinsky, E., and Diamond, E. L. (1955). Evaluation of 1954 Field Trials of Poliomyelitis Vaccine. In *The Challenge of Epidemiology: Issues and Selected Readings*, C. Buck, A. Llopis, E. Najera, and M. Terris, eds. Washington, DC: Pan American Health Organization, 1988, pp. 838–854.
4. White, H. D., Simes, R. J., Anderson, N. E., Hankey, G. J., Watson, J. D., Hunt, D., Colquhoun, D. M., Glasziou, P., MacMahon, S., Kirby, A. C., West, M. J., and Tonkin, A. M. (2000). Pravastatin Therapy and the Risk of Stroke. *New England Journal of Medicine* 343 (5): 317–326.
5. Day, S. (1999). *Dictionary for Clinical Trials*. Chichester: John Wiley & Sons, Ltd.
6. Hennekens, C. H., and Buring, J. E. (1987). *Epidemiology in Medicine*. Boston: Little, Brown and Company.
7. Meinert, C. L. (1986). *Clinical Trials: Design, Conduct, and Analysis*. New York: Oxford University Press.
8. Hulley, S. B., Cummings, S. R., Browner, W. S., Grady, D., Hearst, N., and Newman, T. B. (2001). *Designing Clinical Research: An Epidemiologic Approach*, 2nd ed. Philadelphia: Lippincott Williams & Wilkins.
9. Malone, R. P., Delaney, M. A., Luebbert, J. F., Cater, J., and Campbell, M. (2000). A Double-blind Placebo-controlled Study of Lithium in Hospitalized Aggressive Children and Adolescents with Conduct Disorder. *Archives of General Psychiatry* 57 (7): 649–654.
10. Wassertheil-Smoller, S. (1990). *Biostatistics and Epidemiology: A Primer for Health Professionals*. New York: Springer-Verlag.
11. Rothman, K. J. (2002). *Epidemiology: An Introduction*. New York: Oxford University Press.
12. Elwood, M. (1998). *Critical Appraisal of Epidemiological Studies and Clinical Trials*, 2nd ed. Oxford: Oxford University Press.
13. Zelen, M. (1974). The Randomization and Stratification of Patients to Clinical Trials. *Journal of Chronic Diseases* 27: 365–375.
14. Miller, F. G., and Kaptchuk, T. J. (2004). Sham Procedures and the Ethics of Clinical Trials. *Journal of the Royal Society of Medicine* 97: 576–578.
15. World Medical Association (2004). *Declaration of Helsinki; Ethical Principles for Medical Research Involving Human Subjects*. Available: http://www.wma.net/e/policy/pdf/17c.pdf (Access date: June 18, 2006).

16. Rothman, K. J., Michels, K. B., and Baum, M. (2000). For and Against: Declaration of Helsinki Should be Strengthened. *British Medical Journal* 321: 442–445.

17. The Editors (2002). What Is a Clinical Trial? in Clinical Trials: A Cornerstone of Biomedical Research and Innovation. *The Pfizer Journal, Global Edition* III (1): 10–18.

18. Miller, F. G., and Brody, H. (2002). What Makes Placebo-Controlled Trials Unethical? *American Journal of Bioethics* 2 (2): 3–9.

19. Food and Drug Administration, Department of Health and Human Services (2005). Adequate and Well Controlled Studies, 21 Code of Federal Regulations, Section 134.126. Available: http://www.accessdata.fda.gov/scripts/cdrh/cfdocs/cfcfr/CFRSearch.cfm?fr=314.126 (Access date: June 22, 2006).

20. Woodward, M. (1999). *Epidemiology: Study Design and Data Analysis*. Boca Raton, FL: Chapman and Hall/CRC.

21. Hennekens, C., and Eberlein, K. (1985). A Randomized Trial of Aspirin and Beta-carotene Among U.S. Physicians. *Preventive Medicine* 14 (2): 165–168.

22. Lewis, R. J. (1993). An Introduction to the Use of Interim Data Analyses in Clinical Trials. *Annals of Emergency Medicine* 22 (9): 1463–1469.

23. U.S. Food and Drug Administration, Center for Biologics Evaluation and Research (2006). *Guidance for Clinical Trial Sponsors: Establishment and Operation of Clinical Trial Data Monitoring Committees*. Available: http://www.fda.gov/cber/gdlns/clintrialdmc.htm (Access date: July 6, 2006).

24. Brower, R. G., Lanken, P. N., MacIntyre, N., Matthay, M. A., Morris, A., Ancukiewicz, M., Schoenfeld, D., Thompson, B. T.; National Heart, Lung, and Blood Institute ARDS Clinical Trials Network (2004). Higher Versus Lower Positive End-expiratory Pressures in Patients with the Acute Respiratory Distress Syndrome. *New England Journal of Medicine* 351 (4): 327–336.

25. Jadad, A. R. (1998). *Randomised Controlled Trials: A User's Guide*. London: BMJ Books.

26. Physicians' Health Study (2006). Available: http://phs.bwh.harvard.edu/index.html (Access date: July 7, 2006).

27. Greenberg, R. S., Daniels, S. R., Flanders, W. D., Eley, J. W., and Boring, J. R. III (2001). *Medical Epidemiology*, 3rd ed. New York: Lange Medical Books/McGraw-Hill.

28. Motulsky, H. (1995). *Intuitive Biostatistics*. New York: Oxford University Press.

29. Oxman, A. D., and Guyatt, G. H. (1992). A Consumer's Guide to Subgroup Analyses. *Annals of Internal Medicine* 116: 78–84.

30. Sleight, P. (2000). Debate: Subgroup Analyses in Clinical Trials—Fun to Look At, But Don't Believe Them. *Current Controlled Trials in Cardiovascular Medicine* 1: 25–27.

31. Altman, D. G., and Matthews, J. N. S. (1996). Statistics Notes: Interaction 1: Heterogeneity of Effects. *British Medical Journal* 313: 486.

32. Gebski, V. J., and Keech, A. C. (2003). Statistical Methods in Clinical Trials. *Medical Journal of Australia* 178 (4): 182–184.

33. Kelsey, J. L., Petitti, D. B., and King, A. C. (1998). Key Methodologic Concepts and Issues. In *Applied Epidemiology: Theory to Practice*, R. C. Brownson and D. B. Petitti, eds. New York: Oxford University Press, pp. 58–69.

34. Glass, G. V. (1976). Primary, Secondary, and Meta-analysis of Research. *Educational Researcher* 5 (10): 3–8.

35. Egger, M., and Smith, G. D. (1997). Meta-analysis: Potentials and Promise. *British Medical Journal* 315: 1371–1374.

36. Cook, D. J., Mulrow, C. D., and Haynes, R. B. (1997). Systematic Reviews: Synthesis of Best Evidence for Clinical Decisions. *Annals of Internal Medicine* 126 (5): 376–380.

37. Evans, L. T., Saberi, S., Kim, H. M., Elta, G. H., and Schoenfeld, P. (2006). Pharyngeal Anesthesia During Sedated EGDs: Is "The Spray" Beneficial? A Meta-analysis and Systematic Review. *Gastrointestinal Endoscopy* 63 (6): 761–766.

38. Stoup, D. F., Berlin, J. A., Morton, S. C. et al. for the Meta-analysis of Observational Studies in Epidemiology (MOOSE) Group (2000). Meta-analysis of Observational Studies in Epidemiology: A Proposal for Reporting. *Journal of the American Medical Association* 283 (15): 2008–2012.

39. LeLorier, J., Gregoire, G., Benhaddad, A., Lapierre, J., and Derderian., F. (1997). Discrepancies Between Meta-analyses and Subsequent Large Randomized, Controlled Trials. *New England Journal of Medicine* 337 (8): 536–542.

40. The Cochrane Collaboration (2005). Newcomers' Guide. Available: http://www.cochrane.org/docs/newcomersguide.htm (Access date: July 25, 2006).

41. The Cochrane Collaboration (1999). Prospective Meta-analysis Methods Group. Available: http://www.cochrane.org/docs/pma.htm (Access date: July 25, 2006).

42. Pogue, J., and Yusuf, S. (1998). Overcoming the Limitations of Current Meta-analysis of Randomised Controlled Trials. *The Lancet* 351: 47–52.

43. Helfenstein, U. (2002). Data and Models Determine Treatment Proposals—An Illustration from Meta-analysis. *Postgraduate Medicine* 78: 131–134.

44. Egger, M., Smith, G. D., and Phillips, A. N. (1997). Meta-analysis: Principles and Procedures. *British Medical Journal* 315: 1533–1537.

45. The Cochrane Collaboration (2002). Module 13: Diversity and Heterogeneity. Available: http://www.cochrane-net.org/openlearning/HTML/mod13.htm (Access date: July 31, 2006).

46. Higgins, J. P. T., Thompson, S. G., Deeks, J. J., and Altman, D. G. (2003). Measuring Inconsistency in Meta-analysis. *British Medical Journal* 327: 557–560.

47. Lewis, S., and Clarke, M. (2001). Forest Plots: Trying to See the Woods and the Trees. *British Medical Journal* 322: 1479–1480.

48. Murphy, C. C., Schei, B., Myhr, T. L., and DuMont, J. (2001). Abuse: A Risk Factor for Low Birth Weight? A Systematic Review and Meta-analysis. *Canadian Medical Association Journal* 164 (11): 1567–1572.

49. Centre for Reviews and Dissemination, University of York (2005). Introduction to Systematic Reviews and Critical Appraisal. Available: http://www.york.ac.uk/inst/crd/09metaanalysis.pdf (Access date: August 1, 2006).

50. Higgins, J. P. T., and Green, S., eds. (2005). Heterogeneity. *Cochrane Handbook for Systematic Reviews of Interventions 8.7.* Available: http://www.cochrane.org/resources/handbook/hbook.htm (Access date: August 1, 2006).

51. Thompson, S. G. (1994). Systematic Review: Why Sources of Heterogeneity in Meta-analysis Should Be Investigated. *British Medical Journal* 309: 1351–1355.

52. Khan, N., and McAlister, F. A. (2006). Re-examining the Efficacy of β-blockers for the Treatment of Hypertension: A Meta-analysis. *Canadian Medical Association Journal* 174 (12): 1737–1742.

53. Murray, D. M. (1998). *Design and Analysis of Group-randomized Trials.* New York: Oxford University Press.

54. Murray, D. M., Varnell, S. P., and Blitstein, J. L. (2004). Design and Analysis of Group-randomized Trials: A Review of Recent Methodological Developments. *American Journal of Public Health* 94 (3): 423–432.

55. Wagenaar, A. C., Murray, D. M., and Toomey, T. L. (2000). Communities Mobilizing for Change on Alcohol (CMCA): Effects of a Randomized Trial on Arrests and Traffic Crashes. *Addiction* 95 (2): 209–217.

56. Ukoumunne, O. C., Gulliford, M. C., Chinn, S., Sterne, J. A. C., and Burney, P. G. J. (1999). Methods for Evaluating Area-wide and Organisation-based Interventions in Health and Health Care: A Systematic Review. *Health Technology Assessment* 3 (5). Available: http://www.hta.nhsweb.nhs.uk/fullmono/mon305.pdf (Access date: August 10, 2006).

57. Cummings, P., and Koepsell, T. D. (2002). Statistical and Design Issues in Studies of Groups. *Injury Prevention* 8: 6–7.

58. Donner, A., and Klar, N. (2004). Pitfalls of and Controversies in Cluster Randomization Trials. *American Journal of Public Health* 94 (3): 416–422.

59. Roberts, C., and Sibbald, B. (1998). Randomising Groups of Patients. *British Medical Journal* 316: 1898–1900.

60. Medical Research Council (2002). Cluster Randomised Trials: Methodological and Ethical Considerations. Available: http://www.mrc.ac.uk/index/publications/pdf-cluster_randomised_trials-link (Access date: August 10, 2006).

61. Zyzanski, S. J., Flocke, S. A., Dickinson, L. M. (2004). On the Nature and Analysis of Clustered Data. *Annals of Family Medicine* 2 (3): 199–200.
62. Wears, R. L. (2002). Statistical Methods for Analyzing Cluster and Cluster-randomized Data. *Academic Emergency Medicine* 9 (4): 330–341.
63. Campbell, M. K., and Grimshaw, J. M. (1998). Cluster Randomized Trials: Time for Improvement. *British Medical Journal* 317: 1171–1172.
64. Killip, S., Mahfoud, Z., and Pearce, K. (2004). What Is an Intracluster Correlation Coefficient? Crucial Concepts for Primary Care Researchers. *Annals of Family Medicine* 2 (3): 204–208.
65. Kerry, S. M., and Bland, J. M. (1998). Sample Size in Cluster Randomisation. *British Medical Journal* 316: 549.
66. Grimshaw, J., Eccles, M., Campbell, M., and Elbourne, D. (2005). Cluster Randomized Trials of Professional and Organizational Behavior Change Interventions in Health Care Settings. *The Annals of the American Academy of Political and Social Science* 599: 71–93.
67. Campbell, M. K., Mollison, J., Steen, N., Grimshaw, J. M., and Eccles, M. (2000). Analysis of Cluster Randomized Trials in Primary Care: A Practical Approach. *Family Practice* 17 (2): 192–196.
68. Kerry, S. M., and Bland, J. M. (1998). Analysis of a Trial Randomized in Clusters. *British Medical Journal* 316: 54.
69. Bingenheimer, J. B., and Raudenbush, S. W. (2004). Statistical and Substantive Inferences in Public Health: Issues in the Application of Multilevel Models. *Annual Review of Public Health* 25: 53–77.
70. Diez-Roux, A. V. (2002). A Glossary for Multilevel Analysis. *Journal of Epidemiology and Community Health* 56: 588–594.
71. Woods, A. (2004). Multilevel Modelling in Primary Care Research. *British Journal of General Practice* 54 (504): 560–561.
72. Turner, R. M., White, I. R., and Croudace, T. (2006). Analysis of Cluster Randomized Crossover Trial Data: A Comparison of Methods. *Statistics in Medicine* (Abstract ahead of print). Available: http://www3.interscience.wiley.com/cgi-bin/abstract/112478383/ABSTRACT?CRETRY=1&SRETRY=0 (Access date: September 1, 2006).
73. Simpson, J. M., Oldenberg, B., Owen, N. et al. (2000). The Australian National Workplace Health Project: Design and Baseline Findings. *Preventive Medicine* 31: 249–260.
74. Donner, A. (1998). Some Aspects of the Design and Analysis of Cluster Randomization Trials. *Applied Statistics* 47 (Part 1): 95–113.
75. Koepsell, T. D. (1998). Epidemiologic Issues in the Design of Community Intervention Trials. In *Applied Epidemiology: Theory to Practice*, R. C. Brownson and D. B. Petitti, eds. New York: Oxford University Press, pp. 177–211.
76. Hutton, J. L. (2001). Are Distinctive Ethical Principles Required for Cluster Randomised Controlled Trials? *Statistics in Medicine* 20: 473–488.
77. Eccles, M., Grimshaw, J., Campbell, M., and Ramsay, C. (2003). Research Designs for Studies Evaluating the Effectiveness of Change and Improvement Strategies. *Quality & Safety in Health Care* 12: 47–52.
78. Campbell, D. T., and Stanley, J. C. (1963). *Experimental and Quasi-experimental Designs for Research*. Chicago: Rand McNally College Publishing Company.
79. Vogt, W. P. (1999). *Dictionary of Statistics & Methodology: A Nontechnical Guide for the Social Sciences*, 2nd ed. Thousand Oaks, CA: Sage Publications.
80. Gilbody, S., and Whitty, P. (2002). Improving the Delivery and Organization of Mental Health Services: Beyond the Conventional Randomised Controlled Trial. *British Journal of Psychiatry* 180: 13–18.
81. Dimsdale, T., and Kutner, M. (2004). *Becoming an Educated Consumer of Research: A Quick Look at the Basics of Research Methodologies and Designs*. Meeting of the Minds Practitioner-Researcher Symposium. Available: http://www.air.org/publications/documents/Becoming%20an%20Educated%20Consumer%20of%20Research.pdf (Access date: September 15, 2006).

CHAPTER THIRTEEN

Screening for Disease and Other Conditions

This chapter covers principles of screening for disease and other conditions, including types of screening, validity and reliability of screening tests, guidelines for screening, and methods of assessing the effectiveness of screening programs.

Learning Objectives

- Explain the fundamental purposes and values of screening.
- Compare and contrast the four common types of screening.
- Describe how the validity of a screening test is usually determined.
- Describe the interrelationships among sensitivity, specificity, positive predictive value, negative predictive value, and prevalence.
- Calculate, compare, and interpret a screening test's sensitivity, specificity, positive and negative predictive values, and the prevalence of the disorder for which screening is being used.
- Compare and contrast the potential consequences of false positive and false negative screening results.
- Calculate, interpret, and appraise the overall accuracy of a screening test.
- Define and describe likelihood ratios in the context of screening.
- Determine and interpret a likelihood ratio and posttest probability for a screening test using calculations as well as a nomogram.
- Distinguish among method variability, subject variability, and observer variability.
- Calculate and interpret observer reliability using percent agreement, positive percent agreement, percent negative agreement, and Cohen's kappa.
- Identify the strengths and limitations of percent agreement and effective percent agreement measures.
- Identify the major strengths and limitations of Cohen's kappa.
- Explain and give examples of the major guidelines for screening.
- List common disorders for which screening is generally accepted and for which its acceptance is more controversial.

- Describe and explain the four major types of bias that may threaten evaluations of screening program effectiveness.
- Clarify the basic approaches to overcoming the four major types of bias that may threaten evaluations of screening program effectiveness.
.- Define Bayes' theorem; bias effect; critical point; detectable preclinical phase; false negative rate; false positive rate; false negative, false positive, true negative, and true positive; interobserver and intraobserver reliability; interobserver and intraobserver variability; interrater and intrarater reliability; likelihood ratio for a negative test result; likelihood ratio for a positive test result; nominal; observer; ordinal; precision of a screening test; prevalence effect; prevalence-adjusted bias-adjusted kappa; pseudodisease; reliability; screening level; slippery-linkage bias; sticky-diagnosis bias; true negative rate; true positive rate; weighted kappa; yield; and zero-time shift.

INTRODUCTION

Screening for disease or other disorders is very common in our culture. For example, over 98 percent of all infants born in the United States are screened for phenylketonuria, hypothyroidism, and sickle cell disease.[1] Phenylketonuria (PKU), a congenital, hereditary disorder in amino acid metabolism, and hypothyroidism can cause severe mental retardation if untreated. Sickle cell disease can cause chronic anemia and other significant health problems. School children in the U.S. are often screened for vision and hearing problems and sometimes for other conditions as well. Adults routinely receive screening from their physicians for a number of conditions at appropriate life stages and when they are members of certain high risk groups. In fact, screening is so pervasive in our society that free blood pressure screening is available at many public health departments and pharmacies. In addition, health fairs and mobile units usually offer a variety of low-cost or free screening tests, and some large corporations and public institutions offer their employees periodic screening for various diseases and other conditions.

Screening can be defined as a relatively quick means of identifying individuals who *may* have a given disorder that is not clinically apparent at the time. Screening does not establish a diagnosis but helps to differentiate those who are likely to have the disorder from those who are unlikely to have it. Those who screen positive for a specific disorder should undergo further testing to determine if the disorder is actually present. A positive blood sugar test for diabetes, for instance, does not necessarily mean someone has diabetes. Further testing would be required to establish a definitive diagnosis. In order for screening to be considered valuable, it should at a minimum result in earlier than usual detection when treatment is more effective. Specifically, early treatment should produce a better prognosis than if the disorder were detected and treated later when clinical signs or symptoms are apparent. Examples of some diseases and conditions for which screening is commonly accepted include breast, colorectal, and cervical cancer; hypertension, diabetes, and lipid disorders; and hepatitis B, HIV infection, and tuberculosis. More examples are provided later in the chapter.

Depending on intent, screening can take place at different stages in the natural history of disease and can represent different levels of prevention (chapter 3). Screening for preclinical disease has the objective of identifying individuals in the *stage of presymptomatic disease*. Thus, it is a mode of *secondary prevention* (see figure 3-5). Screening can also be used to identify individuals with risk factors for disease. Typically, this type of screening is aimed at those in the *stage of susceptibility*. Hence, it represents a method of *primary prevention*. Cholesterol screening, for example, is used routinely to identify persons who may be at increased risk of heart disease so that appropriate steps may be taken to reduce their risk. Screening may also be performed during the *stage of clinical disease* to detect complications of a disorder, which if confirmed can then be promptly treated to improve a patient's survival or quality of life. In this application, screening takes the form of *tertiary prevention*.

The chief focus of this chapter is on basic principles associated with screening for diseases or other conditions during the stage of presymptomatic disease, which, as noted above, represents a form of secondary prevention and is the most common application of screening. The concepts and principles discussed in the chapter should also apply to screening aimed at identifying risk factors in healthy individuals (primary prevention) as well as identifying complications in diseased individuals (tertiary prevention). Before discussing some of the more technical aspects of screening, we will first review the various types of screening commonly practiced in public health and medicine.

TYPES OF SCREENING

Screening can be categorized into one of the following four types depending on objectives, target group, or setting. These are:

- **Mass screening**. This form of screening is aimed at large, generally diverse, populations where the probability of individuals having a preclinical form of the disorder of interest is likely to be variable. Screening for PKU is an example of mass screening directed at all newborns. Vision screening at an elementary school is another example of mass screening. In both instances everyone in the defined population is screened regardless of his or her probability of having the disorder of interest.

- **Selective screening**. This form of screening, also known as **targeted screening**, is applied only to select groups with a *greater than average probability* of having a preclinical form of the disorder of interest. Screening for elevated levels of lead in the blood among inner-city children is an example of selective screening. So is screening for tuberculosis among prison inmates. Selective screening can be expected to result in the detection of more positive cases of a given disorder than mass screening because of the higher probability that members of the group have preclinical forms of the disorder.

- **Opportunistic screening**. This type of screening usually occurs in a physician's office when patients come in for unrelated problems, and the physician *takes the opportunity* to perform or order one or more screening tests. This form of screening has also been called **case finding**.[2] Unlike mass or selective screening where individuals with positive screening results are referred for follow-up testing, opportunistic screening places the responsibility for follow up on the physician performing or supervising the screening test. Therefore, opportunistic screening is more likely to result in follow up than other types of screening.[3] Many individuals identified as having elevated blood pressure during a mass screening, for example, may not seek the recommended follow up, but a physician finding elevated blood pressure during a routine examination will ordinarily schedule additional testing. Examples of opportunistic screening include screening for cervical cancer using a Pap test, heart disease using a stress test, and diabetes using a blood glucose or urine test. In addition, optometrists and ophthalmologists routinely screen patients for glaucoma.

- **Multiphasic screening**. This type of screening is not independent of the other three but is designated multiphasic because it involves screening for several disorders on the same occasion.[2] Pre-military exams, for example, often employ multiphasic screening to test for possible disorders such as diabetes, hypertension, and hearing impairment in prospective soldiers.

Accuracy of Screening Tests

As discussed in chapter 8, accuracy has two major components—validity and precision. Thus, screening tests are *accurate* to the extent that they demonstrate *both* validity and precision. In this context, the **validity of a screening test** refers to the degree to which the screening test does what it is designed to do (i.e., detect those who have a given preclinical disorder and those who do not). The **precision of a screening test** refers to its reliability, that is, its consistency from one application to another. Each of the two components of accuracy is discussed in more detail in the sections that follow.

Validity of a Screening Test

Many screening tests are designed to produce positive or negative results based on a predetermined standard. A positive result implies that the disorder is *likely* to be present, and a follow-up diagnostic test is therefore advised. A negative result implies that the disorder is *unlikely* to be present, and a follow-up diagnostic test is therefore not indicated. Unfortunately, screening tests vary in how well they detect the presence or absence of preclinical disorders. The primary way to measure the validity of a screening test is to give a representative group of volunteers the screening test to determine who tests positive and who tests negative and then to give the same group a definitive diagnostic test (i.e., a *gold standard*; see chapter 1) to determine who actually has and does not have the disorder. The results of the screening test are then compared for congruence with the gold standard.* This can lead to four possible outcomes:

- **True positives** (TP). These are individuals who test positive on the screening test and who have the disorder based on the gold standard.
- **False positives** (FP). These are individuals who test positive on the screening test but do not have the disorder based on the gold standard.
- **False negatives** (FN). These are individuals who test negative on the screening test but have the disorder based on the gold standard.
- **True negatives** (TN). These are individuals who test negative on the screening test and who do not have the disorder based on the gold standard.

For simplicity, a 2 × 2 table, such as the one shown below, can be used to summarize the four possible outcomes of a screening test based on the results of a gold standard representing the true status with regard to the disorder of interest.

	True Disorder Status		
Screening Test	Positive	Negative	**Total**
Positive	TP	FP	TP + FP
Negative	FN	TN	FN + TN
Total	TP + FN	FP + TN	TP + FP + FN + TN

Although all four possible outcomes (TP, FP, FN, and TN) are used in evaluating the validity of a screening test, two of these outcomes (FP and FN) are key. If there are no false positives or false negatives, the screening test will have 100 percent validity. Therefore, increasing the validity of screening tests has to do with minimizing the number of false positives and false negatives.

Traditionally, four common measures have been used in validating screening tests.[4-6] These measures are:

- Sensitivity
- Specificity
- Positive predictive value
- Negative predictive value

*An option is to apply the screening test to a group and follow up to determine who develops the disorder.

The first two measures can be broadly conceived as *measures of discrimination* between those who have and do not have the disorder of interest. The latter two measures can be viewed as *measures of prediction* of the probability of having or not having the disorder of interest given the screening test result.[7] Each of these measures is discussed in more detail in the following segments. Some other indicators of validity are also described.

Sensitivity and specificity.   The fundamental measures of the validity of a screening test are *sensitivity* and *specificity*. **Sensitivity** is a measure of the ability of a screening test to identify those with the disorder, while **specificity** is a measure of the ability of a screening test to identify those without it.[4] Statistically speaking, sensitivity is the proportion of those with the disorder of interest who screen positive, while specificity is the proportion of those without the disorder who screen negative. Sensitivity and specificity are usually stated as percents and, as implied previously, are generally determined by comparing the screening results with those of a definitive diagnostic test or gold standard. For example, in principle, the sensitivity and specificity of a new screening test for coronary heart disease could be measured by comparing the screening results on a sample of volunteers to the results obtained by angiograms, which represent the gold standard for the diagnosis of coronary heart disease. Drawing on the above 2 × 2 table, sensitivity and specificity are calculated using the following formulas:

(13.1) $\text{Sensitivity (\%)} = [\text{TP} / (\text{TP} + \text{FN})] \times 100$

(13.2) $\text{Specificity (\%)} = [\text{TN} / (\text{FP} + \text{TN})] \times 100$

Note that the denominator for sensitivity (TP + FN) is equivalent to the number of individuals in the screened population *with* the disorder of interest, and for specificity the denominator (FP + TN) is the same as the number of individuals in the screened population *without* the disorder of interest. Sensitivity and specificity are sometimes referred to as the **true positive rate** (TPR) and the **true negative rate** (TNR), respectively. Other less familiar measures related to the validity of a screening test are the **false negative rate** (FNR) and the **false positive rate** (FPR), which are described in table 13-1. These measures are the counterparts of the true positive rate (sensitivity) and the true negative rate (specificity). Hence, FNR + TPR = 100 percent, and FPR + TNR = 100 percent.

Ideally, we would like to have screening tests with 100 percent sensitivity and 100 percent specificity. This way, the screening test would be able to identify correctly all those with the disorder of interest as well as those without the disorder. Unfortunately, this is usually not possible because many screening tests are based on continuous measures that rely on relatively arbitrary cutoff points known as **screening levels**. These are used to classify participants as positive or negative.[2] Screening questionnaires designed to detect clinical depression, for example, often depend on an overall score to indicate the likelihood of depression. The score used as the cutoff can affect the sensi-

Table 13-1 False Negative and False Positive Rates

The *False Negative Rate* (FNR) is the percent of those with the disease that are false negatives (i.e., those who test negative but have the disease). This is calculated as follows:

$$\text{FNR (\%)} = \frac{\text{No. of False Negatives}}{\text{No. of True Positives} + \text{No. of False Negatives}} \times 100$$

The *False Positive Rate* (FPR) is the percent of those without the disease that are false positives (i.e., those who test positive but do not have the disease). This is calculated as follows:

$$\text{FPR (\%)} = \frac{\text{No. of False Positives}}{\text{No. of False Positives} + \text{No. of True Negatives}} \times 100$$

tivity and specificity of the test. If a relatively *low* score is used to classify someone as clinically depressed, then the test will have very high sensitivity but only by sacrificing some specificity. In other words, most clinically depressed individuals will be classified correctly because of the low standard, but many who are not clinically depressed will be misclassified as depressed. Mathematically, the number of false negatives will be low thereby increasing sensitivity (see formula 13.1), but the number of false positives will be high thus decreasing specificity (see formula 13.2). Similarly, if the screening level is set too *high*, the test will have low sensitivity because many clinically depressed individuals will be misclassified, but the specificity will be very high because most people without clinical depression will be classified correctly. Mathematically, the number of false negatives will be high decreasing sensitivity (see formula 13.1), but the number of false positives will be low increasing specificity (see formula 13.2). This concept is illustrated graphically in figure 13-1. Screening level C in the diagram represents a compromise that minimizes losses in both sensitivity and specificity. This would be an appropriate screening level where sensitivity and specificity are considered of equal importance in a screening application. If sensitivity is considered more important than specificity, however, then screening level A would be a better choice. If, on the other hand, specificity is considered more important than sensitivity, screening level B would be the best choice. In general, increasing the sensitivity of a screening test tends to decrease its specificity and vice versa.

As should be clear from the preceding discussion and an examination of formulas 13.1 and 13.2, the number of *false negatives* affects the *sensitivity* of a screening test, and the number of *false positives* affects its *specificity*. As implied earlier, sensitivity would be 100 percent if there were no false negatives, and specificity would be 100 percent if there were no false positives. Therefore, in deciding whether sensitivity may be more or less important than specificity in a particular screening application, one should weigh the potential conse-

Figure 13-1   Selecting the Screening Level for a Screening Test

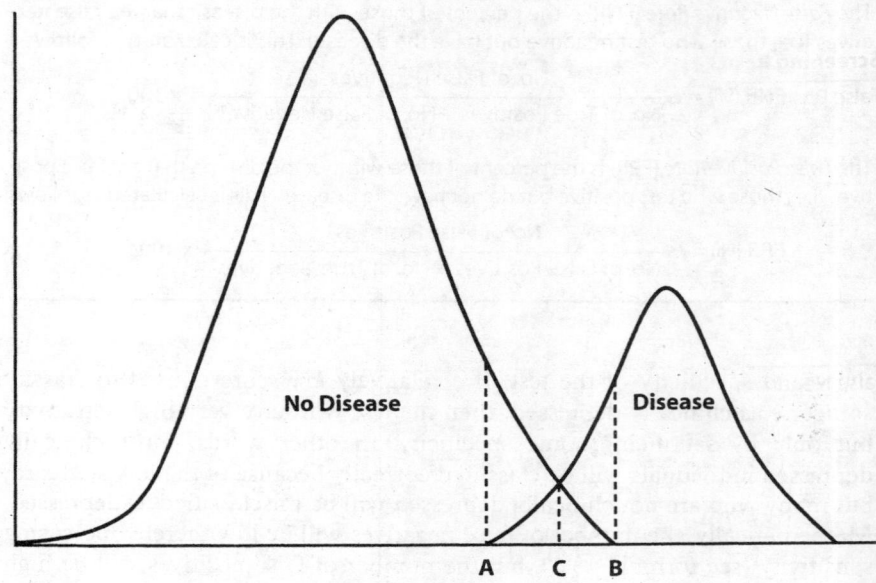

Which Screening Level Is Best?
A: Maximizes sensitivity but reduces specificity
B: Maximizes specificity but reduces sensitivity
C: Minimizes losses in both sensitivity and specificity

quences of identifying more false negatives than false positives and vice versa. Table 13-2 lists some of the potential consequences.

As indicated earlier, determining the actual status of a disorder requires a *definitive* diagnostic test or gold standard. Therefore, screening tests are *presumptive* only; they are not definitive. Nevertheless, screening that results in early detection of a disorder, which in turn leads to more effective treatment and a better prognosis, can be a valuable tool for public health and medical professionals. The qualities of an effective screening program are discussed later in this chapter.

Positive predictive value and negative predictive value. The predictive value of a screening test has two components—*positive predictive value* (also known as **predictive value of a positive test** or **predictive value positive**) and *negative predictive value* (also known as **predictive value of a negative test** or **predictive value negative**). Specifically, **positive predictive value** (PPV) is the probability that those who test positive on a screening test have the disorder in question, and **negative predictive value** (NPV) is the probability that those who test negative do *not* have the disorder in question (see formulas 13.3 and 13.4).

Table 13-2   Potential Consequences of False Positives and False Negatives in a Screening Program

Screening Results	Potential Consequences
False Positives	• Overuse of health care resources due to increased referrals for follow-up diagnostic testing
	• Anxiety associated with the fear of a having a serious disease (e.g., cervical cancer)
	• Inconvenience due to the additional time, expense, or annoyance associated with follow-up diagnostic tests (e.g., breast cancer screening)
	• Increased health risks from some diagnostic tests (e.g., angiograms, surgical biopsies)
False Negatives	• False sense of being free from a serious disease
	• Delayed medical attention that for some diseases could result in permanent disability or death (e.g., PKU, colon cancer)
	• Increased disease transmission when the disease is communicable (e.g., tuberculosis)

Predictive values can be valuable adjuncts to measures of sensitivity and specificity, which are the main measures of validity. They provide an indication of the practical utility of a screening test or program.[8] From a health practitioner's point of view, sensitivity and specificity are stable properties of a screening test that should to be considered *before* deciding whether or not to use a particular screening test. Predictive values, on the other hand, are what practitioners need to know *after* receiving the test results since this knowledge can affect the interpretation of the findings.[3, 4] Positive predictive value, for example, answers the question, if the screening result is positive for a given individual, what is the likelihood that the individual really has the disorder in question? In practice, positive predictive value tends to be considered a more important measure to health practitioners than negative predictive value, although you should be familiar with both measures. When the term "predictive value" is used in screening applications without a modifier the reference is usually to positive predictive value.

Theoretically, a perfectly effective screening test would have positive and negative predictive values of 100 percent each. The actual values, however, depend on the prevalence (P) of the disease or condition in the population being screened (formula 13.5) as well as the sensitivity and specificity of the screening test. The relationship of these factors to positive and negative predictive values are shown mathematically in formulas 13.6 and 13.7, respectively. These formulas are based on **Bayes' theorem**,[9] which is a proposition in probability theory that is commonly used in clinical epidemiology to estimate the probability of a specific diagnosis based on a screening test result.[2]

Based on this relationship, we know, for example, that for fixed levels of sensitivity and specificity, the higher the prevalence of the disorder, the greater the positive predictive value. Likewise, the lower the prevalence, the lower the positive predictive value. In terms of negative predictive value, the higher the prevalence, the lower the negative predictive value, and the lower the prevalence, the greater the negative predictive value. Prevalence then is a very important factor in determining positive or negative predictive values. Sensitivity and specificity can also be significant factors. In general, the greater the specificity of a screening test, the greater its positive predictive value, and the greater the sensitivity of a screening test, the greater its negative predictive value and vice versa.[3] These relationships are summarized in table 13-3. It is important to note that because predictive values are *not* stable properties of a screening test like sensitivity and specificity, they are best seen as population-specific indicators of validity. Therefore, they should not be compared indiscriminately among different populations since large differences in prevalence between populations could lead to disparate predictive values.

(13.3) $$PPV (\%) = [TP / (TP + FP)] \times 100$$

(13.4) $$NPV (\%) = [TN / (FN + TN)] \times 100$$

(13.5) $$P (\%) = [(TP + FN) / (TP + FP + FN + TN)] \times 100$$

As you can see from the above equations, the denominator for positive predictive value (PPV) is equivalent to *all those testing positive* (TP + FP) in the screened population, while the denominator for negative predictive value

Table 13-3   Effects of Changes in Sensitivity, Specificity, and Prevalence on Predictive Values and Other Measures

Increasing ...	Main Effects
Sensitivity	• Increases negative predictive value
	• Decreases false negative rate
Specificity	• Increases positive predictive value
	• Decreases false positive rate
Prevalence	• Increases positive predictive value
	• Decreases negative predictive value

Note: Not all the relationships indicated here are as simple as they may appear. For example, all other factors being equal, increases in prevalence have a more profound effect on positive predictive value when the prevalence is well below 50 percent and on negative predictive value when the prevalence is well above 50 percent. Also, all other factors being equal, increasing sensitivity tends to increase positive predictive value but not to the same extent as it tends to increase negative predictive value. Likewise, increasing specificity tends to increase negative predictive value but not to the same extent as it tends to increase positive predictive value.

(NPV) is equal to *all those testing negative* (FN + TN) in the screened population. The denominator for the prevalence (P) of the disorder corresponds to the *total number of individuals screened* (i.e., the size of the screened population). The data used to calculate formulas 13.3 through 13.5 can be conveniently placed in a 2 × 2 table equivalent to that shown earlier. All of this will be illustrated later in problems 13-1 and 13-2.

(13.6)
$$PPV(\%) = \frac{P \times Sensitivity}{[P \times Sensitivity] + [(1-P) \times (1-Specificity)]} \times 100$$

(13.7)
$$NPV(\%) = \frac{(1-P) \times Specificity}{[(1-P) \times Specificity] + [P \times (1-Sensitivity)]} \times 100$$

The prevalence (P) in formulas 13.6 and 13.7 is usually estimated based on the literature, local databases, or expert clinical judgment.[3] In using these formulas prevalence, sensitivity, and specificity should be stated as proportions versus percents. As one can see from formula 13.6, when specificity is one the PPV will be 100 percent. Also, as shown in formula 13.7, when sensitivity is one the NPV will be 100 percent. Moreover, when the prevalence is one the PPV will be 100 percent, and the NPV will be zero.

Since even a test with relatively high sensitivity and specificity may have poor positive predictive value if the prevalence of the disorder is low, it may not be advisable to use such a test in these circumstances. In general, the same screening test is more likely to have a higher positive predictive value in applications involving *selective screening* than those involving *mass screening* simply because select populations are more likely to have a higher prevalence of the disorder. Negative predictive value, on the other hand, will tend to be higher in applications involving mass versus selective screening due to an expected lower prevalence of the disorder in general populations.

Positive and negative predictive values are important indicators of the usefulness of a screening test, especially positive predictive value. Sometimes new screening tests with high levels of sensitivity and specificity show good positive predictive value in clinical settings but very poor positive predictive value when they are used in general populations. This is due to the difference in the prevalence of the disorder of interest between the two populations. Unless a screening test has a relatively high positive predictive value, it may be questionable for health professionals to order potentially risky and expensive follow-up tests based on a positive screening result. This is because many of those testing positive will turn out not to have the disorder (i.e., will be false positives). As revealed by the formulas for positive and negative predictive value (formulas 13.3 and 13.4), when the number of false positives is high, the positive predictive value will be low, and when the number of false negatives is high, the negative predictive value will be low. As indicated previously, some of the potential consequences of false positives and false negatives are shown in table 13-2.

Overall accuracy.   Sensitivity and specificity are properties of a screening test that give us an indication of its validity. A measure that seeks to combine these two factors into a single summary estimate of overall validity has been referred to by several names, such as **accuracy of the test,**[10] **accuracy,**[11] and **overall accuracy,**[12] even though it only measures one component of accuracy as defined in this text.* Of the three terms, *overall accuracy* seems the most descriptive since the measure represents a weighted average. Mathematically, overall accuracy is the weighted average of the sensitivity and specificity of a screening test: (sensitivity × proportion with the disorder) + (specificity × proportion without the disorder). The standard equation for overall accuracy is given in formula 13.8. While the measure represents the average percent of those correctly classified by a given screening test, it does not present the detail provided by separate calculations of sensitivity and specificity. In fact, it can conceal a low sensitivity or specificity since it depends on the proportion of those with or without the disorder in the population being screened. Indeed, overall accuracy becomes more inaccurate the more sensitivity and specificity differ from each other or the more the prevalence of the disorder deviates from 50 percent in either direction.[12] Therefore, overall accuracy is not recommended as a measure of test validity. If used, it should be considered a supplemental measure that should always be accompanied by separate measures of sensitivity and specificity. Like sensitivity and specificity, its basic calculation is derived from a combination of the four possible screening outcomes shown in the 2 × 2 table referred to earlier in this chapter.

(13.8)

Overall Accuracy (%) = [(TP + TN) / (TP + FP + FN + TN)] × 100

Likelihood ratios.   Other indicators of the validity of screening tests include **likelihood ratios**, which in the context of screening can be expressed as the probability of a particular value of a screening test result in those with the disorder of interest divided by the probability of the same value in those without the disorder.[3] Unlike more traditional measures of validity, likelihood ratios do not require that test results be dichotomized into positive or negative findings. Therefore, they are useful with screening (or diagnostic) tests that are measured on *ordinal* (ordered; defined more specifically later in the chapter) or continuous scales. At the same time, they may still be used when the screening results are dichotomous (i.e., positive or negative).[13] In addition, there are other advantages to likelihood ratios: (a) unlike predictive values, they are not dependent on the prevalence of the disorder, and (b) they can be applied directly to individuals.[14] Hence, they should remain stable in different populations, and they should be useful to clinicians who work with individual patients. In describing likelihood ratios in the following paragraphs we will assume that the screening test results are dichotomous. This will simplify our discussion while still allowing us to explore pertinent aspects of this impor-

*Some authors use the term accuracy in a narrower sense than that used in this textbook, namely to refer specifically to validity.

tant measure. Some descriptions, however, will be true only for dichotomous outcomes. More detail can be found in more advanced resources.

There are two basic types of likelihood ratios. The **likelihood ratio for a positive test result** (LR^+) is the probability of a positive test result in those with the disorder divided by the probability of a positive test result in those without the disorder.[15] For example, an LR^+ of 7.0 means that a positive test result is seven times as likely to be found in those with the disorder than those without the disorder. Similarly, the **likelihood ratio for a negative test result** (LR^-) is the probability of a negative test result in those with the disorder divided by the probability of a negative test result in those without the disorder.[15] For example, an LR^- of 0.20 indicates that a negative test result is only 0.20 times as likely to be found in those with the disorder compared to those without the disorder. Technically, a likelihood ratio is an *odds* as defined in chapter 5.

Though not commonly reported in the literature, some have advocated the use of an additional likelihood ratio that measures the ratio of the probability of a negative test result in those *without* the disorder to the probability of a negative test result in those with the disorder. They argue that this measure, which is the reciprocal of LR^-, is a more logical measure than LR^- since clinicians are more likely to associate a negative test result with the absence of the disorder.[16] In the above example where LR^- was 0.20, this measure would be its reciprocal or $1 / 0.20 = 5.0$. Hence, a negative test result would be five times as likely to be found in those *without* the disorder than in those with the disorder.

The likelihood ratio for a positive test result can be calculated by dividing the true positive rate (sensitivity) by the false positive rate (1 – specificity) as shown in formula 13.9. Likewise, the likelihood ratio for a negative test result can be calculated by dividing the false negative rate (1 – sensitivity) by the true negative rate (specificity) as shown in formula 13.10. You may recall that the false positive rate is the complement of specificity, and the false negative rate is the complement of sensitivity (see the paragraph immediately following formula 13.2). In essence, LR^+ is the ratio of something clinicians desire (sensitivity) to something they do not desire (false positives), and LR^- is the ratio of something clinicians do not desire (false negatives) to something they desire (specificity). Therefore, the larger LR^+ and the smaller LR^-, the better the screening test.[17]

(13.9) $LR^+ = \text{Sensitivity} / (1 - \text{Specificity})$

(13.10) $LR^- = (1 - \text{Sensitivity}) / \text{Specificity}$

Sensitivity and specificity when used in the above formulas should be stated as proportions versus percents.

As measures of odds, the values of both LR^+ and LR^- may range from zero to a value that theoretically has no specific upper limit (see chapter 5). A value of one indicates that the screening test is not useful in separating those who have and do not have the disorder of interest since the probability of the screening outcome is the same in both those with and without the disorder. For LR$^+$, values greater than one indicate an association between a positive screening test result and having the disorder of interest. For LR$^-$, values less than one indicate an association between a negative test result and *not* having the disorder.[15] In general, the more extreme the values (above one for LR$^+$ or below one for LR$^-$), the stronger the associations and the more valuable the screening test because of its predictive power. Rule of thumb guidelines suggest that an LR$^+$ of 5.0 to 10.0 represents a moderate level of association, while a ratio greater than 10.0 implies a strong association. Likewise, an LR$^-$ of 0.1 to 0.2 is indicative of a moderate association, and a ratio of less than 0.1 implies a strong association.[18] Strong associations provide support for the validity of a screening test.

With a small amount of mathematical manipulation (not shown here), it can be demonstrated that LR$^+$ is equivalent to the odds of the disorder among those with a positive screening test divided by the odds of the disorder *in the study population as a whole.* Likewise, LR$^-$ is equivalent to the odds of the disorder among those with a negative screening test divided by the odds of the disorder *in the study population as a whole.*[17] These forms of the likelihood ratios are therefore *odds ratios* (chapter 6). LR$^+$ reveals how much the odds of the disorder are increased when the test result is positive, and LR$^-$ reveals how much the odds of the disorder are decreased when the test result is negative, relative to the odds in the population.[17] For example, an LR$^+$ of 6.0 implies that the odds of having the disorder of interest, *given a positive test result,* are six times the odds of the disorder in the study population. This represents a 500 percent increase in odds. Similarly, an LR$^-$ of 0.25 implies that the odds of having the disorder, *given a negative test result,* are only 0.25 times the odds of the disorder in the study population. This represents a 75 percent decrease in odds. To reiterate previous points, we can say, in general, that a screening test with a very high LR$^+$ and a very small LR$^-$ is likely to be valid.

From a practical point of view, individual clinicians tend to be more interested in *posttest probabilities* (defined below) than likelihood ratios per se. That is, they often want to know what the probability is that someone in their care has the disorder of interest given his or her test result.* Calculating this probability requires first determining the *posttest odds* of the disorder (also defined below). This can be calculated using Bayes' theorem, which was mentioned earlier in this section. The applicable equation is:

(13.11)   Posttest Odds = Pretest Odds × Likelihood Ratio

The **pretest odds** in formula 13.11 are the odds that someone has the disorder of interest prior to the administration of the screening (or diagnostic) test. The pretest odds are usually based on the **pretest probability** of the dis-

---

*The test result can be from a screening test or a diagnostic test. Often clinicians are more concerned with diagnostic tests. The principles, however, are the same.

order, which is an estimate of the chance of the disorder prior to testing. It may be determined based on clinical judgment or on the prevalence of the disorder in the broader population.[13] The pretest probability must be converted from a probability to an odds, however, in order to use formula 13.11. This can be done quite simply in the following manner:

(13.12)   Pretest Odds = Pretest Probability / (1 – Pretest Probability)

In this formula the pretest probability is stated as a proportion (i.e., decimal fraction). If prevalence is used to estimate the pretest probability, it is best derived from a population with characteristics similar to those of the individual of interest. For instance, if one wanted to estimate the pretest probability of prostate cancer for a 50-year-old African American, it would be best to find an estimate of the prevalence of prostate cancer among African Americans of roughly the same age. This should be fairly easy to obtain.

Once the pretest odds are estimated, they are multiplied by the appropriate likelihood ratio (LR^+ or LR^-) to obtain the **posttest odds**, which are the odds that someone has the disorder following the administration of the screening (or diagnostic) test (see formula 13.11). As a final step, the posttest odds are converted into the desired **posttest probability** of the disorder, which is an estimate of the chance of the disorder following the administration of the test. This can be done using formula 13.13.

(13.13)   Posttest Probability = Posttest Odds / (1 + Posttest Odds)

Sample calculations are presented in problems 13-1 and 13-2. Keep in mind that the referents (chapter 6) for the pretest and posttest odds and probabilities are those without the disorder of interest.

A method of simplifying the process of calculating posttest probabilities is to use a **nomogram** (see figure 13-2). This is a "chart showing scales for the variables involved in a particular formula in such a way that corresponding values for each variable lie on a straight line intersecting all the scales."[2(p123)] To employ the nomogram for estimating posttest probabilities, one uses a ruler or other straightedge to connect the predetermined value of the pretest probability with the predetermined value of the likelihood ratio. The point at which the ruler or straightedge crosses the third vertical line is the posttest probability. For example, assume the pretest probability in a particular application is 20 percent and the likelihood ratio for a positive test result is 10. A ruler connecting these two points on the nomogram will cross the third vertical line at a point representing a posttest probability of 70 percent (see figure 13-2). This is the same value we would arrive at if we did the calculation manually.

Figure 13-2   Nomogram for Converting Pretest Probabilities to Posttest Probabilities

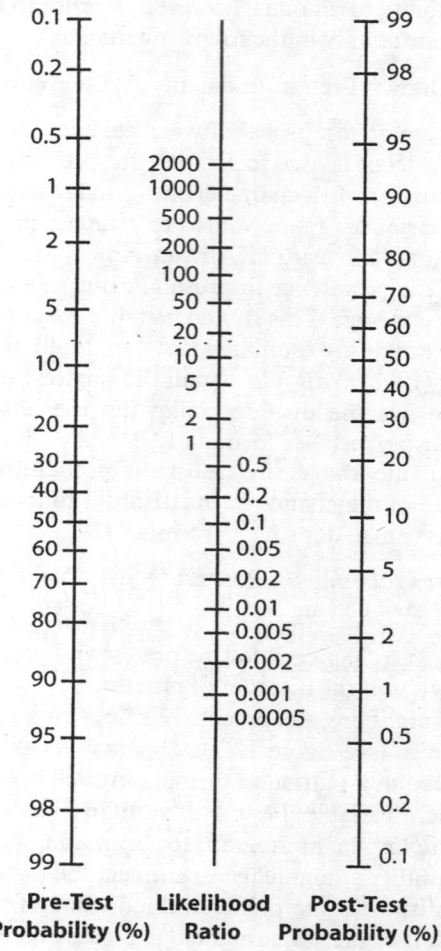

Pre-Test   Likelihood   Post-Test
Probability (%)   Ratio   Probability (%)

Source: Centre for Evidence-Based Medicine, Institute of Health Sciences (No date). Likelihood Ratios. Available: http://www.cebm.net/likelihood_ratios.asp (Access date: October 6, 2006). Permission granted by the Centre for Evidence-Based Medicine.

Problem 13-1: Measures Used in Validating Screening Tests, Part I

A newly developed screening test for the detection of depression was administered to 1,000 adult volunteers attending a large medical clinic in New York. The results of the screening revealed that 152 out of 160 diagnosed cases of depression were correctly identified by the screening test. Also, of the 840 individuals without depression, the screening test correctly identified 714. Based on this information, calculate the test's sensitivity, specificity, overall accuracy, and positive and negative predictive values. Also calculate the posttest probability of depression based on the likelihood ratio for a positive test result. Interpret each of the calculated measures.

Solution:

Step 1: To assist in calculating the requested measures, it is helpful to first place the data into a 2 × 2 contingency table as follows:

True Disorder Status

Screening Test	Positive	Negative	Total
Positive	152 (TP)	126 (FP)	278
Negative	8 (FN)	714 (TN)	722
Total	160	840	1,000

Note that the data provided in the problem are sufficient to complete the above contingency table. There were 160 *diagnosed* cases of depression. This number is placed at the bottom of the left-hand column since it represents the number of actual cases. Since 152 of these cases were correctly identified by the screening test, they represent the number of true positives. This number is placed in the upper left-hand cell of the contingency table. Likewise, there were 840 individuals who did not have depression. This number is placed at the bottom of the right-hand column since it represents the number of noncases. A total of 714 people were correctly identified by the screening test as not having depression. These individuals represent the true negatives. This number is placed in the lower right-hand cell of the contingency table. The remaining numbers for the open cells and marginal totals can be computed using simple subtraction or addition. For example, the number of false negatives is not given in the problem but can be easily determined by subtracting the number of true positives from the total number with depression (i.e., 160 − 152 = 8). This number is then placed in the lower right-hand cell in the table. Note that the column totals and the row totals both equal the total number of persons screened (the grand total), which in this case is 1,000 (i.e., 160 + 840 = 1,000, and 278 + 722 = 1,000).

Step 2: Using the applicable formulas in the chapter and the data in the above 2 × 2 contingency table, calculate the initial list of measures requested in the problem.

Sensitivity = [TP / (TP + FN)] × 100 = (152 / 160) × 100 = 95.0%

Specificity = [TN / (FP + TN)] × 100 = (714 / 840) × 100 = 85.0%

Overall Accuracy = [(TP + TN) / (TP + FP + FN + TN)] × 100 = (866 / 1,000) × 100 = 86.6%

Positive Predictive Value = [TP / (TP + FP)] × 100 = (152 / 278) × 100 = 54.7%

Negative Predictive Value = [TN / (FN + TN)] × 100 = (714 / 722) × 100 = 98.9%

Step 3: To calculate the posttest probability of depression based on the likelihood ratio for a positive test result, a multi-step approach is necessary. First, using the data supplied in the problem and formula 13.5, calculate the baseline prevalence of depression in the study population as an estimate of the pretest probability of the condition for a typical subject in the population. Second, based on this value, calculate the pretest odds of the condition using formula 13.12. Third, use formula 13.9 to calculate the likelihood ratio for a positive test result using the applicable values of sensitivity and specificity previously calculated in step 2. Finally, calculate the posttest odds of the condition using formula 13.11 and convert this to a posttest probability of depression using formula 13.13.

$$\text{Prevalence} = [(TP + FN) / (TP + FP + FN + TN)] \times 100 = (160 / 1,000) \times 100 = 16.0\%$$

$$\text{Pretest Odds of the Disorder} = P / (1 - P) = 0.16 / 0.84 = 0.19$$

$$\text{Likelihood Ratio for a Positive Test Result} = \text{Sensitivity} / (1 - \text{Specificity}) =$$
$$0.95 / 0.15 = 6.33$$

$$\text{Posttest Odds} = \text{Pretest Odds} \times \text{Likelihood Ratio} = 0.19 \times 6.33 = 1.20$$

$$\text{Posttest Probability} = \text{Posttest Odds} / (1 + \text{Posttest Odds}) = 1.20 / 2.20 = 0.545$$

Answer: The sensitivity of the screening test is 95.0 percent. This means that the screening test was able to identify correctly 95 percent of those who have depression in the study population. The specificity of the test is 85.0 percent. This means that the test was able to identify correctly 85 percent of those who do not have depression in the study population. The overall accuracy of the test is 86.6 percent. This indicates that on average the screening test identified correctly 86.6 percent of the depression classifications (i.e., present or absent). The positive predictive value of the test is 54.7 percent. This indicates that of those who tested positive for depression only 54.7 percent actually had the condition. The negative predictive value of the test is 98.9 percent. This means that almost 99 percent of those who tested negative for depression did not have it. The posttest probability of depression is 0.545. This suggests that a representative subject in the study population who screens positive for depression has a 54.5 percent chance of having the condition.

Comments:
1. Based on the screening test results, this is a very sensitive test. It is able to identify correctly 95 percent of those in the study population with depression. Consequently, the false negative rate is only five percent (i.e., sensitivity or the true positive rate + the false negative rate = 100 percent). The specificity of the test is not quite as good, however, since the test is only able to identify correctly 85 percent of those without depression. Consequently, the false positive rate is 15 percent (i.e., specificity or the true negative rate + the false positive rate = 100 percent). In considering whether or not to use the screening test in similar populations, one should consider, among other factors, the validity of existing screening tests for depression.

2. The overall accuracy of the screening test is 86.6 percent. This represents a weighted average of the sensitivity and specificity of the test where the weights are, respectively, the proportions with and without diagnosed depression. Note that the weight applied to specificity (840 / 1000 = 0.84) is much greater than that applied to sensitivity (160 / 1000 = 0.16). Therefore, the overall accuracy is closer to the value of the specificity than it is to the sensitivity of the test. This illustrates why it is important to report sensitivity and specificity along with overall accuracy.

3. The positive predictive value of the screening test appears to be low when compared to the test's sensitivity and specificity. Of those who tested positive for depression on the screening test, only 54.7 percent actually have the condition. This means that many false positives were identified. The negative predictive value, however, appears very high. Of those who tested negative for depression, 98.9% do not have the condition. Thus, less than two percent of those who tested negative for depression are false negatives. More is said about predictive values in problem 13-2.

4. Based on Bayes' theorem, the positive predictive value (PPV) can be expressed in terms of sensitivity, specificity, and prevalence (P) as shown below.[19] This is equivalent to formula 13.6.

$$PPV = \frac{P(\text{Sensitivity})}{P(\text{Sensitivity}) + (1-P)(1-\text{Specificity})}$$

It can be demonstrated mathematically that this is equivalent to the *posttest probability* of the condition based on the likelihood ratio for a positive test result (LR$^+$).

$$\text{Posttest Odds} = \text{Pretest Odds} \times LR^+$$

$$\text{Pretest Odds} = P / 1 - P$$

$$LR^+ = \text{Sensitivity} / (1 - \text{Specificity})$$

$$\text{Therefore, Posttest Odds} =$$

$$\frac{P(\text{Sensitivity})}{(1-P)(1-\text{Sensitivity})}$$

However, Posttest Probability = Posttest Odds / (1 + Posttest Odds)

Therefore, Posttest Probability =

$$\frac{P(\text{Sensitivity})}{(1-P)(1-\text{Specificity})} \times \frac{1}{1 + \dfrac{P(\text{Sensitivity})}{(1-P)(1-\text{Specificity})}} =$$

$$\frac{P(\text{Sensitivity})}{(1-P)(1-\text{Specificity}) + P(\text{Sensitivity})} = \frac{P(\text{Sensitivity})}{P(\text{Sensitivity}) + (1-P)(1-\text{Specificity})}$$

The last expression on the right is exactly the same as that for the positive predictive value. Therefore, the positive predictive value and posttest probability calculated in this problem should yield the same results except for rounding error. This is, in fact, the case (PPV = 54.7 percent and Posttest probability = 0.545 or 54.5 percent). Though not calculated here, the posttest probability based on a likelihood ratio for a negative test result (LR$^-$) is equal to one minus the negative predictive value. The negative predictive value was 98.9 percent (see step 2). Therefore, the posttest probability should be: $1 - 0.989 = 0.011$, which is what a direct calculation of the posttest probability based on LR$^-$ reveals. In short, posttest probability based on LR$^+$ is equivalent to the positive predictive value expressed as a proportion, and posttest probability based on LR$^-$ is equivalent to one minus the negative predictive value expressed as a proportion.

5. We could have estimated the posttest probability in this problem using the *nomogram* in figure 13-2. To do so, we would take the pretest probability and likelihood

ratio calculated in step 3 and connect them on the first two vertical lines using a straightedge. The point at which the straightedge crosses the third vertical line is the posttest probability expressed as a percent.

6. Finally, note that in terms of validity the likelihood ratio for a positive test result suggests only a modest level of validity based on the rule of thumb guidelines presented earlier. Though not calculated in this problem, the likelihood ratio for a negative test result would be 0.059. Based on the same guidelines, this suggests a high level of validity. Stated differently, the calculated LR$^+$ of 6.33 indicates that among those testing positive on the screening test the odds of having depression are about six times the odds of having depression in the study population as a whole. Likewise, an LR$^-$ of 0.059 indicates that among those testing negative on the screening test the odds of having depression are only about 0.06 times the odds of having depression in the study population as a whole. In other words, testing positive increases the odds that one has depression, and testing negative substantially decreases the odds. Therefore, the screening test is helpful, though more so for negative than positive findings based on this measure.

Problem 13-2: Measures Used in Validating Screening Tests, Part II

The same screening test for depression described in problem 13-1 was repeated among 1,000 adult volunteers at a large clinic in Pittsburgh, Pennsylvania. This time, of 40 diagnosed cases of depression, 38 were detected by the screening test. Of 960 persons without depression, the screening test correctly identified 816. Based on these data, calculate the test's sensitivity, specificity, overall accuracy, and positive and negative predictive values. Also calculate the posttest probability of depression based on the likelihood ratio for positive a test result.

Solution:

Step 1: As in problem 13-1, a 2 × 2 contingency table showing frequencies of the outcomes can be developed directly or indirectly from the data provided in the problem.

True Disorder Status

Screening Test	Positive	Negative	Total
Positive	38 (TP)	144 (FP)	182
Negative	2 (FN)	816 (TN)	818
Total	40	960	1,000

Step 2: Using the applicable formulas in the chapter and the data in the above contingency table, calculate the initial list of measures requested in the problem.

Sensitivity = [TP / (TP + FN)] × 100 = (38 / 40) × 100 = 95.0%

Specificity = [TN / (FP + TN)] × 100 = (816 / 960) × 100 = 85.0%

Overall Accuracy (%) = [(TP + TN) / (TP + FP + FN + TN)] × 100 =
(854 / 1,000) × 100 = 85.4%

Positive Predictive Value = [TP / (TP + FP)] × 100 = (38 / 182) × 100 = 20.9%

Negative Predictive Value = [TN / (FN + TN)] × 100 = (816 / 818) × 100 = 99.8%

Step 3: As in problem 13-1, to calculate the posttest probability of depression based on the likelihood ratio for a positive test result, a multi-step approach is necessary. First, using the data supplied in the problem and formula 13.5, calculate the baseline prevalence of depression as an estimate of the pretest probability of the condition for a representative subject in the study population. Second, based on this value, calculate the pretest odds of the condition using formula 13.12. Third, use formula 13.9 to calculate the likelihood ratio for a positive test result using the applicable values of sensitivity and specificity previously calculated in step 2. Finally, calculate the posttest odds using formula 13.11 and convert this to a posttest probability of depression using formula 13.13.

Prevalence = [(TP + FN) / (TP + FP + FN + TN)] × 100 = (40 / 1,000) × 100 = 4.0%

Pretest Odds of the Disorder = P / (1 − P) = 0.040 / 0.96 = 0.042

Likelihood Ratio for a Positive Test Result = Sensitivity / (1 − Specificity) =
0.95 / 0.15 = 6.33

Posttest Odds = Pretest Odds × Likelihood Ratio = 0.042 × 6.33 = 0.266

Posttest Probability = Posttest Odds / (1 + Posttest Odds) = 0.266 / 1.266 = 0.210

Answer: The sensitivity of the screening test is 95.0 percent, and its specificity is 85.0 percent. The overall accuracy of the test is 85.4 percent. Its positive predictive value is 20.9 percent, and its negative predictive value is 99.8 percent. The posttest probability of depression based on the likelihood ratio for a positive test result is 0.210.

Comments:

1. Since sensitivity and specificity are stable measures of the validity of a screening test, it is not surprising that they are the same in problems 13-1 and 13-2 even though the screening test was used in two different study populations (i.e., one in New York and one in Pittsburgh) with different prevalences of depression. In fact, the prevalence of depression was four times as great in the study population represented in problem 13-1 as that represented in this problem (16.0 percent versus 4.0 percent). This stability from population to population is one reason why sensitivity and specificity have traditionally been the preferred measures of the validity of a screening test.

2. While the overall accuracy in this problem (85.4 percent) is close to that in problem 13-1 (86.6 percent), there is a notable difference. This is because the difference in the proportions of those with and without diagnosed depression varies between the two study populations. In problem 13-1, the proportion of depressed subjects was 0.16, and the proportion of non-depressed subjects was 0.84. Therefore, the overall accuracy was equivalent to: (95% × 0.16) + (85% × 0.84) = 86.6%. In this problem, the respective proportions are 0.04 and 0.96. Therefore, the overall accuracy in this problem is even more heavily weighted toward the specificity of the test than in problem 13-1. Specifically, the overall accuracy is: (95% × 0.04) + (85% ×

0.96) = 85.4%. Note that the proportion of those with the disorder of interest is the same as the prevalence of that disorder expressed as a proportion, and the proportion of those without the disorder of interest is one minus the prevalence expressed as a proportion.

3. As mentioned previously in this chapter, the predictive values of a screening test are affected by the prevalence of the disorder for which screening is undertaken. In this problem, the prevalence of depression is only one-fourth that in problem 13-1 (4.0 percent vs.16.0 percent). For the same values of sensitivity and specificity, a smaller prevalence means a lower positive predictive value and a higher negative predictive value. Likewise, a higher prevalence means a higher positive predictive value and a lower negative predictive value. In practice, the differences can be quite dramatic, especially in the case of positive predictive value. Going from a prevalence of 16.0 percent to 4.0 percent in the two problems resulted in a reduction of the positive predictive value from 54.7 percent to just 20.9 percent. This represents a decrease of over 60 percent in the positive predictive value. The inverse effect on negative predictive value is not nearly as dramatic. The four-fold decrease in prevalence resulted in an increase in the negative predictive value from 98.9 percent to 99.8 percent (i.e., an increase of less than one percent). The reason for the smaller effect on negative predictive value is the relatively large number of people without depression in the study populations. Since in both populations the vast majority of the participants do not have depression, most people testing negative on the screening test will be true negatives. Thus, the ratio of true negatives to all individuals testing negative (i.e., the negative predictive value) will be high in both populations.

4. Though not examined in this problem, generally speaking, the greater the sensitivity of a screening test, the greater its negative predictive value. Likewise, the greater the specificity of a screening test, the greater its positive predictive value[3] (see table 13-3). Therefore, increasing sensitivity and specificity of a screening test will increase both its positive and negative predictive values, all other factors being equal. Sensitivity and specificity can be modified by altering the screening level of a test where appropriate.

5. As indicated in the comments for problem 13-1, the value of the posttest probability based on the likelihood ratio for a positive test result is the same as the positive predictive value after allowing for rounding error. In this problem, the posttest probability of depression for a representative subject in the study population is 0.210 or 21.0 percent. The positive predictive value by comparison is 20.9 percent. As with positive predictive value, the posttest probability is a quantity that varies depending on the prevalence (i.e., pretest probability) of the disorder. Likelihood ratios, which depend on the sensitivity and specificity of a screening test, are *not* affected by prevalence. Therefore, the likelihood ratio in this problem (LR^+) is the same as that in problem 13-1. Like sensitivity and specificity, likelihood ratios are stable properties of a screening test and hence ones that are increasingly being used in the validation of screening tests.

Precision of Screening Tests

The concept of precision was discussed in chapter 8. In short, a precise screening test is one in which there is little variability due to random error. It is also important to note that one cannot have a valid screening test unless it is also precise, since precision is a prerequisite to validity. Precise tests, however, are not necessarily valid.[20]

The precision of a screening test is measured by its **reliability**, which is an indicator of the degree of consistency or stability of test results from one administration to another.[21] Thus, a reliable screening test is one that produces the same results when repeated on the same person under similar circumstances. A screening test for prostate cancer that is sometimes positive and sometimes negative for the same person when there has been no change in disease status or other relevant factors would *not* be considered a reliable test. The most common threats to the reliability (precision) of a screening test may be referred to as:

• Method variability
• Subject variability
• Observer variability

Method variability has to do with inconsistencies in test results due to the screening test itself. If the test produces inconsistent results under similar circumstances, it may be due to method variability. This can result from several factors such as chemical changes in the reagents used to produce the test results. Some screening tests, for example, rely on chemicals that are sensitive to temperature and humidity extremes. In these situations the test results may be erratic and therefore unreliable. Also, some chemicals used in screening tests may have a limited shelf life. Once beyond the shelf life, the test may produce unpredictable results. Mechanical tests can also be sensitive to environmental conditions. In some cases, method variability may be reduced by closely following the manufacturer's instructions or by recalibrating the tests at appropriate intervals.

Subject variability may occur due to physiological changes taking place in the subjects being screened. These can lead to inconsistent results when screening tests are repeated. Screening for hypertension, for example, may be influenced a subject's current level of stress. A normotensive person could have a high blood pressure reading due to high stress levels at the time of measurement. Changes in behaviors, such as dietary modifications, increased alcohol consumption, or use of new medications, may also cause subject variability. Strategies for minimizing subject variability include standardizing test procedures and making multiple measurements and averaging the results.

Observer variability refers to variation in the interpretation of screening test results that are attributable to the observer(s). **Observer** is a generic term for the person who interprets the test results. Depending on the nature of the screening, an observer may actually perform the screening and make a decision (e.g., a physical examination by a physician) or interpret the results of screening tests that have been performed by someone else (e.g., mammograms performed by a nurse). There are two basic types of observer variability:

• Intraobserver variability
• Interobserver variability

Intraobserver variability occurs when a single observer comes to different conclusions about the same or identical test results at different times. It represents inconsistent assessment by the observer. Say a college student is inadvertently exposed to tuberculosis while vacationing in Mexico and has a tuberculin skin test performed when he returns home. When a nurse later observes the site of the student's skin test, she indicates that the result is negative. The student learns later that day that a friend who vacationed in the same area has just been diagnosed with tuberculosis. Feeling anxious, he returns to the nurse who now indicates that the test result is positive (so much for relieving his anxiety!). This is an example of intraobserver variability. This type of variability may be evaluated by giving an observer the same or identical test results to interpret at different times and measuring the consistency of the interpretations. For example, intraobserver variability could be evaluated by randomly interspersing multiple test results from the same individual(s) within a group of test results from different individuals. The observer should be blinded to the identity of the individuals being screened and to the fact that repeat tests are being evaluated so as to avoid bias. Otherwise, an observer may allow his or her memory of test results to influence subsequent assessments. Similarly, just knowing that some test results are repeats may make the observer overly cautious so that the process is qualitatively different from routine assessments.

Interobserver variability occurs when two or more independent observers disagree on test results for the same person(s). If the vacationing college student after initially receiving a negative test result went to another nurse who concluded that the test was positive, interobserver variability would have occurred. Obviously, intraobserver and interobserver variability are threats to the precision of a screening test. Theoretically, there should be no observer variability if the results can be determined in an entirely objective manner. A blood test based on an easily detected chemical biomarker using an automated process, for example, should be less subject to observer variability than a sonogram of the liver that requires expert evaluation by a specially trained physician. The automated process for detecting the biomarker, however, may still be subject to method variability, and the levels of the biomarker may be affected by subject variability. Hence, even an apparently objective screening test may not always be reliable (precise).

Quantitative assessment of observer reliability. Whereas observer variability is a measure of *inconsistency* between observations, **observer reliability** is a measure of their *consistency*. The greater the observer reliability, the less the observer variability and vice versa. Therefore, observer reliability and observer variability are related measures that move in opposite directions. For an illustration see figure 13-3.

The two types of observer reliability—**intraobserver reliability** (also known as **intrarater reliability** or similar names) and **interobserver reliability** (also known as **interrater reliability** or similar names)—can be assessed quan-

|Figure 13-3   Observer Reliability versus Observer Variability

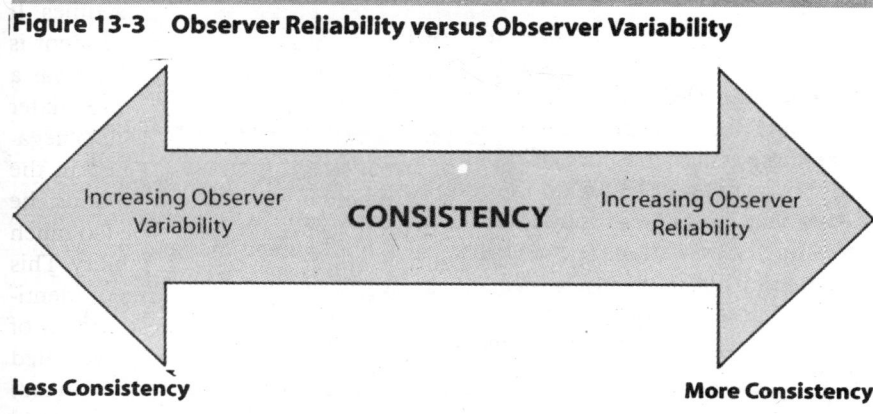

titatively by several methods. The specific methods depend in part on whether the test results represent categorical or continuous measures. To facilitate the discussion we will focus primarily on methods for categorical measures that are also dichotomous. These methods can generally be applied to polychotomous measures as well. In addition, for convenience, we will focus on assessment of *interobserver reliability*. It is important to stress, however, that *the methods described here can be applied to intraobserver reliability as well.* A standard 2 × 2 template will be used in describing methods based on dichotomous measures.*

Observer A

Observer B	Positive	Negative	**Total**
Positive	a	b	a + b
Negative	c	d	c + d
Total	a + c	b + d	a + b + c + d

The simplest method of assessing interobserver reliability is to determine **percent agreement** (sometimes referred to as **overall percent agreement** or **percentage of agreement**) between two observers of the same set of test results. In this method, the number of individuals where each observer agrees on the results is divided by the total number of individuals observed. Based on the above 2 × 2 template, this is expressed as shown in formula 13.14.

*For intraobserver reliability, "Observer A" would be designated as "Observation 1," and "Observer B" would be designated as "Observation 2." Everything else is the same.

(13.14)
$$\text{Percent Agreement} = \frac{a+d}{a+b+c+d} \times 100$$

For example, assume that two dermatologists performed independent total-body skin examinations on the same group of 100 individuals to determine the possible presence of skin cancer. The results of their classifications are shown in table 13-4A on the following page. Both dermatologists determined that the same 41 individuals had evidence of skin cancer based on the screening examinations (a = 41). They also both agreed that another 41 individuals did not have any evidence of skin cancer (d = 41). They disagreed with each other, however, on the other 18 subjects. Based on these findings, the percent agreement is calculated as:

$$[(41 + 41) / (41 + 9 + 9 + 41)] \times 100 = (82 / 100) \times 100 = 82.0\%$$

Thus, the dermatologists agreed on 82 percent of the examinations performed. Percent agreement can range from 0 to 100 percent. Zero percent indicates no agreement on test results, while 100 percent indicates complete agreement. Generally speaking, the higher the percent agreement, the greater the interobserver reliability.

While simple to calculate and interpret, percent agreement has significant limitations as an indicator of interobserver reliability. Most importantly, it does not take chance agreement into account. Even if the dermatologists made their determinations of probable skin cancer completely at random, we would still expect some percent agreement strictly by chance. Therefore, percent agreement tends to be an *inflated* indicator of interobserver reliability.[22] The measure is also misleading when the levels of agreement on positive and negative results (cells a and d) are very dissimilar. For example, the results depicted in table 13-4B produce the same percent agreement as those in table 13-4A (82.0%), but the situations are very different. In table 13-4A, the levels of agreement on positive and negative results are identical, while they are extremely disparate in table 13-4B. In table 13-4B, most of the agreement is on negative findings. The amount of agreement on positive findings is poor by comparison. If the prevalence of the disorder is low in the study population, it can be easier to achieve a high level of agreement on negative versus positive findings. This can conceal a low level of agreement on positive findings. This is the case for the results depicted in table 13-4B. Chance agreement can be a factor here when both observers are aware that the prevalence of the disorder is low, for example, so that they both tend to report more negative than positive results.[23] A high prevalence of the disorder can also produce disparate levels of agreement between positive and negative results with more agreement occurring on positive than negative findings. The effects are the same as those just described.

Alternate measures of percent agreement have been developed in an attempt to overcome the problem of dissimilar levels of agreements on positive and negative results resulting from low or high prevalence of the disorder

Table 13-4   Percent Agreement between Two Dermatologists on the Possible Presence of Skin Cancer Based on Whole-Body Screening

A. High Risk Population

	Dermatologist A		
Dermatologist B	Positive	Negative	Total
Positive	41	9	50
Negative	9	41	50
Total	50	50	100

$$\text{Percent Agreement} = \frac{41 + 41}{100} \times 100 = 82.0 \text{ percent}$$

B. Low Risk Population

	Dermatologist A		
Dermatologist B	Positive	Negative	Total
Positive	2	8	10
Negative	10	80	90
Total	12	88	100

$$\text{Percent Agreement} = \frac{2 + 80}{100} \times 100 = 82.0 \text{ percent}$$

in the study population. These measures are known collectively as **effective percent agreement** (or **effective percentage agreement**). They are intended to be more "sensitive" indicators of interobserver reliability by eliminating the cell with the high level of agreement (cell a or d) whose frequency of agreement, as indicated earlier, may be due in part to chance.[24]

One measure of effective percent agreement is **percent positive agreement**. A common method of calculating this measure is shown below in formula 13.15.

(13.15) $$\text{Percent Positive Agreement} = \frac{a}{a+b+c} \times 100$$

In this equation, the numerator represents the number of paired observations in which the two observers agree that the result is positive, and the denominator is the number of paired observations in which at least one observer classifies the result as positive. The values a through c are based on the 2 × 2 template shown previously. This formula thus eliminates cell d from the calculations. Using the data in table 13-4B, the percent positive agreement is equivalent to:

$$[2 / (2 + 8 + 10)] \times 100 = (2 / 20) \times 100 = 10.0 \text{ percent}$$

Note that the value of percent positive agreement is substantially below the value of percent agreement (10.0% vs. 82.0%). Even a cursory view of table 13-4B makes it clear that most of the percent agreement is due to the agreement among the negative findings. By comparison, there is little agreement among positive findings.

An analogous measure of effective percent agreement is **percent negative agreement** (see formula 13.16). This measure might be considered when the prevalence of the outcome is high, and the number of positive agreements (cell a) is disproportionately higher than the number of negative agreements (cell d) in a standard 2 × 2 table. Ultimately, selection of percent positive or negative agreement statistics will depend on the objectives of the investigators.

(13.16)
$$\text{Percent Negative Agreement} = \frac{d}{b+c+d} \times 100$$

Note that the numerator consists of the number of paired observations in which the two observers agree that the result is negative, and the denominator is the number of paired observations in which at least one observer classifies the result as negative. This formula thus eliminates cell a from the calculations. Percent negative agreement based on the data in table 13-4B is:

$$[80 / (8 + 10 + 80)] \times 100 = (80 / 98) \times 100 = 81.6 \text{ percent}$$

This result reflects the relatively high proportion of agreement in cell d compared to cell a in table 13-4B.

Although effective percent agreement statistics "adjust" for chance due to large variations in agreement between positive and negative results, they do not completely correct for chance agreements.[25, 26] Therefore, percent agreement, percent positive agreement, and percent negative agreement are not recommended as stand-alone indicators of interobserver reliability. They may be of use, however, along with other appropriate indicators of interobserver reliability such as *kappa* (see below) so as to provide a more complete picture of the particular circumstances.

Kappa (or **Cohen's kappa**, as named after its developer) measures the proportion of *nonrandom* agreement between two independent observers. Kappa is considered a measure of the proportion of agreement *above and beyond* the agreement expected by chance alone.[27] Thus, kappa "adjusts" for agreements due to chance. The equation for calculating kappa, based on the 2 × 2 template referred to earlier, is given in formula 13.17. It should be clear from this formula that kappa represents an adjustment of *percent agreement*, stated as a proportion, which is the first entry in the equation.

(13.17)

$$\kappa = \frac{P_o - P_e}{1 - P_e}$$

where,

$$P_o = (a+d)/(a+b+c+d)$$

$$P_e = \left[(a+b)(a+c)\right] + \left[(b+d)(c+d)\right]/(a+b+c+d)^2$$

P_o is the proportion of agreement *observed* between the observers, and P_e is the proportion of agreement *expected* between the observers due to chance alone. The denominator, $1 - P_e$, "reflects the maximum agreement beyond chance that would have been possible given the marginal distributions . . ."[28(p128)]

Kappa can range from a high of +1.0 to a low of −1.0. A value of +1.0 indicates perfect agreement between the observers, and a value of −1.0 indicates perfect disagreement between the observers.[25, 27] A value of zero indicates a level of agreement that is equal to that expected by chance alone, and a value between 0 and −1.0 implies a level of agreement less than that expected by chance alone. Guidelines for interpreting kappa have been developed by several authors. The scales used are arbitrary but may be helpful in providing a general sense of the level of agreement beyond random expectations. One commonly used scale is shown in table 13-5. An example of the calculation and interpretation of kappa appears in table 13-6 on the following page.

Table 13-5   Suggested Guidelines for Interpreting Kappa

Value	Interpretation
0.81–0.99:	Almost perfect agreement
0.61–0.80:	Substantial agreement
0.41–0.60:	Moderate agreement
0.21–0.40:	Fair agreement
0.01–0.20:	Slight agreement

Other Less Common Values of Kappa:
A kappa value of 1.00 indicates perfect agreement between the observers. A value of 0.00 indicates a level of agreement between the observers that is equivalent to that expected by chance alone. A value less than 0.00 indicates a level of agreement between the observers that is less than that expected by chance alone. Finally, a value of -1.00 indicates perfect disagreement between the observers.

Note: In the unusual situation where both observers agree 100 percent that the outcome is present or absent, kappa will have a denominator equal to zero. Mathematically, this is not interpretable. In these rare instances, the kappa should be seen as representing perfect agreement or perfect disagreement as applicable.

References: Bryington, A. A., Palmer, D. J., and Watkins, M. W. (2002). The Estimation of Interobserver Agreement in Behavioral Assessment. *The Behavior Analyst Today* 3 (3): 323–328; Landis, J. R., and Koch, G. G. (1977). The Measurement of Observer Agreement for Categorical Data. *Biometrics* 33: 159–174.

Table 13-6   Illustration of the Measurement of Interobserver Reliability Using Kappa

Problem:

Assume that as part of a quality control program a gynecologist in Sweden sends the results of all routine Papanicolaou screening tests (Pap tests) to a specific clinical laboratory in Stockholm. At the laboratory two pathologists independently read the Pap tests to determine if the screening results are positive or negative for cervical cancer. The results of their independent assessments over a one-year period are analyzed based on the results in the following 2 x 2 contingency table.

Results from Pathologist B	Results from Pathologist A Positive	Negative	Total
Positive	25 (a)	12 (b)	37 (a + b)
Negative	15 (c)	230 (d)	245 (c + d)
Total	40 (a + c)	242 (b + d)	282 (a + b + c + d)

Solution:

$$\kappa = (P_o - P_e) / (1 - P_e)$$
$$P_o = [(a + d) / (a + b + c + d)]$$
$$P_e = [(a + b) (a + c) + (b + d) (c + d)] / (a + b + c + d)^2$$

Using the appropriate cell and marginal totals in the 2 x 2 table, κ is calculated as follows:

$$P_o = [(25 + 230) / 282] = (255 / 282) = 0.90$$
$$P_e = [(37) (40) + (242) (245)] / 282^2 = (1480 + 59,290) / 79,524 = 60,770 / 79,524 = 0.76$$
$$\text{Therefore, } \kappa = (0.90 - 0.76) / (1 - 0.76) = 0.14 / 0.24 = 0.58$$

Interpretation:

The *percent agreement* between the pathologists is 90 percent. However, a significant amount of this agreement is probably due to chance alone. The proportion of agreement after chance is taken into consideration is just 0.58, which, based on the guidelines in table 13-5, represents a moderate level of agreement. Specifically, this indicates that the agreement between the two pathologists is 58 percent above and beyond that predicted by chance alone. In other words, the pathologists accounted for 58 percent of the agreement in the Pap tests after taking chance agreements into consideration. For quality control purposes, a kappa of 0.58 would indicate that the interobserver reliability could be improved.

While kappa is a popular measure that has been used frequently in the assessment of observer reliability, it has a number critics, many of whom have suggested the use of alternate methods. The reasons for the concerns about kappa can be complex, and, therefore, will not be discussed in great detail here. Some pertinent issues with the kappa statistic relate to: (a) limitations on its applicability, and (b) the effects of prevalence and bias on its magnitude. Each of these is discussed briefly in the following paragraphs. It is assumed in these discussions that the observations between observers are independent of each other, which is a fundamental assumption underlying the kappa statistic. It is also assumed that we are only talking about dichotomous results except where indicated.

In terms of limited applicability, Cohen's kappa is only appropriate for **nominal** test results, that is, those representing *unordered* qualitative categories.* These categories may be dichotomous (e.g., positive or negative results) or polychotomous. An example of the latter is reflected in a British study designed to measure interobserver and intraobserver variability in the classification of fractures of the distal humerus.[30] One of the simpler comparisons in the study involved three types of fractures (extra-articular fractures, partial articular fractures, and complete articular fractures). The observers were required to classify the fractures depicted on radiographs according to these three types. The authors reported a kappa of 0.661, implying substantial agreement among the observers (see table 13-5 regarding interpretation of kappa). Kappas based on polychotomous results may be less precise than those based on dichotomous results when differences between certain categories are not considered the same as those between other categories. In other words, some observer disagreements may be regarded as more serious than others.[31] For example, in the classification of fractures of the distal humerus, disagreement between an extra-articular fracture and a complete articular fracture may be considered more a serious error than a disagreement between a partial and complete articular fracture. In this case, a variation of kappa, known as **weighted kappa**, is a more appropriate indicator of interobserver reliability. When the test results are **ordinal**, that is, when they represent *ordered* qualitative categories, such as positive, suspect, and negative, Cohen's kappa should *not* be used. Weighted kappa, however, is an appropriate alternative. Weighted kappa provides some credit for agreements that are close but not perfect.[17] It has been described in the literature as follows:

> Weighted kappa is an appropriate chance adjusted measure of agreement between two observers when there are more than two ordered categories of classification. The statistic . . . gives partial credit for partial agreement in accordance with a . . . weighting scheme. Weighted kappa is obtained by giving weights to the frequencies in each cell of the table according to their distance from the diagonal that indicates agreement.[32(p728)]

Table 13-7 illustrates the calculation of a weighted kappa for a screening test with three possible outcomes assumed to represent an ordinal scale of measurement. The "diagonal" referred to in the above quotation is illustrated in the example by the shaded cells in the 3 × 3 table. The weights chosen for a weighted kappa tend to be subjective but should be based on the potential public health or clinical consequences of accepting a given level of disagree-

---

*Interestingly, percent agreement is suitable for use with all types of measurement scales, categorical or continuous.[29]

Table 13-7 Illustration of the Calculation of a Weighted Kappa

	Observer A			
Observer B	Category 1	Category 2	Category 3	Total
Category 1	32	8	2	42
Category 2	12	25	1	38
Category 3	2	3	15	20
Total	46	36	18	100

Note: The shaded cells forming a diagonal represent perfect agreement between the observers. The weights arbitrarily assigned to the frequencies in each cell are:

Perfect Agreement (i.e., shaded cells) = 1.0

Disagreement by One Category = 0.5

Disagreement by Two Categories = 0.0

Calculation:

A weighted kappa (κ_w) is calculated as shown below. The basic formula is the same as formula 13.17 in the text except that weights have been applied to frequencies in the cells.

$$\kappa_w = (P_{ow} - P_{ew}) / (1 - P_{ew})$$

P_{ow} is the weighted proportion of the agreement observed, and P_{ew} is the weighted proportion of the agreement expected. The basic steps in calculating a weighted kappa based on the data presented in the above 3 x 3 table can be summarized as follows:

Step 1: Calculate P_{ow}

For frequencies with weights other than zero, (a) multiply the sum of the frequencies in the cells showing perfect agreement by the designated weight, (b) add this result to the sum of the frequencies in the cells showing disagreement by one category multiplied by the designated weight, and (c) divide the value obtained from steps a and b by the total number of observations.

$$P_{ow} = [(32 + 25 + 15) (1.0) + (8 + 12 + 1 + 3) (0.5)] / 100 = 84 / 100 = 0.84$$

Step 2: Calculate P_{ew}

For frequencies with weights other than zero, (a) multiply the marginal totals corresponding to each cell showing perfect agreement and sum the products, (b) multiply the result by the designated weight, (c) multiply the marginal totals corresponding to each cell showing disagreement by one category and sum the products, (d) multiply the result by the designated weight, and (e) sum all of the above and divide it by the square of the total number of observations.

$$P_{ew} = \{[(42 \times 46) + (38 \times 36) + (20 \times 18)] (1.0) + [(42 \times 36) + (38 \times 46) + (38 \times 18) + (20 \times 36)] (0.5)\} / 100^2 = 0.60$$

Step 3: Calculate κ_w

$$\kappa_w = (P_{ow} - P_{ew}) / (1 - P_{ew}) = (0.84 - 0.60) / (1 - 0.60) = 0.24 / 0.40 = 0.60$$

Interpretation:
Weighted kappa is interpreted in the same manner as kappa. Therefore, we can say that the observers have accounted for 60 percent of the agreement above and beyond that expected by chance alone. According to the guidelines in table 13-5, this implies moderate agreement, although there is still significant room for improvement.

Reference: Szklo, M., and Nieto, F. J. (2000). *Epidemiology: Beyond the Basics*. Gaithersburg, MD: Aspen.

---

ment.[33] For example, exact agreement could be weighted as one, and "partial" agreement could be weighted somewhere between zero and one with higher weights reflecting more "acceptable" disagreements. Unacceptable disagreements would be weighted as zero. Cohen's kappa, by the way, may be conceived as a weighted kappa with weights of one for agreement and zero for disagreement. A weakness of weighted kappa is that the magnitude of its value depends on the weights chosen.[31] Therefore, weighted kappas cannot be meaningfully compared across different study populations unless the same weighting systems are used. One suggestion for overcoming this problem is to use standardized weights.[31]

Another limitation of kappa is that its magnitude is sensitive to low or high prevalence of the disorder in the study population. This has been described as the **prevalence effect** and exists when the proportion of agreement between observers on positive findings differs from the proportion of agreement on negative findings.[34] This is reflected in differences in the frequencies in cells a and d of the standard 2×2 table referred to earlier. The prevalence effect is due to the fact that observers are more likely to conclude that screening results are negative when the prevalence of the disorder is low and positive when the prevalence of the disorder is high. In either case, the prevalence effect decreases the value of kappa, sometimes substantially. The data in table 13-4B illustrate the prevalence effect as seen by the imbalance in frequencies between cells a and d. In this case it is apparently due to a low prevalence of the disorder. The consequence is a value of kappa that is unexpectedly small considering the relatively high observed agreement (P_o). For example, the kappa for the data in table 13-4A is 0.64 where there is no imbalance but only 0.08 in table 13-4B where there is considerable imbalance. This substantial difference in kappas exists even though the levels of observed agreement are the same ($P_o = 0.82$). If we use the guidelines in table 13-5, we have gone from "substantial agreement" to "slight agreement" after accounting for expectations due to chance. The small kappa for the data in table 13-4B can be attributed to the high degree of chance agreements expected (P_e) when the prevalence effect is large as it is here. It has been argued that kappa is just doing what it is supposed to do in these situations (i.e., correct for expectations due to chance).[35] Nevertheless, this apparent "overcorrection" makes kappa difficult to interpret and can hinder comparisons of kappas across studies with different prevalences of the disorder. It has been demonstrated that when the ratio of positive agreement to negative agreement (frequency in cell a / frequency in cell d) departs substantially from 1.0, kappa decreases precipitously. For ratios between 0.5 and 1.0 or between 1.0 and 2.0, however, the decrease in kappa is relatively modest.[36]

The magnitude of kappa is also influenced by an imbalance due to disagreements between observers. This has been referred to as the **bias effect**, which is the extent to which observers disagree on the proportion of positive or negative results.[34] In general, the greater the difference in levels of disagreement between cells b and c in the standard 2 × 2 table (i.e., the greater the bias effect), the larger the value of kappa. Thus, kappa should be interpreted not only in light of the prevalence effect but also in light of the bias effect.[34] The former phenomenon decreases kappa, while the latter one increases it compared to more balanced findings. These statistical phenomena associated with prevalence and bias effects have been represented in the literature as paradoxes.[37]

Different methods have been proposed for dealing with prevalence and bias effects on kappa, but there is no universally agreed upon method for resolving these issues. One possible solution is to provide appropriate 2 × 2 tables that show the actual distributions of agreement and disagreement between the observers along with the value of kappa. Percent positive and percent negative agreement statistics might also be reported for comparison purposes. Another possible solution is to report the **prevalence-adjusted bias-adjusted kappa** (PABAK) in addition to Cohen's kappa. PABAK is kappa adjusted for any prevalence and bias effects. If there are none, the values of kappa and PABAK should be the same. PABAK is calculated in the following manner:[34]

1. Average the frequencies in cells a and d, and substitute the average value for the existing values in the standard 2 × 2 table.

2. Average the frequencies in cells b and c, and substitute the average value for the existing values in the standard 2 × 2 table.

3. Calculate kappa in the usual manner using the substituted values.

Using the data in table 13-4B, the standard "unadjusted" kappa is 0.08, and the PABAK is a substantially higher 0.64. This difference indicates a significant prevalence effect as noted by the substantially reduced kappa and the substantial imbalance in cells a and d in the contingency table.

In summary, percent agreement is advantageous in that it is simple to calculate and interpret, but it is limited by the fact that it does not account for chance agreement and can be misleading when the levels of agreement on positive and negative results are very different. Effective percent agreement, as measured by percent positive agreement or percent negative agreement, partly overcomes these limitations, but it is not completely immune to inflated values due to chance agreement. Kappa fully corrects for agreements expected by chance alone, but its magnitude can be affected dramatically by prevalence or bias effects as reflected in unbalanced levels of agreement or disagreement in a standard 2 × 2 table. This can make kappa difficult to interpret, especially across study populations. Also, kappa is only appropriate for use with nominal data. Weighted kappa, however, may be used when the data are ordinal or with polychotomous nominal data where not all disagreements are considered equally serious. Finally, it should be reiterated that intraobserver reliability can be assessed in the same manner as interobserver reliability, all other factors being equal.

When the data from screening tests are continuous, an *intraclass correlation coefficient* (ICC; first referred to in chapter 12) may be used as an indicator of interobserver reliability between two or more observers.[38] The formula for the ICC may vary depending on the purpose for which it is being used. In the context of interobserver reliability, it may take the following form:

(13.18)
$$ICC = \frac{SD_S^2}{SD_S^2 + SD_O^2 + SD_E^2}$$

In this equation, SD_S^2 is the variance between the subjects, SD_O^2 is the variance between the observers, and SD_E^2 is the variance due to residual error. Together, these terms represent the total variance, which is the denominator in the equation. The ICC may calculated using analysis of variance (ANOVA) or other techniques.[33, 39] Generally speaking, the ICC reflects the amount of variability in mean scores that is due to true differences between the subjects and the amount that is due to differences between the observers.[28] In studies of interobserver reliability, the ICC is preferred over the *Pearson correlation coefficient* (r; chapter 9), which is not sensitive to systematic biases in the data.[28] For instance, scores by one observer that are consistently five points higher than those by the other observer would have a Pearson correlation coefficient of 1.0, while the ICC would be less than one. Both r and ICC have a range of –1.0 to +1.0, although in practice the ICC normally ranges from zero to one. An ICC of 1.0 is indicative of perfect interobserver reliability. As a general rule of thumb, an ICC of 0.7 is the minimum necessary for "sufficient reliability."[40] A limitation of both r and ICC is that they are affected by the range of values in the study population. In general, when SD_S^2 is small, the ICC will also be small.[33]

Other quantitative indicators of observer reliability based on either categorical or continuous data have been developed but are not discussed here. In general, they tend to be used less frequently in epidemiologic applications. Additional information about these measures can be found in biostatistical or more specialized epidemiologic texts.

SCREENING PROGRAMS: TO SCREEN OR NOT TO SCREEN?

The benefits of screening can be reduced morbidity and mortality and improved quality of life. Nevertheless, screening, especially mass screening, can be expensive and time consuming. Screening programs may require scarce resources for marketing, training, test administration, referral for follow-up examinations, and program evaluation. In addition, there may be other drawbacks, such as having little or no impact on disease outcomes, missing serious cases of disease due to too many false negatives, and unnecessary referrals as a consequence of false positives. This latter problem can place a burden on an already overly burdened health care system as well as produce stress and anxiety in those referred. Table 13-2 summarizes some of the problems associated with identifying too many false negatives or false positives in a screening program. Exhibit 13-1 provides two examples of screening programs with different objectives currently being conducted in the U.S.

Exhibit 13-1
Examples of Two Screening Programs in The United States

The Sage Screening Program
The Sage Screening Program is Minnesota's statewide screening program for breast and cervical cancer. It was established in 1991 and is funded by the Centers for Disease Control and Prevention, the State of Minnesota, and the Twin Cities Race for the Cure. The primary program objective is to promote screening for breast and cervical cancer among age-appropriate women. This objective is accomplished through: (a) the provision of free screening and follow-up services for uninsured and underinsured women, (b) outreach to women without regular health care providers, (c) public education about the importance of screening, (d) information sharing with health professionals, and (e) the development of statewide partnerships to promote screening. Since 1991, the program has served over 91,000 women by providing over 280,000 mammograms and Pap tests. These have resulted in the detection of over 930 breast and cervical cancers in Minnesota and about 3,400 precancerous cervical lesions that have been treated.

New England Newborn Screening Program
The New England Newborn Screening Program is a comprehensive screening program for newborns serving five states in New England, including Massachusetts, Maine, New Hampshire, Rhode Island, and Vermont. The program provides low-cost laboratory screening, clinical follow up, and research to prevent or minimize a number of specific treatable disorders in newborns that can lead to mental retardation, death, and other serious health complications. For testing purposes, blood is taken from the baby's heel when he or she is about two days old. Since 1999, the program has been conducting two pilot studies. One is for DNA risk markers for cystic fibrosis. The objective is to develop the best test for the early detection of cystic fibrosis in newborns. The other pilot study is designed to examine new technology to evaluate risk markers for 19 other metabolic disorders in newborns. These disorders can lead to serious health complications or death but may be treatable if discovered early enough. The disorders include those caused by faulty fat or amino acid metabolism and the buildup of toxic organic acids in the body.

References: Minnesota Department of Health (2006). SAGE: Minnesota's Cancer Screening Program. Available: http://www.health.state.mn.us/divs/hpcd/ccs/mbcccp.htm (Access date: November 3, 2006); University of Massachusetts Medical School (No date). Welcome to the New England Newborn Screening Program. Available: http://www.umassmed.edu/nbs (Access date: November 3, 2006).

Guidelines for Screening

Because there are both potential benefits and potential risks to screening, several factors need to be considered before implementing a screening program in a community (e.g., city, workplace, school) or within a clinical practice. Ethically, the benefits of screening should outweigh the risks. Some of the more important factors to consider are outlined below.

Nature of the disorder. The disease or condition for which screening is being considered should be an *important* public health problem that the targeted population is concerned enough about to submit to screening. It must also be one that can be detected *before* signs or symptoms of the disorder develop. The preclinical period during which a disorder is detectable by screening is referred to as the **detectable preclinical phase** (DPCP)[41] or, especially in regard to cancer screening, the **sojourn time**[42] (see figure 13-4). It occurs during the presymptomatic stage of the natural history of a disease (chapter 3) when the disorder is still occult (i.e., not evident) but detectable by screening. The DPCP should have a high enough prevalence and be long enough that early detection is feasible through periodic screening. This will also help to ensure that an appropriate screening test *yields* enough cases for the screening program to be cost-effective. The **yield** of a screening program can be defined as the number of new cases diagnosed and treated as a result of screening.[43] Depending on the relative prevalence of the disorder in its presymptomatic stage, either mass screening or selective screening may be the more appropriate objective.

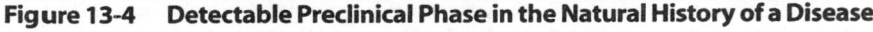

Figure 13-4   Detectable Preclinical Phase in the Natural History of a Disease

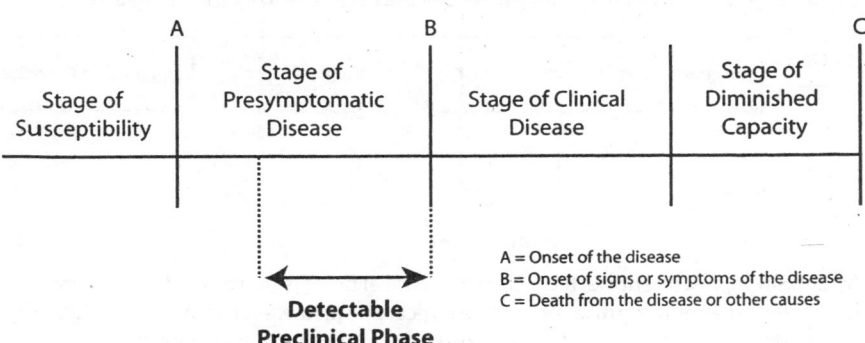

Nature of the screening test. The screening test itself should be accurate (valid and precise), relatively quick and simple to apply, easily interpreted, generally safe, acceptable to those being screened and those providing the screening, widely available, and relatively inexpensive. Good examples are blood pressure tests for hypertension and the fecal occult blood test for colorectal cancer. Some screening tests, however, are not inexpensive (e.g., colonoscopy) but are usually covered, at least in part, by health insurance and may in some instances be available at reduced cost to those meeting certain income guidelines.

Nature of the follow-up tests.   Appropriate follow-up tests must be available to confirm the suspected finding based on screening. These tests should be readily accessible, accurate, safe, and acceptable to those with the presumed disorder from the standpoint of relative comfort and cost. Follow-up tests for tuberculosis, for example, generally meet these guidelines. It should be noted that standards of comfort and cost may be slightly more flexible for high risk individuals identified by selective screening than for generally lower risk individuals identified in mass screening.

Nature of the treatment.   The treatment for the disorder must be readily available, acceptable to patients, and it must be more effective than if it or another treatment were initiated at a later stage of the disorder. In other words, the treatment should result in a significantly better prognosis for those who are identified early in the disease process by screening than those who are diagnosed later when signs or symptoms of the disorder are apparent. In technical terms, there must be a **critical point** during the DPCP. This is a point in the natural history of the disorder *before which* treatment is more effective than if applied later (see figure 13-5). With cancers the critical point is the time at which metastasis occurs.[44] An example of a disease that meets all of the above guidelines is cervical cancer. There is an appropriate critical

Figure 13-5   The Critical Point in the Natural History of a Disease

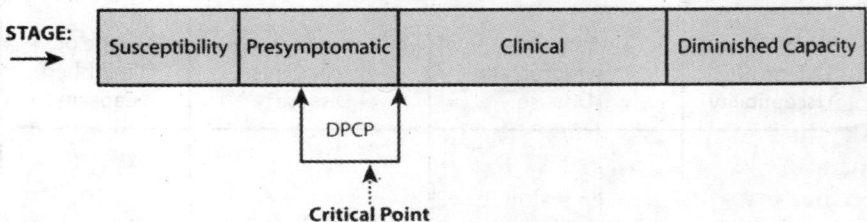

By definition, treatment started before the critical point is more effective than treatment started after the critical point. The critical point, however, must occur within the detectable preclinical phase (DPCP) in order for screening to be useful. If it occurs before the DPCP, screening will not be effective since the disease is not yet detectable. If it occurs in the clinical stage, screening will not be necessary since the disease will be detectable by signs or symptoms of the disease.

Reference: Black, W. C., and Welch, H. G. (1997). Screening for Disease. *American Journal of Roentgenology* 168: 3–11.

point in the DPCP during which early treatment results in a much better prognosis than late treatment. The treatment is also readily available and considered acceptable given the diagnosis. In addition to the other criteria for treatment, a treatment should not cause more injury or harm to the patient than the disorder itself. For example, coronary angioplasty for severe coronary artery disease detected by a cardiac stress test and confirmed by an angiogram can be lifesaving and allow an individual to pursue a relatively normal lifestyle compared to the potential alternatives (e.g., angina pectoris or sudden death).

There may be instances where a screening program makes sense even though not all of the above guidelines have been fully satisfied. For example, screening for phenylketonuria (PKU) in newborns is unlikely to produce a high yield because of its relatively low prevalence in the population. Nevertheless, the consequences of untreated PKU are serious and costly, and yet, it can be easily detected using a simple, accurate, and inexpensive screening test.[45] Therefore, for these and other reasons, screening for PKU has been adopted by all states in the United States, including the District of Columbia.[46]

Screening Applications

There are numerous diseases or conditions (some of which have already been mentioned) for which mass, selective, or opportunistic screening may be appropriate based on the above guidelines. Specific examples are provided in table 13-8. In addition, screening is routinely conducted for congenital hypothyroidism, phenylketonuria, and galactosemia in newborns; tuberculosis and lead poisoning in high risk groups; and hearing impairment in school children. Screening for other disorders, such as abdominal aortic aneurysms, is also performed but in more limited circumstances. Screening for disorders like prostate cancer, glaucoma, lung cancer, skin cancer, and dementia is conducted by many health care professionals, but all have received an "I" grade from the U.S. Preventive Services Task Force (USPSTF; see table 13-8 for an explanation of the grading system).[47] Based on its findings, the USPSTF makes no recommendations for or against screening for these disorders. The American Cancer Society (ACS), however, recommends that prostate cancer screening be offered to men annually beginning at age 50 if they have a life expectancy of at least 10 years. Both the prostate-specific antigen (PSA) blood test and the digital rectal examination (DRE) are recommended. Guidelines for high-risk groups (e.g., men of sub-Saharan African descent) call for screening starting at age 45 or 40 if they have even higher risk based on family history. The ACS recommendations for prostate cancer screening emphasize shared decision making between patients and clinicians given the current uncertainties about the effectiveness of prostate cancer screening.[48] Recommended screening procedures have also been developed for such varied conditions as alcohol misuse, bacteriuria, chlamydial infection, and Rh (D) incompatibility.[47]

Table 13-8 Examples of Disorders for Which Screening Tests Are Recommended in the United States*

Disorder	Main Targeted Population	USPSTF Recommendation[†]
Breast cancer	Women, 40 years and older	B
Cervical cancer	Sexually active women with a cervix	A
Colorectal cancer	Adults, 50 years and older	A
Depression	Adults if systems in place to diagnose and treat	B
Diabetes (type 2)	Adults with hypertension or hyperlipidemia	B
Gonorrhea	Sexually active women at increased risk	B
Hepatitis B infection	Pregnant women at first prenatal visit	A
HIV infection	Adolescents and adults at increased risk	A
Hypertension	Adults, 18 years and older	A
Iron deficiency anemia	Pregnant women	B
Lipid disorders	Males, 35+ years; females, 45+ years	A
Obesity	All adults	B
Osteoporosis	Women, 65 years and older	B
Syphilis	Persons with increased risk	A
Visual impairment	Children less than 5 years	B

A: Strongly recommended for eligible patients. Benefits substantially outweigh harms.
B: Recommended for eligible patients. Benefits outweigh harms.
C: No recommendation. Benefits and harms too close to justify a general recommendation.
D: Not recommended. Procedure appears ineffective or harms appear to outweigh benefits.
I: Insufficient evidence to recommend for or against the procedure.

*Screening tests for these disorders have been critically evaluated by the U.S. Preventive Services Task Force (USPSTF), which is an independent panel of private sector experts in prevention and primary care. The USPSTF is sponsored by the Agency for Healthcare Research and Quality in the U.S. Department of Health and Human Services. A complete list of recommendations can be accessed from the first reference listed at the end of this table.

†The recommendations of the USPSTF are graded according to five classifications, which are summarized above. The grades reflect the strength of the available evidence and the net benefits of screening for the disorder. A grade of A or B is necessary for USPSTF to recommend screening for a particular disorder.

References: Agency for Healthcare Research and Quality (No date). U.S. Preventive Services Task Force, Active Topic Index: A-Z. Available: http://www.ahrq.gov/clinic/uspstf/uspstopics.htm (Access date: November 1, 2006); Agency for Healthcare Research and Quality (No date). Task Force Ratings. Available: http://www.ahrq.gov/clinic/3rduspstf/ratings.htm (Access date: November 1, 2006).

New screening procedures continue to be developed and promoted. For example, electron-beam computed tomography (EBCT), which detects calcification in the coronary arteries and the potential for coronary heart disease (CHD), has been touted by some hospitals in recent years as a screening test for CHD. The procedure has received a "D" grade from the USPSTF, however, which indicates that it is not recommended for routine screening of asymptomatic patients.[47, 49] Though the technology with regard to CT scanning for CHD continues to advance rapidly, the most recent recommendations emanating from the American Heart Association regarding EBCT are similar to those of the USPSTF. However, the Association did leave the door open by suggesting that EBCT scanning may be appropriate for individuals at intermediate risk of coronary artery disease, though not for those at low or high risk.[50] It is important to point out that the recommendations of the USPSTF and other authoritative bodies are subject to change as new data become available. Screening is an evolving science, and some formerly questionable procedures have gained credibility as new data have become available. Likewise, some screening tests have fallen out of favor.

Before leaving this topic, it may be interesting to comment briefly on one other screening procedure that has been aggressively marketed to the public in recent years. This is whole-body computed tomography (CT) scanning. Unlike CT scanning for coronary heart disease, lung cancer, or colon cancer (i.e., virtual CT colonoscopy), which continues to be studied for appropriate use, whole-body CT scanning is not designed to screen for a specific disease and could cause more harm than benefit to those undergoing the procedure. The U.S. Food and Drug Administration, Center for Devices and Radiological Health, provided the following warning to the public regarding whole-body computed CT scanning:

> [W]hen possible risks are compared to the possible benefits, the harms currently appear to be both far more likely and in some cases may not be insignificant. These harms are: (1) radiation exposure which has a small risk of cancer induction for an individual CT procedure, and (2) the possibility of either a false finding of an abnormality or a true finding of an insignificant abnormality, either of which could lead to further harm.[51]

Unfortunately, whole-body CT scanning at this point in time has not sufficiently demonstrated that it meets the guidelines for screening as outlined near the beginning of this section. Clearly, the benefits of the procedure do not outweigh the potential risks.

Other screening tests, both those accepted and those still considered experimental, are frequently marketed to the public through various media sources. One advertisement in a local newspaper, for example, advertises 16 screening tests (not all of which meet the guidelines described in this chapter) ranging from $17.00 to $95.00 each along with the slogan, "It's your health—take control of it!"[52] Perhaps this is a just an early sign of the future of health care.

EVALUATING SCREENING PROGRAMS

In general, screening programs should be adequately evaluated *before* being implemented and, if feasible, periodically *after* being implemented. The purpose in both cases is to assure that the programs meet acceptable standards, such as those in the guidelines described in the previous section. Poorly conceived screening programs can do more harm than good by causing emotional and physical distress, inconvenience, unnecessary expenses, overtreatment, and wasted resources, while never achieving their primary objective, which "is to prevent or delay the development of advanced disease and its adverse effects."[41(p6)] Although evaluations of screening programs may address several program aspects, including process (e.g., number of people screened), cost-effectiveness, efficiency, etc., the most important aspect is the degree to which the programs meet their primary objective as just noted. The remainder of this chapter summarizes some of the basic issues associated with evaluating the effectiveness of screening programs.

Approaches to Evaluation

The most common epidemiologic approach to evaluating the success of a screening program is to use an observational or quasi-experimental study design. Basically, these evaluations involve a comparison of outcomes among those who have undergone screening and those who have not. The outcomes may include survival time, disease incidence, mortality, or other measures. For example, medical researchers in Italy conducted a study to evaluate the impact of a legally mandated pre-participation screening program to reduce sudden cardiovascular deaths among athletes. The screening program, which was started in Italy in 1982, involves a clinical examination and electrocardiogram to detect cardiovascular abnormalities. Trends in sudden cardiovascular deaths in the athletic (screened) and nonathletic (unscreened) populations, 12–35 years of age, were examined between 1979 and 2004. The authors reported that the annual incidence of sudden cardiovascular deaths in athletes decreased by 89 percent from 1979–1980 to 2003–2004 (p < 0.001), while there was no significant change in the incidence for nonathletes over the same period. They concluded that the screening program is an effective strategy for reducing sudden cardiovascular deaths among athletes.[53]

Less common approaches to evaluating screening programs involve randomized controlled trials or group randomized trials. Although these designs are generally considered superior to observational or quasi-experimental studies in terms of internal validity, they are less frequently employed due to generally large sample size requirements, high costs of implementation, and ethical concerns (see chapter 12). Where feasible, however, randomized controlled trials using mortality rates as the outcome measure are widely regarded as the best means of evaluating the effectiveness of screening programs where the intention of screening is to prevent premature death, that is, to prolong life. More is said about this later following a description of the major types of bias potentially involved in comparisons of screened and unscreened populations.

Major Forms of Bias

Evaluation of screening programs using nonrandomized designs such as observational studies (e.g., ecological, case-control, cohort studies) or quasi-experimental studies (e.g., before and after studies) may be subject to several forms of bias. The most important types are listed below and are described in the following paragraphs. Essential to understanding the first three of these biases is the concept of the *natural history of disease* (chapter 3). For convenience, we will focus on screening for disorders where the goal is to prevent premature death. The basic concepts will be the similar for disorders that are not usually life threatening but which can result in serious morbidity if not diagnosed and treated early in their natural history. A good example is glaucoma, which untreated can lead to blindness.

• Lead-time bias

• Length bias

• Overdiagnosis bias

• Volunteer bias

Lead-time bias.   To comprehend *lead-time bias* one has to first understand the concept of **lead time**, which is the time gained by diagnosing a disorder in its presymptomatic stage as a consequence of screening versus diagnosing it in the usual way during the clinical stage when signs or symptoms are apparent.[2] Stated simply, it is the length of time between early diagnosis and usual diagnosis of a disorder. **Lead-time bias**, also known as **zero-time shift**, is "a spurious increase in longevity associated with screening."[4(p884)] It occurs when the survival time from diagnosis to death is not adjusted for lead time when comparing the survival of cases detected by screening with those diagnosed clinically.[41] To illustrate, assume that a proposed screening test for lung cancer will allow physicians to diagnose the disease one year earlier than when it is usually diagnosed clinically upon presentation of signs and symptoms. When diagnosed clinically say patients typically survive an average of 18 months from diagnosis. Also assume that earlier diagnosis does not increase one's life expectancy. In this scenario, patients diagnosed as a result of screening appear to live a year longer than those diagnosed clinically. This difference, however, is illusionary and results because survival time is measured from the time of diagnosis to death. Since early diagnosis does not improve prognosis, the survival times from *disease onset* to death are actually the same for those diagnosed early and at the usual time. This is demonstrated and explained further in figure 13-6 on the following page.

As another example, consider two patients of the same age who presumably contracted lung cancer at the same time. One patient is diagnosed at age

Figure 13-6   An Illustration and Explanation of Lead-Time Bias

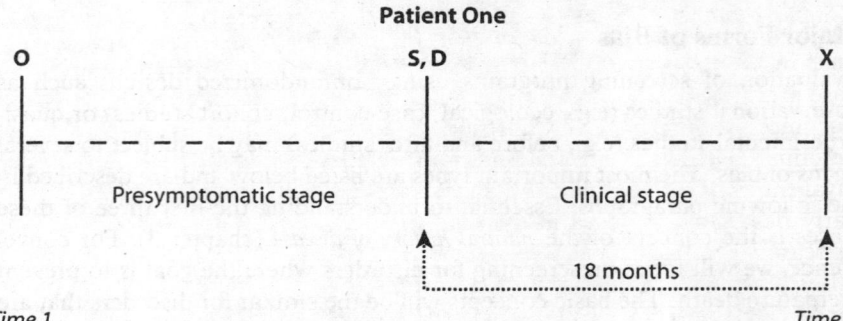

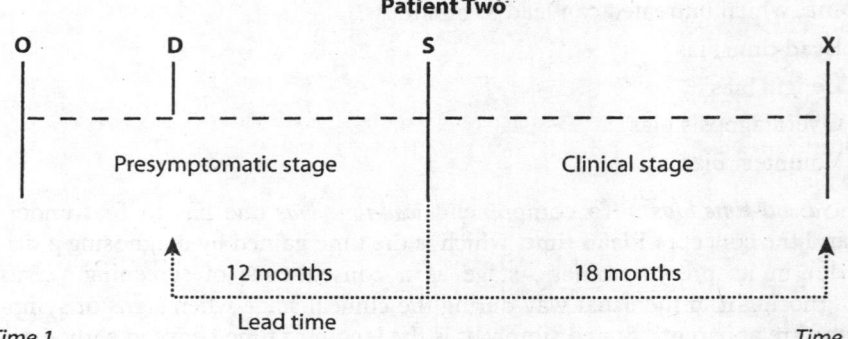

Key
O = Onset of disease
S = Development of signs or symptoms
D = Diagnosis of disease
X = Death

Explanation
Two patients develop the same disease at the same time (Time 1). In the first diagram, Patient One is diagnosed with the disease (D) at the beginning of the clinical stage when signs or symptoms of the disease (S) are apparent. This patient survives 18 months following diagnosis, which is the usual survival time for this disease. In the second diagram, Patient Two is diagnosed with the disease (D) during the presymptomatic stage before signs or symptoms of the disease (S) develop. More specifically, diagnosis is made during the detectable preclinical phase, which is only a portion of the presymptomatic stage of the disease. This early diagnosis is the result of screening. The *lead time* is 12 months, so Patient Two survives a total of 30 months following diagnosis (D): 12 months + 18 months = 30 months. However, Patient Two dies (X) at the same time as Patient One (Time 2). Thus, the lead time falsely implies greater longevity for Patient Two (30 months) than Patient One (18 months). In reality, both patients live the same amount of time from disease onset (O) to death (X). The apparent gain in survival for Patient Two is a result of *lead-time bias*, which results from diagnoses at different times in the disease's natural history.

49 with the help of the proposed screening test but still dies from lung cancer at age 51½. The other patient is diagnosed with lung cancer at age 50 after reporting symptoms to her physician. She later dies from the cancer also at age 51½. Though the first patient was diagnosed earlier, there was no difference in life span between the two patients. Both patients contracted the disease at the same age and died at the same age. In other words, screening did not improve the prognosis. It is important to note that lead-time bias exists any time cases in screened and unscreened populations are compared for survival times from the point of diagnosis to death *regardless* of whether or not early detection improves prognosis.[41] This is because lead time gives the appearance of longer survival in screened cases compared to unscreened (clinically diagnosed) cases. In other words, it produces a positive bias (chapter 8). The consequence is that screening programs appear to be more effective than they really are.

As a side note, screening that does not improve prognosis can be harmful. This is because asymptomatic persons are now identified with a disorder without any reasonable expectations of a more favorable outcome than if they had been diagnosed later when signs or symptoms develop. The additional anxiety, stress, and stigma due to being labeled "sick" can be significant for individuals as well as their family and friends. It can also be expensive. The lead time gained from early detection is only beneficial if a more effective treatment is available that either prolongs life or increases the quality of life compared to treatment provided after a later detection time.

Length bias.   A second type of bias that may occur in the evaluation of screening programs is **length bias**, also known as **length-time bias** or **length-biased sampling**. Like lead-time bias, length bias may cause a screening program to appear more effective than it really is due to positive bias. To comprehend length bias it is helpful to keep three points in mind: (a) a given disorder, such as breast or prostate cancer, may progress at different rates, (b) slowly progressing forms of the disorder tend to have longer detectable preclinical phases than rapidly progressing forms, and (c) individuals with slowly progressing forms of the disorder tend to have a better prognosis than those with rapidly progressing forms. Because of the second factor, slowly progressing forms of a disorder are more likely to be detected by periodic screening than rapidly progressing forms. Since these cases also tend to have a better prognosis, this can have the effect of making screening programs appear more effective than they really are when screened and unscreened populations are compared in terms of survival rates. Breast cancer, for example, progresses at different rates, and slow-growing, nonaggressive breast tumors, which present a more favorable prognosis than fast-growing, aggressive tumors, appear to be more easily detected by mammography. Therefore, women whose breast cancers are detected early by mammography are more likely to survive longer than women whose breast cancers are detected later in the clinical stage. This increased survival is not due to early detection and treatment alone but also to the fact that the cancers detected by mammographic screening tend to be less aggressive than those not detected by screening (i.e., those detected in the clinical stage).[54] Hence, the population undergoing mammography may appear to have a better five-year survival rate, for example, than the population not undergoing the procedure. This is because less aggressive cases of breast cancer, which have a better prognosis, are overrepresented in the screened population, and more aggressive cases, which have a worse prognosis, are overrepresented in the unscreened population.[44] The apparent difference in survival rates between the populations can therefore be at least partially attributed to length bias.

Overdiagnosis bias.   Another type of bias that can affect the evaluation of screening programs is **overdiagnosis bias**. This form of bias, which may be viewed as an extreme form of length bias, can occur when screening leads to the detection of subclinical forms of a disorder that would *not* have been diagnosed clinically during an individual's lifetime.[55] These subclinical forms are often referred to as **pseudodisease**. When individuals with pseudodisease eventually die, death is due to causes other than the disorder of interest.

The inclusion of pseudodisease in a comparison of screened and unscreened populations can lead to a spurious increase in the survival rate in the screened population that may make screening appear effective even when it is not.[41] Thus, like lead-time and length bias, overdiagnosis bias may result in an overly optimistic evaluation of a screening program due to positive bias. Pseudodisease includes early forms of a disorder that do not progress or progress so slowly that they never become clinically apparent.[56] The existence of pseudodisease, therefore, is nearly impossible to document in living human beings. First, most cases of a given disorder that are detected by screening are treated and "cured" with subsequent survival being attributed to the treatment.[55] Some of these cases may be pseudodisease, although they are not recognized as such. Second, since pseudodisease is inapparent, any untreated pseudodisease will not be detected during a person's lifetime. It can, however, be documented at autopsies.[55] Consider, for example, screening for prostate cancer in middle-aged to older men. Screening may detect some pseudodisease that is treated and apparently cured, but these cases will not normally be distinguishable from other early cases of prostate cancer detected by screening. The pseudodisease, however, will increase the survival rate in the screened group. Cases of pseudodisease in the unscreened group will not be diagnosed since their disease never becomes clinically apparent. Therefore, these persons will not influence the survival rate in the unscreened population. The result is an overstatement of survival in the screened versus the unscreened group that is due to overdiagnosis bias.

A concept similar to pseudodisease in infectious disease epidemiology is a *carrier* of disease. For example, the infamous Typhoid Mary (chapter 3), apart from her unsanitary habits in the kitchen, is unlikely to have ever come to the attention of health authorities since she had no signs or symptoms of typhoid fever even though she harbored the causative organism *Salmonella typhi*. It should be also be mentioned that overdiagnosis has other serious consequences for screening. It spuriously increases the sensitivity, specificity, and positive predictive value of screening tests as well as the incidence of the disease.[41, 55] Furthermore, when screening detects pseudodisease in individuals those individuals are subjected to unnecessary treatment that may be costly and potentially dangerous.

Volunteer bias. A fourth type bias that can occur in the evaluation of screening programs is *volunteer bias*, a common type of selection bias (chapter 8). Those who participate in screening programs tend to differ systematically from those who do not in terms of factors that may affect their survival time. For example, volunteers as a group have been reported to be better educated, less likely to smoke, and more concerned about their health than nonvolunteers.[57] If this is true, it could introduce a positive bias into a comparison of screened and unscreened populations due to the fact that those in the screened population may tend to have a better prognosis than those in the unscreened population due to their generally better overall health and life expectancy as a group. On the other hand, it is conceivable that some people who participate in screening programs do so because of a known family history of the disorder or because of the presence of other risk factors for the disorder. We might expect that these participants are less healthy as a group, and, therefore, more prone to premature mortality than their unscreened counterparts. This could introduce negative bias into the evaluation. Unfortunately, investigators are not likely to know the direction or impact of volunteer bias on the results of a screening program evaluation.

Overcoming the Major Forms of Bias

Early detection biases (i.e., lead-time bias, length bias, and overdiagnosis bias) can be prevented in properly designed nonrandomized studies of screening effectiveness by: (a) effectively controlling for the timing of diagnosis, the rate of disease progression, and the detection of pseudodisease, or (b) using an appropriate outcome measure.[58] Since the former may be difficult to achieve, a less demanding approach is to employ an appropriate outcome measure, namely, the *disease-specific mortality rate* (i.e., cause-specific mortality rate; see chapter 5).[58] Outcome measures based on survival from diagnosis to death, such as survival rates or their complement case fatality (chapter 5), are influenced by early detection biases,[59] and therefore, are not appropriate outcome measures for evaluating the effectiveness of screening programs. Disease-specific mortality, on the other hand, is not affected by early detection biases and thus is a suitable outcome measure. Nonetheless, nonrandomized studies are still subject to volunteer bias as well as to confounding by unanticipated, and hence uncontrolled, variables. Consequently, the most commonly accepted standard for evaluating screening programs is a randomized controlled trial using disease-specific mortality rates as the outcome measure. If properly conducted, this design has the potential to show convincingly whether or not a particular screening program is effective. This design should not be affected by any of the four biases previously described and should also be protected from confounding by both anticipated and unanticipated variables (see chapter 12). It is important to note, however, that a randomized controlled trial using survival rates or case fatality as the outcome measure is not automatically protected from all early detection biases. The combination of a well designed randomized controlled trial and an appropriate outcome measure, however, makes this approach most suitable for evaluating the effectiveness of screening programs.

Typically, the evaluation of a new screening program involves a comparison of mortality rates between an experimental group that is offered screening for the target disorder and a control group that is not offered screening. The control group usually receives the standard care upon clinical diagnosis. When this is not feasible due to ethical considerations (e.g., the intervention is already known to be beneficial), alternative designs that offer limited screening to controls might be used. For example, the **split screen design** is one that offers controls the usual care up until the *n*th screen of the experimental group at which time both groups are screened for the disorder of interest.[42]

Common measures of effect in randomized trials using disease-specific mortality rates include the rate ratio, the rate difference (excess rate), or derivative measures such as the percent relative effect or an attributable fraction (see chapter 6). If the screening program is effective, the rate ratio, for example, should be less than one (i.e., $RR < 1.0$). Risk ratios and differences are also sometimes used as well as other measures such as the number of subjects needed to be screened to prevent just one death.[41]

While a randomized controlled trial using disease-specific mortality as the outcome measure has generally been considered the accepted standard for evaluating the effectiveness of screening programs, it is not a perfect standard. There are several limitations to using disease-specific mortality rates as well as limitations to using randomized controlled trials. These and a possible solution are described briefly as follows:

Limitations of disease-specific mortality. The most important limitation of using disease-specific mortality rates as an outcome measure relates to misclassification of the cause of death. Accurate determination of the cause of death is extremely important because the target disorder is usually uncommon in the study population, and misclassifying even a small number of deaths can make a screening program appear beneficial when it is not or vice versa.[60] In fact, this appears to have been the case in several studies.[61] Therefore, standardized methods for ascertaining the cause of death should be used, and those making the classifications should be blinded to study group assignments so as to minimize bias.[60] It may also be helpful to take other precautions such as using an expert monitoring committee that can settle any disputed diagnoses among those determining the causes of death.

Two possible biases in determining the cause of death have been referred to in the screening literature as *sticky-diagnosis bias* and *slippery-linkage bias*.[61] **Sticky-diagnosis bias** occurs when deaths in the screened group are more likely to be attributed to the target disorder than not due to the fact that the target disorder is more likely to be diagnosed in the screened versus the control group. Consider a subject who screens positive for colon cancer, which is subsequently diagnosed and treated. The subject dies later during follow up from an unrelated bowel disease, which is classified as colon cancer based on knowledge of his screening history. In other words, his original diagnosis "sticks." This represents a negative bias that understates the effectiveness of screening. **Slippery-linkage bias** occurs when a positive screening test leads to subsequent diagnostic procedures or treatments that in turn lead to death, but the cause of death is not attributed to the screening, and hence, the target disorder. For instance, consider a subject who screens positive for breast cancer and is subsequently diagnosed and treated for the disease using chemotherapy and radiation. The subject later dies of heart disease induced by the treatment received. Since the heart disease is secondary to the treatment for breast cancer, its attribution to heart disease "slips away" from the screening and introduces positive bias, that is, an overstatement of the effectiveness of screening. In other words, the death from heart disease, although a consequence of screening for breast cancer, is never attributed to the screening. Conversely, this might be viewed as an understatement of the harm of screening. In chapter 2 (exhibit 2-1) we referred to death certificates where the underlying cause of death is indicated along with antecedent and immediate causes. In this case, screening (or breast cancer) may be considered the underlying cause, while heart disease may be considered a subsequent antecedent cause that was a consequence of the breast cancer.

Limitations of randomized controlled trials.   In addition to limitations arising from the use of disease-specific mortality, there are limitations to using randomized controlled trials to evaluate screening programs. One has to do with ethical concerns. It has to be asked in a particular situation whether or not it is ethical to offer the screening to some but to withhold or limit its use with others according to the principle of equipoise (chapter 12). Another problem has to do with compliance. Subjects in the experimental arm of a randomized controlled trial where screening is being offered may refuse to follow the study protocol. At the same time, subjects in the control arm where screening is not being offered may seek it out through other channels. Noncompliance in the experimental group or contamination (chapter 12) in the control group reduces the likelihood of finding any differences in outcomes between the study groups.[60] Nevertheless, an intention-to-treat analysis is usually preferred over a per protocol analysis (chapter 12). Finally, randomized controlled trials where the endpoints (outcomes) are chronic disorders like cancer generally require large sample sizes and long follow-up periods and may not be practical. Disease-specific mortality rates for cancer, for example, tend to be relatively low. Therefore, the power of a study may be low unless the number of subjects is substantial, perhaps as many as 100,000 in each arm of the study.[61] Other limitations of randomized controlled trials in general are discussed in chapter 12.

A possible solution. As a result of the limitations related to disease-specific mortality, some have advocated using *all-cause mortality rates* as the appropriate outcome measures in randomized controlled trials of screening effectiveness. This endpoint represents the crude death rate (chapter 5), which may be adjusted for age, sex, or other relevant factors. All-cause mortality has the advantage of not depending on the classification of deaths according to specific disorders. Therefore, it is not subject to misclassification due to sticky-diagnosis or slippery-linkage bias. Instead, it only depends on accurately determining the number of deaths in the screened and control populations and when they occur.[62] All-cause mortality rates have an additional advantage of capturing deaths that may be side effects of screening or subsequent diagnosis and treatment (e.g., deaths due to perforation of the intestines during colonoscopy). A disadvantage of using all-cause mortality is the extremely large sample sizes needed to provide sufficient power to detect meaningful differences between the study groups when the target disorder is a relatively rare condition (e.g., breast cancer). Since the target disorder is likely to represent only a very small portion of the deaths from all causes, even an apparently effective screening program that reduces disease-specific mortality is unlikely to lower the all-cause mortality rate sufficiently in the experimental group so as to demonstrate a significant difference in all-cause mortality between the study groups.[62] As a compromise of sorts, it has been recommended that all-cause mortality "be considered in conjunction with disease-specific mortality to reduce the possibility that a major harm (or benefit) from screening is hidden by misclassification in cause of death."[63, 41] William C. Black and H. Gilbert Welch[41] also add:

> [A]ll-cause mortality provides an important perspective on the magnitude of benefit. It puts disease-specific mortality reduction in the context of other competing risks and helps the prospective screened individual focus on the overall benefit to be reasonably expected. Although statistically significant changes should not be expected in all-cause mortality (given sample size constraints), its role in generating hypotheses about unexpected risks and in providing perspective should not be ignored. (p. 9)

Concluding Remarks

At the start of the discussion regarding screening programs the question, "To screen or not to screen?" was raised. Given that there are potentially serious physical and psychological risks that can result from screening and given that the total costs of screening can be substantial, new screening programs should not be entered into lightly. There are already many screening programs in place that have not yet been shown to be effective. One might speculate whether or not these programs would be eliminated even if solid evidence was presented that they are not effective. For these and other reasons, the authors of a cancer screening glossary proposed that the following updated criteria be considered in deciding whether or not new cancer screening programs are worthwhile. Their simple and succinct recommendations are general enough to apply to all types of disease screening, and, therefore, they have been rephrased as follows: (a) there should be evidence from randomized controlled trials that the proposed screening is beneficial in terms of mortality reduction or improved quality of life, (b) the extent of inconsequential disease (pseudodisease) that will be generated by the program should be estimated and carefully considered, and (c) the benefits of the program should be weighed against the harms in order to determine that there is likely to be a net benefit.[64] Public health and medical professionals involved in screening would be wise to keep these points in mind along with those outlined earlier in the chapter.

SUMMARY

- Screening is a very common practice in modern society. It is a relatively quick means of identifying those who are likely to have a given disorder and those who are not. To be valuable screening should result in earlier than usual detection of a disorder that leads to more effective treatment. This in turn should result in a better prognosis than if the disorder were to be detected and treated later when clinical signs or symptoms are apparent. Screening is generally considered a form of secondary prevention since the usual objective is to identify individuals in the stage of presymptomatic disease. It can also be used, however, to identify risk factors in healthy individuals (primary prevention) or complications in patients with existing disorders (tertiary prevention).

- There are four basic types of screening. In mass screening everyone in the defined population is screened regardless of risk of the disorder. Selective or targeted screening is applied only to high risk groups and therefore can be expected to yield more cases than mass screening. Opportunistic screening or case finding usually occurs in a physician's office when patients come in for unrelated problems, and the physician takes the opportunity to perform or order one or more screening tests. Multiphasic screening involves screening for several diseases or conditions on the same occasion. It may be a part of mass, selective, or opportunistic screening.

- The validity of a screening test is the degree to which it is able to detect those who have a given preclinical disorder and those who do not. The primary way to measure the validity of a screening test is to give a representative group the screening test followed by a definitive diagnostic test or gold standard. The results are then compared for congruence. Four outcomes are possible—true positives, false positives, true negatives, and false negatives. Only the false positives and false negatives, however, decrease the validity of a screening test.

- Traditionally, four common measures have been used to validate screening tests. These are sensitivity, specificity, positive predictive value, and negative predictive value. Sensitivity is a measure of the ability of a screening test to identify those with the disorder, while specificity is a measure of the ability of a screening test to identify those without the disorder. Statistically, sensitivity is the proportion of those with the disorder who screen positive, and specificity is the proportion of those without the disorder who screen negative. An ideal screening test would have 100 percent sensitivity and specificity, although this is usually not possible since increasing sensitivity tends to decrease specificity and vice versa.

- Positive predictive value is the probability that those who test positive on a screening test actually have the disorder, and negative predictive value is the probability that those who test negative on a screening test really do not have the disorder. Predictive values can be helpful adjuncts to sensitivity and specificity in assessing the validity of a screening test. Their values, however, depend on the sensitivity and specificity of the test as well as the prevalence of the disorder in the population being screened. For given levels of sensitivity and specificity, the higher the prevalence, the greater the positive predictive value and the lower the negative predictive value. Thus, while sensitivity and specificity are considered stable properties of a screening test, predictive values are best seen as population-specific indicators of validity and measures of the usefulness of a screening test.

- A measure that combines sensitivity and specificity to produce a single summary estimate of validity is overall accuracy. It can be misleading, however, when either sensitivity or specificity is disproportionate to the other. Therefore, it should only be used in conjunction with these measures. Other indicators of validity include likelihood ratios, which have several advantages as indicators of validity. For example, they are not limited to use with screening tests based only on dichotomous measures (i.e., positive or negative test results), and they are not dependent on the prevalence of the disorder like predictive values. Two commonly cited likelihood ratios are the likelihood ratio for a positive test result (LR^+) and the likelihood ratio for a negative test result (LR^-). Generally speaking, an LR^+ greater than 10.0 or an LR^- of less than 0.1 suggests a high degree of validity. Clinicians are often interested in the probability that someone in their care has the disorder given his or her screening test result. This can be determined by calculating the posttest probability of the disorder, which is based on the product of the pretest odds and the likelihood ratio. The posttest probability based on the LR^+, for example, is equivalent to the positive predictive value.

- The precision of a screening test is measured by its reliability, that is, its consistency from one application to another. Valid screening tests must also be precise, but precise tests are not always valid. Screening test reliability is affected by method, subject, and observer variability. Method variability has to do with inconsistencies in the test itself. Subject variability may be due to physiological changes occurring in the subjects being screened. Observer variability is the variation in the interpretation of test results attributable to the observer(s). Intraobserver variability occurs when a single observer comes to different conclusions about the same or identical test results at different times. Interobserver variability occurs when independent observers disagree on test results for the same person(s).

- Observer reliability is a measure of consistency between observations and the opposite of observer variability. Like the latter, there are two forms—intraobserver and interobserver reliability. Either form can be quantified in several ways, including percent agreement, effective percent agreement (percent positive and percent negative agreement), and kappa. Unlike kappa, the first two options do not completely correct for chance agreements. Kappa, however, measures the proportion of agreement between observers above and beyond that expected by chance alone. It is only applicable to nominal test results, however, and is susceptible to prevalence and bias effects. The prevalence effect decreases kappa, sometimes dramatically, and the bias effect can increase kappa. Both effects can make the measure difficult to interpret, especially across different populations. Weighted kappa can be used with ordinal test results and provides some credit for agreements that are close but not perfect. For test results based on continuous data an intraclass correlation coefficient is an appropriate option for measuring observer reliability.

- There are potential benefits and risks to screening. Therefore, several factors must be considered before implementing a screening program. These relate to the nature of the disorder (e.g., Is it an important public health problem, and can it be detected before signs or symptoms develop?), the nature of the screening test (e.g., Is it accurate as well as quick, easily interpreted, and safe to use?), the nature of the follow-up tests (e.g., Are they accessible, accurate, and safe?), and the nature of the treatment (e.g., Is it readily available, acceptable to patients, and effective?).

- The evaluation of screening programs using nonrandomized designs may be subject to lead-time, length, overdiagnosis, and volunteer bias. Lead-time bias is a spurious increase in longevity associated with earlier than usual detection of a disorder. Length bias results when cases having a better prognosis are overrepresented in the screened versus the unscreened population. Overdiagnosis bias can occur when screening leads to the detection of subclinical forms of a disorder (pseudodisease) that would not have been diagnosed clinically during an individual's lifetime. Volunteer bias can occur when those who choose to participate in screening programs are systematically different from those who do not. All of these biases can result in an overestimation of the effectiveness of a screening program. These biases can be effectively eliminated using a well designed randomized controlled trial with disease-specific mortality as the outcome measure. This design should also control for confounding from both anticipated and unanticipated variables.

- While a randomized controlled trial using disease-specific mortality is generally recommended for evaluating the effectiveness of a screening program, it is not a perfect standard. One problem is misclassification of the cause of death, which can introduce serious error. Disease-specific mortality rates are also subject to sticky-diagnosis and slippery-linkage biases. Furthermore, ethics may limit the use of randomized controlled trials of screening effectiveness when screening has already been shown to be beneficial. Even when feasible, noncompliance and contamination may be problems. Large sample size requirements and long follow-up periods may be other detractors. All-cause mortality has been proposed as an alternative to disease-specific mortality as an outcome measure since it is not affected by misclassification nor sticky-diagnosis or slippery-linkage biases. A major disadvantage, however, is the extremely large sample size required to detect significant differences between the experimental and control groups. Nevertheless, it has been suggested that both disease-specific and all-cause mortality be reported together in randomized controlled trials of screening effectiveness so as to provide a more comprehensive depiction of the results.

New Terms

- accuracy (validity measure)
- accuracy of the test
- Bayes' theorem
- bias effect
- case finding
- Cohen's kappa
- critical point
- detectable preclinical phase
- early detection biases
- effective percent agreement
- effective percentage agreement
- false negative
- false negative rate
- false positive
- false positive rate
- interobserver reliability
- interobserver variability
- interrater reliability
- intraobserver reliability
- intraobserver variability
- intrarater reliability

- kappa
- lead time
- lead-time bias
- length bias
- length-biased sampling
- length-time bias
- likelihood ratio
- likelihood ratio for a negative test result
- likelihood ratio for a positive test result
- mass screening
- method variability
- multiphasic screening
- negative predictive value
- nominal
- nomogram
- observer
- observer reliability
- observer variability
- opportunistic screening

- ordinal
- overall accuracy
- overall percent agreement
- overdiagnosis bias
- percent agreement
- percent negative agreement
- percent positive agreement
- percentage of agreement
- positive predictive value
- posttest odds
- posttest probability
- precision of a screening test
- predictive value negative
- predictive value of a negative test
- predictive value of a positive test
- predictive value positive
- pretest odds
- pretest probability
- prevalence effect
- prevalence-adjusted bias-adjusted kappa
- pseudodisease
- reliability
- screening
- screening level
- selective screening
- sensitivity
- slippery-linkage bias
- sojourn time
- specificity
- split screen design
- sticky-diagnosis bias
- subject variability
- targeted screening
- true negative
- true negative rate
- true positive
- true positive rate
- validity of a screening test
- weighted kappa
- yield
- zero-time shift

Study Questions and Exercises

1. A new screening test for glaucoma produced the following results:

True Glaucoma Status

Screening Test	Positive	Negative
Positive	87	14
Negative	16	362

Based on these data, calculate the test's sensitivity, specificity, positive predictive value, negative predictive value, and overall accuracy, respectively. Also, calculate the posttest probability of glaucoma based on the likelihood ratio for positive a test result. Interpret each of the calculated measures. Do you consider this a valid screening test, and why or why not?

2. Each of the following statements refers directly or indirectly to a particular indicator of the validity of a screening test. Identify the measure being referred to in each item using the following key:

A. Sensitivity
B. Specificity
C. Positive Predictive Value
D. Negative Predictive Value

E. False Positive Rate
F. False Negative Rate
G. Overall Accuracy
H. Likelihood Ratio

___ a. Eighteen percent of those with diagnosed depression tested negative on a new screening test for the disorder.

___ b. Of a 125 individuals testing positive for colon cancer, 91.2% had the disease.

___ c. Seventy-five percent of those with diabetes had positive blood sugar tests.

___ d. Three thousand women were screened for cervical cancer. Of these, follow-up diagnostic tests revealed that 75 of those testing positive had cervical cancer, and 2,600 of those testing negative did not have cervical cancer.

___ e. Public health investigators found that a negative screening test was 0.05 times as likely to be found in those with HIV infection as those without HIV infection.

___ f. Seven percent of those without breast cancer had positive mammographic screening tests for breast cancer.

___ g. Only 36 percent of those with positive blood tests for *Helicobacter pylori*, a presumptive cause of gastric ulcers, had diagnostic evidence of gastric ulcers.

___ h. Sixty-three percent of the men testing negative on the prostate specific antigen test for prostate cancer were free of prostate cancer.

___ i. Four hundred children without hearing impairments were tested using a standard screening test for hearing. Eighty-seven percent tested negative for hearing impairments.

3. Indicate whether each of the following statements is true or false (T or F). For each false statement, indicate why it is false.

___ a. The sensitivity of a screening test is directly affected by the number of false positives in the population.

___ b. Screening is most commonly performed as a means of secondary prevention.

___ c. For given levels of sensitivity and specificity, the smaller the prevalence of the disorder, the smaller the negative predictive value.

___ d. The yield of a screening program is equal to the number of individuals screened.

___ e. Targeted screening is more likely to result in follow-up diagnostic testing than other types of screening.

___ f. Kappa tends to be decreased by the prevalence effect but increased by the bias effect.

___ g. A screening test with a sensitivity and specificity of 90 percent each will have a likelihood ratio for a positive test result of 11.

___ h. The screening test referred to in item g will have a likelihood ratio for a negative test result of 0.11.

___ i. The shorter the detectable preclinical phase of a disorder the less likely the disorder is to be detected by periodic screening.

___ j. Mass screening is more likely to produce a higher yield than selective screening, all other factors being equal.

___ k. The critical point is the earliest point in the natural history of a disease at which a disorder can be detected by screening.

___ l. Lead-time bias only results when treatment in the presymptomatic stage of disease is more effective than treatment during the clinical stage of disease.

___ m. Length bias is possible when evaluating screening programs based on survival rates if the target disorder progresses at different rates and if individuals with less aggressive forms of the disease tend to have a better prognosis.

___ n. Sticky-diagnosis bias is a positive bias that can occur in studies of screening effectiveness when survival time is used as the outcome measure.

___ o. Volunteer bias is a type of early detection bias.

4. Two radiologists were assigned independently to review the results of mammograms on a group of women attending a public health clinic in Ohio. The results of their assessments are shown in the 2 × 2 table below.

Observer A

Observer B	Positive	Negative
Positive	16	14
Negative	21	95

Based on these data, calculate the percent agreement, percent positive agreement, percent negative agreement, and kappa, respectively. Interpret each of the calculated measures. Do you consider this a reliable screening test, and why or why not?

5. Comment on the following statement using principles discussed in this chapter: "If we could just develop an accurate screening test capable of detecting lung cancer early in its presymptomatic stage we could have a great impact on reducing lung cancer deaths."

References

1. Centers for Disease Control and Prevention, Division of Laboratory Sciences (2006). Newborn Screening: Quality Assurance and Proficiency Testing for Newborn Screening. Available: http://www.cdc.gov/nceh/dls/newborn_screening.htm (Access date: September 26, 2006).
2. Last, J. M., ed. (2001). *A Dictionary of Epidemiology*, 4th ed. New York: Oxford University Press.
3. Fletcher, R. H., Fletcher, S. W., and Wagner, E. H. (1988). *Clinical Epidemiology: The Essentials*, 2nd ed. Baltimore: Williams and Wilkins.
4. Grimes, D. A., and Schultz, K. F. (2002). Uses and Abuses of Screening Tests. *The Lancet* 359: 881–884.
5. Waisman, Y., Zerem, E., Amir, L., and Mimouni, M. (1999). The Validity of the Uriscreen Test for Early Detection of Urinary Tract Infection. *Pediatrics* 104: 41–44.
6. Fritschi, L., Dye, S. A., and Katris, P. (2006). Validity of Melanoma Diagnosis in a Community-based Screening Program. *American Journal of Epidemiology* 164 (4): 385–390.
7. Irwig, L., Bossuyt, P., Glasziou, P., Gatsonis, C., and Lijmer, J. (2002). Evidence Base of Clinical Diagnosis: Designing Studies to Ensure That Estimates of Test Accuracy Are Transferable. *British Medical Journal* 324: 669–671.
8. Marks, M. C., Alexander, J., Sutherland, D. H., and Chambers, H. G. (2003). Clinical Utility of the Duncan-Ely Test for Rectus Femoris Dysfunction During the Swing Phase of Gait. *Developmental Medicine & Child Neurology* 45: 763–768.
9. Gaeta, T. (2005). Screening and Diagnostic Tests. *eMedicine*. Available: http://www.emedicine.com/emerg/topic779.htm (Access date: October 2, 2006).
10. Wassertheil-Smoller, S. (1990). *Biostatistics and Epidemiology: A Primer for Health Professionals*. New York: Springer-Verlag.
11. Friis, R. H., and Sellers, T. A. (1999). *Epidemiology for Public Health Practice*, 2nd ed. Gaithersburg, MD: Aspen.
12. Alberg, A. J., Park, J. W., Hager, B. W., Brock, M. V., and Diener-West, M. (2004). The Use of 'Overall Accuracy' to Evaluate the Validity of Screening or Diagnostic Tests. *Journal of General Internal Medicine* 19: 460–465.
13. Sonis, J. (1999). How to Use and Interpret Interval Likelihood Ratios. *Family Medicine* 31 (6): 432–437.
14. Attia, J. (2003). Moving Beyond Sensitivity and Specificity: Using Likelihood Ratios to Help Interpret Diagnostic Tests. *Australian Prescriber* 26 (5): 111–113.
15. Greenberg, R. S., Daniels, S. R., Flanders, W. D., Eley, J. W., and Boring, J. R. III (2001). *Medical Epidemiology*, 3rd ed. New York: Lange Medical Books/McGraw-Hill.
16. Weissler, A. M., and Bailey, K. R. (2004). A Critique on Contemporary Reporting of Likelihood Ratios in Test Power Analysis. *Mayo Clinic Proceedings* 79: 1317–1318.
17. Jekel, J. F., Katz, D. L., and Elmore, J. G (2001). *Epidemiology, Biostatistics, and Preventive Medicine*, 2nd ed. Philadelphia: W. B. Saunders Company.
18. University of Washington, Department of Medicine (No date). Advanced Physical Diagnosis: Learning and Teaching at the Bedside, Edition I—Epidemiology Glossary. Available: http://depts.washington.edu/physdx/eglossary.html (Access date: October 3, 2006).
19. Ahlbom, A., and Norell, S. (1990). *Introduction to Modern Epidemiology*, 2nd ed. Chestnut Hill, MA: Epidemiology Resources, Inc.
20. Engel, R. J., and Schutt, R. K. (2005). Conceptualization and Measurement. In *The Practice of Research in Social Work*. Thousand Oaks, CA: Sage Publications, pp. 63–100.

21. Vogt, W. P. (1999). *Dictionary of Statistics and Methodology: A Nontechnical Guide for the Social Sciences*, 2nd ed. Thousand Oaks, CA: Sage Publications.
22. Watkins, M. W., and Pacheco, M. (2000). Interobserver Agreement in Behavioral Research: Importance and Calculation. *Journal of Behavioral Education* 10 (4): 205–212.
23. McGinn, T., Wyer, P. C., Newman, T. B., Keitz, S., Leipzig, R., Guyatt, G., for the Evidence-Based Medicine Teaching Tips Working Group (2004). Tips for Teachers of Evidence-based Medicine: 3. Understanding and Calculating Kappa. *Canadian Medical Association Journal* 171 (11): Online-1 to Online-9. Available: http://www.cmaj.ca/cgi/data/171/11/1369/DC1/1 (Access date: October 23, 2006).
24. Hartmann, D. P. (1977). Considerations in the Choice of Interobserver Reliability Estimates. *Journal of Applied Behavior Analysis* 10 (1): 103–116.
25. Bryington, A. A., Palmer, D. J., and Watkins, M. W. (2002). The Estimation of Interobserver Agreement in Behavioral Assessment. *The Behavior Analyst Today* 3 (3): 323–328.
26. Hopkins, B. L., and Hermann, J. A. (1977). Evaluating Interobserver Reliability of Interval Data. *Journal of Applied Behavior Analysis* 10: 121–126.
27. Cohen, J. (1960). A Coefficient of Agreement for Nominal Scales. *Educational and Psychological Measurement* 20: 37–46.
28. Hunt, R. J. (1986). Percent Agreement, Pearson's Correlation, and Kappa as Measures of Inter-examiner Reliability. *Journal of Dental Research* 65 (2): 128–130.
29. Goodwin, L. D. (2001). Interrater Agreement and Reliability. *Measurement in Physical Education and Exercise Science* 5 (1): 13–34.
30. Wainwright, A. M., Williams, J. R., and Carr, A. J. (2000). Interobserver and Intraobserver Variation in Classification Systems for Fractures of the Distal Humerus. *Journal of Bone and Joint Surgery (Br)* 82-B: 636–642.
31. Maclure, M., and Willett, W. C. (1987). Misinterpretation and Misuse of the Kappa Statistic. *American Journal of Epidemiology* 126 (2): 161–169.
32. Viswanathan, A. C., Crabb, D. P., McNaught, A. I., Westcott, M. C., Kamal, D., Garway-Heath, D. F., Fitzke, F. W., and Hitchings, R. A. (2003). Interobserver Agreement on Visual Field Progression in Glaucoma: A Comparison of Methods. *British Journal of Ophthalmology* 87: 726–730.
33. Szklo, M., and Nieto, F. J. (2000). *Epidemiology: Beyond the Basics.* Gaithersburg, MD: Aspen.
34. Sims, J., and Wright, C. C. (2005). The Kappa Statistic in Reliability Studies: Use, Interpretation, and Sample Size Requirements. *Physical Therapy* 85 (3): 257–268.
35. Vach, W. (2005). The Dependence of Cohen's Kappa on Prevalence Does Not Matter. *Journal of Clinical Epidemiology* 58 (7): 655–661.
36. McCall, W. D., Jr. (2003). Effect of "Prevalence" on Kappa. Available: http://www.acsu.buffalo.edu/~wdmccall/os512d/KappaBaseRate2.html (Access date: October 27, 2006).
37. Feinstein, A. R., and Cicchetti, D. V. (1990). High Agreement but Low Kappa: I. The Problems of Two Paradoxes. *Journal of Clinical Epidemiology* 43 (6): 543–549.
38. McDowell, I., and Newell, C. (1996). *Measuring Health: A Guide to Rating Scales and Questionnaires*, 2nd ed. New York: Oxford University Press.
39. Kasner, S. E., Chalela, J. A., Luciano, J. M., Cucchiara, B. L., Raps, E. C., McGarvey, M. L., Conroy, M. B., and Localio, A. R. (1999). Reliability and Validity of Estimating the NIH Stroke Scale Score From Medical Records. *Stroke* 30: 1534–1537.
40. Hripcsak, G., and Heitjan, D. F. (2002). Measuring Agreement in Medical Informatics Reliability Studies. *Journal of Biomedical Informatics* 35 (2): 99–110.
41. Black, W. C., and Welch, H. G. (1997). Screening for Disease. *American Journal of Roentgenology* 168: 3–11.
42. Warwick, J., and Duffy, S. W. (2005). A Review of Cancer Screening Evaluation Techniques, With Some Particular Examples in Breast Cancer Screening. *Journal of the Royal Statistical Society* 168 (Part 4): 657–677.
43. Mausner, J. S., and Kramer, S. (1985). *Mausner & Bahn Epidemiology—An Introductory Text*, 2nd ed. Philadelphia: W. B. Saunders Company.

44. Gates, T. J. (2001). Screening for Cancer: Evaluating the Evidence. *American Family Physician* 63: 513–522.

45. New York State Department of Health (1999). Chronic Disease Teaching Tools—Disease Screening. Available: http://www.nyhealth.gov/diseases/chronic/discreen.htm (Access date: November 7, 2006).

46. U.S. General Accounting Office (2003). Report to Congressional Requesters: Newborn Screening—Characteristics of State Programs (No. GAO-03-449). Washington, DC: U.S. General Accounting Office.

47. Agency for Healthcare Research and Quality (No date). U.S. Preventive Services Task Force, Active Topic Index: A-Z. Available: http://www.ahrq.gov/clinic/uspstf/uspstopics.htm (Access date: November 1, 2006).

48. Smith, R. A., Cokkinides, V., and Eyre, H. J. (2006). American Cancer Society Guidelines for the Early Detection of Cancer, 2006. *CA: A Cancer Journal for Clinicians* 56 (1): 11–25.

49. Agency for Healthcare Research and Quality (No date). Task Force Ratings. Available: http://www.ahrq.gov/clinic/3rduspstf/ratings.htm (Access date: November 1, 2006).

50. Budoff, M. J., Achenbach, S., Blumenthal, R. S. et al. (2006). Assessment of Coronary Artery Disease by Cardiac Computed Tomography: A Scientific Statement from the American Heart Association Committee on Cardiovascular Imaging and Intervention, Council on Cardiovascular Radiology and Intervention, and Committee on Cardiac Imaging, Council on Clinical Cardiology. *Circulation* 114: 1761–1791.

51. U.S. Food and Drug Administration, Center for Devices and Radiological Health (2002). Whole-Body CT Screening—Should I or Shouldn't I Get One? Available: http://www.fda.gov/cdrh/ct/screening.html (Access date: November 2, 2006).

52. Crown Diagnostics (November 29, 2006). *Daily Chronicle* 128 (265): A3, DeKalb, Illinois.

53. Corrado, D., Basso, C., Pavei, A., Michieli, P., Schiavon, M., and Thiene, G. (2006). Trends in Sudden Cardiovascular Death in Young Competitive Athletes After Implementation of a Preparticipation Screening Program. *Journal of the American Medical Association* 296 (13): 1593–1601.

54. Moody-Ayers, S. Y., Wells, C. K., and Feinstein, A. R. (2000). "Benign" Tumors and "Early Detection" in Mammography-screened Patients of a Natural Cohort with Breast Cancer. *Archives of Internal Medicine* 160 (8): 1109–1115.

55. Black, W. C. (2000). Overdiagnosis: An Underrecognized Cause of Confusion and Harm in Cancer Screening. *Journal of the National Cancer Institute* 92 (16): 1280–1282.

56. American College of Physicians (March/April, 1999). Primer on Lead Time, Length and Overdiagnosis Bias. *Effective Clinical Practice.* Available: http://acponline.org/journals/ecp/primers/marapr99.htm (Access date: November 10, 2006).

57. American Heart Association (1980). The National Diet-Heart Study: Final Report. AHA Monograph No. 18. New York: American Heart Association. (Reported in Streiner, D. L., Norman, G. R., and Blum, H. M. (1989). *PDQ Epidemiology.* Toronto: B. C. Decker).

58. Patz, E. F., Jr., Black, W. C., and Goodman, P. C. (2001). CT Scanning for Lung Cancer: Not Ready for Routine Practice. *Radiology* 221: 587–591.

59. Strauss, G. M., Gleason, R. E., and Sugarbaker, D. J. (1997). Screening for Lung Cancer: Another Look; A Different View. *Chest* 111: 754–768.

60. Welch, H. G., and Black, W. C. (1997). Evaluating Randomized Trials of Screening. *Journal of General Internal Medicine* 12: 118–124.

61. Gotway, M. B., and Webb, W. R. (2002). CT for Lung Cancer Screening. *Applied Radiology* 31 (8): 21–33.

62. Black, W. C., Haggstrom, D. A., and Welch, H. G. (2002). All-cause Mortality in Randomized Trials of Cancer Screening. *Journal of the National Cancer Institute* 94 (3): 167–173.

63. National Cancer Institute (2006). Cancer Screening Overview (PDQ), Health Professional Version. Available: http://www.cancer.gov/cancertopics/pdq/screening/overview/healthprofessional/allpages (Access date: November 20, 2006).

64. Barratt, A., Mannes, P., Irwig, L., Trevena, L., Craig, J., and Rychetnik, L. (2002). Cancer Screening. *Journal of Epidemiology and Community Health* 56: 899–902.

CHAPTER FOURTEEN

Disease Outbreaks, Disease Clusters, and Public Health Surveillance

This chapter covers the basic principles of disease outbreak investigations, the problems and issues in detecting noncommunicable disease clusters, and the fundamentals of public health surveillance.

Learning Objectives

- Explain the meaning and the differences among the terms epidemic, disease outbreak, and disease cluster.

- Describe the primary and secondary purposes of disease outbreak investigations.

- Discuss the steps involved in disease outbreak investigations.

- Interpret epidemic curves as to the probable type of outbreak, and for common source outbreaks, the probable time of exposure.

- Construct and interpret attack rate tables using the appropriate statistical measures.

- Differentiate among spatial, temporal, space-time, and time-cohort clusters.

- Discuss the problems in substantiating noncommunicable disease clusters and their causes, including the role of chance.

- List at least four diseases and their causes that have been identified from disease clusters.

- Describe the major objectives, uses, and sources of data for public health surveillance systems.

- Compare and contrast active surveillance, passive surveillance, sentinel surveillance, and syndromic surveillance.

- Identify at least six questions to ask in determining whether a surveillance system is likely to be effective.

- Recognize the National Notifiable Diseases Surveillance System, the Behavioral Risk Factor Surveillance System, the National Electronic Injury Surveillance System, the Early Aberration Reporting System, and the National Electronic Disease Surveillance System.

- Define attack rate difference and ratio, attributable risk, cancer cluster, emerging and reemerging infectious disease, hot-spot cluster, index case, public health surveillance, sentinel event, vector, and vehicle.

INTRODUCTION

Many epidemiologists, along with a cadre of other health professionals, are involved in a number of practical activities at the local, state, national, or international levels with the primary aim of protecting public health. These activities include the investigation and control of *disease outbreaks* or *epidemics* (chapter 1) as well as the detection of *disease clusters*. Closely allied to these and other public health activities are the collection, analysis, and use of pertinent data, which encompass the practice of *public health surveillance*. This chapter addresses these three common applications of epidemiology—the investigation of disease outbreaks, the detection of disease clusters, and the practice of public health surveillance. Public health authorities frequently become aware of potential disease outbreaks or epidemics through observations and reporting by physicians, nurses, or laboratory workers who notice abnormal numbers of cases of a disease or unusual symptoms or clinical findings.[1] Suspected disease clusters are usually reported by members of the general public who become aware of an apparent grouping of generally uncommon diseases thought to have a shared environmental cause. Public health surveillance is an essential element of public health practice and the means by which diseases and other health-related conditions are recorded, tracked, and monitored to detect potential disease outbreaks or clusters, for example, and, ultimately, to protect and improve public health.

DISEASE OUTBREAK INVESTIGATION

Disease outbreaks were referred to in chapter 1 along with a similar term *epidemics*. Before defining disease outbreak, we will first clarify epidemic, which may be a more recognizable term. Both terms are closely related and are often used interchangeably. Technically, an **epidemic** is the occurrence of a specific disease or other health-related outcome at a frequency that is *clearly in excess* of normal expectations for a given population and time.[2] The *usual* (or normal) frequency is referred to as the *endemic* level (chapter 2). Therefore, in order to determine if an outcome is epidemic or not, we compare its frequency with the endemic level in the same population during a similar time period. If the occurrence is "clearly in excess" of the endemic level, the disease is said to be epidemic. A logical question is, what constitutes "clearly in excess?" While there is no definitive answer to this question, one must recognize that even the frequency of an endemic disease fluctuates somewhat in a population over time, and *expected* increases based on past experience do not constitute epidemics. Instead, the presence of an epidemic implies that something *unusual* is occurring in a population and that there is a detectable cause for the sudden increase in the incidence of the outcome. An investigation is the usual way of determining the cause and its appropriate management. Sometimes a suspected epidemic will turn out to be due to sporadic, unrelated cases of the disease, different diseases with similar signs or symptoms, changes in reporting procedures, new diagnostic criteria for the disease, population changes that affect the incidence, or other factors.[3] These situations do not represent epidemics. For example, we expect influenza rates in the midwest to rise substantially in the late fall and early winter months and to be at relatively low levels at other times of the year. Influenza is not, however, considered epidemic in the fall and winter months unless its cumulative incidence is "clearly in excess" of that anticipated for that time of year (i.e., the endemic level). Instead, influenza is following an *expected* cyclic pattern (chapter 1) that is seasonal. Finally, it is worth mentioning that "clearly in excess" does not necessarily mean statistically different from expected levels. Even one case of smallpox in a population would be considered epidemic, since the World Health Organization has certified this disease to be globally eradicated.[4]

The term **disease outbreak** properly refers to an epidemic confined to a localized area, such as a village or town or within an institutional setting like a day-care center or hospital.[2] Epidemics, on the other hand, are not limited to localized areas. In fact, very large epidemics (those that generally traverse international borders and affect large numbers of people) are known as *pandemics*[4] (see chapter 2). Disease outbreak investigations may be more limited in scope than some epidemic investigations, but the procedures will be similar. In addition, they usually involve communicable diseases or other acute conditions, such as poisonings. Epidemics are also largely confined to acute outcomes but may also include chronic conditions such as obesity and certain noncommunicable diseases. In summary, a disease outbreak can be conceived as a localized epidemic of limited scope, while a pandemic is a broad-based epidemic generally crossing international borders. Thus, an epidemic can be relatively small or large or any size in between.

Major Objectives

The primary objectives of investigating a disease outbreak are to: (a) identify the cause of the outbreak so that effective controls can be initiated to prevent further spread of the disease, and (b) prevent similar outbreaks from occurring in the future. Since by the time a disease outbreak is investigated it may be nearly or completely over, the second purpose is often dominant. Disease outbreak investigations also provide opportunities for research, training, and program improvement,[3] which may be considered secondary objectives. Disease outbreaks can present opportunities to learn more about the natural history of a disease, to identify important risk factors, and to test control procedures. In addition, the investigation of disease outbreaks presents an opportunity to train new and aspiring epidemiologists. The Centers for Disease Control and Prevention (CDC), for example, operates a number of training programs. Furthermore, local and state public health departments can benefit from disease outbreak investigations by identifying program weaknesses or gaps that may have led to an outbreak. Sometimes outbreak investigations are initiated because of public demands or political pressure even when the existence of an outbreak is highly doubtful. This chapter focuses on the primary objectives of disease outbreak investigation, which have the ultimate goal of protecting public health.

General Guidelines

The investigation of a disease outbreak can be a time-intensive and laborious process depending on the nature of the disease, its distribution, and the need for answers. Michael B. Gregg and others have outlined the major tasks that should be completed in investigating a disease outbreak.[5] The most basic steps are described briefly in exhibit 14-1. These steps are not always followed sequentially, and some may be completed simultaneously; therefore, they are best perceived as guidelines. The investigation of a disease outbreak rarely proceeds in an orderly fashion from step one to step two and so on. In many cases the next step begins before the previous step has been completed. This is due to the fact that data are continually being collected and evaluated during the investigative process. Just as a homicide detective may revisit the scene of the crime several times during an investigation or interview suspects and witnesses on more than one occasion, the epidemiologists performing an investigation of a disease outbreak may go back and forth among the steps as new information comes to light.

One of the most revealing steps in the investigation of a disease outbreak comes when one characterizes the data by person, place, and time variables (step four in exhibit 14-1). This step can provide specific information about potential risk factors that is helpful in generating hypotheses about the nature and cause of the outbreak. This information is enhanced when it can be presented in graphic form. For example, when cases are plotted on a spot map (chapter 2) by *place* of occurrence or residence, along with other geographic features, one may get visual clues that suggest the possible source of the outbreak. Figure 14-1, immediately following exhibit 14-1, for instance, is a spot map showing a hypothetical distribution of cases from an outbreak of histoplasmosis.* The grouping of the cases near an abandoned amusement park strongly suggests that the park may have been the source of the infection. As mentioned in chapter 2, one must be careful in interpreting spot maps if the population at risk is not evenly distributed over the mapped area.[2] In these instances area-specific disease rates should be used instead of the number of

---

*Histoplasmosis is a respiratory disease caused by inhalation of dusts contaminated by the droppings of infected pigeons and other birds.

Exhibit 14-1

Basic Steps in Investigating a Disease Outbreak

1. Verify the Existence of an Outbreak

It is important to be reasonably sure that one is dealing with an outbreak before committing valuable resources to an investigation. The existence of a disease outbreak (or epidemic) is established by determining if the rate of reported cases of the disease exceeds expected levels.* Most local or state health departments should have ongoing surveillance systems that track reportable diseases over time and that can be used to verify an outbreak. Other sources of morbidity or mortality data may be necessary, however, especially if the disease is not reportable. Verifying the existence of an outbreak might involve telephone surveys of physicians, hospitals, or clinics and examination of absentee records from schools or places of work. Community surveys or data from similar areas may also be necessary to establish background levels of the disease. The cases may be unconfirmed at this point, and one should also be aware of factors that might artificially increase the rate of reported cases (e.g., recent changes in reporting procedures, new diagnostic methods, increased awareness).

2. Confirm the Diagnosis of the Disease

Some outbreaks may be due to familiar diseases, and others may be due to unrecognized diseases or other health-related problems. In either case, it is important to confirm the diagnosis early in the investigation. Sometimes this can be accomplished in the first step. Confirming the diagnosis should keep the investigation on track and help in identifying the cause of the outbreak. The diagnosis should be established by standard or specialized laboratory procedures wherever possible, although it is not always necessary or even possible to confirm every case of the disease by laboratory findings. Clinical diagnosis may be the norm. Moreover, it is helpful at this point to talk with some cases to understand the problem better and to help confirm the diagnosis.

3. Prepare a Case Definition and Count Cases

Once the diagnosis has been established, it is important to develop a working case definition using acceptable criteria. The criteria will include signs and symptoms of the disease and any necessary restrictions by person, place, or time variables. The purpose of the criteria is to differentiate cases from noncases, and the goal is to include all cases of the disease. The criteria should be kept as simple and objective as possible (e.g., presence of fever, bloody diarrhea, elevated white blood cell counts). For convenience, cases may be classified as *suspect* (those meeting some of the criteria), *probable* (those meeting most of the criteria), and *definite* (those with laboratory confirmation). Cases may be moved along the suspect-to-definite spectrum as additional evidence becomes available. This helps to minimize false positives. Once the case definition has been prepared, one needs to find and record the number of cases. This may involve contacting or visiting health care providers, laboratories, schools, and businesses or conducting community surveys. Since the initial cases probably represent only a small fraction of the total affected, it is important to search for additional cases that may

*The CDC defines a foodborne-disease outbreak, however, as "an incident in which two or more persons experience a similar illness resulting from the ingestion of a common food." (See References.)

(continued)

be more dispersed from the initial geographic area. In addition, one should collect as much information on the cases as possible (personal and demographic data, time of disease onset, clinical features of the disease, possible exposures or other risk factors, recent contacts, etc.).

4. **Characterize the Data by Person, Place, and Time Variables**

   Characterizing the data that were collected in the third step by person, place, and time variables is equivalent to performing a descriptive epidemiologic study. The purpose is to provide a comprehensive profile of the cases that will suggest hypotheses as to the cause of the outbreak. The profile should be updated during the course of the investigation as necessary. Person variables include personal characteristics, like age, sex, race/ethnicity, and occupation, as well as personal behaviors that may be related to exposure (e.g., needle sharing, eating raw shellfish, drinking from a particular water supply). Place variables can reveal the geographic distribution of cases and clustering around potentially important factors (e.g., a river, a wooded area, a farm). A spot map may be useful in this regard. Time factors usually refer to time of onset of the disease. When plotted against the number of cases, this can reveal the likely mode of transmission of the disease and other clues that may be helpful in identifying the cause of the outbreak.

5. **Formulate and Test Hypotheses**

   The results of the previous steps should be sufficient to develop specific hypotheses about the cause of the outbreak. These hypotheses should be testable and should address the possible source and mode of transmission of the disease as well as other pertinent factors. Knowledge of the disease should help in formulating hypotheses as should the description of the disease by person, place, and time factors. Often those affected with the disease may be able to provide important clues to its etiology. Testing hypotheses may be as simple as comparing the hypotheses with the known facts or may involve analytic epidemiologic studies, such as case-control or retrospective cohort studies, to confirm the suspected cause. When even these studies are inconclusive, additional steps may be necessary. This may involve the formulation of new hypotheses and additional investigations, including laboratory and environmental studies.

6. **Apply Control and Preventive Measures**

   Control measures should be applied as soon as possible in a disease outbreak investigation in order to help curtail the outbreak if it is still in progress. Preventive measures are important to preclude additional cases or similar outbreaks in the future. Control and preventive measures may involve "breaking" the chain of infection (chapter 3) or instituting policies designed to do so. Disinfection of a contaminated water supply or elimination of breeding areas for mosquitoes are examples of controls aimed at an infectious agent and a reservoir, respectively. In general, it is not essential to understand fully the cause of a disease outbreak to institute effective control measures. Therefore, control and preventive measures can begin early in a disease outbreak investigation. However, the better the cause of an outbreak is understood, the more effective the controls are likely to be. Hence, this step is listed at this point in the investigation.

7. **Prepare a Final Report**

   The final report of a disease outbreak investigation should be written and should follow the typical scientific format which includes an introduction, background, methods, results, discussion, and recommendations. It is important that the report contain definitive conclusions where possible and specific, detailed recommendations for future action. If it is not possible to come to definitive conclusions, it may be necessary to extend the investigation as was the case with the 2006 outbreak involving *E. coli* O157:H7 contamination of prepackaged fresh spinach produced in California (see References). A definitive conclusion as to the cause of the outbreak eliminates alternative explanations and helps to elicit cooperation in implementing future prevention and control efforts. The final report is also important in that it becomes the official record of the outbreak and may be consulted in legal proceedings or as an educational tool. In addition to a final report, a final oral briefing is commonly conducted for the local health authorities and those involved in the investigation. In general, communication about the progress of an outbreak investigation should be an ongoing effort that is directed to all concerned parties, including the media.

References: Centers for Disease Control and Prevention (March 17, 2000). Appendix B: Guidelines for Confirmation of Foodborne-disease Outbreaks. *Morbidity and Mortality Weekly Report* 49 (SS01): 54–62; Gregg, M. B. (1996). Conducting a Field Investigation. In *Field Epidemiology* (Gregg, M. B., ed.). New York: Oxford University Press, pp. 44–59; Centers for Disease Control and Prevention (1992). *Principles of Epidemiology: An Introduction to Applied Epidemiology and Biostatistics*, 2nd ed. Atlanta: The Centers; U.S. Food and Drug Administration (October 20, 2006). Nationwide *E. Coli* O157:H7 Outbreak: Questions & Answers. Available: http://www.cfsan.fda.gov/~dms/spinacqa.html (Access date: December 5, 2006).

Figure 14-1   Spot Map Showing a Grouping of Cases of Histoplasmosis Near an Abandoned Amusement Park Along a River

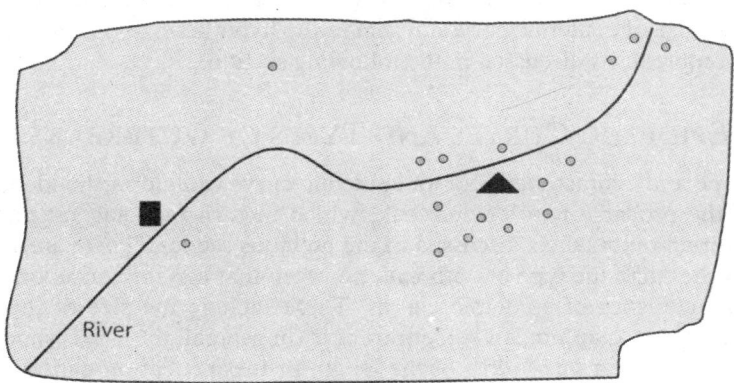

■ **Elementary School**   ▲ **Abandoned Amusement Park**   ● **Histoplasmosis Case**

cases to account for differences in population density among the areas being compared.[3] As indicated in chapter 1, unless the denominators (e.g., the populations at risk) are the same, we should always confine our comparisons to rates and not to numerators alone (i.e., raw numbers).

The appropriate measures to use in investigating disease outbreaks are *attack rates* (chapter 5), which are measures of cumulative incidence applied to a narrowly but well-defined population being observed over a limited time period.[5] The calculation of attack rates (formula 14.1) proceeds in the same manner as cumulative incidence, but the results are usually reported as percentages. Attack rates are ordinarily calculated by age, sex, race, occupation, and other relevant *person* variables to reveal potentially high-risk groups.

(14.1)

$$\text{Attack rate} = \frac{\text{Number of new cases occurring among a specified population during a given time period}}{\text{Population at risk at the beginning of the time period}} \times 100$$

When the distribution of cases is plotted by *time* of disease onset, a wealth of information is revealed about a disease outbreak, including its magnitude, its likely source and mode of transmission, its possible duration, and the nature of the disease, including its probable etiologic agent and incubation period.[5] This information is useful in generating hypotheses about the cause of the disease outbreak. A graphic representation of the case distribution by time of onset in the form of a histogram is known as an **epidemic curve**. Usually, epidemic curves are constructed for the outbreak as a whole, but they can also be constructed for specific person or place variables to determine how these variables influence the time of disease onset or exposure.[5] The use of epidemic curves in generating hypotheses about the types of disease outbreaks is discussed in the following section.

EPIDEMIC CURVES AND TYPES OF OUTBREAKS

The shape and characteristics of an epidemic curve can aid in the identification of the probable type of outbreak, which in turn may suggest possible causes for an outbreak as discussed in the previous section. There are several factors other than the type of outbreak, however, that can influence the shape and characteristics of epidemic curves. These include the size of the time intervals used in graphing an epidemic curve (in general, the x-axis should be in time units about one-fourth of the length of the incubation period of the disease or less),[3, 5] the thoroughness of case finding, the certainty of the diagnosis, the length of the incubation period of the disease, the number of susceptible individuals, and the point one is at in the outbreak. Because of these factors, epidemic curves should not be used in isolation to draw conclusions about the type of outbreak. The accumulated data should always be viewed as a whole.

There are three basic types of disease outbreaks (or epidemics): (a) *common source*, (b) *propagated*, and (c) *mixed*. Each of these exhibits a characteristic epidemic curve as described in the following sections.

Common Source Outbreaks

A **common source outbreak** is a disease outbreak that results from exposure of a susceptible group of people to a common agent of disease (e.g., pathogenic organism, toxic substance). An outbreak of salmonellosis resulting from the consumption of contaminated egg salad during a church-sponsored buffet luncheon is an example of a common source outbreak. In this example, the egg salad is considered the **vehicle*** that supports the growth and transmission of the salmonella, which represent the common agent of the disease. Common source outbreaks can be further classified as: (a) *point source outbreaks,* (b) *continuing source outbreaks,* or (c) *intermittent source outbreaks.*[5] The differences have to do with the duration of exposure to the common agent of disease, which in turn affects the duration of the outbreak.

A **point source outbreak** is a type of common source outbreak where the duration of exposure to the common agent of disease is relatively brief and virtually simultaneous among those exposed. The epidemic curve typically shows a rapid rise in the number of cases to a peak level followed by a more gradual decline as illustrated in figure 14-2 on the following page. Point source outbreaks are relatively short-lived and normally conclude within a time frame equal to the range of the incubation period of the disease (i.e., maximum incubation period – minimum incubation period + 1).

A **continuing source outbreak** is a common source outbreak where the exposure to the common agent of disease is prolonged beyond a brief period, and the exposure is not simultaneous among all those exposed. For example, a continuing source outbreak might occur when visitors at a park consume contaminated water at different times over a period of several days. Three visitors may consume the water on day one, four more may consume it on day two, and so on. The epidemic curve usually shows a rapid rise in the number of cases to a plateau followed by a gradual decline. Continuing source outbreaks are expected to last longer than the time range of the incubation period of the disease because the exposure period is protracted, and not all are exposed at the same time. Figure 14-3 on p. 517 shows an example of a continuing source outbreak.

An **intermittent source outbreak** is a common source outbreak where the exposure to the common source of disease is irregular. An epidemic curve for this type of outbreak may show small clusters of individual cases spread out over a relatively protracted time period.[5] An intermittent source outbreak might occur, for example, in a cafeteria when contaminated roast

---

*In the context of epidemiology, a *vehicle* is an inanimate substance or object, such as food, water, bedding, or surgical equipment, that is capable of transmitting an agent of disease to a susceptible host. The vehicle serves as an intermediary in disease transmission, and the mechanism of transmission is considered indirect. A vehicle may or may not support the growth of the agent.[3, 4]

Figure 14-2   Example of an Epidemic Curve Representing a Point Source Outbreak*

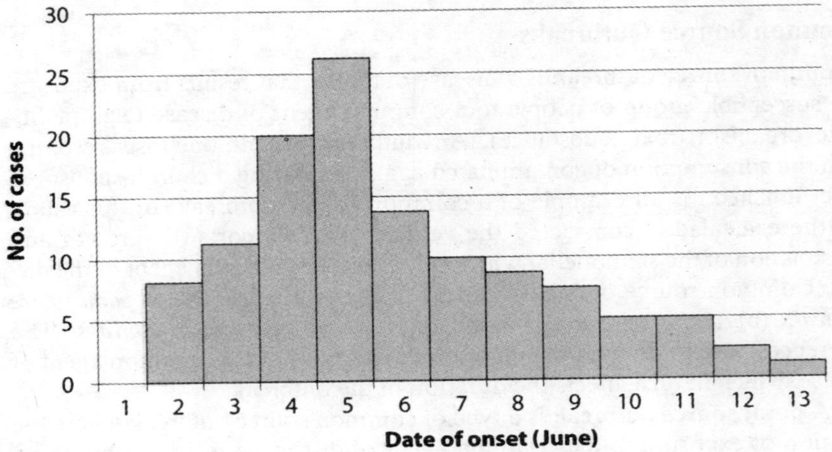

*Hypothetical outbreak of cryptosporidiosis, a waterborne parasitic disease, with an approximate incubation period of 1–12 days. Notice that the outbreak shows a rapid rise in the number of cases to a peak level followed by a more gradual decline, and that it lasts for a duration equal to the range of the incubation period of the disease (i.e., 12 days).

Reference: Chin, J., ed. (2000). *Control of Communicable Diseases Manual*, 17th ed. Washington, DC: American Public Health Association.

beef is served as an entree on Monday, in sandwiches on Wednesday, and as a component of soup on Friday. The intermittent exposure should leave gaps in the epidemic curve. Because of the variety of epidemic curves that might be produced by intermittent source outbreaks, this type of outbreak is not illustrated here.

If one knows the specific disease responsible for a common source outbreak, it is easy to estimate the probable time of exposure to the common source that may have caused the outbreak. Using the epidemic curve, and assuming the outbreak is already over, one simply goes to the first case of the disease in the outbreak and counts backwards the minimum length of the incubation period of the disease. Then one goes to the last case of the disease in the outbreak and counts backwards the maximum length of the incubation period of the disease. The time range created by this process is the probable time of exposure to the common source. For example, if the disease has an incubation period of four to eight days, one would go to the first case of the disease represented on the epidemic curve and count backwards four days (i.e., the minimum incubation period). He or she would then go to the last case of the disease on the curve and count backwards eight days (i.e., the maximum incubation period). If the first case occurred on November 6, one

Figure 14-3   Example of an Epidemic Curve Representing a Continuing Source Outbreak*

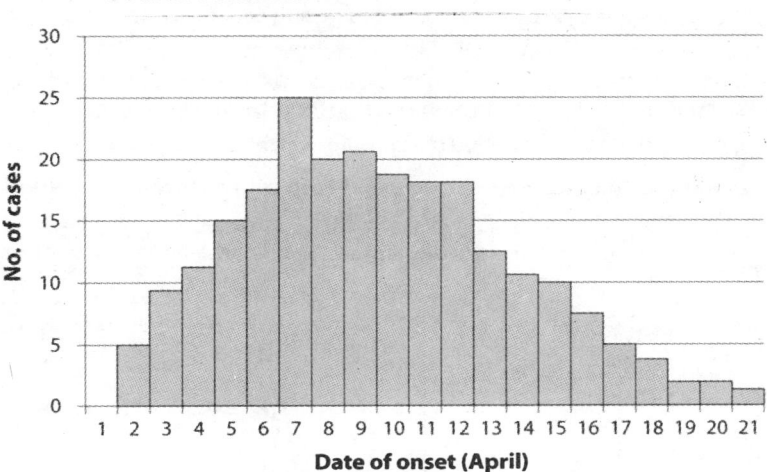

Date of onset (April)

*Hypothetical outbreak of cryptosporidiosis, a waterborne parasitic disease, with an approximate incubation period of 1–12 days. Notice that the outbreak shows a rapid rise in the number of cases to a plateau followed by a gradual decline, and that it lasts for a duration longer than the range of the incubation period of the disease (i.e., greater than 12 days).

Reference: Chin, J., ed. (2000). *Control of Communicable Diseases Manual,* 17th ed. Washington, DC: American Public Health Association.

would count back four days to November 2. If the last case occurred on November 18, one would count back eight days to November 10. Thus, one would expect that the common source exposure occurred from November 2–10. This would likely imply a continuing source outbreak, since the presumed exposure was not brief but protracted, and the duration of the outbreak exceeded the range of the disease's incubation period, which was five days.

The procedure described above is illustrated using two examples in exhibit 14-2. The first outbreak likely represents a point source since the exposure was brief (i.e., on April 1), and the duration of the outbreak did not exceed the range of the incubation period (i.e., 12 days). Also, the epidemic curve is characteristic of a point source outbreak. The second outbreak likely represents a continuing source since the exposure was prolonged (i.e., from March 1–9), and the duration of the outbreak exceeded the range of the incubation period or 12 days. In addition, the epidemic curve is representative of a continuing source outbreak. The incubation periods for most communicable diseases are available in the *Control of Communicable Diseases Manual* available from the American Public Health Association[4] or from many other sources. If you know the probable time of exposure, but not the disease, and hence not the

Exhibit 14-2
Estimating the Probable Time of Exposure in Common Source Outbreaks

Step 1: Go to the first case on the epidemic curve and count backwards the length of the minimum incubation period of the disease from, but not including, the first case.

Step 2: Go to the last case on the epidemic curve and count backwards the length of the maximum incubation period of the disease from, but not including, the last case.

Step 3: Record the probable period of exposure, which is the resulting time interval.

Examples: Common Source Outbreaks Each with an Incubation Period of 1–12 days

Count back 1 day from first case on April 2 and 12 days from the last case on April 13

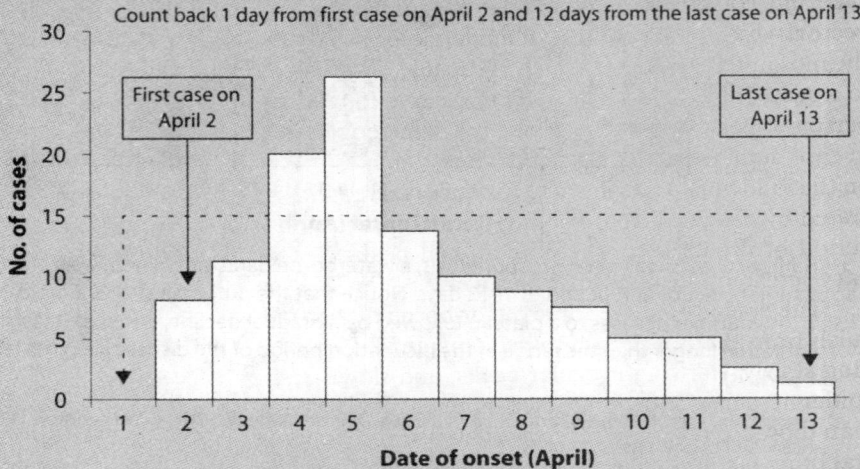

Probable time of exposure in the above example is April 1.

Count back 1 day from first case on March 2 and 12 days from last case on March 21

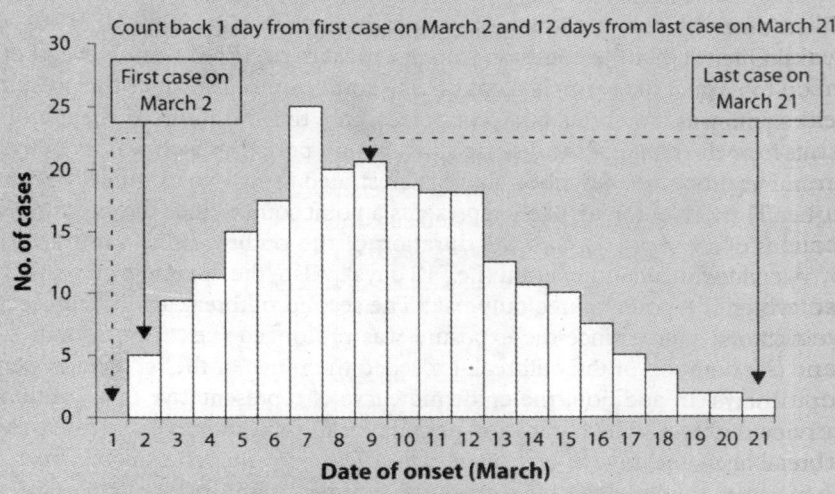

Probable time of exposure in the above example is from March 1 to 9.

incubation period, you can reverse the process by counting forward from the first point of exposure to the first case of the disease on the epidemic curve and from the last point of exposure to the last case of the disease on the epidemic curve to determine the probable incubation period of the disease and perhaps from this and other information determine the likely identity of the disease.

Propagated Outbreaks

A **propagated outbreak** is a progressive disease outbreak that usually is due to direct person-to-person transmission of the disease (e.g., via touching, sneezing, coughing, or sexual relations) or by indirect transmission through a **vector**, which in the context of epidemiology is an animate source, such as a fly, mosquito, or rodent, which is capable of transmitting an agent of disease to a susceptible host.* The epidemic curve for a propagated outbreak due to person-to-person spread is typically characterized by a relatively gradual rise in case numbers and a steeper decline,[5] such as that illustrated in figure 14-4 on the following page. In some instances there may be two or three peaks separated by distances approximately equal in length to the average incubation period of the disease. These additional peaks represent secondary and tertiary spread of the disease, respectively.[3]

The epidemic curve for a vector-borne disease may be difficult to distinguish from that for person-to-person spread. It has been described as beginning slowly, showing irregular peaks, and slowly tailing off.[5] In general, the epidemic curves for propagated outbreaks tend to show a longer duration than those for common source outbreaks, although, as stated previously, several other factors can affect the shape of epidemic curves.

Mixed Outbreaks

Mixed outbreaks are a combination of common source and propagated outbreaks. Often these begin with a common source exposure that is followed by person-to-person spread of the disease. An example is a common source outbreak of shigellosis, an acute bacterial disease causing diarrhea and fever, that results from a contaminated community well and proceeds to spread among the community residents by direct person-to-person contact. The epidemic curve frequently shows a single large peak and subsequent smaller peaks.[6] Other combinations of common source and propagated outbreaks are also possible.

A concept that can be useful in disease outbreaks of all types is the **index case**, which is the first case in a defined group to come to the attention of the investigators.[2] Often the index case is the one who introduced the causative agent (e.g., an infected food handler, an elementary school student with streptococcal sore throat, an employee with hepatitis A). Discovering and interviewing the index case may be helpful in discovering how and why the outbreak began.

*The *vector* serves as an intermediary in disease transmission, and the mechanism of transmission is considered indirect. The vector may be infected with the disease organism or may be simply a mechanical carrier.[3, 4]

Figure 14-4 Example of an Epidemic Curve Representing a Propagated (Person-to-Person) Outbreak*

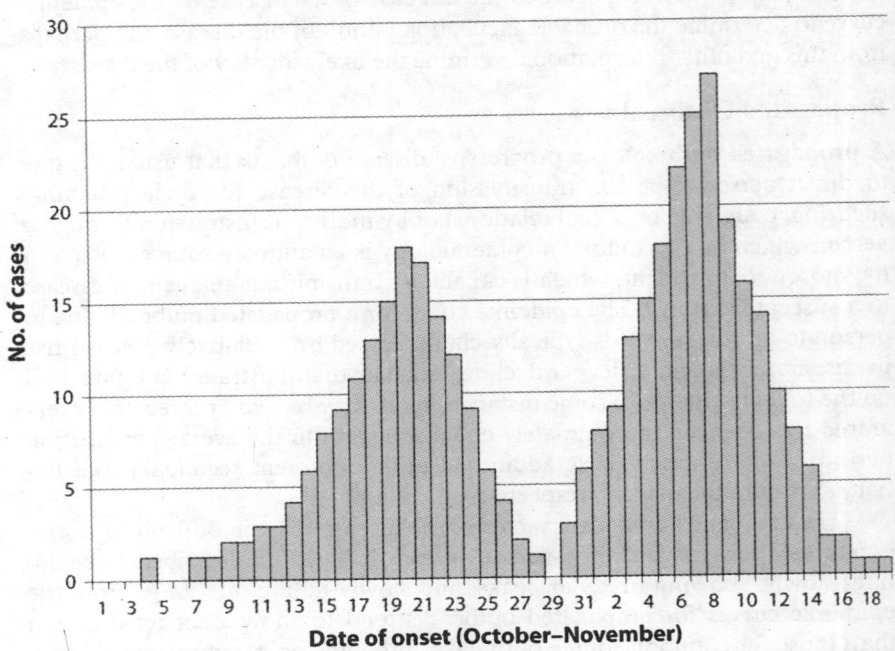

Date of onset (October–November)

*Hypothetical outbreak of an unspecified viral disease causing fever, malaise, and rash with an incubation period of 15–23 days. Notice that the outbreak shows a relatively gradual rise in case numbers and a steeper decline. Also note that there are two peaks separated by a distance approximately equal to the average incubation period of the disease (i.e., 19 days). The average incubation period can be estimated as follows: [(15 + 23) / 2] = 19.

TESTING HYPOTHESES USING ANALYTIC STUDIES

As indicated in the fifth step of investigating disease outbreaks (see exhibit 14-1), it is sometimes necessary to carry out analytic epidemiologic studies to substantiate a given hypothesis about the cause of a disease outbreak. These investigations commonly involve case-control studies (chapter 10) or retrospective cohort studies (chapter 11). Both designs are especially useful since they can be performed "after the fact" (retrospectively) and because they involve controlled comparisons. Their purpose is to determine if a given exposure is linked to the disease implicated in the outbreak.

Case-Control Studies

Case-control studies are appropriate when the source population; that is, the "cohort" that generated the cases, can be easily identified and queried about suspected exposures. In practice, case-control studies are usually used in disease outbreak investigations when a complete cohort *cannot* be easily defined and enumerated.[7] For example, in a disease outbreak on an international flight where the cases are hospitalized at the destination point, the other passengers may have dispersed to various locations around the globe by the time the investigation is underway. Even if the cases can be identified, it may be difficult or expensive to get cooperation from even a randomly selected sample of eligible controls in the source population. In these circumstances, controls may be selected from other groups for convenience. Investigators need to be cautious, however, in choosing controls based on convenience since this could introduce selection bias into the study.[3]

Once the case and control groups have been defined, it is necessary to solicit information about exposures suspected of causing the disease. Common methods of collecting appropriate data include questionnaires, interviews, and examinations. The methods used should be identical for both case and control groups to avoid potential information biases (chapter 8). Because case-control studies cannot normally produce attack rates, the usual measure of association is the odds ratio (see formula 6.7 in chapter 6), which can be calculated using a contingency table for each exposure to be examined. A confidence interval for the odds ratio can be calculated from formula 10.3 in chapter 10, and statistical significance, if preferred, can be calculated using a chi-square test for independence (see formula 9.7 in chapter 9 or 10).

Retrospective Cohort Studies

The retrospective cohort design also works well when a specific cohort can be easily defined and enumerated. For example, in the common source outbreak of salmonellosis referred to earlier in this chapter, the cohort would be all those who attended the church-sponsored buffet luncheon. This cohort could be enumerated easily and followed up to determine who ate what foods. Another example would be an outbreak of norovirus disease (e.g., viral gastroenteritis) among passengers of a cruise ship. In general, epidemics where the initial population at risk is relatively small and localized are most suitable for this design. A summary of the major advantages and disadvantages of using case-control or retrospective cohort studies in disease outbreak investigations appears in table 14-1.

Typically, in a retrospective cohort analysis of a disease outbreak several exposures are examined simultaneously using an **attack rate table**. This is very common in outbreaks due to foodborne illnesses. Specifically, the attack rate table is used to determine which food(s) is likely to be responsible for the outbreak. The use of a food attack rate table is illustrated in problem 14-1. The table divides the cohort into exposed persons (i.e., those who ate the suspected foods) and unexposed persons (i.e., those who did not eat the suspected foods). Attack rates are then calculated in each group using formula 14.1. That is, for each item being examined, the number ill (the cases) is divided by the number of ill *and* well (equivalent to the population at risk), and the result is multiplied by 100.

Table 14-1   Major Advantages and Disadvantages of Case-Control and Retrospective Cohort Studies in Disease Outbreak Investigations

Study Type	Advantages	Disadvantages
Case-Control Studies	• Relatively quick to perform • Relatively inexpensive • Does not require complete ascertainment of cohort (i.e., can use a representative sample of cases and controls)	• Generally cannot measure attack rates • Potential for bias in measuring exposures and selecting controls • Cannot normally measure multiple outcomes simultaneously
Retrospective Cohort Studies	• Can measure attack rates directly • Less opportunities for bias • Can measure multiple outcomes simultaneously	• Relatively time-consuming to conduct • Relatively expensive • Requires complete ascertainment of the cohort

Reference: Brownson, R. C. (1998). Outbreak and Cluster Investigations. In *Applied Epidemiology: Theory to Practice*, R. C. Brownson and D. B. Petitti, eds. New York: Oxford University Press, pp. 83–84.

To determine which food is most likely to have served as a vehicle for the outbreak, one could calculate an **attack rate ratio**, a type of risk ratio or relative risk, for each suspected food item by dividing the attack rate among those who ate a specified food by the attack rate among those who did not eat the specified food. The food with the highest attack rate ratio will be suspect. A confidence interval for the relative risk can be calculated using formula 11.4 in chapter 11 and substituting the attack rate ratio for the CIR. If preferred, a test of statistical significance using a chi-square test for independence can be used (see formula 9.7 in chapter 9 or 10). As an alternative, one could determine the **attack rate difference**, a type of risk difference, for each suspected food by subtracting the attack rate among those who did not eat the food from the attack rate among those who did eat the food. This measure is commonly referred to in disease outbreak investigations as the **attributable risk**, the risk of the disease attributable to eating the particular food. In this case one would be looking for the food with the highest attributable risk. A confidence interval for the attributable risk can be calculated using formula 11.6 in chapter 11 and substituting the appropriate attack rate measures for the cumulative incidence measures. Statistical significance of the attributable risk, if desired, can be calculated using the same chi-square test as for the attack rate ratio (formula 9.7).

In analyzing attack rate tables, it is also beneficial to calculate the *attributable fraction among the exposed* (chapter 6) using formula 6.16, but substituting attack rates for cumulative incidence, or formula 6.17. This will reveal the percent of the risk of the disease in the exposed group that is attributable to the exposure. The closer this measure is to 100 percent, the more likely a suspected food accounted for the outbreak. An attributable fraction among the exposed of 85 percent, for example, says that 85 percent of the risk of the disease among those who ate the suspected food was attributable to eating the suspected food. The other 15 percent of the risk is presumed to be due to reasons other than eating the food, assuming the reporting is accurate. An attributable fraction among the exposed of less than 100 percent will always result when some of those who report not eating the suspected food contract the disease. This can be due to cross-contamination between foods, the presence of other contaminated foods, or other sources related or unrelated to the disease outbreak. It can also be due to faulty recall, as when one reports not eating a particular food when in fact he or she did eat it. A low attributable fraction among the exposed for a particular food suggests that the food may not be the source of the outbreak.

Problem 14-1: Retrospective Cohort Analysis of a Foodborne Outbreak Using an Attack Rate Table

An investigation of an outbreak of staphylococcal food poisoning occurred during the first week of November 2007. The case definition was acute onset of nausea, cramps, and vomiting between 9:00 PM and 4:00 AM, November 2-3, among members and spouses of the Order of the Elephant Lodge who attended an annual banquet at the Hungry Horse restaurant in Fremont City, Texas, on the evening of November 2. As part of a retrospective cohort study to test their hypotheses about which foods were involved in the outbreak, the investigators began developing an attack rate table. A partially completed table showing the number of individuals who came down with food poisoning as defined above and the number who did not is provided for each food investigated. Complete the attack rate table, including the attack rates for each suspected food, and determine the most likely food responsible for the outbreak. Justify your response.

Attack Rate Table								
	Exposed Persons *Those who ate suspected foods*				Unexposed Persons *Those who did not eat suspected foods*			
Suspected Food	Ill	Well	Total	Attack Rate (%)	Ill	Well	Total	Attack Rate (%)
Ham	36	5			2	11		
Potato Salad	40	4			9	6		
Peas	16	15			10	13		

Solution:

Step 1: For each food item in each exposure category (i.e., those who ate the suspected food and those who did not eat the suspected food) add the number of ill and well persons together to obtain the total. This is the applicable population at risk. Next, calculate the food-specific attack rates by dividing the number of ill persons by the applicable population at risk. Place this information in the cells marked attack rate (%).

Food-specific attack rates for the exposed group:
Ham: [36 / (36 + 5)] × 100 = (36 / 41) × 100 = 87.8%
Potato salad: [40 / (40 + 4)] × 100 = (40 / 44) × 100 = 90.9%
Peas: [16 / (16 + 15)] × 100 = (16 / 31) × 100 = 51.6%

Food-specific attack rates for the unexposed group:
Ham: [2 / (2 + 11) × 100 = (2 / 13) × 100 = 15.4%
Potato salad: [9 / (9 + 6)] × 100 = (9 / 15) × 100 = 60.0%
Peas: [10 / (10 + 13)] × 100 = (10 / 23) × 100 = 43.5%

The completed attack rate table appears below. The figures added to the original table are in italics.

Attack Rate Table							
	Exposed Persons *Those who ate suspected food*				**Unexposed Persons** *Those who did not eat suspected foods*		
Suspected Food	**Ill**	**Well**	**Total**	**Attack Rate (%)**	**Ill**	**Well**	**Total**	**Attack Rate (%)**
Ham	36	5	*41*	*87.8*	2	11	*13*	*15.4*
Potato Salad	40	4	*44*	*90.9*	9	6	*15*	*60.0*
Peas	16	15	*31*	*51.6*	10	13	*23*	*43.5*

Step 2: The next step in determining the most likely food responsible for the outbreak of staphylococcal food poisoning is to calculate the attack rate ratio (ARR) of food poisoning, or the attributable risk (AR), for each suspected food.

Ham: ARR = 87.8% / 15.4% = 5.7, or AR = 87.8% − 15.4% = 72.4%

Potato salad: ARR = 90.9% / 60.0% = 1.5, or AR = 90.9% − 60.0% = 30.9%

Peas: ARR = 51.6% / 43.5% = 1.2, or AR = 51.6% − 43.5% = 8.1%

Based on the high ARR or the large AR, the ham appears to be the most likely food involved in the outbreak. The 95 percent confidence interval for the ARR using formula 11.4 (calculation not shown) is 1.6 to 20.5. This broad confidence interval implies that the ARR for ham is relatively imprecise, probably due to small numbers, but statistically significant. In fact, the chi-square value is 24.8, p < 0.001 (formula 9.7; calculation not shown).

Step 3: We can next determine the attributable fraction (risk) among the exposed (AR_e) in each case using either formula 6.16 (using attack rates) or 6.17 (using attack rate ratios). We will use formula 6.17, which is [(ARR − 1) / ARR] × 100. Both formulas should yield the same results.

Ham: AR_e = [(5.7 − 1) / 5.7] × 100 = 82.5%

Potato salad: AR_e = [(1.5. − 1) / 1.5] × 100 = 33.3%

Peas: AR_e = [(1.2 − 1) / 1.2] × 100 = 16.7%

These results support the suspicion that eating the ham is responsible for the outbreak. A high percentage of the risk of staphylococcal food poisoning among those consuming the ham was attributable to eating the ham (82.5%) and not to other factors.

Answer: Contaminated ham eaten at the Hungry Horse restaurant on the evening of November 2, 2007, appears to be the most likely explanation for the staphylococcal food poisoning outbreak that occurred among the members of the Order of the Elephant Lodge and their spouses in Fremont City, Texas on November 2 and 3. Those individuals who ate the ham were 5.7 times more likely to get staphylococcal food poisoning than those who did not eat the ham (95% CI = 1.6 to 20.5). Also, 82.5% of the risk of food poisoning among those who ate the ham was attributable to eating the ham.

Comments:

1. An attack rate table is a convenient method of determining which exposures are likely to be responsible for a disease outbreak. Though frequently used in point source outbreaks involving vehicles, such as food, beverages, or water supplies, attack rate tables may be used in any retrospective cohort analysis of an outbreak, including propagated outbreaks. In propagated outbreaks involving person-to-person spread of disease, for example, one may develop an attack rate table based on the characteristics of the individuals involved in the outbreak (e.g., by age, sex, or racial/ethnic group). Also, the factors examined in an attack rate table do not need to be dichotomous. One could look at the amount of food eaten, for instance.

2. While the attack rate ratio or the attributable risk is the most important measure in identifying the probable "cause" of a disease outbreak, the attributable fraction among the exposed provides an important perspective. The relatively high attributable fraction among the exposed found in this problem helps to confirm that eating the ham is the likely source of the outbreak. It indicates that among those who ate the ham, only 17.5 percent (100% − 82.5% = 17.5%) of the risk of food poisoning could not be explained by eating the ham. It is possible that some of the cases that occurred in the unexposed group were due to faulty memory (e.g., forgetting that one tasted the ham) or eating foods that contained or were contaminated by the ham, possibly through the use of common utensils. In general, when the attributable risk percent is low, say less than 50%, one would want to search for other factors that might explain an outbreak.

3. Another measure that can be useful in assessing the role of a factor in an outbreak is the population attributable fraction (formula 6.18 in chapter 6 but using attack rates). This measure tells us how many of the cases might not have occurred had the ham not been contaminated at the banquet. The population attributable fraction (PAF) for ham is calculated as follows:

[(Overall attack rate − attack rate in those not eating ham) / overall attack rate] × 100

Based on the data in the attack rate table, the overall attack rate for the ham is:

$$[(36 + 2) / (41 + 13)] \times 100 = (38 / 54) \times 100 = 70.4\%$$

Therefore,

$$PAF = [(70.4\% - 15.4\%) / 70.4\%] \times 100 = 78.1\%$$

This implies that about 78% of the cases of staphylococcal food poisoning in this outbreak could have been prevented if the ham had not been contaminated. To the extent that other cases were due to cross-contamination by the ham, the use of ham in other foods, etc., the percent of cases that could be prevented would be even higher, perhaps 100 percent.

4. To support a conclusion that contaminated ham was responsible for the outbreak, it would be helpful to have laboratory confirmation that the ham was indeed contaminated with staphylococcal toxin and that those who developed food poisoning were affected by the same toxin. This may not always be possible, however (e.g.,

the ham may have been completely consumed or the leftovers may have been discarded, and the cases may have already recovered). It may be useful at this point to reemphasize that a foodborne disease investigation, like any other disease outbreak investigation, depends on going through all the applicable procedures involved in disease outbreak investigation (see exhibit 14-1).

5. While it has been implied that the ham was responsible for, or the "cause" of, the outbreak, it is really only a *proxy* for the real cause, which is the staphylococcal organisms that produced the enterotoxin that causes staphylococcal food poisoning. This distinction is critical to preventing similar outbreaks in the future. After all, suggesting that ham not be served at future banquets will not be sufficient to prevent additional outbreaks of staphylococcal food poisoning at the Hungry Horse restaurant. What epidemiologists need to know is how the ham became contaminated, and what might be done to prevent a similar occurrence in the future. This is a part of step six in exhibit 14-1. Identifying the ham as the "cause" of the outbreak then is not the final step. One needs to find out where the breakdown occurred in the restaurant. Was the ham undercooked, and why? Did someone with a staphylococcal infection prepare the ham in an unsanitary manner? Is hand washing strictly enforced? Was the ham improperly stored? These and other questions need to be answered before the outbreak investigation can be concluded. The final step in disease outbreak investigation, the final report (step seven in exhibit 14-1), should include specific, detailed recommendations for preventing future outbreaks of a similar nature.

DISEASE CLUSTERS

The National Cancer Institute defines a **disease cluster** as, "the occurrence of a greater than expected number of cases of a particular disease within a group of people, a geographic area, or a period of time."[8] There are four possible types of disease clusters: (a) *spatial clusters*, (b) *temporal clusters*, (c) *space-time clusters*, and (d) *time-cohort clusters*.[7] **Spatial clusters** are localized areas within a larger area showing an increased incidence of a given disease. They are also sometimes referred to as **hot-spot clusters**.[9] **Temporal clusters** occur when disease incidence is higher at certain times than at other times. **Space-time clusters** are combinations of spatial and temporal clusters where an increased incidence of a given disease occurs in a localized area during a given time period. Finally, **time-cohort clusters** are those in which an increased incidence of a given disease occurs in a group of people who share a common characteristic in addition to place of residence. An example is an occupational disease cluster among residents of a given community.[7]

It is important to recognize that disease clusters of all types may be either *real* or *perceived*.[10] To be considered a *real* disease cluster, the "increased incidence" of the disease should be: (a) greater than expected for the specific group, geographic area, or time period, and (b) unlikely to be the result of random variation or chance alone. Although disease clusters may involve either communicable or noncommunicable diseases (chapter 3), the most controversial and difficult disease clusters to substantiate are those involving noncommunicable conditions such as cancer, birth defects, or neurological disorders. Generally speaking, these **noncommunicable disease clusters** may be differentiated from *disease outbreaks* not only because of their noncommunicability but because they also tend to represent relatively uncommon disorders in proportionately smaller numbers. For these reasons, perceived noncommunicable disease clusters do not usually require an immediate investigation like most suspected disease outbreaks or epidemics.

Investigating Noncommunicable Disease Clusters

In most cases, perceived noncommunicable disease clusters in a community come to the attention of health authorities by reports from concerned residents. Often these represent perceived **cancer clusters**, that is, clusters in which the disease is cancer. It has been estimated, for example, that over 1,000 perceived cancer clusters are reported to state health departments in the United States each year.[11] Typically, someone, who may have cancer, knows of family members, relatives, friends, or acquaintances that have cancer in their neighborhood or community. The person or persons often suspects that these cancers are related and may be due to a known source of environmental contamination in the area such as a hazardous waste site, a cellular tower, or industrial pollution. The task of the health department is to determine the extent to which the perceived cluster should be investigated. Specifically, the objectives are to determine if a real disease cluster is likely to exist, and if so, to determine its potential cause. Before we describe guidelines for investigating noncommunicable disease clusters, it is important to understand the problems inherent in these investigations.

Difficulties in substantiating noncommunicable disease clusters. There are many reasons it is difficult to substantiate noncommunicable disease clusters and their causes, especially in community settings. Ross C. Brownson[7] has summarized several, which are elaborated upon below.

- *Rare outcomes.* Most noncommunicable disease clusters tend to involve relatively rare disorders. Therefore, standard statistical procedures that usually depend on a normal distribution and relatively large sample sizes are generally inadequate to determine incidence measures and whether or not they are greater than expected. Alternate statistical procedures, though widely available, are generally more complex and have limitations that make it difficult to demonstrate causal associations. Also, health agency personnel may be less familiar with these methods.

- *Imprecise case definitions.* Reports of perceived clusters are often based on imprecise definitions of the outcome. Different types of cancers, for example, may be inappropriately grouped together when they are likely to have different etiologies. This makes it very unlikely that one will find a common cause for the cluster. In addition, failure to differentiate between primary and secondary (metastasized) cancers may confound possible relationships with environmental factors.

- *Uncertain populations at risk.* It may be difficult or impossible to identify the appropriate population at risk or other denominator from which to develop incidence measures. This is because the area in which the perceived cluster exists is often poorly defined and may not represent specific geographical units for which data are available. If a perceived spatial disease cluster exists in part of a community, for example, does that mean that only those who live in that part are at risk of the disease, or are others in the community also at risk? What about those in the surrounding county? In other words, how does one determine the precise population at risk when the cluster it not circumscribed by a well-defined unit? Furthermore, if the suspected cause of the cluster is not limited to the area affected, it may be questionable whether that area represents the population at risk. A dangerous tendency is to determine the population at risk based strictly on when and where the cases occur. This has the effect of making random clustering appear to be real.[12] According to the National Cancer Institute: "One of the greatest problems in defining clusters is the tendency to expand the geographic borders of the cluster to include additional cases of the suspected disease as they are discovered."[8] This has the effect of creating clusters. One should instead first define the population at risk and then determine if the incidence is excessive.[8] Another consideration is that data for small geographic areas or population subgroups tend to be less accurate than those for entire communities or counties, especially during intercensal years.[12]

- *Long induction and latency periods.* It may be difficult to associate specific exposures with diseases like cancer because of their long induction and latency periods (chapter 3). Most cancers, for example, have induction and latency periods that span many years or decades. This makes it a virtual impossibility that a recent exposure (e.g., a newly constructed chemical plant) could be responsible for a perceived cancer cluster. Long induction and latency periods require careful consideration of exposure-outcome relationships to ensure that cancer induction is even possible in a given situation. In individually-based studies (e.g., case-control studies) it will be necessary to conduct a thorough history on subjects and to account for gaps in exposure due to residential mobility.

- *Weak associations and multifactorial etiology.* In general, any associations found in disease clusters between noncommunicable diseases and environmental exposures are likely to be weak, making it difficult say with any certainty that the results are not due to systematic or nonsystematic errors. Part of the problem is that noncommunicable diseases, especially chronic ones like cancer, have multifactorial etiologies (chapter 2). This makes it unlikely that a strong association will be found between the disease and any specific exposure.

- *Low exposures.* Environmental exposures suspected as causes of disease clusters are generally too low, too varied, and too short to account for many chronic, noncommunicable diseases such as multiple sclerosis or leukemia.

The discontinuous nature of most human exposures to environmental agents also tends to result in lower overall doses than continuous exposures.

The role of chance. An underappreciated factor by the public with regard to perceived disease clusters is the role of chance. This is illustrated in the following example. A Sunday morning newspaper provides the following winning state lottery numbers from Saturday night: 12-13-14-15-16-35. Notice that the first five numbers are consecutive and appear to have clustered in a nonrandom fashion. Because the lottery process is random, however, we know this "clustering" must be due to chance. In fact, this sequence is as likely an occurrence as any other combination of six lottery numbers, much to the surprise of the average person. As another example, say you are to take 400 evenly sized marbles, 200 black and 200 white, place them in a large, oversized container with a lid. You shake them vigorously to be sure they are well mixed and then dump them on a smooth, unobstructed floor. You would likely find that the overall distribution of the marbles would be well dispersed, but there would be some small clusters of black or white marbles that occurred strictly by chance. Something similar can be operating when several cases of leukemia are reported on the same block in a neighborhood. This distribution might be just a chance occurrence in the overall expected pattern of leukemia for the entire neighborhood, community, county, or state. The number of cases on the block may be like the cluster of black or white marbles in the overall distribution of marbles on the floor. As mentioned earlier, to substantiate a real cluster it is necessary to show that the incidence of the disease is greater than that expected for the group, place, or time and that chance is an unlikely explanation for the difference. These can be significant hurdles to overcome when considering low incidence noncommunicable disorders. According to the National Cancer Institute, perceived cancer clusters are more likely to be real if at least one of the following conditions is met: (a) the cancers are of one type rather than several different types, (b) the type of cancer is rare rather than common, and (c) the incidence of the cancer is higher in an age group that is not usually affected by the cancer.[8] The unusualness of these characteristics makes it more likely that any observed differences are real. Even if these conditions are met, however, it still may not be possible to identify a common cause of the cluster.

Historical disease clusters. Although most investigations of disease clusters in community or occupational settings do not result in findings of causal associations with environmental contaminants, in the rare instances that they do, the benefits to public health can be significant.[13] As far back as 1775, Percival Pott, an English physician, noticed a clustering of scrotal cancer cases among young chimney sweeps in England. The habit at the time was for young boys to be lowered into the chimneys naked so they could remove the accumulated ash without ruining their clothes. Due to poor hygienic practices at the time, the soot accumulated in the ridges of their scrota where over the years it increased their rate of scrotal cancer. Today we know the cause of the cancer was benzo(α)pyrene, a potent environmental carcinogen and a component of soot.[14] Other environmental agents that have been identified as causes of noncommunicable diseases from studies of disease clusters include coal dust (black lung disease), asbestos (mesothelioma), vinyl chloride (angiosarcoma of the liver), radium (osteosarcoma of the jaw), the pesticide dibromochloropropane or DBCP (male infertility), diethylstilbestrol (adenocarcinoma of the vagina), and thalidomide (phocomelia or "seal-limb disorder"). These and similar discoveries have saved numerous lives and have advanced the effectiveness of public health practice. Based on these and other success stories, why are so many perceived noncommunicable disease clusters never substantiated as being real? As indicated earlier, the answer has a lot to do with probability. Many perceived clusters are actually just random variations of expected patterns of disease.

It should be noted that most of the associations that have been discovered historically have come from investigations of disease clusters in occupational *versus* community settings. This is not surprising considering that in occupational settings there is an easily identifiable population at risk and common, well-defined environmental exposures that are typically higher and more prolonged than those experienced by members of the general public.[7, 12] In terms of community settings, a well-known example of a cluster investigation was one that took place in Woburn, Massachusetts in the 1980s. It was here that cases of childhood leukemia were thought to be associated with certain wells contaminated by industrial chemicals.[15, 16] While a causal link was not demonstrated conclusively, the investigation did identify prenatal chemical exposures as potential risk factors for childhood leukemia. It also resulted in the clean up of an existing hazardous waste site.[13] This incident became the subject of a popular book and film entitled, *A Civil Action*. Another disease cluster of 20 deaths from mesothelioma, a rare form of cancer of the lining of the pleural cavity in the thorax, occurred during a four-year period in a small village in Turkey. The disease was linked to erionite, a fibrous mineral found in high concentrations in the village's soil.[17] This is one of the few community-based cancer clusters to be linked conclusively to an environmental carcinogen.

Few noncommunicable disease cluster investigations result in identifying real clusters and even fewer result in linking these clusters to common environmental causes whether the clusters are discovered in occupational or community settings. Nevertheless, the investigation of suspected clusters can still "help public health officials target resources for disease prevention and treatment, spur the discovery and cleanup of existing environmental hazards, and enable researchers to develop and test hypotheses about the possible links between environmental exposures and chronic disease."[13(p5)] Most real clusters where environmental causes have been established are those where the exposure has been persistently high in the affected population but rare in other populations. Also, the usual relative risk of the disease has been extremely high (e.g., RR $\geq$ 20).[17]

Guidelines for cluster investigations.   The investigation of disease clusters can be very time consuming and expensive. Therefore, a number of state and other health agencies have developed policies and procedures for dealing with reports of perceived disease clusters. Almost two decades ago, the Centers for Disease Control and Prevention (CDC) developed guidelines that have been the basis for many program protocols. These guidelines contain four major stages: (a) Initial Contact and Response, (b) Assessment, (c) Major Feasibility Study, and (d) Etiologic Investigation.[10] There are also a number of steps within each stage. Each of the stages is outlined in detail in exhibit 14-3. As with disease outbreak investigations, not all of the steps need to be followed sequentially within a stage. Depending upon the circumstances, some steps may be performed simultaneously or in a different order. The CDC has recommended that while a systematic approach is crucial, agencies should maintain appropriate flexibility.[10] Additional resources and support for responding to concerns about clusters have been developed by the CDC since the original guidelines were developed.[18]

One very important component of cluster investigation is the establishment and use of an advisory committee, which can guide the agency through the sometimes complex and difficult decisions that must be made during the evaluation of perceived clusters. Also, the responsible agency needs to be cognizant of the fact that it operates within a broader community with social, political, scientific, legal, and other interests. Therefore, communication and interaction with stakeholders is of vital concern. Following basic guidelines for improving risk communication with regard to issues of public health can significantly improve trust and cooperation among concerned parties and facilitate the success of cluster evaluation programs.[19]

So, how well are we doing regarding noncommunicable disease cluster investigations in the United States? A report of the Johns Hopkins Center for Excellence in Environmental Public Health Tracking surveyed the 50 states with the purpose of developing a profile of the state public health agency capacity to address noncommunicable disease clusters.[20] The main findings were less than encouraging.

- There was no consistent identifiable individual or agency division responsible for addressing reports of perceived disease clusters.
- The training and expertise of those responsible for addressing perceived disease clusters was widely variable.
- Not all professionals addressing perceived disease clusters worked in traditional public health agencies.
- States generally lacked the dedicated personnel to address perceived or reported disease clusters.

Moreover, it was found that only 15 states had protocols for reporting perceived noncommunicable disease clusters to the state health agency, and only 16 states had protocols for responding to perceived disease clusters. In addition, only eight states had protocols for communicating with the public

Exhibit 14-3
Summary of CDC Guidelines for Investigating Disease Clusters

Step 1: Initial Contact and Response

• Gather contact information from the reporting party.

• Gather initial information on the perceived cluster.
  – Suspected disease and suspected exposure
  – Number of cases, geographic area, time period of concern
  – How the reporting party learned about the perceived cluster

• Obtain information on the persons affected.
  – Age, sex, occupation, race/ethnicity
  – Diagnosis, date of diagnosis, date of death, length of time at site
  – Contact information, physician contact information

• Discuss initial impressions with reporting party, for example:
  – A variety of diagnoses (versus one diagnosis) is unlikely to represent a real cluster.
  – Length of time in residence may need to be substantial to implicate an environmental cause.

• Request further information on cases and plan to obtain more complete enumeration.

• Assure reporting party that a written response will be forthcoming.

• Maintain a log of initial contacts and contact public affairs or other appropriate office.

• Decide whether or not to proceed to Step 2.
  – If not, stop and prepare a written summary for the reporting party and for the agency.
  – If so (e.g., the cluster represents a single and rare disease, there is a plausible exposure or plausible clustering), proceed to Step 2.

Step 2: Assessment

Step 2a: Preliminary Evaluation

• Using data from Step 1, and possibly other sources, perform an in-house calculation of observed versus expected occurrence.
  – Determine the appropriate geographic area and the time period in which to study the cluster.
  – Determine which cases will be included in the analysis. Though all cases should be assumed to be real at this point, some may need to be excluded from analysis because they occurred outside the geographic area or the time period decided upon or because the outcome for a given case differs from that of the other cases.
  – Determine an appropriate reference population. Measures of occurrence (or other statistics) calculated for the cluster should be compared with those for the reference population in order to determine if there is an excess number of cases.
  – If the number of cases is sufficient, and if an appropriate denominator is available (e.g., population of the community, number of children in the school, or number of employees in the workplace), calculate measures of occurrence, standardized morbidity or mortality ratios, or proportionate mortality ratios.
  – Compare the calculated statistics with those of the reference population to assess significance. Chi-square tests and Poisson regression are commonly used techniques for comparing proportions.

– If the number of cases is not large enough to obtain meaningful measures, or if the denominator data are unavailable, use a statistical test developed to assess space, time, or space-time clustering.

• If the preliminary evaluation suggests an excess occurrence, proceed to Step 2b.

• If the preliminary evaluation suggests no excess, respond to the reporting party, indicating findings and advising that no further investigation is needed.

• If the preliminary evaluation shows no excess but the data suggest an occurrence of biologic and public health importance, decide if further assessment is warranted. A decision to proceed further at this point should not be based solely on an arbitrary criterion for statistical significance.

Step 2b: Case Evaluation

• Verify the diagnosis by contacting the responsible physicians or by referring to the appropriate outcome registry if available. Verification is often a multi-step process, involving initial contact with the patient, family, or friends and subsequent referral to the responsible physicians to obtain permission to examine the records.

• If possible, obtain copies of relevant pathology reports or the medical examiner's reports.

• Obtain histological reevaluation if needed. Often, however, confirmation and reevaluation are difficult to obtain.

• If cases are verified and an excess is confirmed, proceed to Step 2c.

• If some (or all) of the cases are not verified and an excess is not substantiated, respond to the reporting party, outlining the findings and advising that further evaluation is not warranted.

• If some of the cases are not verified but biologic plausibility persists and the data are suggestive, consider proceeding with Step 2c.

Step 2c: Occurrence Evaluation

• Determine the most appropriate geographic (community) and temporal boundaries for the apparent cluster.

• Ascertain all potential cases within the defined space-time boundaries.

• Identify the appropriate data bases for both the numerator and denominator and their availability.

• Identify statistical and epidemiologic procedures to be used in describing and analyzing the data.

• Perform an in-depth review of the literature, and consider the epidemiologic and biologic plausibility of the purported association.

• Assess the likelihood that an event-exposure relationship may be established.

• Assess community perceptions, reactions, and needs.

• Complete the proposed descriptive investigation.

• If an excess is confirmed and the epidemiologic and biologic plausibility are compelling, proceed to Step 3.

• If an excess is confirmed but no relationship to an exposure is apparent, terminate the investigation, and inform the persons concerned of the possible level of risk involved.

(continued)

- If an excess is not confirmed, terminate the investigation and present the findings to the reporting party and other concerned parties.

Step 3: Major Feasibility Study

- Review the detailed literature search with particular attention to known and presumed causes of the outcome(s) of concern.

- Consider the appropriate study design and potential costs and expected outcomes. Also consider sample size, the appropriateness of using previously identified cases, the geographic area and time period concerned, and the selection of a comparison group.

- Determine what data should be collected on cases and controls, including physical and laboratory measurements.

- Determine the nature, extent, and frequency of and the methods used for environmental measurements.

- Delineate the logistics of data collection and processing.

- Determine the appropriate plan of analysis, including hypotheses to be tested and power to detect differences. Assess the epidemiologic and policy implications of alternative results.

- Assess the current social and political ambiance, giving consideration to the impact of decisions and outcomes.

- Assess the resource implications and requirements of both the study and alternative findings.

- If the feasibility study suggests that an etiologic investigation is warranted, proceed to Step 4. The investigation may require extensive resources, however, and the decision to proceed will be related to the allocation of resources.

- If the feasibility study suggests that little will be gained from an etiologic investigation, summarize the results of this process for the reporting party and all other concerned parties. In some circumstances the public or media may continue to demand further investigation regardless of cost or biologic merit of an investigation. The effort devoted to community relationships, media contacts, and advisory committee interaction will be critical for an appropriate public health outcome.

Step 4: Etiologic Investigation

- Using the major feasibility study as a guide, develop a protocol, and implement the study. The circumstances of most epidemiologic studies tend to be unique; therefore, more specific guidance is not appropriate for inclusion in these guidelines.

- The results of an etiologic investigation are expected to contribute to epidemiologic and public health knowledge. This contribution may take a number of forms, including the demonstration that an association does or does not exist between exposure and disease, or the confirmation of previous findings.

Source: Centers for Disease Control and Prevention (1990). Guidelines for Investigating Clusters of Health Events. *Morbidity and Mortality Weekly Report* 39 (RR-11): 1–16.

about perceived clusters. The investigators concluded: "There is a broad diversity of expertise and preparedness to address disease clusters, with the majority of states lacking sufficient resources, expertise, and prescribed protocols."[20] They offered a number of recommendations for developing a cohesive national approach to disease clusters, strengthening disease cluster programs, and advancing scientific methods of disease cluster evaluation.[20] Unfortunately, it seems that the CDC or other guidelines have not been followed by a number of states.

As a final note, another particularly good source of guidelines for investigating disease clusters was published by the New Zealand Ministry of Health more than a decade ago.[21] In addition, to a good discussion of the stages of investigation, it provides helpful flowcharts as well as forms for gathering data.

PUBLIC HEALTH SURVEILLANCE

Definition, Objectives, and Applications

More than 20 years ago the Centers for Disease Control and Prevention adopted a comprehensive definition of *public health surveillance* that has remained virtually unchanged since that time.[22] According to the CDC, **public health surveillance** is the:

> Ongoing, systematic collection, analysis, and interpretation of health-related data essential to the planning, implementation, and evaluation of public health practice, closely integrated with the timely dissemination of these data to those responsible for prevention and control.[23]

This definition illustrates several key elements of modern public health surveillance: (a) it is a continuous process, (b) it is more than simple data collection and use, and (c) it is intimately interwoven into public health practice (see figure 14-5). The historical roots of modern public health surveillance can be traced back to John Graunt and the "Bills of Mortality" and his successor William Farr (see chapter 2). Its scope has expanded significantly since those times. Today, modern public health surveillance "can be viewed as extending far beyond the narrow confines of disease reporting and registers to include surveillance of behavioral risk factors, of health care utilization and quality, of adverse events from drugs and medical devices, and of knowledge, attitudes, and beliefs concerning health."[24(p385)]

Public health surveillance has at least four major objectives related to public health practice: (a) determining the status of public health, (b) defining public health priorities, (c) evaluating public health programs, and (d) stimulating public health research.[23] While the ongoing collection, analysis, and interpretation of appropriate health-related data are the bedrock of public health surveillance, these activities have little meaning if the data are not disseminated and used appropriately. Some common applications of public health surveillance are listed in table 14-2. These include, for example, detecting disease outbreaks and clusters, which have previously been discussed.

Figure 14-5   Public Health Surveillance

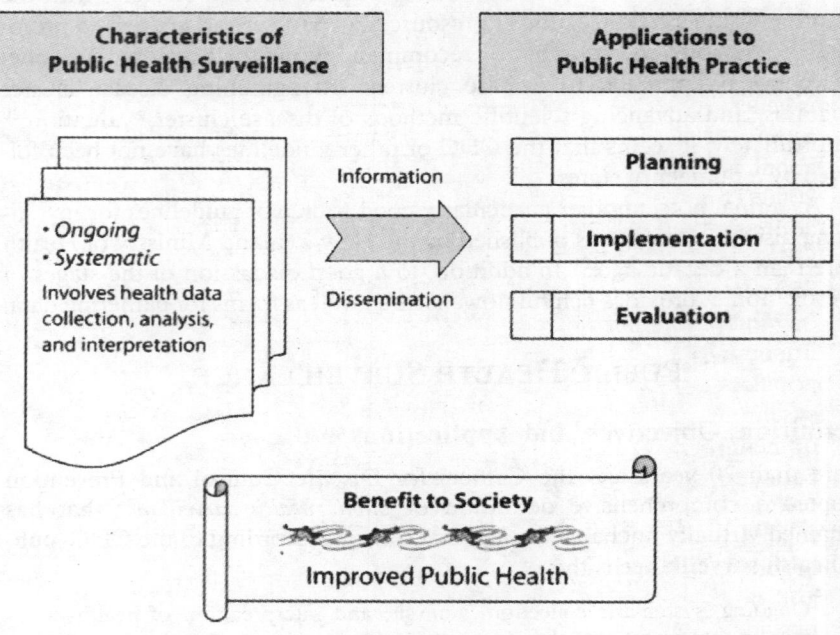

Reference: Centers for Disease Control (August, 1986). *Comprehensive Plan for Epidemiologic Surveillance: Centers for Disease Control, August, 1986.* Atlanta: The Centers.

Table 14-2   Common Applications of Public Health Surveillance

- Estimating the Magnitude of Health-Related Problems
- Determining the Distribution of Health-Related Problems
- Understanding the Natural History of Diseases
- Documenting Trends in Health-Related Problems
- Detecting Disease Outbreaks and Clusters
- Monitoring Changes in Infectious Agents
- Discovering Changes in Health-Related Practices
- Facilitating the Health Planning Process
- Generating Hypotheses for Research

Reference: Centers for Disease Control and Prevention (2006). Public Health Surveillance Slide Set. Available: http://www.cdc.gov/epo/dphsi/phs/overview.htm (Access date: December 9, 2006).

The contributions of public health surveillance to our understanding of public health issues are illustrated in the following brief account of childhood asthma. Based on public health surveillance we know that childhood asthma is a significant public health problem in the United States affecting millions of children. The prevalence of asthma remains at historically high levels and is generally higher in the Northeast region of the U.S. While death rates from asthma appear to have declined recently following an upward trend from about 1980 to 1995, ambulatory care for asthma has been increasing since 2000. This increase may reflect increasing prevalence, severity, or progress in addressing the disease. Racial differences in the prevalence of this disorder are extensive, and the cause-specific mortality rate among black children is 350 percent higher than that among white children.[25]

Public health surveillance in the U.S. provides health professionals with important data on nearly every major aspect of health and health care of the population. Good public health surveillance also serves as an early warning system for identifying public health emergencies.[26] In recent years, the development of international monitoring systems for the early warning of potential pandemic influenza and other potentially serious diseases have been a high priority of public health organizations around the world. The variety of health-related data generated by public health surveillance is used by a wide spectrum of individuals and organizations in the U.S. concerned with health promotion and disease prevention. Included are public health practitioners; health care providers, such as hospitals, physicians, and allied health professionals; members of affected communities; government officials at the local, state, and federal levels; and professional and private nonprofit organizations.[27]

Types of Public Health Surveillance

The two most basic types of public health surveillance are active and passive surveillance. **Active surveillance** requires that the health authority formally responsible for surveillance (e.g., the public health department) obtain the health-related data being sought on a regular basis directly from health care providers (e.g., physicians and hospitals) and laboratories. This may require telephone calls, faxes, e-mails, or personal visits to these sources. Active surveillance must be frequent enough to provide useful data, and it is usually very expensive and time consuming. This is a reason why it is infrequently practiced, and when it is, it is usually practiced for only a limited time to deal with a specific problem or continuously for only one or a small number of diseases or conditions. Active surveillance systems may be helpful in detecting and monitoring **emerging infectious diseases** or **reemerging infectious diseases,*** such as severe acute respiratory syndrome (SARS) or cholera,

*Emerging infectious diseases are infectious diseases, previously unknown or virtually unknown in a population, that have been increasing or threatening to increase in recent years. Reemerging infectious diseases are once familiar infectious diseases in a population that were thought to be decreasing or disappearing but are now on the rise. These diseases need to be monitored closely because they can quickly become established in a population.

respectively, because of their epidemic potential. FoodNet is the Foodborne Diseases Active Surveillance Network, which is a collaboration of the U.S. Department of Agriculture, Food Safety and Inspection Service; the Food and Drug Administration; the Centers for Disease Control and Prevention; and several state health departments and local investigators across the country. It has the goal of identifying the incidence of foodborne illness in the United States more accurately by using active surveillance methods.[28]

Passive surveillance does *not* use active means to solicit health-related data. Instead, various health care providers and laboratories are usually required by law to report certain diseases or conditions (i.e., notifiable diseases; chapter 2) using prescribed methods designed by the agency formally responsible for surveillance. In the U.S., physicians and hospitals usually report to local health departments, while laboratories usually report to the state health department. This information is exchanged between the local and state health departments and with the CDC.[27] Systems based on passive surveillance are much less expensive and troublesome to operate than those based on active surveillance, and, hence, most surveillance systems in the world are predominantly passive. Reporting in passive surveillance systems, however, often seriously understates the true incidence of many notifiable diseases, especially those that might not be considered very serious by health care practitioners or that might be embarrassing to patients (e.g., staphylococcal food poisoning and gonorrhea, respectively). In contrast, reporting based on active surveillance systems tends to be more accurate and complete. Many comprehensive surveillance systems, while basically passive, also use active strategies for certain health-related problems. In addition, disease registries (chapter 10) may depend on active, passive, or a combination of these methods of surveillance.

There are other distinguishable types of public health surveillance that depend on either active or passive approaches. One of these is **sentinel surveillance**. This strategy involves prearranging for particular reporting sources to report all cases of the **sentinel events**, that is, the diseases or conditions that are to be reported under the sentinel surveillance system. The reporting sources are usually a select sample of health care providers or employers who are likely to see the sentinel events and who have agreed to report them to the appropriate health authority.[3] Sentinel events are typically those that alert public health authorities to potential problems (e.g., epidemics, failure of preventive measures) and may require some type of public health response when reported. Emerging and reemerging infectious diseases fit this description. An example of a sentinel surveillance system is the Sentinel Event Notification System for Occupational Risks (SENSOR), which is supported by the National Institute for Occupational Safety and Health (NIOSH). This system, which involves several state agencies that have cooperative agreements with NIOSH, is involved in conducting surveillance of certain targeted work-related conditions, including amputations, carpal tunnel syndrome, noise-induced hearing loss, silicosis, and others.[29] A shortcoming of sentinel surveillance systems is that the number of cases reported may understate the true number of cases in the population at risk, and, therefore, incidence measures or attack rates estimated from sentinel surveillance may be negatively biased. An advantage is that the rate of reporting for sentinel events is generally better than that from purely passive surveillance systems.[5] The Centers for Disease Control and Prevention has summarized major characteristics as well as key advantages and disadvantages of sentinel surveillance systems in the context of the surveillance of antibiotic resistance. The aspects described are generally applicable to other sentinel surveillance systems relying on select hospitals and laboratories as the reporting sources. This summary is reproduced in table 14-3.

Sentinel surveillance has also been used to describe *surrogate reporting systems* such as the testing of dead crows or other targeted birds for West Nile virus, the virus causing West Nile disease, a mosquito-borne, fever-producing illness that can lead to encephalitis. In the midwest, testing for West Nile virus is usually done in the spring by local health departments. Deaths of the targeted birds generally precede human cases by several weeks, thereby permitting local public health departments to intensify prevention efforts as appropriate.[27]

Another more recently developed type of surveillance is known as **syndromic surveillance**, which is a type of surveillance that seeks to detect disease outbreaks "earlier and more completely than might otherwise be possible with traditional public health methods."[30] To better understand syndromic surveillance a little bit of history may be helpful. In 1993 a massive

Table 14-3   CDC's Summary of Sentinel Surveillance

System Definition	Key Advantages	Key Disadvantages
Limited case ascertainment area	Can easily collect individual patient-related data	Although less costly than population-based surveillance, sentinel system may still require significant financial investments in personnel and resources
Surveillance network comprised of selected hospitals and laboratories out of all possible hospitals/laboratories in surveillance area	Less costly and burdensome on resources	
	Flexible system design	
	Useful for documenting trends	Data may have biased or skewed findings
Traditionally includes largest hospitals in geographic area	Allows for routine monitoring of antibiotic non-susceptibility	Data is not generalizable to geographic population
Should do pre-evaluation to select appropriate sentinel sites		This method does *not* collect incidence data

Source: Centers for Disease Control and Prevention (2006). Sentinel Surveillance Method. In *Antibiotic Resistance Surveillance Toolkit for Streptococcus pneumoniae.* Atlanta: The Centers. Available: http://www.cdc.gov/drspsurveillancetoolkit/ (Access date: December 14, 2006).

outbreak of cryptosporidiosis occurred in Milwaukee, Wisconsin (see chapter 1). Following the outbreak it was discovered that over-the-counter sales of anti-diarrheal medications had more than tripled weeks before health authorities became aware of the outbreak. This led to speculation that if over-the-counter sales of these medications had been monitored, thousands of cases might have been prevented.[31] Concerns following the terrorist attack on the United States on September 11, 2001, and the finding of envelopes containing anthrax spores in the mail later that year accelerated the development of syndromic surveillance systems for the early detection of both bioterrorism attacks and emerging and reemerging infectious disease threats.[31, 32]

Syndromic surveillance systems are designed to detect potential disease outbreaks before diagnosis of the disease is confirmed (see figure 14-6). As such, they rely on continuous monitoring of key indicators of potential disease outbreaks, such as trends in certain symptoms, the sale of certain medications, or school or work absenteeism (see table 14-4 for examples of potential data sources). Contrary to what the name implies, syndromic surveillance does not always monitor *syndromes* (i.e., well-defined constellations of signs and symptoms).[32, 33] For example, to detect bioterrorism events early on, syndromic surveillance systems may be designed to focus on the collection and analysis of data of trends in "flu-like symptoms" reported by hospitals, urgent care centers, and other health care providers as well as on drug store sales of "flu-like" medications. The reasoning is that infection with biologic agents of terrorism, such as smallpox, anthrax, or plague, usually manifest "flu-like" symptoms in their early stages.[34] The primary objective is early detection and rapid response so as to minimize morbidity and mortality.[32] Traditional methods of disease outbreak investigation, including development of epidemic curves, are applicable but modified so that disease diagno-

Figure 14-6   Rationale for Syndromic Surveillance Based on Release of a Biologic Agent

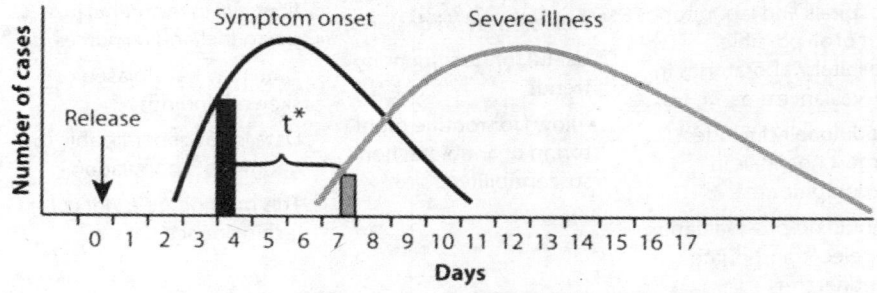

* t = time between detection by syndromic (prediagnostic) surveillance and detection by a traditional (diagnosis-based) surveillance.

Source: Henning, K. J. (2004). Overview of Syndromic Surveillance, What Is Syndromic Surveillance? *Morbidity and Mortality Weekly Report* 53 (Supplement): 5–11.

Table 14-4   Potential Data Sources for Syndromic Surveillance

Clinical Data Sources
Emergency department (ED) or clinic total patient volume
Total hospital or intensive-care-unit admissions from ED
ED triage log of chief complaints
ED visit outcome (diagnosis)
Ambulatory-care clinic/HMO outcome (diagnosis)
Emergency medical system (911) call type
Provider hotline volume, chief complaint
Poison control center calls
Unexplained deaths
Medical examiner case volume, syndromes
Insurance claims or billing data
Clinical laboratory or radiology ordering volume

Alternative Data Sources
School absenteeism
Work absenteeism
Other-the-counter medication sales
Health-care provider database searches
Volume of Internet-based health inquiries by the public
Internet-based illness reporting
Animal illnesses or deaths

Source: Henning, K. J. (2004). Overview of Syndromic Surveillance, What is Syndromic Surveillance? *Morbidity and Mortality Weekly Report* 53 (Supplement): 5–11.

sis is not necessary to identify and characterize a potential outbreak. Syndromic surveillance systems also rely on electronic transmission of data in an effort to expedite the investigational process. In fact, where feasible, the emphasis is on transmitting pre-existing health data so as to provide immediate accessibility to the desired information while limiting the need for health care providers to collect and manually enter additional new types of data.[32]

Syndromic surveillance holds considerable promise and has been the focus of much research and funding. According to Michael A. Stoto of the RAND Corporation:

> In the short time since the idea was conceived, there have been remarkable developments in methods and tools used for syndromic surveillance. Researchers have capitalized on modern information technology, connectivity, and the increasingly computerized medical and administrative databases to develop tools that integrate vast amounts of disparate data, perform complex statistical analyses in real time, and display the results in thoughtful decision-support systems."[31]

Nevertheless, syndromic surveillance continues to be a largely untested method of early outbreak detection that could be wrought with problems, such as those that might be found in a defective smoke alarm—low sensitivity (the alarm does not always detect smoke when a fire is present) or a low specificity (the alarm frequently goes off when no fire is present). Other concerns include how syndromic surveillance should be evaluated, the potential threats to civil liberties and privacy based on the methods and types of data collection, and associated legal issues.[33] Ultimately, these systems, which are being developed at all levels of government—locally, regionally, and nationally—must be successfully integrated into the broader public health system to be effective.[34] Syndromic surveillance, sentinel surveillance, and the traditional methods of passive and active surveillance need to be incorporated into a well-functioning system of public health surveillance that meets the objectives enumerated earlier.

Sources of Data

Public health surveillance is a multifaceted activity that depends on numerous types and sources of data. The CDC, for example, maintains over 100 surveillance systems that deal with over 200 infectious and noninfectious diseases.[27] The data for these surveillance systems come from a long list of sources, including medical and hospital records, pharmacy records, laboratory reports, vital records (chapter 2), vaccine utilization records, disease registries, disease outbreak and epidemic investigations, population-based surveys (appendix B), school and employment records, police records, information on animal reservoirs and vectors, environmental monitoring systems, and other sources. Examples of major surveillance systems in the U.S. are listed in table 14-5, some of which are described below. An overview of the general flow of information in a surveillance system is illustrated in figure 14-7 on p. 543. This represents a passive system.

The **National Notifiable Diseases Surveillance System** is a national surveillance system based on mandated reporting of certain diseases and conditions at the state level. The diseases or conditions that must be reported may vary from state to state. The CDC receives data from these reporting systems

---

Table 14-5   Examples of National Surveillance Systems in the U.S.

- National Notifiable Diseases Surveillance System
- Behavioral Risk Factor Surveillance System
- Youth Risk Behavior Surveillance System
- National Electronic Injury Surveillance System
- The Early Aberration Reporting System
- National Oral Health Surveillance System
- Pregnancy Nutrition Surveillance System
- Pregnancy Risk Assessment Monitoring System
- Pediatric Nutrition Surveillance System
- Hazardous Substances Emergency Events Surveillance System

Figure 14-7   Basic Steps in a Surveillance System

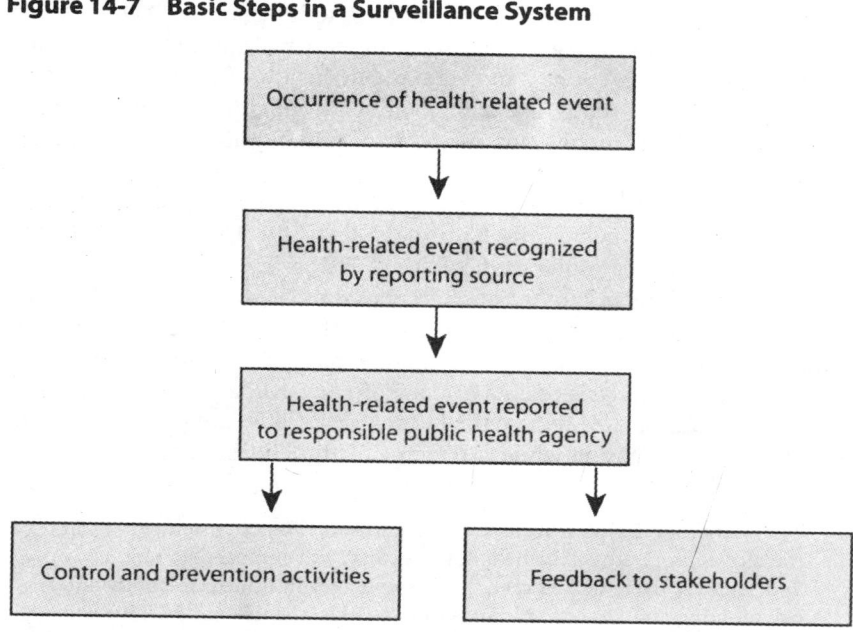

Source: German, R. R. et al. (2001). Updated Guidelines for Evaluating Public Health Surveillance Systems: Recommendations from the Guidelines Working Group. *Morbidity and Mortality Weekly Report* 50 (RR-13): 1–35.

on a voluntary basis each week and publishes them in the *Morbidity and Mortality Weekly Report (MMWR)*, a CDC publication. An annual summary report is also published. State health department officials and the CDC determine which diseases should be nationally notifiable. The list of nationally notifiable diseases is revised periodically based on recommendations of the Council of State and Territorial Epidemiologists in collaboration with the CDC.[35]

The **Behavioral Risk Factor Surveillance System** (BRFSS) "is the world's largest, on-going telephone health survey system, tracking health conditions and risk behaviors in the United States yearly since 1984. Conducted by the 50 state health departments as well as those in the District of Columbia, Puerto Rico, Guam, and the U.S. Virgin Islands with support from the CDC, BRFSS provides state-specific information about issues such as asthma, diabetes, health care access, alcohol use, hypertension, obesity, cancer screening, nutrition and physical activity, tobacco use, and more."[38]

The **National Electronic Injury Surveillance System** is operated by the Consumer Product Safety Commission and collects injury data from 100 emergency departments randomly selected from all U.S. hospitals with emergency departments. The system has the flexibility to gather other related data as needed.[37] Finally, the **Early Aberration Reporting System** (EARS) of the

CDC originated as a "method for monitoring bioterrorism during large-scale events. Its evolution to a standard surveillance tool began in New York City and the national capitol region following the terrorist attacks of September 11, 2001. Various city, county, and state public health officials in the United States and abroad currently use EARS on syndromic data from emergency departments, 911 calls, physician office data, school and business absenteeism, and over-the-counter drug sales."[38]

Recent efforts by CDC in cooperation with various states to integrate surveillance systems include the **National Electronic Disease Surveillance System** (NEDSS). According to the CDC, NEDSS "is an initiative that promotes the use of data and information system standards to advance the development of efficient, integrated, and interoperable surveillance systems at the federal, state, and local levels."[39] A fundamental goal "is the ongoing, automatic capture and analysis of data that are already available electronically."[39] A successful NEDSS will reduce the burden on health care providers in supplying needed information while enhancing the timeliness and quality of data provided. The CDC has stated the following regarding its goal for NEDSS.

> The vision of NEDSS is to have integrated surveillance systems that can transfer appropriate public health, laboratory, and clinical data efficiently and securely over the Internet. NEDSS will revolutionize public health by gathering and analyzing information quickly and accurately. This will help improve the nation's ability to identify and track emerging infectious diseases and potential bioterrorism attacks as well as to investigate outbreaks and monitor disease trends.[40]

Population data normally are combined with surveillance data to generate relevant prevalence, incidence, or mortality measures that can then be used to compare health problems by person, place, or time variables. The major source of population data in the United States is the U.S. Census Bureau located in the Department of Commerce. It has been conducting comprehensive counts and profiles of the U.S. population every ten years since 1790. The agency also collects less comprehensive data during intercensal periods.

In addition to the CDC, there are several other agencies responsible for public health surveillance. The major agencies at the state and local levels are usually public health departments or their equivalent, while at the international level it is the World Health Organization. The principal health statistics agency within the U.S. government is the National Center for Health Statistics (NCHS), which is located in the CDC. This agency is a major resource for information on the health status of the nation. It is legally responsible for the collection, analysis, and dissemination of a wide range of health-related data. It also provides technical assistance to state and local authorities.[41] A summary of the major surveys and data systems administered by the NCHS are presented in appendix B. Significant sources of health and safety statistics in the work environment are generated and maintained by the Bureau of Labor Statistics in the U.S. Department of Labor.

Characteristics of Effective Surveillance Systems

Public health surveillance is a vital component of comprehensive public health practice. Ideally, it provides valid, reliable, and useful information for decision making that helps public health agencies achieve their objectives. At the same time, surveillance systems require scarce resources and can be expensive to operate. They also require a significant time commitment by trained personnel. Therefore, public health surveillance systems need to be evaluated on a periodic basis to determine if they are fulfilling their intended purposes. The major characteristics of effective surveillance systems are incorporated in the following ten questions. These questions do not cover every aspect of surveillance systems and, some questions may be more important than others depending on the objectives of the specific surveillance system being reviewed.[42] Nevertheless, affirmative responses to each of the questions are generally indicative that the surveillance system being reviewed is on the right track.

1. Does the system detect important health events?
2. Are the health events detected in a valid and reliable manner?
3. Does the system provide data that are representative of the population served?
4. Is the system easy to use?
5. Is the system acceptable to those who use it?
6. Is the reporting of health information timely?
7. Is the system efficient in terms of flexibility and costs?
8. Does the system provide adequate protection of individual privacy?
9. Is the system secure so as to protect confidential data and the integrity of the system as a whole?
10. Does the system make a qualitative difference in public health practice?

SUMMARY

- Technically speaking, an epidemic is the occurrence of a specific event at a frequency that is clearly in excess of normal expectations for a given population and time period. The presence of an epidemic implies that something unusual is happening in a population. A disease outbreak is generally defined as an epidemic confined to a localized area or within an institutional setting such as a hospital.

- The primary objectives for investigating disease outbreaks are to identify the cause so as to prevent any further spread of the disease and to prevent similar outbreaks from occurring in the future. Disease outbreak investigations also provide opportunities for research, training, and program improvement, which may be considered secondary objectives.

- The investigation of a disease outbreak can be a laborious process and normally requires completion of multiple steps, including verifying the existence

of an outbreak; confirming the diagnosis of the disease; preparing a case definition and counting cases; characterizing the data by person, place, and time;
formulating and testing hypotheses; applying control and preventive measures;
and preparing a final report. One of the most revealing steps is characterizing
the data by person, place, and time variables. This step may provide help in
identifying potential risk factors and suggesting hypotheses about the nature
and source of the outbreak. Often spot maps and epidemic curves can be developed in this step. Both can provide clues to the potential cause of the outbreak.

- There are three basic types of disease outbreaks or epidemics—common
  source, propagated, and mixed. A common source outbreak results from a
  common source of exposure. This type can be further classified as a point,
  continuing, or intermittent source outbreak depending on the extent and
  consistency of the exposure. Propagated outbreaks are progressive and usually due to direct person-to-person transmission or by indirect transmission
  through a vector.

- A disease cluster is a greater than expected number of cases of a given disease in a particular group of people, geographic area, or period of time.
  There are four possible types of disease clusters—spatial, temporal, space-
  time, and time-cohort. It is important to recognize that disease clusters may
  be real or perceived. Real disease clusters represent those where the incidence of the disease is greater than expected and unlikely to be due to
  chance. The most difficult disease clusters to substantiate are noncommunicable disease clusters, such as cancer clusters.

- Noncommunicable disease clusters usually come to the attention of health
  authorities by reports from residents who have knowledge of several persons with the disease in question. What to do about these reports can be
  perplexing. Options range from a cursory review of the information presented to a full-scale investigation. The adoption of a protocol and use of
  an advisory committee can help health agencies decide which actions to
  take in any given situation.

- There are many difficulties in substantiating noncommunicable disease
  clusters and their causes. These include the need for alternate statistical
  procedures due to rare outcomes as well as problems due to imprecise case
  definitions, uncertain populations at risk, long induction and latency periods, generally weak associations, and low levels of exposure. A frequently
  underappreciated factor by the public is the significant role that chance can
  play in perceived clusters.

- Public health surveillance represents the ongoing, systematic collection,
  analysis, and interpretation of health-related data for planning, implementing, and evaluating public health programs. It has grown in complexity and
  extends well beyond disease reporting. Common objectives of public health
  surveillance include determining the status of public health, defining public
  health priorities, evaluating public health programs, and stimulating public
  health research.

- The most basic types of public health surveillance are active and passive surveillance. Active surveillance requires that the responsible health authority obtain the desired data directly from health care providers and laboratories. Passive surveillance requires the reporting sources to supply the desired data. Since it is usually less expensive, passive surveillance is the dominant system in most countries, including the U.S. Passive surveillance, however, is more likely to understate the incidence of notifiable diseases than active surveillance.

- Two other types of surveillance are sentinel and syndromic surveillance. Sentinel surveillance involves prompt reporting of important health-related events by prearrangement with selective reporting sources. Due to the selective nature of sentinel surveillance, reporting may be negatively biased. Syndromic surveillance has the goal of detecting outbreaks before the disease is diagnosed. Systems based on this method rely on continuous monitoring of key indicators of potential outbreaks such as trends in certain symptoms, sales of medications, or absenteeism from school or work. Surveillance has been used to detect potential outbreaks due to bioterrorism.

- Sources of data for public health surveillance are numerous and include hospital records, laboratory reports, vital records, disease registries, surveys, police records, and a variety of other sources. The evaluation of surveillance systems is costly and time intensive but should be conducted on a periodic basis to ensure that the systems are meeting their intended purposes.

New Terms

- active surveillance
- attack rate difference
- attack rate ratio
- attack rate table
- attributable risk
- Behavioral Risk Factor Surveillance System
- cancer cluster
- common source outbreak
- continuing source outbreak
- disease cluster
- disease outbreak
- Early Aberration Reporting System
- emerging infectious disease
- epidemic
- epidemic curve
- hot-spot cluster
- index case
- intermittent source outbreak
- mixed outbreak
- National Electronic Disease Surveillance System
- National Electronic Injury Surveillance System
- National Notifiable Diseases Surveillance System
- noncommunicable disease cluster
- passive surveillance
- point source outbreak
- propagated outbreak
- public health surveillance
- reemerging infectious disease ·
- sentinel event
- sentinel surveillance
- space-time cluster
- spatial cluster
- syndromic surveillance

- temporal cluster
- time-cohort cluster
- vector
- vehicle

Study Questions and Exercises

1. For a given disease with an incubation period of 2–6 days, what specific type of disease outbreak is most likely represented by the epidemic curve shown below, and why? Also, what is the probable time of exposure for this outbreak?

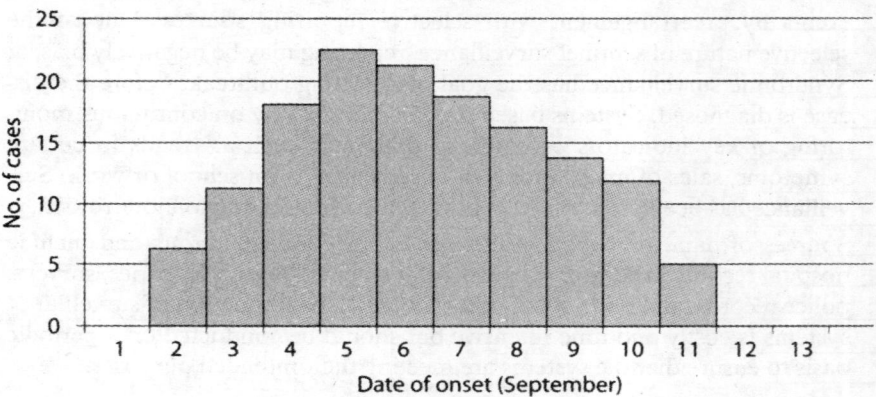

Date of onset (September)

2. For a given disease with an incubation period of 10–18 days, what type of disease outbreak is most likely represented by the epidemic curve shown below, and why? Also, what is the probable mode of transmission for this outbreak?

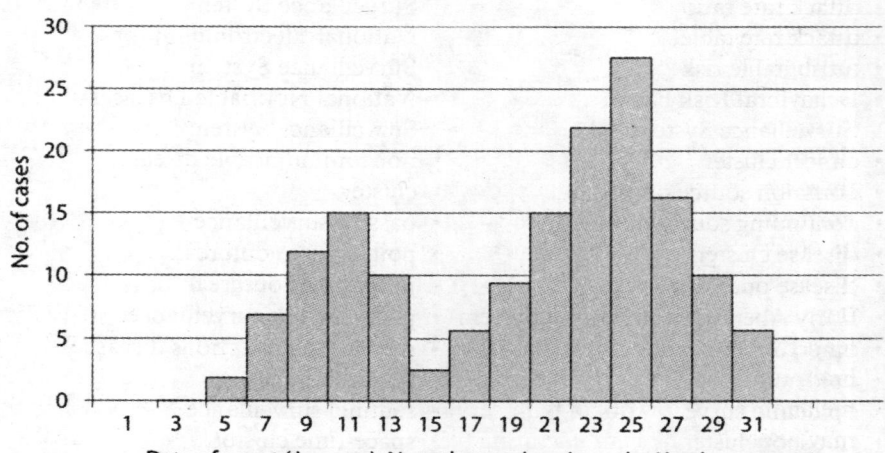

Date of onset (January). Note that each unit on the X-axis represents a two-day period (e.g., January 1 is actually January 1–2).

3. Briefly outline the steps you would follow in investigating an alleged outbreak of viral meningitis on a college campus.

4. On June 1, 13 people became ill after attending a retirement dinner for a colleague. The symptoms were acute gastritis, vomiting, and fever. Using the food histories in the table below for the 20 individuals attending the dinner, construct an attack rate table and determine the most likely source of the outbreak. Justify your response.

Person	Became Ill?	Ate Beef?	Ate Chicken?	Ate Salad?
1	Yes	Yes	Yes	Yes
2	Yes	Yes	Yes	No
3	Yes	No	Yes	Yes
4	No	Yes	No	No
5	Yes	Yes	No	Yes
6	No	Yes	No	No
7	Yes	Yes	Yes	Yes
8	Yes	Yes	No	Yes
9	Yes	No	Yes	No
10	No	No	Yes	No
11	Yes	Yes	Yes	No
12	No	No	No	Yes
13	No	No	No	No
14	Yes	Yes	Yes	Yes
15	No	No	No	Yes
16	No	No	Yes	No
17	Yes	Yes	No	Yes
18	Yes	Yes	No	Yes
19	Yes	Yes	Yes	No
20	Yes	Yes	Yes	No

5. Assume you are working as the chief epidemiologist at the local county health department. You receive a phone call from a woman who believes there is a cancer cluster in her community. She reports that she lives in the northern part of the county in Clayton, a city with a population of about 25,000. She further states that her sister, who lives just two blocks away, was recently diagnosed with non-Hodgkin's lymphoma, and a neighbor of her sister recently died of leukemia. She also relates that she knows of at least five other cases of cancer in the community, including a child with a brain tumor, two cases of prostate cancer, an elderly man with malignant melanoma, and a woman with cervical cancer. She suspects that the cause may be a pesticide manufacturing plant that was built last year just outside the city limits. She demands that the health department investigate immediately. Is it likely the situation described represents a real cancer cluster,

and why or why not? Also, as the chief epidemiologist at the health department, how would you respond to the woman's demand for an immediate investigation of the alleged problem? Explain.

6. Compare and contrast the relative advantages and disadvantages of active, passive, sentinel, and syndromic surveillance systems. Also, provide at least two specific examples of diseases or other health-related conditions that would be most appropriate for each type of surveillance system (i.e., active, passive, sentinel, and syndromic). Indicate briefly why the selected diseases or conditions are appropriate to the specific system.

References

1. Reingold, A. L. (1998). Outbreak Investigations—A Perspective. *Emerging Infectious Diseases* 4 (1): 21–27.
2. Last, J. M., ed. (2001). *A Dictionary of Epidemiology*, 4th ed. New York: Oxford University Press.
3. Centers for Disease Control and Prevention (1992). *Principles of Epidemiology: An Introduction to Applied Epidemiology and Biostatistics*, 2nd ed. Atlanta: The Centers.
4. Chin, J., ed. (2000). *Control of Communicable Diseases Manual*, 17th ed. Washington, DC: American Public Health Association.
5. Gregg, M. B., ed. (1996). *Field Epidemiology*. New York: Oxford University Press.
6. Kelsey, J. L., Thompson, W. D., and Evans, A. S. (1986). *Methods in Observational Epidemiology*. New York: Oxford University Press.
7. Brownson, R. C. (1998). Outbreak and Cluster Investigations. In *Applied Epidemiology: Theory to Practice*, R. C. Brownson and D. B. Petitti, eds. New York: Oxford University Press, pp. 71–104.
8. National Cancer Institute (2006). National Cancer Institute Fact Sheet: Cancer Clusters. Available: http://www.cancer.gov/cancertopics/factsheet/Risk/clusters#p1 (Access date: December 6, 2006).
9. Aamodt, G., Samuelsen, S. O., and Skrondal, A. (2006). A Simulation Study of Three Methods for Detecting Disease Clusters. *International Journal of Health Geographics* 5: 15. Available: http://www.ij-healthgeographics.com/content/5/1/15 (Access date: December 2, 2006).
10. Centers for Disease Control and Prevention (1990). Guidelines for Investigating Clusters of Health Events. *Morbidity and Mortality Weekly Report* 39 (RR-11): 1–16.
11. Trumbo, C. W. (2000). Public Requests for Cancer Cluster Investigations: A Survey of State Health Departments. *American Journal of Public Health* 90 (8): 1300–1302.
12. Thun, M. J., and Sinks, T. (2004). Understanding Cancer Clusters. *CA: A Cancer Journal for Clinicians* 54: 273–280.
13. Dutzik, T., and Baumann, J. (2002). *Health Tracking & Disease Clusters: The Lack of Data on Chronic Disease Incidence and Its Impact on Cluster Investigations*. Washington, DC: U.S. PRIG Education Fund. Available: http://www.environmentillinois.org/uploads/Mr/b9/Mrb9kyAamLXO5pZxi_5gHg/Health_Tracking_and_Disease_Clusters.pdf (Access date: December 6, 2006).
14. Nadakavukaren, A. (2006). *Our Global Environment: A Health Perspective*, 6th ed. Long Grove, IL: Waveland Press, Inc.
15. Cutler, J. J., Parker, G. S., Rosen, S., Prenney, B., Healy, R., and Caldwell, G. G. (1986). Childhood Leukemia in Woburn, Massachusetts. *Public Health Reports* 101 (2): 201–205.
16. Durant, J. L., Chen, J., Hemond, H. F., and Thilly, W. G. (1995). Elevated Incidence of Childhood Leukemia in Woburn, Massachusetts: NIEHS Superfund Basic Research Program Searches for Causes. *Environmental Health Perspectives* 103 (Supplement 6): 93–98.
17. Neutra, R. R. (1990). Counterpoint from a Cluster Buster. *American Journal of Epidemiology* 132 (1): 1–8.

18. Kingsley, B. S., Schmeichel, K. L., and Rubin, C. H. (2007). An Update on Cancer Cluster Activities at the Centers for Disease Control and Prevention. *Environmental Health Perspectives* 115 (1): 165–171.

19. Oleckno, W. A. (1995). Guidelines for Improving Risk Communication in Environmental Health. *Journal of Environmental Health* 58 (1): 20–23.

20. Johns Hopkins Center for Excellence in Environmental Public Health Tracking (2006). State Capacity to Address Non-Communicable Disease Clusters. Available: http://www.jhsph.edu/ephtcenter/Clusters%20Results%20Powerpoint.pdf (Access date: December 12, 2006).

21. New Zealand Ministry of Health (1997). *Investigating Clusters of Non-communicable Disease: Guidelines for Public Health Services*. Wellington: Ministry of Health (Manatu Hauora). Available: http://www.moh.govt.nz/moh.nsf (Access date: December 6, 2006).

22. Thacker, S. B., and Berkelman, R. L. (1988). Public Health Surveillance in the United States. *Epidemiologic Reviews* 10: 164–190.

23. Centers for Disease Control and Prevention (2006). Public Health Surveillance Slide Set. Available: http://www.cdc.gov/epo/dphsi/phs/overview.htm (Access date: December 9, 2006).

24. Rutherford, G. W. (2001). Principles and Practices of Public Health Surveillance, Second Edition. *American Journal of Epidemiology* 154 (4): 385–386. (Book Review of Teutsch S. M., and Churchill R. E., eds. (2000). *Principles and Practices of Public Health Surveillance*. 2nd ed. New York: Oxford University Press.)

25. Akinbami, L. (2006). The State of Childhood Asthma, United States, 1980–2005. *Advance Data from Vital and Health Statistics*, No. 381. Hyattsville, MD: National Center for Health Statistics.

26. World Health Organization (2006). Public Health Surveillance. Available: http://www.who.int/immunization_monitoring/burden/routine_surveillance/en/index.html (Access date: December 9, 2006).

27. Northwest Center for Public Health Practice (2006). Introduction to Public Health Surveillance. Available: http://www.nwcphp.org/training/courses-exercises/courses/introduction-to-public-health-surveillance (Access date: December 9, 2006).

28. United States Department of Agriculture, Food Safety and Inspection Service (1998). Foodborne Diseases Active Surveillance Network (FoodNet). Available: http://www.fsis.usda.gov/OA/background/bfoodnet.htm (Access date: December 9, 2006).

29. National Institute of Occupational Safety and Health (1999). NIOSH Report of Activities for Fiscal Year 1997. DHHS (NIOSH) Publication No. 99–116. Available: http://www.cdc.gov/niosh/pdfs/99–116.pdf (Access date: December 14, 2006).

30. Centers for Disease Control and Prevention Working Group (2004). Framework for Evaluating Public Health Surveillance Systems for Early Detection of Outbreaks. *Morbidity and Mortality Weekly Report* 53 (RR-05): 1–11. Available: http://www.cdc.gov/MMWR/preview/mmwrhtml/rr5305a1.htm (Access date: December 14, 2006).

31. Stoto, M. A. (2005). Syndromic Surveillance. *Issues in Science and Technology*. Available: http://www.issues.org/21.3/index.html (Access date: December 14, 2006).

32. Henning, K. J. (2004). Overview of Syndromic Surveillance, What is Syndromic Surveillance? *Morbidity and Mortality Weekly Report* 53 (Supplement): 5–11.

33. Mostashari, F., and Hartman, J. (2003). Syndromic Surveillance: A Local Perspective. *Journal of Urban Health* 80 (2, Supplement 1): i1–i7.

34. RAND Center for Domestic and International Health Security (2004). Syndromic Surveillance: An Effective Tool for Detecting Bioterrorism? *Research Highlights*. Santa Monica, CA: RAND Corporation.

35. Centers for Disease Control and Prevention (2006). National Notifiable Diseases Surveillance System: History. Available: http://www.cdc.gov/epo/dphsi/nndsshis.htm (Access date: December 15, 2006).

36. Centers for Disease Control and Prevention, National Center for Chronic Disease Prevention and Health Promotion (2006). Behavioral Risk Factor Surveillance System, BRFSS: Turning Information into Health. Available: http://www.cdc.gov/brfss/ (Access date: December 18, 2006).

37. Consumer Product Safety Commission (No date). National Electronic Injury Surveillance System, CPSC Document #3002. Available: http://www.cpsc.gov/cpscpub/pubs/3002.html (Access date: December 18, 2006).

38. Centers for Disease Control and Prevention (2006). EARS: Early Aberration Reporting System. Available: http://www.bt.cdc.gov/surveillance/ears/ (Access date: December 18, 2006).
39. Centers for Disease Control and Prevention (No date). An Overview of the NEDSS Initiative. Available: http://www.cdc.gov/nedss/About/overview.html (Access date: December 18, 2006).
40. Centers for Disease Control and Prevention (No date). National Electronic Disease Surveillance System. Available: http://www.cdc.gov/nedss (Access date: December 18, 2006).
41. U.S. Department of Health and Human Services, Centers for Disease Control and Prevention, National Center for Health Statistics (1999). *National Center for Health Statistics . . . Monitoring the Nation's Health: Programs and Activities.* DHHS Publication No. (PHS) 99–1200. Hyattsville, MD: The Centers.
42. German, R. R. et al. (2001). Updated Guidelines for Evaluating Public Health Surveillance Systems: Recommendations from the Guidelines Working Group. *Morbidity and Mortality Weekly Report* 50 (RR-13): 1–35.

Practical Resources in Epidemiology

FREE STATISTICAL SOFTWARE

OpenEpi

OpenEpi provides free statistical tools for calculating common epidemiologic measures. These can be used at the OpenEpi Web site or can be downloaded for use on a personal computer.

According to its developers, "OpenEpi provides statistics for counts and person-time rates in descriptive and analytic studies, stratified analysis with exact confidence limits, matched pair analysis, sample size calculations, random numbers, chi-square for dose-response trend, sensitivity, specificity and other evaluation statistics, R x C tables, and links to other useful sites."

URL: http://www.OpenEpi.com

Epi Info

Epi Info was developed by the Centers for Disease Control and Prevention (CDC) and can be used to conduct disease outbreak investigations, manage databases for public health surveillance, and perform statistical calculations. With Epi Info users can quickly develop study questionnaires, design specific databases, and analyze data. Epi Map, a feature of Epi Info, allows one to displays maps based on data entered into Epi Info. Other related features are also available. The latest version can be downloaded for use on a personal computer.

URL: http://www.cdc.gov/EpiInfo

Other Statistical Software

There is a wide variety of free statistical software available on the World Wide Web. For example, check out the following site, which provides links to various statistical packages and other statistical tools.

URL: http://statpages.org/javasta2.html

MAJOR JOURNALS IN EPIDEMIOLOGY (ENGLISH LANGUAGE)

In addition to the journals listed here, there are many journals in public health and medicine that also publish epidemiologic studies.

American Journal of Epidemiology
Annals of Epidemiology
Cancer Epidemiology Biomarkers
  and Prevention
Community Dentistry and Oral
  Epidemiology
Controlled Clinical Trials
Emerging Infectious Diseases
Emerging Themes in Epidemiology
Epidemiologic Perspectives and
  Innovations
Epidemiologic Reviews
Epidemiology
Epidemiology and Infection

European Journal of Epidemiology
Genetic Epidemiology
Infection Control and Hospital
  Epidemiology
International Journal of Epidemiology
Journal of Clinical Epidemiology
Journal of Epidemiology and
  Community Health
Journal of Pharmacoepidemiology
Ophthalmic Epidemiology
Paediatric and Perinatal Epidemiology
Pharmacoepidemiology and Drug Safety
Social Psychiatry and Psychiatric
  Epidemiology

OTHER USEFUL PUBLICATIONS

The Epidemiology Monitor

This is a lively and useful newsletter about events and resources in epidemiology. It is available by subscription but portions are available free at the Web site, including a feature referred to as EpiMonday.
URL: http://www.epimonitor.net

Morbidity and Mortality Weekly Report

This is a weekly publication of the Centers for Disease Control and Prevention providing provisional data on morbidity and mortality, reports of disease outbreak investigations, public health recommendations and announcements, and other articles on other topics of epidemiologic interest.
URL: http://www.cdc.gov/mmwr

Weekly Epidemiological Record

This is a weekly publication of the World Health Organization providing information, announcements, and reports on communicable diseases.
URL: http://www.who.int/wer/en

Eurosurveillance

This is a weekly and monthly online journal of the European Centre for Disease Prevention and Control that publishes reports and analyses related to epidemiology, surveillance, and prevention and control of communicable diseases. There is also a quarterly print edition containing material from the weekly and monthly editions.
URL: http://www.eurosurveillance.org/index-02.asp

COMPREHENSIVE INFORMATION ON EPIDEMIOLOGY

Supercourse: Epidemiology, the Internet and Global Health

The Supercourse is an evolving collection of free PowerPoint lectures on topics related to epidemiology and public health. According to the Web site, there are over 3,000 lectures in over 26 languages.

URL: http://www.pitt.edu/~super1

The WWW Virtual Library: Medicine and Health: Epidemiology

This resource site, which is maintained by the Department of Epidemiology and Biostatistics at the University of California, San Francisco, contains links to links to U.S. and international organizations concerned with aspects of epidemiology as well as a host of other resource links of interest to epidemiologists.

URL: http://www.epibiostat.ucsf.edu/epidem/epidem.html

Surveys and Data Systems
National Center for Health Statistics

Name	Data Source/Methods	Selected Applications of the Data Produced	Planned Sample	Planned Periodicity
Vital Statistics Cooperative Program (VSCP)	• State vital registration • Linked Birth/Infant Death Program • Matched multiple data sets	• Life expectancy • Causes of death • Infant mortality • Prenatal care and birth weight • Birth rates • Non-marital births • Pregnancy outcomes • Occupational mortality • Teenage pregnancy • Method of delivery • Preterm delivery • Multiple births • Perinatal mortality • Maternal smoking	• All births (4 million records annually) • All deaths (about 2.4 million records annually) • Reported fetal deaths of 20+ weeks gestation (about 30,000 annually) • Counts of marriages and divorces	Annual
National Health and Nutrition Examination Survey (NHANES)	• Personal interview • Physical examination • Laboratory tests • Nutritional assessment • DNA repository	• Total prevalence of disease or conditions including those unrecognized or undetected • Nutrition monitoring • Heart disease • Diabetes • Osteoporosis • Iron deficiency anemia and other nutritional disorders • Environmental exposures monitoring • Children's growth and development • Infectious disease monitoring • Overweight/physical fitness	• Approximately 5,000 persons per year, all ages • Oversample adolescents • Oversample 60+ years • Oversample Blacks and Mexican Americans • Pregnant women	Annual with capability for longitudinal follow up

Name	Data Source/Methods	Selected Applications of the Data Produced	Planned Sample	Planned Periodicity
National Health Interview Survey (NHIS)	• Personal interviews	Annual data on: • Health status and limitations • Utilization of health care • Injuries • Family resources • Health insurance • Access to care • Selected conditions • Health behaviors • Functioning • HIV/AIDS testing • Immunization	• Approximately 40,000 households • Oversample Blacks and Hispanics	Annual
National Hospital Discharge Survey (NHDS)	• Hospital records • Computerized data sources	• Patient characteristics • Hospital characteristics • Length of stay • Diagnosis and multiple diagnoses • Surgical and diagnostic procedures	• 500 hospitals • 300,000 discharges	Annual
National Ambulatory Medical Care Survey (NAMCS)	• Encounter forms completed by physicians practicing in private offices • Physician-level personal interviews	• Characteristics of patients' visits • Diagnoses and treatment • Prescribing patterns • Characteristics of practice	• 3,000 physicians in office-based practices • 25,000 patient visits	Annual
National Hospital Ambulatory Medical Care Survey (NHAMCS)	• Encounter forms completed by physicians and other hospital staff • Facility and personal interviews	• Characteristics of patients' visits to hospital outpatient departments and emergency departments • Diagnoses and treatment • Prescribing patterns • Characteristics of facility	• 600 hospitals • 70,000 patient visits	Annual

Name	Data Source/Methods	Selected Applications of the Data Produced	Planned Sample	Planned Periodicity
National Survey of Family Growth (NSFG)	• Personal interviews	• Contraception and sterilization • Teenage sexual activity and pregnancy • Family planning and unintended pregnancy • Adoption • Breastfeeding • Infertility • Marriage, divorce, and cohabitation	• 12,500 men and women • Oversample Blacks, Hispanics, and teens	Periodic, transition to continuous
National Immunization Survey (NIS) (in partnership with CDC/NIP)	• Telephone interviews • Provider record check component • Weighting adjustment for non-telephone households	• Evaluation of immunization status of preschool population (NIS) • Demographic characteristics • Family resource data • Health care utilization	• 900,000 households screened to find NIS sample of households, with children 19–35 months • 400 completed NIS interviews in each of 78 non-overlapping areas • Option allows for additional data collection on other topics from the households screened for the NIS sample	Continuous with quarterly 12 month moving averages

Name	Data Source/Methods	Selected Applications of the Data Produced	Planned Sample	Planned Periodicity
National Survey of Children with Special Health Care Needs	• Conducted using the State and Local Area Integrated Telephone Survey (SLAITS) mechanism • Telephone interviews • Statistical adjustments for households without telephones • Utilizes NIS sample frame • Sponsored and funded by Maternal and Child Health Bureau, HRSA • Additional funding by OASPE	• Children with special health care needs • Health care utilization and barriers • Performance partnership initiatives • Health insurance coverage • State Children's Health Insurance Program (SCHIP) attitudes and experience • Characteristics of SCHIP eligible but unenrolled children	• State-based samples of children 0–17 years of age • All 50 states plus DC • Detailed interview for children identified with special needs • Detailed interview for low-income uninsured children	Periodic implementation (every 4 years)
National Asthma Survey	• Conducted using the SLAITS mechanism • Telephone interviews • Statistical adjustments for households without telephones • Utilizes NIS sample frame • Sponsored and funded by National Center for Environmental Health, CDC	• Asthma prevalence rates • Health care utilization and barriers • Asthma management and medication use	• State-based samples of adults and children • Four States and national sample in 2003	Unspecified periodic implementation in all 50 States subject to funding by sponsors

Name	Data Source/Methods	Selected Applications of the Data Produced	Planned Sample	Planned Periodicity
National Survey of Children's Health	• Conducted using the SLAITS mechanism • Telephone interviews • Statistical adjustments for households without telephones • Utilizes NIS sample frame • Sponsored and funded by the Maternal and Child Health Bureau, HRSA	• Physical, emotional, and dental health • Health insurance coverage • Health care utilization and barriers • Medical home • Child, family, and neighborhood well-being • Children with special health care needs • Performance partnership initiatives	• State-based samples of children 0–17 years of age • All 50 States plus DC	Periodic implementation (every 4 years) subject to funding by sponsors
National Home and Hospice Care Survey (NHHCS)	• Home health agencies and hospices • Interviews with administrators and staff familiar with agency/medical records	• Characteristics of home health agencies and hospices • Number and characteristics of patients and discharges • Medical diagnoses and functional status	• 1,800 home health agencies and hospices • 10,800 current patients • 10,800 discharged patients	Bi-annual (Last conducted in 2000)
National Survey of Early Childhood Health	• Conducted using the SLAITS mechanism • Telephone interviews • Statistical adjustments for households without telephones • Utilizes NIS sample frame • Sponsored by American Academy of Pediatrics (AAP) • Funded by Gerber Foundation, Maternal and Child Health Bureau, and AAP	• Parents' perceptions of the quality of pediatric care • Content of anticipatory guidance • Health care utilization and barriers • Home safety measures • Health insurance coverage	• National sample of children 4–35 months of age • Oversample of Black non-Hispanic and Hispanic children	Unspecified periodic implementation subject to funding by sponsors

Name	Data Source/Methods	Selected Applications of the Data Produced	Planned Sample	Planned Periodicity
National Survey of Ambulatory Surgery (NSAS)	• Abstract forms completed by facility staff	• Patient characteristics • Diagnosis and multiple diagnoses • Surgical and diagnostic procedures	• 750 facilities • 120,000 surgery visits	Annual through 1996; periodic thereafter
National Health Interview Survey on Disability (NHIS-D)	• Personal interviews • Follow-up interviews	• Sensory, mobility, and communication impairments • Functional limitations • Personal assistance • Special education • Mental health conditions • Employment and transportation limitations • Therapeutic services • Children with special health needs • Post polio syndrome	• Phase 1 screens 90,000 households • Phase 2 is a follow up of those persons with moderate to severe disabilities • Phase 2: approximately 20,400 children and adults in 1994 and approximately 12,400 children and adults in 1995	Special 2-year study (1994–1995)
Second Supplement on Aging (SOAII)	• Personal interviews • Administrative match data; NDI cause-of-death and CMS Medicare files	• Functional status • Living arrangements • Use of hospitals and nursing homes • Death rates by social, economic, family, and health characteristics	• 9,447 persons age 70 and over at the time of Phase 2 of NHIS-D (1994–1996)	Cross-sectional survey, serves as a baseline to the LOSA II

Name	Data Source/Methods	Selected Applications of the Data Produced	Planned Sample	Planned Periodicity
Second Longitudinal Study of Aging (LSOA II)	• Telephone interviews • Administrative match data; NDI cause-of-death and CMS Medicare files	• Changes in functional status, chronic conditions, co-morbidity • Causes and consequences of change • Living arrangements, social support • Health care coverage and utilization • Death rates by social, economic, family, and health characteristics	• 9,447 persons age 70 and over at the time of Phase 2 of NHIS-D (1994–1996)	Baseline plus 2 follow-up waves, each at 2-year intervals
National Death Index (NDI)	• State registration-death certificates	• Facilitates epidemiological follow-up studies • Verification of death for individuals under study • Optional release of coded causes of death available to users upon request • Most NCHS surveys are linked to NDI	• All deaths	Annual
Joint Canada/United States Survey of Health (JCUSH)	• Same questionnaire administered by telephone in 2003 in both countries, in English or French in Canada, in English or Spanish in the United States	• Directly compare U.S. and Canadian estimates of health status, chronic conditions, utilization of health care services, etc.	• 5,200 U.S. adults • 3,500 Canadian adults	One time, in 2003

Name	Data Source/Methods	Selected Applications of the Data Produced	Planned Sample	Planned Periodicity
National Nursing Home Survey (NNHS)	• Long-term care providers • Interviews with facility administrators and staff familiar with facility/medical records	• Characteristics of nursing homes • Number and characteristics of residents and discharges • Medical diagnoses and functional status	• 1,500 nursing homes • 9,000 current residents • 9,000 discharges	Last conducted in 1999

Source: U.S. Department of Health and Human Services, Centers for Disease Control and Prevention (No date). Summary of Surveys and Data Systems, National Center for Health Statistics, June 2004. Available: http://www.cdc.gov/nchs/data/NCHS_Survey_Matrix.pdf (Access date: April 2, 2007).

Ten Common Health and Population Indices Used in Epidemiology

Ten Common Health and Population Indices Used in Epidemiology*

1. Crude Birth Rate	$\dfrac{\text{Number of live births during a specified time period}}{\text{Mid-interval population}}$	× 1,000
2. Fertility Rate	$\dfrac{\text{Number of live births during a specified time period}}{\text{Mid-interval population of women aged 15–44 years}}$	× 1,000
3. Crude Death Rate (CDR)	$\dfrac{\text{Number of deaths during a specified time period}}{\text{Mid-interval population}}$	× 1,000 (or 100,000)
4. Cause-specific Mortality Rate	$\dfrac{\text{Number of deaths from a specific cause during a specified time period}}{\text{Mid-interval population}}$	× 100,000
5. Proportionate Mortality Ratio (PMR)	$\dfrac{\text{Number of deaths from a specific cause during a specified time period}}{\text{Total number of deaths in the same time period}}$	× 100
6. Infant Mortality Rate	$\dfrac{\text{Number of deaths in infants aged 0–1 year during a specified time period}}{\text{Number of live births in the same time period}}$	× 1,000
7. Neonatal Mortality Rate	$\dfrac{\text{Number of deaths in infants aged less than 28 days during a specified time period}}{\text{Number of live births in the same time period}}$	× 1,000
8. Perinatal Mortality Rate	$\dfrac{\text{Number of fetal deaths after 28 weeks or more of gestation + Number of infant deaths within 7 days of birth during a specified time period}}{\text{Number of live births + Number of fetal deaths after 28 weeks or more of gestation}}$	× 1,000
9. Fetal Death Rate	$\dfrac{\text{Number of fetal deaths after 20 weeks or more of gestation during a specified time period}}{\text{Number of live births + Number of fetal deaths after 20 weeks or more of gestation}}$	× 1,000
10. Maternal Mortality Rate	$\dfrac{\text{Number of deaths due to childbirth during a specified time period}}{\text{Number of live births in the same time period}}$	× 100,000

*Most of these indices are routinely reported on a calendar basis. The population bases are those in most common use.

Glossary

A

a posteriori **comparison** An "after the fact" statistical comparison. The term generally refers to a comparison that is made after the study results are already available and for which no study hypothesis has been previously developed. Such a comparison is unplanned and may be biased.

a priori **hypothesis** A predetermined hypothesis, that is, one that is formulated before initiating an analytic or experimental epidemiologic study.

absolute risk A synonym for **risk**. Absolute risk is sometimes used to differentiate risk from relative risk.

accuracy (of a study) A measure of the degree to which a study is free from errors. The accuracy of a study has two major components—validity and precision. Also see **validity; precision.**

accuracy (validity measure) A synonym for **overall accuracy.**

accuracy of the test A synonym for **overall accuracy.**

active immunity A type of immunity that results when the body produces its own antibodies in reaction to an infection or a vaccine.

active surveillance Surveillance that requires the responsible health authority to obtain the desired health-related data directly from health care providers (e.g., physicians and hospitals) and laboratories. Also see **public health surveillance.**

active treatment In the context of randomized controlled trials, active treatment refers to the use of the standard regimen (e.g., the accepted or customary treatment or procedure) in the control arm of the trial.

actuarial method A synonym for **life table method.** This particular term derives from its historic use in determining life expectancy in the insurance industry.

additive effects In the assessment of effect measure modification or statistical interaction, additive effects are those based on an additive model. Also see **additive model.**

additive interaction Statistical interaction based on an additive model. Also see **additive model.**

additive model A mathematical model based on difference measures of association (e.g., risk differences). In an additive model the combined effect of two or more variables on an outcome is the sum of their separate effects.

adherence A synonym for **compliance.**

adjusted odds ratio A summary odds ratio that has been statistically modified to remove the effect of one or more confounding factors. A common type of adjusted odds ratio is the Mantel-Haenszel odds ratio (OR_{MH}). Also see **Mantel-Haenszel odds ratio.**

adjusted rate A summary or overall measure of occurrence that has been statistically modified to remove the effect of one or more confounding factors, such as age, sex, or race/ethnicity.

admission rate bias A form of selection bias that can result from the admission practices of health care facilities. This bias is most often exhibited in hospital-based case-control studies when cases admitted to the facility differ systematically from potential controls on factors other than diagnosis due to the facility's admission practices. A specific type of admission rate bias is Berkson's bias. Also see **Berkson's bias.**

age adjustment A statistical procedure that controls for differences in age distributions when comparing summary measures of occurrence between different populations. Age adjustment provides a way of making fair, unbiased comparisons between summary measures.

age standardization A synonym for **age adjustment**.

alpha level The chance of a type I error that an investigator is willing to take when testing a hypothesis. Alpha levels are commonly preset at 0.05 or sometimes 0.01. Also see **type I error; p-value**.

alternative hypothesis In hypothesis testing, the alternative hypothesis is the one that states an association exists. If the null hypothesis is rejected, the alternate hypothesis is accepted, and it is concluded that the hypothesized association is statistically significant. An alternative hypothesis may be either directional or non-directional. Also see **null hypothesis; directional hypothesis; non-directional hypothesis**.

ambidirectional cohort study A synonym for **mixed cohort study**.

ambispective cohort study A synonym for **mixed cohort study**.

analytic cross-sectional study A cross-sectional study that is designed to test one or more predetermined hypotheses about associations between exposure and outcome. This type of study is usually referred to simply as a cross-sectional study. It is distinguished from a descriptive cross-sectional study, however, by the presence of one or more *a priori* hypotheses. Also see **cross-sectional study**.

analytic ecological study An ecological study that is designed to test one or more predetermined hypotheses about associations between exposure and outcome. This type of study is usually referred to simply as an ecological study. It is distinguished from a descriptive ecological study, however, by the presence of one or more *a priori* hypotheses. Also see **ecological study**.

analytic epidemiology A facet of epidemiology concerned with uncovering the causes of morbidity and mortality using observational methods. Useful in identifying risk factors for disease and explaining disease patterns in a population. This aspect of epidemiology tests *a priori* hypotheses.

analytic study A type of observational epidemiologic study that tests one or more predetermined hypotheses about associations between exposure and outcome. Ecological studies, cross-sectional studies, case-control studies, prospective cohort studies, retrospective cohort studies, and certain hybrid studies may be considered analytic studies when there are *a priori* hypotheses to test.

antagonism Based on a causal model, antagonism occurs when two or more factors acting together in a population result in a smaller frequency of outcomes than would be expected if the factors operated independently. In other words, the combined effects of the factors are less than the sum of the individual effects. Phenobarbital use and occupational exposure to benzopyrene, for example, act in an antagonistic manner.

antecedent cause of death On a death certificate, any disease or condition that led to the immediate cause of death. Also see **immediate cause of death**.

antibody A protein substance or globulin derived from B and T lymphocytes that is formed as a defensive response to a specific antigen.

antigen A foreign substance, such as an infectious organism, that stimulates antibody production when it enters the body.

arm A term commonly used in experimental trials to describe either the experimental or control group. For example, the control arm in a randomized controlled trial refers to the control group, while the experimental arm refers to the experimental group. Experimental trials with multiple experimental or control groups have many arms. A two-arm trial, however, has only one experimental and one control group.

association See **statistical association**.

attack rate Cumulative incidence applied to a narrowly but well-defined population being observed over a limited time period such as during a disease outbreak.

attack rate difference The difference between the attack rate in the exposed group and the attack rate in the unexposed group. This is a type of cumulative incidence difference or risk difference using attack rates. Also see **attributable risk**.

attack rate ratio The ratio of the attack rate in the exposed group to the attack rate in the unexposed group. This is a type of cumulative incidence ratio or risk ratio using attack rates.

attack rate table A table containing attack rates among individuals exposed and unexposed to potential causes of a disease outbreak. Attack rate tables typically are used in retrospective cohort analyses of disease outbreaks where several exposures are examined simultaneously. They help in identifying the potential cause of the outbreak.

attributable fraction among the exposed An epidemiologic measure that indicates the proportion of the risk of a given outcome among the exposed group that is attributable to the exposure of interest. The measure, which is often stated as a percentage, is based on the assumption that the exposure is causative. It provides an indication of the impact of the exposure; that is, it indicates the proportion of outcomes that might be reduced in the exposed group if the exposure were to be eliminated.

attributable risk The risk difference calculated using attack rates. Also see **risk difference**.

B

baseline data Data collected at the beginning of a study. These data may be compared to data collected during or after the study to assess, for example, the impact of an intervention.

Bayes' theorem A proposition in probability theory that is commonly used in clinical epidemiology to estimate the probability of a specific diagnosis based on a screening test result.

before and after studies A category of quasi-experimental studies that involve measurements and comparisons of the study outcomes before and after the intervention. Two common types of before and after studies are the one-group pretest-posttest design and the nonequivalent control group design. Also see **one-group pretest-posttest design; nonequivalent control group design**.

behavioral epidemiology A specialization in epidemiology involving the study of the role of behavioral factors in health, disease, or death in human populations. Typical factors examined include substance use, activity levels, dietary choices, and sexual practices.

Behavioral Risk Factor Surveillance System This surveillance system, which is conducted by state and territorial health departments in the United States, involves ongoing telephone surveys that track health conditions and risk behaviors on an annual basis. The system is supported by the Centers for Disease Control and Prevention and provides state-specific information about issues such as asthma, diabetes, health care access, alcohol use, hypertension, obesity, cancer screening, nutrition and physical activity, tobacco use, and other health-related issues.

Berkson's bias A type of selection bias, named after Dr. Joseph Berkson, that can, for example, occur in hospital-based case-control studies when the combination of the study exposure and outcome increases the chance that exposed cases will be admitted to the hospital. This can result in an artificially higher rate of exposure among hospitalized cases than controls. Also see **admission rate bias**.

beta level The chance of making a type II error when testing a hypothesis. Also see **type II error**.

bias A type of systematic (nonrandom) error in the design or conduct of a study that can lead to erroneous results. In epidemiologic studies bias can cause overestimation of the measure of association or effect (positive bias) or underestimation of the measure of association or effect (negative bias). The two major categories of bias are selection bias and information bias.

bias effect In the context of screening tests, a bias effect is the difference in the extent to which observers disagree on the proportion of positive or negative test results. It tends to increase the value of kappa, which is a measure of observer reliability. Also see **kappa**.

Bills of Mortality A phrase used for the weekly and annual recording of births and deaths in England in the sixteenth and seventeenth centuries. John Graunt used the Bills of Mortality in a 1662 landmark publication that is now considered the forerunner of modern vital statistics.

biological interaction A real effect that represents the combined involvement of two or more factors in disease causation. Both synergism and antagonism are examples of biological interaction. Also see **synergism; antagonism**.

biological plausibility One of several guidelines for evaluating whether an association is likely to be causal or not based on Hill's postulates. In general, plausible associations are more likely to be causal. Biological plausibility focuses on whether or not the association makes biological sense given what is known about the exposure and outcome. For example, the association between cigarette smoking and lung cancer is biologically plausible since we know that cigarette smoke contains numerous chemicals that can harm lung tissue and cellular components.

biomarker A cellular or molecular indicator of exposure to an environmental agent, such as elevated liver enzymes or the presence of toxic residues in the blood, urine, hair, or other body specimens.

blinding A procedure that conceals certain information so as to avoid bias in a study. In analytic and experimental epidemiologic studies blinding keeps the investigators or subjects unaware of subject classifications with regard to exposure or outcome status. The purpose is to minimize the bias that can result from knowing how the subjects are classified by exposure or outcome. Also see **single-blinded study; double-blinded study; triple-blinded study**.

block randomization A randomization technique that effectively assures equal numbers of subjects in the experimental and control arms of a randomized controlled trial. During the recruitment period, subjects are divided into small blocks or groupings of equal size as they enter the trial. Within each block the subjects are then randomly assigned to the experimental or control groups in such a way that equal numbers are assigned to each group. Block randomization thus assures perfect balance in the number of subjects in each study group as long as complete blocks of subjects are assigned.

bubonic plague See **plague**.

C

cancer cluster The occurrence of a greater than expected number of cases of cancer within a group of people, a geographic area, or a period of time. The cancers are generally of the same type and the distribution is believed not to be due to chance alone. Also see **disease cluster**.

carrier An individual who has no overt signs or symptoms of a communicable disease but nevertheless harbors the causative agent, which can be transmitted to others. For example, Typhoid Mary was a carrier of typhoid fever, which she unwittingly transmitted to others.

carryover effects The residual effects of an intervention that can occur in a crossover design during the period after the intervention has been completed. A common method of dealing with carryover effects is to introduce a washout period. Also see **washout period**.

case fatality The proportion of cases of a given disease that die from the disease in a specified time period. Case fatality, which is often stated as a percent, is both an indicator of the seriousness of a disease as well as a measure of prognosis for those with the disease.

case fatality rate A synonym for **case fatality**.

case fatality ratio A synonym for **case fatality**.

case finding A synonym for **opportunistic screening**.

case report A type of descriptive study that presents a detailed description of an individual patient in order to characterize and understand a specific disease or syndrome. This type of study is common in clinical epidemiology, although in the strictest sense it is not an epidemiologic study per se.

case series A type of descriptive study that is an extension of the case report. It describes the characteristics of a group or cluster of individuals with the same disease or symptoms in an attempt to quantify various aspects of the group and thus present a relatively complete profile of the illness. Technically, a case series is not an epidemiologic study per se, although it is commonly used in clinical epidemiology and can suggest hypotheses about causation that can lead to further study.

case-base sampling A type of sampling ordinarily used in case-cohort studies where controls are randomly selected from the subjects in the source population who are free of the study outcome at the beginning of the study period.

case-cohort study A type of hybrid or case-control study that represents a variation of the nested case-control study. A distinguishing feature of this design is that the controls are selected randomly from all members of the cohort, typically at the beginning of the study.

case-control study A type of observational epidemiologic study in which the subjects are selected according to outcome status before exposure status is determined. Cases (those with the disorder) and controls (those without the disorder) are compared with regard to exposure history.

case-crossover study A variation of the case-control study design in which only cases are used. The cases, however, serve as their own controls. Therefore, this is not a case series.

causal association An association between an exposure and outcome such that a change in the frequency of the exposure in a population results in a change in the frequency of the outcome. It is important to recognize that causal associations in epidemiology are population phenomena. Thus, a change in exposure frequency does not mean that every exposed individual in the population develops the outcome but only that the frequency of the outcome changes in the population. A causal association may also be thought of as a statistical association that cannot be readily explained by bias, confounding, or random error and where the purported cause precedes the effect.

causal pie model A causal model conceptualized by Kenneth J. Rothman. Basically, the model purports that outcomes are caused by different combinations of component causes, which may be likened to pieces or slices of a complete pie.

cause See **causal association**. Also see **necessary cause; sufficient cause**.

cause-specific mortality rate A measure of the risk of death due to a specific cause, such as the breast cancer mortality rate. It is sometimes referred to as the disease-specific mortality rate.

censored observations In the context of survival analysis, censored observations represent data on individual subjects who have not yet developed the study outcome. Basically, the data on survival time (time to the study outcome) is incomplete. This is usually due to deaths from other causes, losses to follow up, or early termination of the study (i.e., prior to observing the outcome).

chain of infection The process involved in the transmission of communicable diseases. This process entails six components that include the infectious agent, the reservoir, the portal of exit, the mode of transmission, the portal of entry, and the susceptible host.

chi-square test A test of statistical significance commonly used to test the null hypothesis that two nominal variables (e.g., exposure and outcome status) are independent or not associated by comparing observed and expected frequencies in a contingency table.

clinical diversity A synonym for **clinical heterogeneity**.

clinical epidemiology The application of epidemiologic principles and methods to clinical decision making, such as diagnosis, prognosis, and treatment of disease. Clinical epidemiology is patient oriented, while classical epidemiology is population oriented.

clinical heterogeneity Differences between the component studies of a meta-analysis in terms of variations in the study interventions, outcomes, or subjects.

clinical significance A level of statistical significance that is meaningful from a public health or clinical point of view. Also known as practical significance.

clinical trial An experimental trial involving human subjects, usually in a clinical setting. Unlike a randomized controlled trial, a clinical trial does not always involve randomization of subjects into study groups. Clinical trials are commonly used in testing new drugs prior to marketing.

closed cohort study A cohort study in which no one can be added to the study once follow up begins. Conceptually, all subjects in a closed cohort study not developing the study outcome have the same length of follow up, which is the maximum observation time.

cluster randomized trial A synonym for **group randomized trial**.

clustering effect In the context of group randomized trials, the clustering effect is the tendency for individuals in a group to be similar to each other. This dependency has important implications for the analysis of group randomized trials where the units of inference are individuals, and analyses that do not account for the clustering effect will tend to overstate the significance of the findings.

Cochrane Collaboration An international organization established to ensure that up-to-date, accurate information about the effects of health care interventions is readily available worldwide. The Collaboration prepares, maintains, and disseminates qualitative and quantitative systematic reviews of the effects of health care interventions that are easily accessible.

coefficient of determination In simple linear regression, the coefficient of determination is the proportion of the variance in the dependent variable (i.e., the study outcome) that is explained by the independent variable (i.e., the study exposure). It is measured by the square of the correlation coefficient (r^2) and gives an indication of the magnitude of the effect of the exposure on the outcome. When there are multiple independent variables, as in multiple linear regression, the coefficient of determination is the proportion of the variance in the dependent variable that is explained by all the independent variables considered simultaneously. Here it is measured by the square of the multiple correlation coefficient (R^2).

Cohen's kappa See **kappa**.

cohort A designated group of individuals who are followed over time such as in a cohort study or randomized controlled trial.

cohort design (for GRTs) A sampling design in group randomized trials involving follow up in which the same individuals are sampled each time outcome measurements are to be made. This design is most appropriate when the objective is to measure the effects of the intervention on the individuals within the study population. Also see **repeated cross-sectional design** (for GRTs).

cohort study An observational epidemiologic study in which members of the study population are classified by exposure status and then followed over time to determine outcome status in the exposure groups. Cohort studies may be prospective, retrospective, or mixed. Also see **prospective cohort study; retrospective cohort study; mixed cohort study**.

common source outbreak A disease outbreak that results from the exposure of a susceptible group of people to a common agent of disease (e.g., pathogenic organism, toxic substance). Also see **point source outbreak; continuing source outbreak; intermittent source outbreak**.

communicable disease A disease that can be transmitted directly or indirectly to a susceptible person through contact, inhalation, or ingestion. Also known as an infectious disease.

community trial A synonym for a **group randomized trial**.

competing risks Causes that remove a subject from further observation in an epidemiologic study. For example, in a prospective cohort study of the effect of smokeless tobacco on the development of oral cancer, subjects who die from unrelated causes, such as heart disease and stroke, are said to have died from competing risks. In this example, heart disease and stroke are the competing risks, and the deceased subjects are no longer at risk of the study outcome.

completely randomized design Random allocation in which the units of assignment (individuals or groups) are made without any pre-stratification, blocking, or matching. In a randomized controlled trial this is also commonly known as simple randomization. Completely randomized designs work best when the number of units of assignment are large. Also see **simple randomization**.

compliance Subject conformity with the study protocol in an epidemiologic study, especially in regard to randomized controlled trials. Also see **noncompliance**.

component causes In reference to the causal pie model described by Kenneth J. Rothman, component causes are factors that work in combination to cause a particular outcome. A pie symbolizes a sufficient cause of the outcome, while the pieces of the pie symbolize the necessary causes. Without all the pieces of the pie, the pie cannot cause the outcome. Also see **causal pie model**.

concordant pairs In the context of analyzing a case-control study where pair matching is used, concordant pairs are those case-control pairs where exposure status is the same between cases and controls. In this situation, the calculation of the matched-pairs odds ratio depends on ignoring the concordant pairs in the analysis. Also see **discordant pairs**.

concurrent cohort study A synonym for **prospective cohort study**.

conditional logistic regression A method of multivariable analysis commonly used in the analysis of matched case-control studies. In fact, it is the standard multiple logistic regression procedure applied when analyzing matched case-control studies.

confidence interval The probable range in which the true value of a measure lies based on sample data. The most commonly reported confidence interval in epidemiology is the 95% confidence interval. For example, if the 95% confidence interval for a sample risk ratio is 2.0 to 4.0, one can be 95% confident that the true value lies within this range of values. It would only be expected to lie outside this range five percent of the time.

confidence level The level of certainty that the true value of a measure lies within a stated confidence interval. For example, for a 95% confidence interval, the level of certainty (or confidence level) is 95%. For a 90% confidence interval, the confidence level is 90%.

confidence limits The minimum and maximum values of the range represented by a confidence interval. These limits are also referred to as the lower and upper confidence limits, respectively. For example, a 95% confidence interval of 2.0 and 4.0, usually designated as 95% CI = 2.0 to 4.0, has a lower confidence limit of 2.0 and an upper confidence limit of 4.0.

confounder A synonym for **confounding factor**.

confounding A distortion in the magnitude of the true effect of a study exposure on a study outcome due to a mixing of effects between the exposure and an extraneous factor. Confounding is a nuisance that needs to be controlled so as to provide a more accurate representation of the real effect of the exposure on the outcome.

confounding factor An extraneous factor that distorts the magnitude of the effect of a study exposure on a study outcome. Also see **confounding**.

consistency of the association One of several guidelines for evaluating whether an association is likely to be causal or not based on Hill's postulates. An association is said to be consistent, and hence more likely to be causal, when multiple investigators studying the relationship in different populations, at different times, in different places, and using different methodologies obtain similar results.

construct validity The degree to which a variable accurately measures the theoretical phenomenon of interest.

contamination In the context of experimental trials, contamination represents crossovers from the control group to the experimental group. This may happen, for example, when some individuals randomly assigned to the conventional treatment seek out the experimental treatment instead. Contamination tends to reduce the chances of finding differences between the experimental and control groups. In general, contamination is more of a problem in randomized controlled trials than in group randomized trials.

contextual effects The influence of the social or environmental setting on individual risk of health-related outcomes. For example, one might estimate the contextual effects of living in an area where illegal drug trafficking is rampant on the risk of adolescent mortality, controlling for individual drug use.

continuing source outbreak A type of common source outbreak where the exposure to the common agent of disease is prolonged beyond a brief period, and the exposure is not simultaneous among all those exposed. Continuing source outbreaks are expected to last longer than the time range of the incubation period of the disease because the exposure period is protracted, and not all are exposed at the same time.

contributory cause A causative factor that is neither necessary nor sufficient to cause disease. For example, a sedentary lifestyle is a contributory cause of coronary heart disease. Most causes of chronic diseases are contributory causes. Also see **not necessary and not sufficient cause**.

convenience sample A sample of study subjects selected for expedience. Convenience samples are usually chosen because they are readily available. They may be biased, however, and not representative of the population from which they were selected.

correct temporal sequence One of several guidelines for evaluating whether an association is likely to be causal or not based on Hill's postulates. This one states that in order for an exposure to be considered causal it must precede the outcome. Of all the guidelines used to judge whether or not an association is likely to be causal, this is the only one that is considered essential.

count A measure of occurrence that merely represents the number of occurrences of a given exposure or outcome. For example, in saying that there were 14 reported cases of West Nile disease in Illinois during June, one is reporting a count of the number of cases of the disease.

covariate A variable that is possibly predictive of a study outcome such as a confounding factor or an effect modifier.

Cox proportional hazards model A multiple regression technique used in survival analysis that is appropriate when the study outcome represents time-to-event versus the occurrence of an event. Specifically, the Cox proportional hazards model predicts the time to the study outcome for each subject in the study, while controlling for differences in time under observation and differences in subject characteristics. It can be used to assess confounding and interaction.

critical point In the context of screening, the critical point is the point in the natural history of a disorder before which treatment is more effective than if applied later. The critical point must be sometime during the detectable preclinical phase in order for screening to be useful. For cancer, the critical point is the point of metastasis.

critical value The value that a test statistic must equal or exceed to be considered statistically significant at a given alpha level.

cross-level bias Bias introduced by inappropriate inferences from the group to the individual level and vice versa. For example, an ecological fallacy could introduce a cross-level bias.

crossover design A variation of the standard randomized controlled trial in which the intervention is applied at different times to each subject. In the most basic application, the study population is randomized into an experimental and control group and after a specified time period the original experimental group becomes the control group, and the original control group becomes the experimental group. This type of design may also be applied to group randomized trials.

crossovers Subjects in the experimental arm of a randomized controlled trial who do not complete the assigned intervention or subjects in the control arm who seek the intervention or another active treatment or procedure. Crossovers are noncompliant with the study protocol and can cause investigators to come to erroneous conclusions about the efficacy or effectiveness of an intervention.

cross-product ratio A synonym for **odds ratio** in the context of a case-control study.

cross-sectional study An observational epidemiologic study in which exposure and outcome status are assessed simultaneously, that is, at the same point in time or during a brief period of time. Cross-sectional studies can be either descriptive (exploratory) or analytic depending on whether or not predetermined hypotheses are being tested.

crude birth rate The proportion of live births occurring in a defined population during a specified time period. The crude birth rate is a good indicator of population growth.

crude death rate A measure of the risk of death from all causes in a defined population during a specified time period.

crude odds ratio The overall odds ratio without regard to specific classification variables, such as age, sex, or race/ethnicity.

crude prevalence The overall prevalence of the outcome in a study population without regard to exposure status or vice versa.

crude rate An overall (summary) measure of occurrence for a defined population. A common example is the crude death rate.

cumulative incidence The proportion of the population at risk that develops a given outcome in a given period of time. In a cohort study, for example, cumulative incidence measures a subject's average risk of developing the study outcome during the follow-up period. This assumes all subjects begin the study at the same time and follow up is complete for all subjects.

cumulative incidence difference A type of risk difference where the measures of occurrence are cumulative incidence. Specifically, it is the difference between the cumulative incidence for a given outcome among the exposed group and the cumulative incidence for the outcome among the unexposed group.

cumulative incidence rate A synonym for **cumulative incidence**.

cumulative incidence ratio A type of risk ratio where the measures of occurrence are cumulative incidence. Specifically, it is the ratio of the cumulative incidence for a given outcome among the exposed group to the cumulative incidence for the outcome among the unexposed group.

cumulative incidence sampling A method of sampling controls in a case-control study which normally involves selecting the controls from subjects in the source population who are free of the study outcome at the end of the study period.

cumulative meta-analysis A type of meta-analysis that involves repeating a meta-analysis each time a new study meeting the eligibility criteria has been conducted. Rather than being static, this type of meta-analysis is ongoing and therefore always current. In a forest plot of a cumulative meta-analysis each entry represents cumulated data versus data from each component study.

cyclic pattern Periodic, often predictable, increases in the frequency of a particular cause of morbidity or mortality in a specified population. For example, there is a predictable seasonal variation in the frequency of influenza, which peaks in the late fall and winter months.

D

data and safety monitoring board A synonym for **data monitoring committee**.

data and safety monitoring committee A synonym for **data monitoring committee**.

data monitoring committee A committee consisting of various outside experts who regularly review the accumulated data in a sequential trial in order to determine if the trial should be stopped or modified in some way based on interim findings. Also see **stopping rules**.

Declaration of Helsinki A highly regarded and widely adopted policy statement of the World Medical Association that enumerates principles for the ethical practice of medical research involving human subjects. The Declaration is updated periodically.

defined population The population of interest. For example, in a study of breast cancer among adult women, the defined population is adult women. A defined population may be as broad or as narrow as one chooses to define it.

density sampling A synonym for **incidence density sampling**.

density-based sampling A synonym for **incidence density sampling**.

dependent variable The outcome variable in a study (e.g., outcome status). It is dependent on the effect of one or more independent variables. Also see **independent variable**.

descriptive cohort study A cohort study that does not test predetermined hypotheses about associations between exposures and outcomes. Descriptive cohort studies are often used to describe the incidence of one or more outcomes of interest. They may also suggest hypotheses for further study.

descriptive cross-sectional study A cross-sectional study that does not test predetermined hypotheses about associations between exposures and outcomes. This type of study is usually referred to simply as a cross-sectional study. It is distinguished from an analytic cross-sectional study, however, by the absence of one or more *a priori* hypotheses. Also see **cross-sectional study**.

descriptive ecological study An ecological study that does not test predetermined hypotheses about associations between exposures and outcomes. This type of study is usually referred to simply as an ecological study. It is distinguished from an analytic ecological study, however, by the absence of one or more *a priori* hypotheses. Also see **ecological study**.

descriptive epidemiology A facet of epidemiology concerned with describing the frequency and distribution of morbidity or mortality in a population by person, place, or time variables. Useful in planning health programs and services, identifying potential health issues or trends, and suggesting hypotheses for further study. This aspect of epidemiology involves observation and description of what exists in a population and does not test *a priori* hypotheses.

descriptive study An observational epidemiologic study that does not test predetermined hypotheses. A descriptive study simply describes what exists in a population by person, place, or time variables. Descriptive studies are useful in demonstrating trends and generating hypotheses about disease causation.

design effect In the context of group randomized controlled trials, the design effect is the ratio of the number of subjects needed in a group randomized trial to the number of subjects needed in a comparable randomized controlled trial in order to achieve the same level of statistical efficiency or power, all other factors being equal. It can be thought of as a correction factor for the clustering effect. Also see **clustering effect**.

detectable preclinical phase The preclinical period during which a disorder is detectable by screening. In terms of the natural history of disease, this occurs during the presymptomatic stage.

diagnostic suspicion bias A form of information bias that can occur when knowledge of subject exposure status influences how the outcome is diagnosed.

differential misclassification A consequence of information bias that occurs when subjects in a study are incorrectly classified with respect to exposure or outcome status in a disproportionate manner. In other words, there is a different proportion of incorrect classifications on exposure status between the outcome groups or of outcome status between the exposure groups. Differential misclassification can lead to overestimation or underestimation of the measure of association or effect. Also see **nondifferential misclassification**.

direct causal association A causal association in which the cause leads directly to the effect without any intervening steps. For example, fire is a direct cause of burns, and *Yersinia pestis* is a direct cause of bubonic plague. Also see **indirect causal association**.

direct cause A synonym for **direct causal association**.

direct method A method of rate adjustment that is often used when the specific rates in each population being compared are available and stable. Also see **indirect method**.

directional hypothesis In hypothesis testing, an alternate hypothesis that indicates the expected direction of the association. For example, if H_O is OR equals 1.0, then H_A may be OR is greater than 1.0, where H_O is the null hypothesis, and H_A is the alternate hypothesis.

discordant pairs In the context of analyzing a case-control study where pair matching is used, discordant pairs are those case-control pairs where exposure status differs between cases and controls. In this situation, the calculation of the matched-pairs odds ratio is simply the ratio of the discordant pairs. Also see **concordant pairs**.

disease A physiological or psychological dysfunction. Also see **morbidity**.

disease cluster The occurrence of a greater than expected number of cases of a particular disease within a group of people, a geographic area, or a period of time. Disease clusters may be either real or perceived. Also see **noncommunicable disease cluster**.

disease iceberg concept An analogy that explains the clinician's often distorted view of the severity or frequency of certain diseases in a population due to the fact that only a small portion of those who have the disease seek treatment. This term derives from the fact that four-fifths of an iceberg is submerged or out of view.

disease odds ratio The odds ratio calculated by taking the odds of the study outcome among the exposed group to the odds of the study outcome among the unexposed group. Also see **exposure odds ratio**.

disease outbreak An epidemic confined to a localized area, such as a village or town, or within an institutional setting like a day-care center or hospital. Sometimes the terms disease outbreak and epidemic are use synonymously.

disease registry See **population-based disease registry**.

disease-specific mortality rate See **cause-specific mortality rate**.

dose-response relationship One of several guidelines for evaluating whether an association is likely to be causal or not based on Hill's postulates. The presence of a dose-response relationship increases the likelihood that an association is causal. A dose-response relationship is one where increasing levels of the exposure (dose) are associated with increases in the frequency of the outcome (response). For example, there is a dose-response relationship between the amount of alcohol consumed and the number of unintended injuries.

dot map A synonym for **spot map**.

double-blinded study In the context of randomized controlled trials, a double-blinded study is one in which neither the subjects nor the investigators (technically, the assessors) are aware of the subjects' group assignments. This design helps to overcome bias on the part of both the subjects and the investigators.

double-masked study See **double-blinded study**.

dynamic cohort study A synonym for **open cohort study**.

E

e A synonym for **exp**.

Early Aberration Reporting System A surveillance software system operated by the Centers for Disease Control and Prevention that can be used with syndromic surveillance data for the early detection of bioterrorism and other disease outbreaks.

early detection biases A term referring collectively to lead-time, length, and overdiagnosis bias. Also see **lead-time bias; length bias; overdiagnosis bias**.

ecological fallacy An error of reasoning that occurs when associations among groups of people are used to draw conclusions about associations among individuals. Ecological fallacies are often committed based on the results of ecological studies, although they can be made in certain other types of studies as well (e.g., group randomized trials).

ecological model A model that attempts to explain disease causation as an imbalance of the interaction among host, agent, and environmental factors.

ecological study An observational epidemiologic study in which the units of analysis are groups of people versus individuals and where summary measures of exposure or outcome are investigated. Ecological studies can be descriptive (exploratory) or analytic depending on whether or not predetermined hypotheses are being tested. Both descriptive and analytic ecological studies include multiple-group comparison studies, time-trend studies, and mixed studies.

ecological unit An aggregate of individuals that comprises a unit of analysis in an ecological study. Typically ecological units represent groups defined by geographical areas, such as cities, states, or countries, or by time periods.

effect measure modification A real effect that occurs in a study when a third factor (the effect modifier) influences the magnitude or direction of a causal association between a study exposure and outcome. For example, cigarette smoking modifies the effect of radon exposure on the development of lung cancer. Individuals exposed to radon who smoke cigarettes have a much higher risk of lung cancer than individuals exposed to radon who do not smoke cigarettes. Thus, cigarette smoking is an effect modifier of the causal association between radon exposure and lung cancer. The word "measure" is included in the term because effect measure modification depends on the measure of association or effect used.

effect modification See **effect measure modification**.

effect modifier The factor that modifies or alters the effect of an exposure on an outcome. Also see **effect measure modification**.

effect size Technically, a measure of the difference in outcomes between two groups. It is often measured, however, as a standardized difference, such as the difference in mean outcomes between the experimental and control groups in a randomized controlled trial divided by the standard deviation of the outcome in the control group or both groups. In this text, it is defined simply as the size of an association one would like to detect in a study if the association exists.

effective percent agreement A term referring collectively to percent positive agreement and percent negative agreement. These are alternate measures of percent agreement that are more sensitive measures of observer reliability. Also see **percent positive agreement; percent negative agreement**.

effective percentage agreement A synonym for **effective percent agreement**.

effective sample size In general, effective sample size refers to sample size after taking into account subject losses, such as those due to deaths, withdrawals, or losses to follow up. In the context of group randomized trials, effective sample size also refers to the sample size after adjusting for the clustering effect. Also see **clustering effect**.

effectiveness A measure of the degree to which an intervention is beneficial under ordinary, real life situations. It is a measure of the benefits of a treatment, procedure, or program to whom it is offered whether or not they use it. It is best determined in randomized trials.

efficacy A measure of the degree to which an intervention is beneficial under ideal conditions. It is a measure of the benefits of a treatment, procedure, or program among those who use it compared to those who do not. It is best determined in randomized trials.

efficacy analysis A synonym for **per protocol analysis**.

efficiency See **statistical efficiency**.

eligibility criteria The criteria used to define who is to be included and excluded from a study. In randomized controlled trials, the goal of the eligibility criteria is to optimize the conditions for successful testing of the intervention. Also see **inclusion criteria; exclusion criteria**.

emerging infectious disease An infectious disease previously unknown or virtually unknown in a population that has been increasing or threatening to increase in recent years. Also see **reemerging infectious disease**.

endemic The constant presence or usual frequency of a specific disease in a given population. The endemic level represents the expected level of the disease in the population at a given time.

endpoints This term has different meanings. In the context of epidemiologic studies, particularly randomized trials, endpoints refer to study outcomes. In reference to the measure known as years of potential life lost, an endpoint is the age considered not to constitute premature or untimely death. Several endpoints, such as 65, 70, and 75 years, have been used with this measure.

environmental epidemiology A specialization in epidemiology that focuses on the effects of environmental exposures on health-related outcomes. Environmental exposures include numerous physical, chemical, and biological agents carried through air, land, water, or food. Examples include indoor and outdoor air contaminants, hazardous wastes, waterborne pathogens, and foodborne toxins.

epidemic The occurrence of a specific disease at a frequency that is clearly in excess of normal expectations for a given population and time.

epidemic curve A graphic representation of the distribution of disease cases by time of onset and frequency in the form of a histogram. Epidemic curves are commonly used in the investigation of disease outbreaks and may provide clues to the source or mode of transmission of the disease.

epidemiologic triangle See **ecological model**.

epidemiology The study of the distribution, determinants, and deterrents of morbidity or mortality, broadly defined, in human populations.

equal effects model In the context of meta-analysis, there are two major approaches to integrating the findings of individual studies. One of these is based on an equal effects model, which is a model based on the assumption that the underlying effect is equal in all studies included in the meta-analysis. Therefore, it is assumed in this model that the reported effects for each component study differ only because of random error. The equal effects model is more commonly referred to as a fixed effects model, although this term can be misleading. Also see **random effects model**.

equipoise An ethical principle applicable to the conduct of randomized controlled trials that states that there should be genuine uncertainty about the benefits or harms of the regimens being offered. This principle is important so that individuals randomized to experimental and control groups are not subject to a regimen that is known to be inferior to an alternative based on their assignments.

error The discrepancy between a measured value and its true value. This can be represented as: error = measured value − true value.

excess odds ratio A statistical measure of effect that can be computed as OR − 1, where OR is the odds ratio. For example, if the odds ratio is 1.8, the excess odds ratio is 0.8.

excess prevalence The prevalence of a given outcome in the exposed group that is associated with the exposure, all other factors being equal. It is equivalent to the prevalence difference. Also see **prevalence difference**.

excess rate The rate of a given outcome in the exposed group that is associated with the exposure, all other factors being equal. For example, if the rate in the exposed group is 3.0 per 100 person-years, and the rate in the unexposed group is 1.0 per 100 person-years, then the excess rate is 2.0 per 100 person-years. The excess rate is equivalent to the rate difference. Also see **rate difference**.

excess risk The risk of a given outcome in the exposed group that is associated with the exposure, all other factors being equal. For example, if the risk in the exposed group is

3.0 per 100, and the risk in the unexposed group is 1.0 per 100, then the excess risk is 2.0 per 100. The excess risk is equivalent to the risk difference. Also see **risk difference**.

exclusion criteria The criteria used to define who is to be excluded from a study, for example, in a randomized controlled trial. Also see **eligibility criteria**.

exp The exponential or e, which is the base used in natural logarithms. The value of exp is approximately 2.71828. The expression exp (x) is equivalent to e^x; thus, exp (2) is e^2, which is 2.71828^2 or approximately 7.38905. Also see **ln**.

experimental epidemiology A facet of epidemiology concerned with determining the efficacy or effectiveness of various interventions using experimental or quasi-experimental methods. Useful in evaluating a health treatment, procedure, or program. This aspect of epidemiology tests *a priori* hypotheses.

experimental evidence One of several guidelines for evaluating whether an association is likely to be causal or not based on Hill's postulates. Confirmation of an association by a randomized controlled trial, for example, provides strong evidence that an association is causal.

experimental study An epidemiologic investigation in which the investigators control the conditions of the experiment, including the subjects' exposure status. Experimental studies can be recognized by a planned intervention, which involves the introduction of an investigational treatment, procedure, or service so as to determine its efficacy or effectiveness with regard to a desirable outcome (e.g., longevity, pain reduction). There are two major types of planned experimental studies in epidemiology—randomized controlled trials and group randomized trials.

exploratory case-control study A descriptive case-control study in which there are no specified *a priori* hypotheses about associations between exposure and outcome. Cases and controls are selected, and a variety of factors are examined to determine if any are related to the outcome of interest. Exploratory case-control studies can be useful in identifying potential risk factors and possible causes of disease outbreaks or epidemics.

exploratory study A term used in reference to some descriptive studies, especially where the purpose is to generate hypotheses. In this type of study the investigators literally search for possible relationships that can be examined later using analytic or experimental studies.

exposure The potential risk factor in an epidemiologic study, whether that factor represents an actual exposure (e.g., radon gas), a behavior (e.g., not wearing a seat belt), or an individual attribute (e.g., race/ethnicity). Also see **outcome**.

exposure odds ratio The odds ratio in a case-control study calculated by taking the ratio of the odds of the study exposure among the cases to the odds of the study exposure among the controls. Also see **disease odds ratio**.

exposure status A term for classifying subjects according to their level of exposure to a potential risk factor. Exposure status may be measured dichotomously as present or absent or may be represented by several levels, such as heavy, moderate, and light, and no alcohol consumption. Also see **outcome status**.

exposure suspicion bias A form of information bias that can occur when knowledge of subjects' outcome status influences how exposure is assessed. It is a potential problem in case-control studies, for example.

external comparison group In the context of a cohort study, an external comparison group is a group outside the study cohort that serves as a control group for comparison purposes. An external comparison group is often composed of a general population sample in the same geographic area with similar demographics as the study cohort. External comparison groups are most often used with special exposure cohorts.

external validity The degree to which the results of a study are relevant for populations other than the study population. Also known as generalizability.

F

factorial design A variation of the traditional randomized controlled trial which is intended to answer two or more research questions at the same time. In this type of study the subjects are randomized into experimental and control groups and then each of these groups is randomized again to test additional study hypotheses. This type of design may also be applied to group randomized trials.

false negative In the context of screening, a false negative is an individual who tests negative on a screening test but has the disorder for which screening was performed.

false negative rate The percent of those with a given disorder who are falsely classified as not having the disorder based on a screening test.

false positive In the context of screening, a false positive is an individual who tests positive on a screening test but does not have the disorder for which screening was performed.

false positive rate The percent of those without a given disorder who are falsely classified as having the disorder based on a screening test.

fertility rate The number of live births occurring in a population during a specified time period in relation to the number of women 15–44 years of age during the same time period. Like the crude birth rate, the fertility rate is a good indicator of population growth.

fetal death rate The number of fetal deaths after 20 weeks or more of gestation during a specified time period in relation to the number of live births plus fetal deaths after 20 weeks or more of gestation during the same time period.

fixed cohort study A synonym for **closed cohort study**.

fixed effects model A synonym for **equal effects model**.

fixed sample design See **fixed sample size design**.

fixed sample size design A type of randomized controlled trial where the sample size is normally fixed before the trial begins, and the findings are not generally analyzed until the conclusion of the trial. Subjects may be enrolled all at once or over time until the specified sample size is reached.

force of morbidity See **incidence density**.

forest plot A diagrammatic representation of the statistical results of a meta-analysis. A forest plot provides readers with a visual representation of the effect estimates and applicable confidence intervals for each component study in the meta-analysis as well as an overall estimate of the effect and its confidence interval.

frequency matching A form of group matching that seeks to make study and comparison groups similar with respect to the frequency of extraneous variables. For example, in a case-control study that uses frequency matching for sex, if 40% of the case group are females, then the investigator seeks to obtain 40% females in the control group. Frequency matching tends to reduce but not eliminate confounding. It does, however, increase study efficiency.

futility One of several reasons that might be used to stop a randomized controlled trial in progress, particularly a sequential or group sequential trial. Specifically, futility is a statistical judgment that no difference is likely to be found between the study groups. Therefore, continuing the study would mean subjecting the study participants to an unproven intervention without any reasonable likelihood of finding a benefit over the standard treatment. Also see **stopping rules**.

G

general cohort A type of cohort used in cohort studies. A general cohort is usually a general population group defined by person, place, or time factors or another broadly based group, such as members of a health maintenance organization, trade union, or school. General cohorts consist of both exposed and unexposed individuals with the exposed individuals serving as the exposed group, and the unexposed individuals serving as the comparison group. Also see **special exposure cohort**.

generalizability A synonym for **external validity**.

genetic epidemiology A specialization in epidemiology that deals with the distribution, causes, and control of health-related outcomes in groups of relatives and with inherited causes of disease in populations. It is concerned with the genetic components of health and disease in human populations. The focus of genetic epidemiology is on complex diseases like coronary heart disease and breast cancer that have multifactorial etiologies.

gold standard A method, test, measure, or procedure that is generally regarded as the best available. In the context of screening, gold standard refers to a diagnostic test that is widely accepted as being the best available. For example, the angiogram is the gold standard for diagnosing coronary heart disease. In the context of epidemiologic study designs, the randomized controlled trial is often referred to as the gold standard of epidemiologic studies.

group randomized trial A planned epidemiologic experiment in which groups of people are randomly allocated to intervention or control conditions in order to evaluate the effectiveness of one or more interventions. A distinctive feature of a group randomized trial is that the units of assignment are intact groups of people versus individual persons.

group sequential design A type of sequential design in which analysis of the accumulated findings is conducted at predetermined intervals following enrollment of a specified number or block of subjects. Generally, only two or three interim analyses are planned in a group sequential design, rather than the continuing analyses that are characteristic of conventional sequential designs. Also see **sequential design**.

H

haphazard sample A synonym for **convenience sample**.

Hawthorne effect The tendency of research subjects to change their behaviors due purely to the fact that they are being studied.

hazard period The time period in a case-crossover study following the exposure during which the risk of the study outcome is increased. This "trigger period" is usually the time just before the occurrence of the outcome. For example, in a case-crossover study of intense exertion and sudden cardiac death, the hazard period is the time immediately following the heavy exertion.

hazard ratio The ratio of the hazard rate in the exposed group to that in the unexposed group. The hazard rate is a time-dependent instantaneous incidence density calculated in the Cox proportional hazards model. The hazard ratio is often interpreted as a relative risk.

health A state of well-being and positive functioning and not just the absence of disease.

healthy worker effect A form of selection bias that can arise when health outcomes among workers are compared to those among the general population. Since workers tend to have better overall health as a group than the general population, the comparison tends to favor the working group, especially when the outcome is mortality. This is because workers must have a certain level of health to work, while the general population includes those who are unable to work because of health problems.

herd immunity The resistance of a group or population to the spread of a disease due to the fact that a high proportion of the group is immune to the disease.

heterogeneity In the context of meta-analysis, heterogeneity, broadly defined, refers to differences among the component studies. Also see **clinical heterogeneity; methodological heterogeneity; statistical heterogeneity**.

heterogeneity of effect A synonym for **effect measure modification** or **interaction**.

hierarchical modeling A synonym for **multilevel analysis**.

Hill's postulates A set of guidelines developed by Austin Bradford Hill in 1965 to determine whether or not a statistical association is likely to represent a causal association. Some of these guidelines are: correct temporal sequence, strength of the association, consistency of the association, dose-response relationship, biological plausibility, and experimental evidence.

historical cohort study A synonym for **retrospective cohort study.**

holistic model of health A comprehensive paradigm that explains health either on the community or individual level. An example is the health field concept, which envisions the environment, lifestyle, human biology, and health care organization as the key factors contributing to a community's health.

homogenous In the context of meta-analysis, homogeneous refers to component studies that are similar in terms of study interventions, outcomes, subjects, design, and quality, so that the results are consistent except for random variation.

hospital admission rate bias A synonym for **admission rate bias.**

hospital controls Subjects comprising the control group of a hospital-based case-control study. Hospital controls are selected from patients admitted to the same clinical facility as the cases but without the study outcome.

hospital-based case-control study A case-control study in which the subjects are selected among patients admitted to one or more clinical facilities, usually, but not necessarily, hospitals.

hot-spot cluster A term sometimes used in reference to a **spatial cluster.**

hybrid study An epidemiologic study that combines features of two or more study designs. Some common types of hybrid studies include nested case-control studies, case-cohort studies, panel studies, and repeated surveys.

I

I^2 A measure that quantifies the degree of inconsistency among the results of the component studies of a meta-analysis. It has been proposed as an alternative to a standard test of heterogeneity. I^2 ranges from zero to 100 percent with zero indicating no heterogeneity and 100 percent indicating maximal heterogeneity.

immediate cause of death On a death certificate, the disease or condition that led directly to death. The immediate cause of death should be an actual disorder (e.g., pneumonia) as opposed to a mode of dying (e.g., respiratory failure).

immunity See **active immunity; passive immunity; herd immunity.**

inactive treatment In the context of randomized controlled trials, inactive treatment refers to the use of a placebo, sham procedure, or no intervention at all in the control arm of the trial. Also see **active treatment.**

incidence The number of new occurrences in a defined population during a specified period of time. In practice, incidence may be used to refer to cumulative incidence or incidence density.

incidence density The rate at which new cases occur in a population expressed in terms of person-time units. For example, researchers reporting 15.0 cases of unintentional injuries per 100 person-years at a particular worksite are reporting the incidence density of unintentional injuries at that site.

incidence density difference The difference between the incidence density in the exposed group and that in the unexposed group. The incidence density difference is a commonly reported rate difference.

incidence density ratio The ratio of the incidence density in the exposed group to that in the unexposed group. The incidence density ratio is a commonly reported rate ratio.

incidence density sampling A method of sampling controls in a case-control study where the controls are selected from the person-time experience that produced the cases. Typically, the controls are randomly selected from those who are at risk of the study outcome at the time each case develops. The method is typically used in nested case-control studies.

incidence odds The ratio of the number of people who develop a new occurrence to the number of people who do not develop the occurrence in a given population during a specified period of time. Also see **prevalence odds.**

incidence proportion A synonym for **cumulative incidence**.

incidence rate A synonym for **incidence density**. It is also sometimes used inappropriately to refer to cumulative incidence.

incidence rate ratio A synonym for **incidence density ratio**.

inclusion criteria The criteria used to define who is to be included in a study, for example, in a randomized controlled trial.

incubation period The time between the invasion of an infectious agent and the development of the first signs or symptoms of the disease. For example, hepatitis A has an average incubation period of 28–30 days.

independent variable A variable that is expected to influence the dependent variable in a study. In epidemiologic studies, the independent variable is typically exposure status, which is used to predict outcome status, the dependent variable. Also see **dependent variable**.

index case The first case of a disease in a defined group to come to the attention of investigators during a disease outbreak. Often the index case is the one who introduced the causative agent into the group.

indirect causal association An association in which the cause leads to the effect through one or more intervening steps. For example, sharing syringes can cause HIV infection, which in turn causes AIDS. Therefore, sharing syringes is an indirect cause of AIDS. Also see **direct causal association**.

indirect cause A synonym for **indirect causal association**.

indirect method A method of rate adjustment that can be used when one or more of the specific rates in one of the populations being compared is either unavailable or unstable. Also see **direct method**.

indirectly standardized rate An "adjusted rate" calculated using the indirect method of adjustment. It is calculated by multiplying the crude rate in the reference population by the standardized mortality or morbidity ratio as appropriate.

individual matching A form of matching where individuals in the study group are matched on selected characteristics with individuals in the comparison group but not necessarily on a one-to-one basis. Also see **pair matching; frequency matching**.

induction period In reference to noncommunicable diseases, it is the period from initial exposure to causative agents to disease initiation. The disease, however, is not apparent at any time during the induction period. Also see **latency period**.

infant mortality rate The number of deaths among infants up to one year of age during a specified time period in relation to the number of live births during the same time period. It is often used as an indicator of the health status of a population.

infectious disease A synonym for **communicable disease**.

information bias A type of systematic error due to measurement flaws that can result in misclassification of subjects with regard to exposure or outcome status. This type of bias occurs during the data collection phase of a study.

informed consent Voluntary assent to participate in a study, such as a randomized controlled trial, after receiving an adequate explanation of its purpose, methods, and procedures as well as the potential risks and benefits of participation.

institutional review board In the United States, a standing committee within the sponsoring institution that reviews research protocols using ethical guidelines designed to protect the safety and well-being of the study participants. Also see **research ethics committee**.

intention-to-treat analysis The analysis of the results of a randomized controlled trial based on the original subject assignments to experimental and control groups as determined by randomization, whether or not all the subjects complied with the study protocol.

interaction The combined effect of two or more independent variables on a dependent variable. For example, interaction occurs when two risk factors together increase or decrease the magnitude of an outcome compared to only one of the factors. Interaction is assessed in statistical modeling. In practice, interaction is often used synonymously with effect measure modification. It is also known as statistical interaction. Also see **effect measure modification**.

intermittent source outbreak A common source outbreak where the exposure to the causative agent is irregular. An intermittent source outbreak might occur, for example, when a contaminated food is served in a restaurant on different days over the course of a week.

internal comparison group In the context of a cohort study, an internal comparison group is the subset of a general cohort that is not exposed to the study factor. This group serves as the control group in the study.

internal validity The degree to which the results of a study, apart from random error, are true for the source population. Internal validity is threatened by sources of systematic error, namely bias and confounding.

interobserver reliability A measure of the level of agreement or consistency between two or more independent observers of the same phenomenon (e.g., a screening test result). High interobserver reliability implies low interobserver variability and vice versa. Also see **interobserver variability**.

interobserver variability A measure of the level of disagreement or inconsistency between two or more independent observers of the same phenomenon (e.g., a screening test result). For example, when two radiologists tend to disagree on the results of chest x-rays for the same individuals, a high level of interobserver variability is said to have occurred.

interrater reliability A synonym for **interobserver reliability**.

interrupted time-series design A type of quasi-experimental study design where multiple measurements of the study outcome are made prior to and following the intervention without the use of a separate control group.

interval estimation A method of assessing the precision of a point estimate of a population parameter using a confidence interval. In general, the wider the confidence interval, the less precise the point estimate and vice versa. Thus, wider confidence intervals suggest more random error in an estimate than narrower confidence intervals.

intervention study A synonym for **experimental study**. The term derives from the fact that in experimental studies investigators "intervene" into the lives of their subjects by manipulating their exposure status with regard to the study variable(s).

interviewer bias A type of information bias that can occur when interviewers' awareness of subject outcome status influences how they assess exposure status or when their knowledge of exposure status influences how they assess outcome status.

intraclass correlation coefficient A measure of the correlation between individual outcomes in a group or cluster. Its magnitude is dependent on the extent of the clustering effect. The intraclass correlation coefficient is commonly used in analyzing data from group randomized trials and in measuring interobserver reliability when the data are continuous. Also see **clustering effect**.

intracluster correlation coefficient A synonym for **intraclass correlation coefficient**.

intraobserver reliability A measure of the level of consistency in the assessments of a single observer of the same phenomenon (e.g., a screening test result) at different times. High intraobserver reliability implies low intraobserver variability and vice versa. Also see **intraobserver variability**.

intraobserver variability A measure of the level of inconsistency in the assessments of a single observer of the same phenomenon (e.g., a screening test result) at different times. For example, if a pathologist tends to interpret the same Pap test as positive on certain days but negative on other days, a high level of intraobserver variability is said to have occurred.

intrarater reliability A synonym for **intraobserver reliability**.

J, K

Kaplan-Meier product limit method A method of survival analysis that uses each subject's exact survival time rather than estimates based on a uniformity assumption. In general, the Kaplan-Meier method is more precise and requires a smaller sample size than the life table method of survival analysis. Also see **life table method**; **survival analysis**.

kappa A statistical measure of the proportion of nonrandom agreement between two observers. Kappa is considered a measure of the proportion of agreement above and beyond the agreement expected by chance alone. It is commonly used, for example, to measure interobserver or intraobserver reliability where the test results are based on nominal data. Also see **weighted kappa**.

L

latency period In reference to noncommunicable diseases, it is the time from disease initiation to the clinical expression of disease (i.e., when disease is diagnosed due to overt signs or symptoms). The latency period follows the induction period, and together they represent the time of disease development.

latent period A synonym for **latency period**.

lead time The time gained by diagnosing a disorder in its presymptomatic stage as a consequence of screening versus diagnosing it in the usual way during the clinical stage when signs or symptoms are apparent.

lead-time bias A type of bias that occurs when survival time is overestimated due to an early diagnosis that does not improve prognosis. Lead-time bias is possible when survival times are compared for two groups where the disease has been diagnosed at different stages in its natural history (e.g., in the presymptomatic versus the clinical stage). Lead-time bias is a type of early detection bias associated with screening.

length bias A type of bias that can occur when comparing survival times among screened and unscreened populations. This type of bias is likely when there is a higher proportion of individuals with slowly progressing forms of a disease in the screened population compared to the unscreened population. Because individuals with slowly progressing forms tend to have a better prognosis, and hence a longer survival time, than those with rapidly progressing forms, this type of bias can lead to overestimation of the effectiveness of a screening program. Length bias is a real possibility when periodic screening is conducted for certain diseases since those with slowly progressing forms of the disease are more likely to be detected than those with rapidly progressing forms.

length-biased sampling A synonym for **length bias**.

length-time bias A synonym for **length bias**.

levels of prevention The various levels at which disease can be prevented or controlled. Also see **primary prevention**; **secondary prevention**; **tertiary prevention**.

life table method A method of survival analysis in which subject survival times are divided into a number of small time intervals. Based on an assumption of uniformity, the proportion of subjects surviving to a given interval is estimated by the product of the proportions surviving each prior interval. This method is used less frequently than other methods of survival analysis, which are more precise. Also see **Kaplan-Meier product limit method**; **survival analysis**.

lifetime prevalence A variant of period prevalence that refers to the proportion of individuals in a defined population who have had a given occurrence (e.g., disease) at any time during their lives. Thus, the time period for lifetime prevalence is the collective lifetimes of the individuals in the population.

likelihood ratio A measure that can be used to assess the validity of a screening test. In this context, it is the probability of a particular value of a test result in those with the disorder of interest divided by the probability of the same value in those without the disorder of interest.

likelihood ratio for a negative test result A type of likelihood ratio equal to the probability of a negative test result in those with the disorder divided by the probability of a negative test result in those without the disorder. It is often abbreviated as LR⁻. For example, an LR$^-$ of 0.10 indicates that a negative test result is only 0.10 times as likely to be found in those with the disorder compared to those without the disorder.

likelihood ratio for a positive test result A type of likelihood ratio equal to the probability of a positive test result in those with the disorder divided by the probability of a positive test result in those without the disorder. It is often abbreviated as LR$^+$. For example, an LR$^+$ of 8.0 indicates that a positive test result is eight times as likely to be found in those with the disorder than those without the disorder.

ln The natural logarithm, or more explicitly, the logarithm in the base e. In the expression exp (x) = Y, x is the natural logarithm of Y; that is, x is the power that e must be raised to get Y. In the expression ln (x) = Y, x is the value of e raised to a power of Y. Also see **exp**.

logistic regression A type of regression analysis in which the outcome is dichotomous. In logistic regression there is only one dependent and one independent variable. Also see **multiple logistic regression**.

longitudinal study A general term referring to an investigation in which subjects are studied over time. Data on the study subjects are collected during successive time periods. An example is a cohort study.

loss to follow-up bias A form of selection bias that can occur in longitudinal studies when significant losses to follow-up result in a sample that is systematically different from the original or study population with regard to exposure and outcome status.

lower confidence limit The minimum value represented by a confidence interval. For example, in the following confidence interval, 2.0 is the lower confidence limit: 95% CI = 2.0 to 4.0. Also see **confidence limits; upper confidence limit**.

M

Mantel-Haenszel chi-square test A type of chi-square test of significance that is used with Mantel-Haenszel measures of association, such as the Mantel-Haenszel odds ratio (OR$_{MH}$). It is also known simply as the Mantel-Haenszel test.

Mantel-Haenszel incidence density difference An adjusted incidence density difference using the Mantel-Haenszel method. It is more commonly referred to as the Mantel-Haenszel rate difference. Also see **Mantel-Haenszel method**.

Mantel-Haenszel incidence density ratio An adjusted incidence density ratio using the Mantel-Haenszel method. It is more commonly referred to as the Mantel-Haenszel rate ratio. Also see **Mantel-Haenszel method**.

Mantel-Haenszel incidence rate difference A synonym for **Mantel-Haenszel incidence density difference**.

Mantel-Haenszel incidence rate ratio A synonym for **Mantel-Haenszel incidence density ratio**.

Mantel-Haenszel method A statistical technique commonly used in stratification to produce a summary measure of association or effect that is adjusted for one or more potentially confounding factors. The technique involves taking a weighted average of the stratum-specific measures of association where the weights depend on the number of observations in each stratum. It is also used in meta-analysis to derive a summary estimate of effect for the component studies based on an equal effects (or fixed effects) model.

Mantel-Haenszel odds ratio An adjusted odds ratio using the Mantel-Haenszel method. Also see **Mantel-Haenszel method**.

Mantel-Haenszel rate difference A term usually used when referring to the **Mantel-Haenszel incidence density difference**.

Mantel-Haenszel rate ratio A term usually used when referring to the **Mantel-Haenszel incidence density ratio**.

Mantel-Haenszel risk difference A measure analogous to the Mantel-Haenszel incidence density difference but based on the cumulative incidence difference.

Mantel-Haenszel risk ratio A measure analogous to the Mantel-Haenszel incidence density ratio but based on the cumulative incidence ratio.

Mantel-Haenszel test See **Mantel-Haenszel chi-square test**.

masking A synonym for **blinding**.

mass screening A form of screening aimed at large, generally diverse, populations where the probability of individuals having a preclinical form of the disorder of interest is likely to be variable. In mass screening, everyone in the defined population is screened regardless of his or her probability of having the disorder of interest. Screening for cholesterol levels at a health fair is an example of mass screening.

matched case-control study A case-control study that uses individual matching. Matched case-control studies are analyzed differently from unmatched studies.

matched pairs odds ratio The odds ratio calculated from a pair-matched case-control study. The matched pairs odds ratio is an adjusted odds ratio and is equivalent to the Mantel-Haenszel odds ratio used in stratification.

matching A procedure that attempts to produce study and comparison groups that are similar with regard to extraneous or potentially confounding factors. Matching may be performed at the individual or group level. Also see **individual matching; pair matching; frequency matching**.

maternal mortality rate The number of deaths due to childbirth during a specified time period in relation to the number of live births during the same time period. The World Health Organization defines the time period as during pregnancy or within 42 days following pregnancy. The maternal mortality rate is a common health status indicator of a population.

maturation A term commonly used in relation to quasi-experimental studies. It refers to processes associated with the passage of time, such as aging of the subjects. Maturation can confound apparent effects found in some quasi-experimental studies and therefore may need to be controlled.

McNemar's chi-square test A type of chi-square test for examining statistical significance when pair matching is used. This test statistic represents a special application of the Mantel-Haenszel chi-square test.

measure of association A quantity that expresses the degree of statistical relationship between an exposure and outcome (e.g., OR, RR). The association may be causal or noncausal depending on the circumstances. The term is most appropriately used in reference to observational studies. Also see **measure of effect**.

measure of effect A measure of association based on a causal association. Although the term may be used in reference to all types of epidemiologic studies, it is most appropriately used in reference to experimental studies.

measures of occurrence Quantitative measures of disease, death, or other attributes. They are usually based on counts, ratios, proportions, or rates. Common examples in epidemiology include cumulative incidence, incidence density, and prevalence.

measurement bias A synonym for **information bias**.

measurement error An error in measuring the value of a variable. Its magnitude is represented by the difference between the true value and the reported value. Measurement errors may be due to inexact measurements, sloppy techniques, bias, and other factors. As long as they are truly random, measurement errors only tend to dilute an association.

membership bias A type of selection bias that results from the fact that those who belong to organized groups (e.g., the military, athletic associations, civic groups, religious organizations) tend to differ systematically from the general population with regard to health status and other factors. For example, members of organized groups tend to be healthier and less susceptible to morbidity and premature mortality than members of the general population, which include those too ill to participate in groups. The healthy worker effect is a type of membership bias.

meta-analysis A method of summarizing the findings of several studies examining similar research questions. A major objective is to pool the results statistically so as to determine the overall effect as well as to identify important trends and develop appropriate policies.

method variability A threat to the reliability of a screening test. Specifically, method variability has to do with inconsistencies in test results due to the screening test itself. It occurs when a screening test produces different results under similar circumstances. Such a screening test is unreliable and not useful for the early detection of disease or other conditions.

methodological diversity A synonym for **methodological heterogeneity**.

methodological heterogeneity Differences among the component studies of a meta-analysis due to differences in trial design or quality.

misclassification bias A synonym for **information bias**.

mixed cohort study A cohort study that involves aspects of both prospective and retrospective cohort studies. Usually, past or historical exposure is assessed and follow up continues from that time up to the present and into the future. Also see **cohort study**.

mixed (ecological) study An ecological study that examines the association between changes in hypothesized exposure levels and outcome rates for several populations over time. A mixed study can be thought of as a combination of a multiple-group and time-trend study.

mixed outbreak A combination of common source and propagated outbreaks. Often a mixed outbreak begins with a common source exposure that is followed by person-to-person spread of the disease.

molecular epidemiology A specialization in epidemiology that uses molecular and biochemical measures to study the contribution of potential genetic and environmental risk factors to the distribution, causes, and prevention of disease and death in families and across populations. For example, molecular epidemiology has been used to improve assessments of exposure and in defining inherited susceptibility to cancers through DNA fingerprinting. It has also been used, for instance, to differentiate new cases of tuberculosis from reactivated cases by subtyping the infectious agent.

morbidity Any departure from physiological or psychological well-being, whether objective or subjective. It is commonly used to describe diseases, injuries, and other nonfatal conditions.

mortality Deaths in a population.

multicollinearity In general terms, a high degree of correlation between independent factors. More precisely, it refers to a situation in multiple regression analysis where multiple independent variables are highly correlated with each other. This makes it difficult, if not impossible, to isolate their independent effects on the dependent variable.

multifactorial etiology Multiple causation, that is, the concept that certain diseases and other conditions have multiple causes, often interrelated. For example, heart disease, which has multiple, interrelated causes, is said to have a multifactorial etiology. Most models of disease causation assume a multifactorial etiology.

multilevel analysis Analysis using advanced statistical modeling techniques that examine the independent and combined effects of individual level and group level variables in order to better explain health-related outcomes.

multilevel modeling A synonym for **multilevel analysis**.

multiphasic screening Screening for several diseases or conditions on the same occasion. Health fairs, for example, may use multiphasic screening to test for possible diabetes, hypertension, hearing impairment, and other potential disorders in individuals at the same time.

multiple logistic regression A type of regression analysis in which the dependent variable is dichotomous (e.g., present or absent) and the independent variables are nominal or continuous. Unlike logistic regression, there are two or more independent variables in this technique. Multiple logistic regression is popular in analyzing data from case-control and other epidemiologic studies because adjusted odds ratios can be easily derived from the regression coefficients, which are part of the regression equation. Also see **logistic regression**.

multiple pretest-posttest design In the context of group randomized trials, a multiple pretest-posttest design is one in which the outcome measurements are made at several different points before and after the intervention. This design allows investigators to examine patterns in the data, which can help to explain any observed differences.

multiple R squared See **coefficient of determination**.

multiple time-series design A type of quasi-experimental study design employing a separate control group where multiple measurements of the study outcome are made prior to and following the intervention in both the intervention and control groups.

multiple-group study An ecological study where the ecological units are places (e.g., countries, states, institutions). Generally, several ecological units are examined at the same time.

multiplicative effects In the assessment of effect measure modification or statistical interaction, multiplicative effects are those based on a multiplicative model. Also see **multiplicative model**.

multiplicative interaction Statistical interaction based on a multiplicative model. Also see **multiplicative model**.

multiplicative model A mathematical model based on ratio measures of association (e.g., risk ratios). In a multiplicative model the combined effect of two or more variables on an outcome is the product of their separate effects.

multivariable method One of several statistical methods used to analyze the effects of more than one independent variable on a dependent variable (e.g., multiple logistic regression).

N

narrative review The type of review found in a traditional research review article. Narrative reviews tend to be subjective in that there are no established rules for the authors to follow with regard to which studies to include or exclude from the review. Also see **systematic review**.

National Electronic Disease Surveillance System A national effort to integrate disease surveillance systems at the national, state, and local levels. A major objective is to promote the rapid exchange of reliable, real-time data in an efficient manner over the Internet that will allow health authorities to identify and track emerging threats while monitoring disease trends.

National Electronic Injury Surveillance System A national surveillance system operated by the Consumer Product Safety Commission. It collects injury data from 100 emergency departments randomly selected from all U.S. hospitals with emergency departments. The system gathers injury data and has the flexibility to gather other related data as needed.

National Notifiable Diseases Surveillance System A national surveillance system based on mandated reporting of certain diseases and conditions at the state level. The diseases or conditions that must be reported may vary from state to state. In general, health care providers report to local health departments which in turn report to the state. The states voluntarily report to the Centers for Disease Control and Prevention.

natural experiment A relatively rare situation in nature that mimics a planned experimental study. Technically, a natural experiment is an observational study that only has the appearance of an experiment. A classic example is John Snow's investigation of cholera deaths in the drinking water supplied by two rival water companies in mid-1800s.

natural history of disease The potentially predictable life cycle of a disease or other disorder from onset to final outcome. The natural history of disease has four stages—stage of susceptibility, stage of presymptomatic disease, stage of clinical disease, and stage of diminished capacity.

natural logarithm See **ln**.

necessary and sufficient cause A cause that is required to produce an outcome and is able to cause the outcome by itself. For example, excess lead exposure is a necessary and sufficient cause of lead poisoning.

necessary but not sufficient cause A cause that is required to produce an outcome but is not able to cause the outcome by itself. In other words, additional factors are necessary for the outcome to occur. A classic example is alcoholism. While alcohol is necessary for the disease to develop, it is not a sufficient cause. Additional factors, including certain genetic, social, behavioral, and environmental factors, also appear to be required.

necessary cause A cause that is always required for a particular outcome to occur.

negative bias Bias that results in an underestimation of the magnitude of a measure of association or effect between an exposure and outcome.

negative confounder A confounding factor that leads to underestimation of the magnitude of the measure of association or effect between an exposure and outcome.

negative interaction Interaction where the observed combined effect of two or more variables is less than the expected combined effect, all other factors being equal.

negative predictive value The probability that those who test negative on a screening test do not have the disorder in question. Negative predictive value is usually stated as a percent and is calculated by dividing the number of true negatives by the number testing negative in the study population.

neonatal mortality rate The number of deaths among infants less than 28 days old during a specified time period in relation to the number of live births during the same time period. The usual time period is one calendar year.

nested case-control study A case-control study embedded (nested) within an existing, defined cohort. The cohort may be part of a prospective or retrospective cohort study, randomized controlled trial, or another source. This type of study may be referred to as a hybrid study since it combines features of two study designs.

neuroepidemiology A specialization in epidemiology that focuses on the study of neurological disorders, such as multiple sclerosis, epilepsy, and Alzheimer's disease.

Neyman's bias A synonym for **prevalence-incidence bias**.

nominal A term referring to nominal data, a nominal variable, or a nominal measurement scale. Nominal represents unordered qualitative categories, such as racial/ethnic groups or religion affiliations.

nomogram In the context of screening, a nomogram is a graphic tool that can be used to simplify the calculation of posttest probabilities.

nonadherence A synonym for **noncompliance**.

noncausal association A real association, but one that is not causal. In other words, a change in the frequency of the exposure in a population does not necessarily result in a change in the frequency of the outcome. Noncausal associations often result from confounding. For example, some studies have found a noncausal association between alcohol consumption and lung cancer that is due to confounding by cigarette smoking.

noncommunicable disease A disease that cannot be transmitted to others, either directly or indirectly. Also known as a noninfectious disease. For example, coronary heart disease and cystic fibrosis are noncommunicable diseases.

noncommunicable disease cluster A disease cluster where the disorder is a noncommunicable disease. Noncommunicable disease clusters tend to represent relatively uncommon disorders such as multiple sclerosis, leukemia, or mesothelioma.

noncompliance Subject nonconformance with the study protocol in an epidemiologic study, especially in regard to randomized controlled trials.

nonconcurrent cohort study A synonym for **retrospective cohort study**.

noncrossover design A synonym for **parallel group design** in reference to randomized controlled trials.

nondifferential misclassification A consequence of information bias that occurs when subjects in a study are incorrectly classified with respect to exposure or outcome status in a uniform manner. In other words, there is a similar proportion of incorrect classifications with regard to exposure status between the outcome groups or with regard to outcome status between the exposure groups. Nondifferential misclassification generally results in a dilution of the magnitude of the measure of association or effect, that is, toward no association. Also see **differential misclassification**.

non-directional hypothesis In hypothesis testing, an alternate hypothesis that does not indicate the expected direction of the association. For example, if H_O is OR equals 1.0, then H_A is OR does not equal 1.0, where H_O is the null hypothesis, and H_A is the alternate hypothesis.

nonequivalent control group design A type a quasi-experimental study design. Specifically, it is a type of before and after study with a separate control group. Also see **before and after studies**.

noninfectious disease A synonym for **noncommunicable disease**.

non-respondent bias A synonym for **non-response bias**.

non-response bias A type of bias that can occur when those who participate in studies differ systematically from those who do not. This type of bias can occur, for example, when those who respond to questionnaires are systematically different from those who do not respond. Volunteer bias is a type of non-response bias. Also known as response bias.

nonsystematic error Random error. Nonsystematic errors are not predictable or reproducible. An example is sampling variation. Also see **systematic error**.

nosocomial infections Infections acquired in a hospital or other health care facility.

not necessary and not sufficient cause A cause that is not required to produce an outcome and when present is not able to cause the outcome by itself. Hence, there are other causes of the outcome. A not necessary and not sufficient cause is known as a contributory cause. Also see **contributory cause**.

not necessary but sufficient cause A cause that is not required to produce an outcome but when present is able to cause the outcome by itself. This means that there are other causes of the outcome. For example, dehydration is a not necessary but sufficient cause of headaches.

notifiable disease A disease or condition that must be reported to the appropriate health authority by law whenever it is diagnosed. Reporting is usually by physicians, laboratories, or hospital personnel. In general, notifiable diseases are important because their presence in excess numbers can have significant public health implications. Notifiable diseases are also known as reportable diseases.

null hypothesis A hypothesis stating that there is no association between an exposure and outcome of interest.

null value The value of a measure of association or effect corresponding to no association or no effect. For example, the null value for a risk ratio is one, and the null value for a risk difference is zero.

O

observation bias A synonym for **information bias**.

observational study A kind of epidemiologic study in which the investigators collect, record, and analyze data on subjects without controlling their exposure status or the conditions of the study. The investigators simply observe the subjects as they naturally divide themselves by potentially significant variables or exposures. Observational studies include descriptive and analytic studies and do not involve planned interventions, which are characteristic of experimental studies.

observer In the context of screening, observer is a generic term for the person who interprets screening test results.

observer reliability An inclusive term referring to interobserver or intraobserver reliability. Also see **interobserver reliability; intraobserver reliability**.

observer variability An inclusive term referring to interobserver or intraobserver variability. Also see **interobserver variability; intraobserver variability**.

occupational epidemiology A specialization in epidemiology that focuses on the effects of workplace exposures on the health and safety of workers. Some concerns of occupational epidemiology include the effects of noise, toxic gases and particulates, and job stress on the development of occupational diseases and injuries. Occupational epidemiology may also be considered a branch of environmental epidemiology. Also see **environmental epidemiology**.

odds The probability of an outcome occurring relative to it not occurring. For example, if 10 people get a disease when exposed to a particular risk factor, and only 5 get the disease when not exposed to the factor, the odds of getting the disease are 10 to 5 or 2 to 1. Technically, this is the incidence odds. Also see **prevalence odds**.

odds ratio The ratio of two odds. In a case-control study, the odds ratio may be expressed as the odds of the exposure among the cases to the odds of the exposure among the controls (exposure odds) or as the odds of the outcome among the exposed to the odds of the outcome among the unexposed (disease odds).

one-group pretest-posttest design A type of quasi-experimental study design. Specifically, it is a type of before and after study without a separate control group. Also see **before and after studies**.

open cohort study A cohort study in which eligible subjects may enter the study at any given time. Subjects may also leave the cohort at any given time. Thus, not all subjects are necessarily observed for the same length of time.

opportunistic screening A type of screening that usually occurs in a physician's office when patients come in for unrelated problems, and the physician takes the opportunity to perform or order one or more screening tests. Opportunistic screening is also known as case finding.

ordinal A term referring to ordinal data, an ordinal variable, or an ordinal measurement scale. Ordinal represents ordered qualitative categories, such as those used to assess job satisfaction as low, moderate, or high. The intervals between the rankings are not necessary the same.

outcome The disease or other health-related occurrence that is being investigated in an epidemiologic study. An example is prostate cancer. Also see **exposure**.

outcome status A term for classifying subjects in an epidemiologic study by whether or not they have the disease or other health-related occurrence under investigation. Outcome status is often measured dichotomously as present or absent, but it may also be measured on several levels, such as severe, moderate, mild, or none. Also see **exposure status**.

overall accuracy An overall summary measure of the validity of a screening test. Overall accuracy is estimated by dividing the number of individuals who are classified correctly by the screening test (i.e., true positives plus true negatives) by the total number of individuals tested. It is usually expressed as a percent. Technically, overall accuracy is a weighted average of the screening test's sensitivity and specificity.

overall percent agreement A synonym for **percent agreement**.

overdiagnosis bias A type of bias that can occur when screening leads to the detection of subclinical forms of a disorder that would not have been diagnosed clinically during an individual's lifetime. These subclinical forms are referred to as pseudodisease, and their inclusion as cases can spuriously increase the apparent effectiveness of screening programs. Also see **pseudodisease**.

overmatching Inappropriate or unnecessary matching. Matching on a factor that is associated with the exposure but not with the outcome is an example of overmatching. Such a factor cannot be a confounder; hence, matching is inappropriate and may significantly reduce the statistical efficiency of the study.

overview A synonym for **meta-analysis**.

P

pair matching A form of individual matching in which subjects from the study and comparison groups are paired together on a one-to-one basis with regard to the variables for which matching is sought.

pandemic An epidemic on grand scale causing illness or death over an extensive area, generally crossing international borders and afflicting large numbers of people. A pandemic of plague, for example, occurred in Western Europe between 1347 and 1351.

panel study A type of hybrid study that combines features of the cross-sectional and prospective cohort designs. Panel studies can be viewed as a series of cross-sectional studies conducted on the same subjects (the panel) during successive time intervals.

parallel group design The most common type of randomized controlled trial in which the subjects are randomly assigned to one of two or more study groups, and no subjects receive more than one study regimen during the course of the experiment.

parallel treatment design A synonym for **parallel group design**.

passive immunity A type of immunity that occurs when one receives antibodies from another host. It can be conferred by injection of a serum, placental transfer, or breast-feeding. The immunity is immediate and occurs without the body producing its own antibodies. Also see **active immunity**.

passive surveillance Surveillance in which various health care providers (e.g., physicians and hospitals) and laboratories are required by law to report certain diseases or conditions using prescribed methods designed by the agency responsible for surveillance. Also see **public health surveillance; active surveillance**.

Pearson correlation coefficient A statistical measure of the magnitude of the linear relationship between two continuous variables. It ranges from -1 to +1, where -1 indicates a perfect inverse relationship, 0 indicates no relationship, and +1 indicates a perfect positive relationship.

Pearson's r See **Pearson correlation coefficient**.

per protocol analysis A method of analysis sometimes used in randomized controlled trials where subjects who did not adequately comply with the study protocol are excluded from the analysis. This method has a number of disadvantages, the chief of which is the loss of the benefits of randomization.

percent agreement In the context of screening, percent agreement is a method of assessing observer reliability. The number of agreements on subjects' outcome status is divided by the total number of subjects observed, and the result is expressed as a percent.

percent negative agreement In the context of screening, a more sensitive measure for assessing observer reliability than percent agreement. It is calculated by dividing the number of paired observations in which there is agreement that the result is negative by the number of paired observations in which at least one observer classifies the result as negative. The measure is expressed as a percent.

percent positive agreement In the context of screening, a more sensitive measure for assessing observer reliability than percent agreement. It is calculated by dividing the number of paired observations in which there is agreement that the result is positive by the number of paired observations in which at least one observer classifies the result as positive. The measure is expressed as a percent.

percent relative effect The percent change in a ratio measure of association or effect from a baseline value of one. For example, a risk ratio of 3.2 represents an increased risk of 220%, and a risk ratio of 0.7 represents a decreased risk of 30%.

percentage of agreement A synonym for percent agreement.

perinatal mortality rate The number of fetal deaths after 28 weeks or more of gestation plus the number of infant deaths within 7 days of birth during a specified time period in relation to the number of live births plus the number of fetal deaths after 28 weeks or more of gestation during the same time period.

period prevalence The proportion of a defined population that has had a given disorder at any time during a specified time interval regardless of whether or not the cases survived. Basically, period prevalence measures prevalence of an occurrence over a span of time.

person-time chi-square test A chi-square test that can be used to determine the statistical significance of a rate ratio or rate difference. It is known as the person-time chi-square because rate ratios and rate differences are based on incidence densities, which are calculated using person-time units.

person-time incidence rate A synonym for **incidence density**.

person-time units Units of measure that combine the number of persons at risk of a specified occurrence with their time at risk. An example is person-years. Person-time units are most often used in follow-up studies, such as cohort studies. They may be calculated by summing each individual's time at risk in a study population and serve as the denominators when determining incidence densities.

person-years The most common type of person-time units used in epidemiologic studies. One hundred person-years is equivalent to 100 persons each being at risk for one year or 50 persons each being at risk for two years or any other combination of persons and time whose ultimate product is 100. Hence, not all persons in a study need to be at risk for the same time period. For example, 25 persons at risk for two years and 50 persons at risk for one year would also total 100 person-years.

Peto method A common technique for producing a summary estimate of effect in a meta-analysis based on an equal effects (fixed effects) model.

pharmacoepidemiology A specialization in epidemiology that involves the application of epidemiologic methods to the study of drug effects and drug utilization patterns.

placebo In a narrow sense, an inert, pharmacologically inactive substance (a so-called "sugar pill") that is made to appear like the experimental treatment in a randomized controlled trial. In a broader sense, any inactive treatment or procedure with no known beneficial effects. This latter definition of placebo includes sham procedures. Placebos are sometimes used in the control arm of a randomized controlled trial. Also see **sham procedure**.

placebo effect The tendency for those receiving a treatment to experience beneficial effects even when the treatment has no known therapeutic value. In order for an experimental treatment to be considered efficacious in a placebo-controlled trial, its beneficial effects must exceed the placebo effect in the control group. Also see **placebo-controlled trial**.

placebo-controlled trial A randomized controlled trial in which the control group receives a placebo or sham procedure. Many drug trials, for example, are placebo-controlled trials.

plague An infectious disease, primarily of historical importance, that is caused by *Yersinia pestis*, a bacterium that is transmitted primarily by the bite of the infected rat flea. Plague has three clinical forms—bubonic, septicemic, and pneumonic.

point estimate An estimated population parameter calculated from a representative sample of a population, ideally a randomly selected sample. A common synonym is sample estimate.

point prevalence The proportion of a defined population that has a specific disease or attribute at a point in time. Point prevalence is calculated by dividing the number of existing occurrences at a given point in time by the total defined population at the same time and multiplying the result by an appropriate population base.

point source outbreak A type of common source outbreak where the duration of exposure to the common agent of disease is relatively brief and virtually simultaneous among those exposed. Point source outbreaks are relatively short-lived and normally conclude within a time frame equal to the range of the incubation period of the disease.

Poisson regression A multiple regression technique that may be used, for example, in open cohort studies to address confounding and interaction. This method is appropriate when the outcome is dichotomous and rare, the independent variables are categorical, person-time units are measured, and the sample size is large.

pooling One of two general approaches to aggregating data so as to produce a summary measure of association or effect (e.g., the Mantel-Haenszel odds ratio). The other method is standardization. Pooling is used with stratification, which controls confounding, and is based on the assumption that the stratum-specific measures of association or effect are uniform. It is also commonly used in meta-analysis as a method of statistically combining the findings of individual component studies into an overall estimate of the measure of effect. This measure is statistically more efficient than the individual findings because of the increased sample size. Also see **standardization**.

population at risk Those in a defined population who are susceptible to a given outcome at a given point in time. In closed cohorts, the population at risk consists of those who are at risk of the outcome at the beginning of the follow-up period. The population at risk is generally followed over time to determine the attack rate or cumulative incidence of the outcome.

population attributable fraction The proportion of the absolute risk of an outcome among an entire defined population that can be attributed to a given exposure. This measure assumes the exposure is causal.

population base A value of 100, 1,000, 10,000, 100,000, etc. that is routinely multiplied by a measure of occurrence, such as cumulative incidence, to avoid reporting a decimal fraction. For example, a cumulative incidence of 0.015 is expressed as 1.5 cases per 100 population using a population base of 100 (i.e., 0.015 x 100 = 1.5 per 100). This is also equivalent to 15 cases per 1,000 population if a population base of 1,000 is used instead.

population controls Subjects comprising the control group of a population-based case-control study. These subjects are usually selected randomly from the source population without the study disease. Also see **source population**.

population prevalence difference The excess prevalence of an occurrence in a defined population that is associated with a given exposure. It is calculated by subtracting the prevalence of the occurrence in the unexposed group from the prevalence of the occurrence in the population as a whole.

population rate difference The excess rate of an occurrence in a defined population that is associated with a given exposure. It is calculated by subtracting the rate of the occurrence in the unexposed group from the rate of the occurrence in the population as a whole.

population risk difference The excess risk of an occurrence in a defined population that is associated with a given exposure. It is calculated by subtracting the risk of the occurrence in the unexposed group from the risk of the occurrence in the population as a whole.

population-based case-control study A case-control study in which the cases and controls are selected from the total or a representative sample of a defined population.

population-based disease registry An ongoing system that collects and registers all cases of a particular disease or class of diseases as they develop in a defined population (e.g., a cancer registry). Not all disease registries, however, are population-based.

positive bias Bias that results in an overestimation of the magnitude of a measure of association or effect between an exposure and outcome.

positive confounder A confounding factor that leads to overestimation of the magnitude of a measure of association or effect between an exposure and outcome.

positive interaction Interaction where the observed combined effect of two or more variables is greater than the expected combined effect, all other factors being equal.

positive predictive value The probability that those who test positive on a screening test have the disorder in question. Positive predictive value is usually stated as a percent and is calculated by dividing the number of true positives by the number testing positive in the study population.

posttest odds The odds that someone has a given disorder following the administration of an appropriate screening (or diagnostic) test. Also see **pretest odds**.

posttest probability The probability that someone has a given disorder following the administration of an appropriate screening (or diagnostic) test. Also see **pretest probability**.

posttest-only design In the context of group randomized trials, a posttest-only design is a type of trial in which the study outcomes are measured in the intervention and control groups only at the conclusion of the trial.

potential confounder A suspected confounding factor, that is, one that may distort the effect of a study exposure on a study outcome. There are several criteria that must be met for a factor to be considered a confounder. In practice, one rarely knows if these criteria have all been met. Therefore, factors known to meet one or more of the criteria may be considered potential confounders. Also see **confounding**.

power In the context of statistics, power is the probability of detecting an association if one really exists. Because power is largely affected by sample size, studies with inadequate sample size have insufficient power to detect real associations.

practical significance A synonym for **clinical significance**.

precision (of a study) The degree to which nonsystematic (random) error is absent in a study. Precision is concerned with the consistency or stability of the study results. For example, results based on small studies tend to be more unstable, and hence less precise, than those based on large studies.

precision of a screening test The reliability of a screening test, that is, the degree to which it provides consistent results from one application to the next.

predictive value negative A synonym for **negative predictive value**.

predictive value of a negative test A synonym for **negative predictive value**.

predictive value of a positive test A synonym for **positive predictive value**.

predictive value positive A synonym for **positive predictive value**.

predisposing or enabling factors Factors that can increase susceptibility or facilitate a specific outcome. The term is used to refer to indirect causes. For example, advanced age is a predisposing factor for Alzheimer's disease. Also, easy access to alcohol is an enabling factor for alcoholism. Sometimes these indirect factors are referred to as risk factors.

pretest odds The odds that someone has a given disorder prior to the administration of an appropriate screening (or diagnostic) test. Also see **posttest odds**.

pretest probability The probability that someone has a given disorder prior to the administration of an appropriate screening (or diagnostic) test. Also see **posttest probability**.

pretest-posttest design In the context of group randomized trials, a pretest-posttest design is a type of trial in which the study outcomes are measured before and after the intervention.

prevalence Two definitions of prevalence are possible: (a) the number of people with a specific outcome or attribute in a defined population at a designated time, or (b) the proportion of a defined population who have a specific outcome or attribute at a designated time. The former definition represents a count, and the latter definition represents a proportion. Also see **point prevalence**; **period prevalence**; **lifetime prevalence**.

prevalence difference The difference between the prevalence in the exposed group and the prevalence in the unexposed group in an epidemiologic study. Also see **excess prevalence**.

prevalence effect In the context of screening tests, the prevalence effect exists when the proportion of agreement between observers on positive findings differs from the proportion of agreement on negative findings. The prevalence effect decreases the value of kappa and tends to be a consequence of either a low or high prevalence of the disorder in the study population. Also see **kappa**.

prevalence odds The ratio of the number of people who have a given occurrence to the number of people who do not have the occurrence in a given population at a point in time. Also see **incidence odds**.

prevalence odds ratio An odds ratio based on prevalent cases versus incident cases. Specifically, it is the ratio of the prevalence odds in the exposed group to the prevalence odds in the unexposed group.

prevalence proportion A synonym for **prevalence** (second definition).

prevalence ratio The ratio of the prevalence of an occurrence in the exposed group to the prevalence of the occurrence in the unexposed group. This measure of association is most commonly used in cross-sectional studies.

prevalence study A term sometimes used to refer to a cross-sectional study since prevalence is the usual measure of occurrence in cross-sectional studies.

prevalence survey A term sometimes used to refer to a cross-sectional study since prevalence is the usual measure of occurrence in cross-sectional studies.

prevalence-adjusted bias-adjusted kappa An adjusted kappa that takes into account both the prevalence effect and the bias effect in screening applications. Also see **prevalence effect; bias effect; kappa**.

prevalence-incidence bias A form of selection bias that can occur when asymptomatic, mild, clinically resolved, or fatal cases are inadvertently excluded from the case group in a study because the cases are examined sometime after the disease process has begun (i.e., looking at prevalent versus incident cases). This bias exists if the association would have been different had the missed cases been included in the sample. Prevalence-incidence bias is most often associated with case-control or cross-sectional studies.

prevention trial See **preventive trial**.

preventive trial A type of randomized controlled trial that focuses on individuals without clinical manifestations of the study outcome. The purpose of a preventive trial is to determine if a particular intervention reduces the clinical occurrence of the outcome. Also see **primary prevention trial; secondary prevention trial**.

primary prevention A level of prevention aimed at preventing new cases of disease or other conditions from developing by controlling their causes. It is applicable to persons in the stage of susceptibility. Examples include efforts to encourage immunizations for communicable diseases and health education about nutritious foods.

primary prevention trial A type of preventive trial that focuses on individuals in the stage of susceptibility. Primary prevention trials seek to test modes of preventing study outcomes before they develop. Unlike preventive trials that may focus on primary or secondary prevention, primary prevention trials focus only on primary prevention.

primary source A source of data collected firsthand by an investigator (i.e., an original data source). Also see **secondary source**.

probability sample A type of sample in which everyone in the sampled population has a known probability of being selected. An example is a randomly selected sample.

prognostic factor A factor that is predictive of a study outcome. The term is especially used in the context of randomized controlled trials.

propagated outbreak A progressive disease outbreak that is usually due to direct person-to-person transmission of the disease or by indirect transmission through a vector. Also see **common source outbreak**.

prophylactic trial A synonym for **preventive trial**.

proportion A ratio where the numerator is included in the denominator. Cumulative incidence, for example, is a proportion as is prevalence.

proportionate mortality ratio The ratio of the number of deaths due to a specific cause to the total number of deaths occurring in a population during a specified time period. The proportionate mortality ratio is a measure of how important a particular cause of death is in relation to all deaths in the population. Unlike the cause-specific mortality rate, it is not a measure of the risk of death.

prospective cohort study An observational epidemiologic study that classifies the study subjects without the study outcome according to exposure status in the present time and then follows them into the future to determine if the rate of development of the study outcome is different in the exposed and unexposed groups. Also see **cohort study**.

prospective meta-analysis A relatively new type of meta-analysis in which the component studies are selected based on criteria developed before the studies have been completed. This avoids certain biases that may be present when studies are selected retrospectively.

protocol See **study protocol**.

pseudodisease In the context of screening, pseudodisease is a subclinical form of disease detected by screening that would not have developed clinically before the individual dies of another unrelated cause. When pseudodisease is included in comparisons of screened and unscreened populations it tends to make the screened population appear to have a better survival rate than the unscreened population. This is due to two factors: (a) individuals with pseudodisease are only detected in the screened group, and (b) they have a better prognosis than those clinically detected in the unscreened group.

psychosocial epidemiology A specialization in epidemiology that can be conceived as a synthesis of social and behavioral epidemiology in that its focus is on the study of psychological, behavioral, and social determinants of health, disease, or death in human populations. Some use the term synonymously with social epidemiology, since social epidemiology is partly rooted in the social sciences, including psychology and sociology. Also see **social epidemiology**; **behavioral epidemiology**.

public health surveillance The ongoing systematic collection, analysis, and interpretation of health-related data essential to the planning, implementation, and evaluation of public health practice, closely integrated with the timely dissemination of these data to those responsible for prevention and control. Also see **active surveillance**; **passive surveillance**; **sentinel surveillance**; **syndromic surveillance**.

publication bias A form of bias that can develop in a meta-analysis when the search for relevant studies is restricted to those that have been published. In general, published studies tend to report positive findings more often than unpublished ones and tend to be different in other ways as well.

p-value The probability of obtaining a measure that is at least as extreme as that obtained in a study given that the null hypothesis is true. The lower the p-value, the less likely that chance alone accounts for an observed association. By convention, associations are usually considered statistically significant when the corresponding p-value is equal to or less than 0.05 and not significant when the p-value is greater than 0.05.

Q

qualitative interaction Statistical interaction where the effects of exposure on the outcome differ in direction across the strata in a stratified analysis. For example, with regard to risk ratios (RRs), some of the RRs are equal to or greater than one, and some of the RRs are less than one.

qualitative systematic review Systematic reviews that summarize studies without combining the results statistically.

quantitative interaction Statistical interaction where the effects of exposure on the outcome differ from stratum to stratum in a stratified analysis, but all are in the same direction. For example, with regard to risk ratios (RRs), all the RRs are greater than one, or all the RRs are less than one.

quantitative systematic review A synonym for a **meta-analysis**.

quasi-experiment A synonym for **quasi-experimental study**.

quasi-experimental study A study where the investigators do not have full control over the assignment or timing of the intervention but where the study is still conducted as if it were an experiment. In many instances, the defining factor is a lack of subject randomization into experimental and control groups.

R

r See **Pearson correlation coefficient**.

r squared Synonym for **coefficient of determination**.

random digit dialing A method of random selection using the telephone. In this method, telephone numbers are dialed randomly within given telephone exchanges for the selected area. It is a popular method of obtaining subjects for telephone surveys.

random effects model In the context of meta-analysis, there are two major approaches to integrating the findings of individual studies. One of these is based on a random effects model, which is a model based on the assumption that the underlying effect varies in each component study due to actual differences in effect as well as random error. Also see **equal effects model**.

random allocation See **randomization**.

random assignment See **randomization**.

random error Variability in a measure due to chance. Random error tends to dilute a measure of association or effect from its true value. Also see **nonsystematic error**.

random selection A method of sampling from a defined population where each person in the defined population has an equal chance of being chosen for the sample.

random variation See **random error**.

randomization The random distribution of study subjects into study groups (e.g., experimental and control groups in a randomized controlled trial). Randomization assures that the subjects have the same probability of being assigned to any of the study groups. Also known as random allocation or random assignment.

randomized community trial A term that may be used synonymously with group randomized trial or more specifically to indicate a group randomized trial where the units of analysis are entire communities.

randomized controlled trial A planned experimental epidemiologic study designed to test the efficacy or effectiveness of one or more interventions. It involves randomization of individuals into experimental and controls groups, application of the intervention(s), and follow up. Also see **clinical trial**; **group randomized trial**.

randomly selected See **random selection**.

rare disease assumption The assumption that the study outcome is "rare." This assumption may be required depending on the sampling method when one uses the odds ratio to estimate the risk or rate ratio. A cumulative incidence of less than 10 per 100 is a rule of thumb for what constitutes a "rare" outcome, although some suggest smaller frequencies.

rate A type of ratio where time is expressed or implied in the denominator. It is a measure of change per unit of time. For example, incidence density is a rate. The term rate is also sometimes used loosely in epidemiology to refer to measures that are technically ratios or proportions as in the crude mortality rate, which is traditionally expressed as a proportion.

rate adjustment A statistical procedure that adjusts for differences in the distribution of factors such as age and sex that may confound a comparison of crude morbidity or mortality rates. Rate adjustment provides a way to make fair, unbiased comparisons between population summary rates. Also known as rate standardization. Also see **age adjustment**.

rate difference The difference between rates of occurrence in the exposed and unexposed groups in an epidemiologic study. An example is incidence density difference. The rate difference is a measure of association or effect between an exposure and outcome.

rate ratio The ratio of rates of occurrence, specifically the rate of occurrence in the exposed group to that in the unexposed group in an epidemiologic study. Rate ratios are commonly reported in follow-up studies where person-time data have been collected. An example is the incidence density ratio. The rate ratio is a measure of association or effect between an exposure and outcome.

rate standardization A synonym for **rate adjustment**.

ratio The relationship of one quantity to another quantity where the quantities are not necessarily measured in the same units. An example is the odds ratio.

recall bias A type of information bias that can occur when recall about past exposure status is different between those who have the outcome and those who do not. It is particularly common in case-control studies. In general, cases tend to recall past exposures better than controls.

recruitment The subject enrollment process in a study, particularly in reference to experimental studies.

recruitment period The time during which recruitment takes place in a study.

reemerging infectious disease A once familiar infectious disease that was thought to be decreasing or disappearing in a population but is now on the rise. Also see **emerging infectious disease**.

referent The comparison or reference group in a study. For example, the unexposed group is the referent in a cohort study.

registry See **population-based disease registry**.

regression equation A mathematical expression that describes the relationship between a dependent and one or more independent variables. A regression equation allows investigators to predict the effect of the independent variable(s) on the dependent variable. A regression equation is sometimes referred to as a prediction equation or a regression model.

regression line The line that best describes the relationship between a dependent and an independent variable. A regression line can be obtained by performing a simple linear regression analysis. It represents the line that best fits the data in a scatter plot.

regression to the mean The tendency for an extreme value in a distribution of measurements to be closer to the mean value upon subsequent measurement. This phenomenon can bias the findings of a study, for example, a quasi-experiment using the nonequivalent control group design.

relative odds A synonym for the **odds ratio** usually in the context of a case-control study.

relative risk A general term that has been used to refer to risk ratios, rate ratios, odds ratios, and prevalence ratios. In a strict sense it is equivalent only to the risk ratio. Relative risk is a measure of association or effect between an exposure and outcome. Also see **risk ratio**.

relative survival rate The ratio of the survival rate for a group of patients with a given disease to the survival rate in a general population sample that has similar characteristics, such as age, sex, race, and calendar year of observation. It is, thus, the ratio of the observed rate to the expected rate. The relative survival rate is usually expressed as a percent.

reliability An indicator of the degree of consistency or stability of a measure from one use to the next. For example, a screening test that produces similar results under similar circumstances is considered reliable. One that produces inconsistent results is considered unreliable.

repeated cross-sectional design (for GRTs) A sampling design in group randomized trials involving follow up in which a new sample of individuals is selected from each group each time outcome measurements are to be made. This design is most appropriate when the objective is to measure the effects of the intervention on the study population as a whole. Also see **cohort design** (for GRTs).

repeated surveys A type of hybrid study where successive cross-sectional studies are performed over time on the same study population, but each sample is selected independently. Therefore, while the samples may be representative of the study population, the actual subjects may not be the same from one survey to the next.

response bias See **non-response bias**.

reportable disease A synonym for **notifiable disease**.

reporting bias A type of information bias that can occur when subjects intentionally or unintentionally underreport or overreport exposures or outcomes. This may be for a variety of reasons, including their social undesirability (e.g., illicit drug use) or desirability (e.g., handwashing).

research ethics committee A committee that reviews research protocols using ethical guidelines designed to protect the safety and well-being of the study participants.

Research ethics committee is a name more commonly applied to groups performing this function outside than within the United States. Also see **institutional review board**.

residual confounding Confounding that persists in a study even after attempts to control it. Three common reasons for residual confounding are failure to consider important confounders, flawed characterization of confounders, and misclassification of confounders.

restricted randomization A modified form of simple randomization designed to achieve certain objectives such as equally sized study groups. Examples are block or stratified randomization. Also see **simple randomization**.

restriction A procedure that limits the subjects in a study to only those with certain characteristics (e.g., Asian females). Restriction is commonly used in all types of epidemiologic studies to control for potential confounding. A study restricted to males, for example, cannot be confounded by differences in sex.

retrospective cohort study An observational epidemiologic study in which the study population (cohort) represents an historical group of individuals reconstructed using available data sources. The members of the historical cohort are classified according to exposure status at the time the cohort existed and then followed up to the present time to determine if the rate of development of the study outcome is different in the exposed and unexposed groups. Also see **cohort study**.

rho A common designation for the intraclass correlation coefficient.

risk The probability that a specified outcome will occur within a given time period. Average risk is commonly measured by cumulative incidence.

risk difference The arithmetic difference between the absolute risk in the exposed and unexposed groups in an epidemiologic study. A common type of risk difference is the cumulative incidence difference. The risk difference is a measure of association or effect between a given exposure and outcome. Also see **excess risk**.

risk factor A behavior, environmental exposure, or inherent human characteristic that increases the probability of the occurrence of a given outcome. It is considered a causal factor for the outcome. For example, a high blood pressure is a risk factor for heart disease.

risk indicator A synonym for **risk marker**.

risk marker A factor that is statistically associated with an increased risk of a given outcome but which is not considered a causal factor for that outcome. Risk markers are noncausal factors that are presumably associated with other causes of the outcome. An example is elevated C-reactive protein, which is a risk marker for coronary heart disease.

risk ratio A measure of association or effect that is calculated by taking the ratio of the risk of a given occurrence among those exposed to a suspected risk factor to those who are not exposed to the same factor. The most commonly reported risk ratio is the cumulative incidence ratio.

risk set The subjects in a study who are at risk of the study outcome at any given point in time.

rumination bias A type of information bias that can occur when those with a given disorder reflect more deeply on past exposures in an effort to identify possible causes of their condition than those without the disease. It can be considered a type of recall bias. Also see **recall bias**.

run-in period In the context of a randomized controlled trial, a run-in period is a pre-trial phase during which eligible subjects are given the control (or sometimes the experimental) regimen for a specified period of time. The primary objective is to increase the potential for compliance in the trial by screening out those subjects who are noncompliant during the run-in period.

S

sample estimate See **point estimate**.

sampling error A synonym for **sampling variation**.

sampling variation The random variation that can result when using sample statistics to estimate population parameters. Sampling variation is a result of using a sample instead of an entire population. No one sample is a perfect representation of the sampled population; therefore, sample statistics vary in their ability to estimate population parameters.

scatter diagram See **scatter plot**.

scatter plot The pattern of points that results when two quantitative variables are plotted on a graph. Each point formed by the intersection of the values of the two variables represents one unit in the analysis. The pattern of the points is indicative of the degree and direction of the relationship between the variables. For example, the more the points cluster along a straight line, the stronger the linear relationship. Also known as a scatter diagram.

screening A relatively quick means of identifying individuals who may have a given disease or condition that is not clinically apparent at the time. Screening does not establish a diagnosis but helps to differentiate those who are likely to have the disorder from those who are unlikely to have it. Those who are likely to have the disorder based on screening should undergo diagnostic testing.

screening level The cutoff point at which the result of a screening test is considered positive. Below the cutoff point the test is considered negative. For example, a blood glucose screening test for diabetes may set the cutoff point at 110 milligrams per deciliter. Those above the 110 mark screen positive for diabetes, and those below the 110 mark screen negative.

secondary prevention A level of prevention aimed at identifying existing cases of disease in an early stage, especially subclinical cases, so as to effect a cure or prevent any complications. It is most appropriately applied to those in the stage of presymptomatic disease or the early stage of clinical disease where treatment is more likely to be effective. Screening for disease is a common example.

secondary prevention trial A type of preventive trial that focuses on individuals in the stage of presymptomatic disease. Secondary prevention trials typically seek to test methods that might impede the development of the study outcome in high risk individuals.

secondary source A source of data that has not been collected firsthand by an investigator. It is a nonoriginal source of data that has been collected by someone else. It is thus secondhand data. Also see **primary source**.

secular trend A long-term change in the pattern of morbidity or mortality for a given disorder in a given population. For example, the mortality rate for septicemia in the U.S. showed a steady increase between 1951 and 1988.

selection bias Systematic error that results from the way in which the subjects are selected or retained in a study. This bias can occur, for example, when the characteristics of the subjects selected for a study differ systematically from those in the source population or when the study and comparison groups are selected from different populations. It can also result from excessive losses where the losses are systematically different from those retained in the study.

selective screening Screening applied only to select groups with a greater than average probability of having a preclinical form of the disease or condition of interest. Also known as targeted screening.

sensitivity A measure of the ability of a screening test to identify those with the disorder of interest. Sensitivity is measured as the percent of those with the disorder whose screening test is positive.

sensitivity analysis A way of ascertaining the robustness of an assessment by performing secondary analyses using different assumptions, methods, etc. For example, sensitivity analysis can be used to examine apparent heterogeneity among the component studies of a meta-analysis.

sentinel event A disease or condition that alerts public health authorities to a potential public health problem (e.g., a developing epidemic, a failure of preventive measures) and that may require some type of public health response when reported. Of the numerous diseases and other conditions that generally must be reported in passive surveillance systems only a small number are considered sentinel events. Also see **sentinel surveillance**.

sentinel surveillance Surveillance that prearranges for certain reporting sources to report all cases of specific predetermined diseases or conditions that may require a public health response (sentinel events). The reporting sources are usually a select sample of health care providers or employers that are likely to see the events and that have agreed to report them to the appropriate health authority. Also see **sentinel event; public health surveillance**.

sequential design A type of randomized controlled trial in which sample size is not fixed but varies depending on the results of repeated analyses of the accumulating data. Basically, before a new subject (or pair of subjects) is enrolled in a sequential trial, the data generated up to that point are analyzed to determine whether or not the study should continue. Inherent in a sequential design is consecutive enrollment of subjects during the recruitment period and repeated analyses of the data in order to reach a decision about the efficacy or safety of the intervention as soon as possible. Also see **group sequential design**.

sham procedure A bogus procedure sometimes used in the control arm of a randomized controlled trial. It is designed to appear like a real procedure but without any anticipated effects. Use of a sham procedure is analogous to the use of a placebo in a drug trial. Also see **placebo**.

short-term fluctuation A relatively brief, unexpected increase in the frequency of a particular disease in a specific population. Short-term fluctuations are commonly manifested in disease outbreaks or epidemics.

significance level A synonym for **alpha level**.

simple randomization Randomization, especially in reference to randomized controlled trials, without any modifications, such as stratification or blocking. This method works best at producing comparable groups when the study population is large. Also see **completely randomized design**.

simple survival rate A measure of the probability that cases of a given disease will survive for a specified period of time. Like case fatality, it is an indicator of the prognosis for those with the disease. An example is the five-year simple survival rate for breast cancer. Some refer to this as the survival rate.

Simpson's paradox A situation where a confounder alters an effect to such an extent that a true positive effect appears negative, or a true negative effect appears positive. In other words, in Simpson's paradox confounding changes the direction of the effect.

single-blinded study A study in which the subjects are kept unaware of their group assignment, although the investigators are still aware. While a single-blinded study can minimize bias introduced by the subjects, it has no effect on bias on the part of the investigators, specifically, those assessing outcome status. Also see **blinding**.

single-masked study See **single-blinded study**.

slippery-linkage bias A form of bias associated with screening. Slippery-linkage bias occurs when a positive screening test leads to subsequent diagnostic procedures or treatments that in turn lead to death, but the cause of death is not attributed to the screening, and hence, the target disorder. As a result, the effectiveness of screening is overstated. Also see **sticky-diagnosis bias**.

social epidemiology A specialization in epidemiology focusing on the study of social determinants of health, disease, or death in human populations. Social epidemiologists examine the roles of societal characteristics such as socioeconomic status, social inequality, poverty, gender, race/ethnicity, and other social and cultural factors on health-related outcomes.

sojourn time A synonym for **detectable preclinical phase**, especially as it relates to cancer.

source population In general, the population from which those eligible for a study are chosen. In the context of a case-control study, the source population is the population that generated the cases for the study. The controls should also be selected from the source population independent of exposure status. Also see **study base**.

space-time cluster A combination of spatial and temporal disease clusters where an increased incidence of a given disease occurs in a localized area during a given time period. Also see **disease cluster; spatial cluster; temporal cluster**.

spatial cluster A disease cluster where a localized area within a larger area shows an increased incidence of a given disease. Also see **disease cluster**.

special exposure cohort A type of cohort used in cohort studies. A special exposure cohort represents only the exposed group. Typically, it is used when the exposure is uncommon or unique. Special exposure cohorts may include certain occupational groups, persons undergoing certain medical treatments, those with specific environmental exposures, or members of organizations with unusual dietary habits or lifestyles. Also see **general cohort**.

specific rate A "rate" for a distinct subgroup within a defined population. The most commonly reported specific rates are those based on age, sex, or race/ethnicity (i.e., age-specific rates, sex-specific rates, and race/ethnicity-specific rates). The term rate is used loosely here and may actually represent a proportion, for example. Also see **rate**.

specificity A measure of the ability of a screening test to identify those without the disorder of interest. Specificity is measured as the percent of those without the disorder whose screening test is negative.

split screen design An approach that is sometimes used to evaluate the effectiveness of a screening program. Instead of not offering the control group screening for the disorder of interest, it is offered the usual care up until the nth screen of the experimental group at which time both the experimental and groups are screened.

spot map A map showing the geographical location of each case of a disease or other attribute, usually by place of occurrence or residence. A spot map is frequently used in disease outbreak investigations to discover where cases aggregate, thus suggesting possible causes of the outbreak.

spurious association A false association found in a study and generally caused by random error or bias.

stable population A population where there is little migration into or out of the population.

stage of clinical disease A stage in the natural history of disease. In this stage signs or symptoms of the disease are apparent. This is the stage where the disease is commonly diagnosed and treated.

stage of diminished capacity A stage in the natural history of disease. This stage is characterized by a convalescent period or a residual disability. In the former case, there is a period following completion of clinical disease during which the individual has not yet returned to his or her former level of well-being. In the latter case, the disease has produced definite complications that compromise a person's health status. The disability may be temporary or permanent.

stage of presymptomatic disease A stage in the natural history of disease. In this stage, the disease process has begun, but no overt signs or symptoms of the disease are yet evident. The individual is in the induction or latency periods for the disease.

stage of susceptibility A stage in the natural history of disease. In this stage, the disease has not yet developed, but the host is susceptible to the disease because of the presence of risk factors, such as high cholesterol for heart disease.

stages of cancer A way of classifying a cancer by the extent of its progression. Stage one cancers are localized and have not yet metastasized to other parts of the body. Stage two cancers have infiltrated underlying tissues more than stage one cancers but have still not metastasized to other parts of the body. Stage three cancers have metastasized to surrounding tissues, and stage four cancers have spread extensively throughout the body. More detailed staging may also be described.

standard error The standard deviation of the sampling distribution of a statistic. It is a measure of sampling error.

standard population A population used for comparison purposes in rate adjustment. It is a stable population whose distribution with regard to the factors being controlled (e.g., age, sex, race/ethnicity) is known. The standard population may be an actual or a derived population. An example is the 2000 U.S. standard million population.

standardization A method used in stratification to produce a summary measure of association or effect that is adjusted for confounding by one or more factors. Unlike pooling, standardization does not require that the stratum-specific measures of association be constant across the strata. Also see **pooling**; **rate adjustment**; **age adjustment**.

standardized incidence ratio A type of standardized morbidity ratio where the cases are incident cases. It is sometimes used as a standardized measure of association in open cohort studies.

standardized morbidity ratio When used in reference to indirect rate adjustment, it is the ratio of the number of observed cases in the study population to the number of expected cases based on the specific rates in the reference population.

standardized mortality ratio When used in reference to indirect rate adjustment, it is the ratio of the number of observed deaths in the study population to the number of expected deaths based on the specific rates in the reference population.

standardized odds ratio A standardized measure of association or effect sometimes employed in closed cohort studies where the fundamental measure of occurrence is odds.

standardized rate A synonym for **adjusted rate**.

standardized rate ratio A standardized measure of association or effect sometimes employed in open cohort studies where the fundamental measure of occurrence is incidence density.

standardized risk difference A standardized measure of association or effect sometimes employed in closed cohort studies where the fundamental measure of occurrence is cumulative incidence expressed as a difference.

standardized risk ratio A standardized measure of association or effect sometimes employed in closed cohort studies where the fundamental measure of occurrence is cumulative incidence expressed as a ratio.

statistical association A statistical relationship between two or more variables. In epidemiologic studies, a statistical association is one where the presence of the study exposure is related to a change in the probability of the study outcome. A statistical association is not necessarily causal, however. Also see **causal association**.

statistical efficiency A measure of the relative degree of precision in an analysis; that is, a measure of the extent to which random error is reduced. A statistically efficient analysis will have greater power, which is the ability to detect an association if it exists, for the same sample size than a statistically inefficient analysis.

statistical heterogeneity Differences in the effect estimates among the component studies of a meta-analysis.

statistical interaction A synonym for **interaction**.

statistical power See **power**.

statistical significance See **statistically significant**.

statistical test A synonym for **test statistic**.

statistically significant An indication that chance alone is an unlikely explanation for an observed association between two variables. An association is usually considered statistically significant when the associated p-value is less than or equal to the preset alpha value, which is usually 0.05.

steady-state conditions Conditions where a population is stable, and the incidence and prevalence under consideration are unchanging.

sticky-diagnosis bias A form of bias associated with screening. Sticky-diagnosis bias occurs when deaths in the screened group are more likely to be attributed to the target disorder than not due to the fact that the target disorder is more likely to be diagnosed in the screened versus the control group. As a result, the effectiveness of screening is understated. Also see **slippery-linkage bias**.

stopping rules Rules for deciding when to terminate an experimental trial. Stopping rules should be determined in advance of a trial and should be based on sound criteria.

stratification A procedure used in the analysis phase of an epidemiologic study to control for confounding or to detect effect measure modification. Stratification involves separating a sample into two or more subgroups according to specified levels of a third variable. For example, the results of a study of the effects of cigarette smoking on the development of cerebrovascular disease might be stratified by blood pressure levels to control for potential confounding by blood pressure or to examine whether or not different blood pressure levels modify the effect of cigarette smoking on cerebrovascular disease.

stratified randomization A modification of simple randomization sometimes used in randomized controlled trials when the sample size is relatively small. This technique increases the probability that the experimental and control groups will be similar with regard to the stratified factor(s). Stratified randomization involves three basic steps: (a) separation of the sample into appropriate strata, (b) random allocation of subjects in each stratum into experimental and control groups, and (c) compilation of the stratum-specific experimental and control groups into final experimental and control groups.

stratum-specific odds ratio An odds ratio that is specific to a stratification subgroup and thus is free of the confounding effect of the variable used in the stratification. For example, with stratification by sex the odds ratio for males is free of confounding by sex as is the odds ratio for females. There are also other stratum-specific measures of association (e.g., the stratum-specific risk ratio).

strength of the association One of several guidelines for evaluating whether an association is likely to be causal or not based on Hill's postulates. This one refers to the fact that, in general, the stronger an association is between an exposure and outcome, the more likely it is a causal association.

study base In the context of a case-control study, study base is often used interchangeably with source population. Technically, it represents the group of persons or person-time experience in which the study outcomes develop. Study base is also used in reference to other types of epidemiologic studies. For example, the study base for a cohort study is often defined as the members of the underlying cohort during the times they are eligible to become cases. This definition accommodates both closed and open cohorts. Also see **source population**.

study efficiency See **statistical efficiency**.

study population The sample selected for an epidemiologic study. It may consist of the entire source population (e.g., a cohort study) or only a part. In a randomized controlled trial, for example, the study population consists of volunteers from the source population who have met the eligibility criteria for participation in the study and have agreed to participate. Also see **source population**.

study protocol The written plan and procedures to be followed in a study. A study protocol should be comprehensive and include a description of the study rationale, design, and analysis as well as other features of the study. While important for all types of epidemiologic studies, the term is most often used in reference to experimental trials.

subclinical disease A disease that is fully developed but produces no overt signs or symptoms in the host. Subclinical disease is also called asymptomatic disease and may be communicable or noncommunicable.

subgroup analyses Analyses that are performed on subcategories of a study population, such as subgroups based on age differences. The purpose of subgroup analyses is to detect effect measure modification. Subgroup analyses in randomized controlled trials and meta-analyses can produce misleading findings for a number of reasons, especially when they are not planned prior to the study.

subject variability A threat to the reliability of a screening test. Specifically, subject variability may occur due to physiological or other changes in the subjects being screened. These changes can lead to inconsistent results when the screening tests are repeated on the same individuals.

sufficient cause A cause that is able to produce a particular outcome by itself. Sufficient causes are rare. Most disorders have a multifactorial etiology.

surveillance See **public health surveillance**.

survival analysis A set of statistical techniques used to characterize survival time in one or more groups. Survival analysis is most often used in follow-up studies and is especially useful when the follow-up periods for subjects vary widely or when the subjects enter the study at different times. The results of survival analysis can be used to make inferences about how various exposures, treatments, or other factors affect survival time. Also see **survival time; survival curve; life table method; Kaplan-Meier product limit method**.

survival curve A graphic presentation of the proportion of subjects in a defined group surviving to successive points in time. Survival curves are generated in survival analysis. Survival may be measured as time to death or as time to some other specified outcome, such as a particular disease or complications of a disease. Also see **survival analysis; survival time**.

survival time The time to occurrence of a specific outcome (e.g., death, disease) from a defined starting point. Survival time is measured in survival analysis. Also see **survival analysis**.

survival rate See **simple survival rate**.

syndromic surveillance A type of surveillance that seeks to detect disease outbreaks earlier and more completely than may be possible with traditional public health methods. To do so, syndromic surveillance relies on continuous monitoring of key indicators of potential outbreaks such as trends in specific symptoms, sales of certain medications, and job or school absenteeism. The focus is on real time data, and systems based on syndromic surveillance collect the data before any disease is diagnosed. This surveillance method has been used in an effort to counter the potential effects of bioterrorism as well as more traditional disease outbreaks. Also see **public health surveillance**.

synergism Based on a causal model, synergism occurs when two or more factors acting together in a population result in a greater frequency of outcomes than would be expected if the factors operated independently. In other words, the combined effects of the factors are greater than the sum of the individual effects. Cigarette smoking and occupational exposure to asbestos, for example, act in a synergistic manner.

systematic error A nonrandom flaw in study design, conduct, analysis, or interpretation that tends to uniformly increase or decrease the true magnitude of the measure of association or effect between an exposure and outcome. Bias and confounding are the two primary reasons for systematic errors.

systematic review A comprehensive, rigorous, and standardized approach to selecting, assessing, and synthesizing all relevant studies on a given topic. Systematic reviews are designed specifically to minimize subjectivity and hence improve the accuracy of the inferences. Also see **qualitative systematic review; quantitative systematic review**.

T

targeted screening A synonym for **selective screening**.

temporal cluster A disease cluster where disease incidence is higher at certain times than at other times. Also see **disease cluster**.

temporal patterns of disease A change in disease frequency over time. Temporal patterns include short-term fluctuations, cyclic patterns, and secular trends. Temporal patterns relate to specific disorders. For example, influenza shows a cyclic pattern in the midwest that is seasonal in nature.

ten percent rule See **10 percent rule.**

10 percent rule A rule of thumb for ratio measures of association or effect stating that a difference of more than 10 percent between the adjusted and crude measures is indicative of confounding.

tertiary prevention A level of prevention that attempts to limit disability and improve functioning where clinical disease or its complications are already well established. It is most applicable in the late stage of clinical disease or the stage of diminished capacity in the natural history of disease. An example is rehabilitation after a stroke.

test of heterogeneity A statistical test sometimes used in the process of stratification to assess whether effect measure modification is likely to be present. Tests of heterogeneity are also sometimes used in a meta-analysis to determine which model is most appropriate for pooling the findings of the component studies.

test of homogeneity A synonym for **test of heterogeneity.**

test of statistical significance See **test statistic.**

test statistic A statistic used to test a null hypothesis. Its value is compared to a set of critical values to determine if an observed association is statistically significant or not based on a preset alpha level. An example of a test statistic is the chi-square test for independence. Also known as a test of statistical significance or statistical test.

therapeutic trial A type of randomized controlled trial that focuses on patients in order to test an intervention that could cure the condition, prevent recurrences, or improve quality of life. Therapeutic trials are commonly used in testing the efficacy of new drugs and medical or surgical procedures.

threshold A level of exposure (dose) that must be reached before any effects become apparent. Below the threshold level there are no observed effects.

time-cohort cluster A disease cluster where an increased incidence of a given disease occurs in a group of people who share a common characteristic in addition to place of residence. Also see **disease cluster.**

time-series studies A category of quasi-experimental studies involving a succession of periodic measurements where an intervention is introduced at some point during the process. Two common variations are the interrupted time-series design and the multiple time-series design. Also see **interrupted time series design; multiple time-series design.**

time-to-event analysis A synonym for **survival analysis.**

time-trend study An ecological study where the ecological units are time periods. Time-trend studies are designed to determine if changes in study exposures are correlated with changes in study outcomes in a single population over time.

triple-blinded study A study in which the subjects, those assessing outcomes, and those analyzing the data are unaware of the subjects' group assignments. Also see **blinding.**

triple-masked study See **triple-blinded study.**

true negative In the context of screening, a true negative refers to an individual who tests negative on a screening test and does not have the disorder for which screening was performed.

true negative rate A synonym for **specificity.**

true positive In the context of screening, a true positive refers to an individual who tests positive on a screening test and has the disorder for which screening was performed.

true positive rate A synonym for **sensitivity.**

2000 U.S. standard million population The 2000 U.S. standard population where the proportions in each age group are applied to an arbitrary population of one million. It is a type of derived standard population. Also see **2000 U.S. standard population.**

2000 U.S. standard population A commonly used standard population in age adjustment. It represents the proportion of the U.S. population in each of 11 age groups based on the projected year 2000 population of the United States. Also see **standard population.**

type I error In statistical hypothesis testing, a type I error is the error that results from rejecting the null hypothesis when it is actually true. The probability of this type of error is measured by the p-value.

type II error In statistical hypothesis testing, a type II error is the error that results from failing to reject the null hypothesis when it is actually false. The probability of this type of error is measured by the beta level.

U

underlying cause of death On a death certificate, the underlying cause of death is the cause that initiated the chain of events that ultimately produced death. It is the official cause of death used in mortality statistics for the United States.

unit of analysis The object of study or what is being studied. The unit of analysis is usually the individual, but it can also be a group of people defined by a geographical area or a time period. For example, the unit of analysis in a cohort study is the individual, and the unit of analysis in an ecological study is the group, commonly known as the ecological unit.

unmatched case-control study A case-control study design in which individual matching is not used. Specifically, individual cases are not matched to individual controls on the basis of potential confounders. Frequency matching, however, may be used in unmatched case-control studies. Also see **frequency matching**.

upper confidence limit The maximum value represented by a confidence interval. For example, in the following confidence interval, 4.0 is the upper confidence limit: 95% CI = 2.0 to 4.0. Also see **confidence limits**; **lower confidence limit**.

V

validity (of a study) The degree to which systematic error is absent in a study. There are two major types of validity—internal validity and external validity. Also see **internal validity**; **external validity**.

validity of a screening test The degree to which a screening test does what it is designed to do (i.e., detect those who have a given preclinical disease or condition and those who do not).

variance inflation factor A synonym for **design effect**.

vector An animate source, such as a fly, mosquito, or rodent, that is capable of transmitting an agent of disease to a susceptible host. The vector serves as an intermediary in disease transmission, and the mechanism of transmission is considered indirect. A vector may be infected with the disease organism or may be a mechanical carrier of the organism. Some limit the term vector to nonvertebrate species only, although it is common practice to apply it to small vertebrate animals as well (e.g., rats, skunks, bats).

vehicle An inanimate substance or object, such as food, water, bedding, or surgical equipment, that is capable of transmitting an agent of disease to a susceptible host. The vehicle serves as an intermediary in disease transmission, and the mechanism of transmission is considered indirect. A vehicle may or may not support growth of the agent.

vital event A registered life event such as a birth, death, marriage, divorce, or certain disease. In the U.S. vital events must be reported by law.

vital record A completed registration form or certificate of a vital event, such as a birth, death, marriage, or divorce certificate. Also see **vital event**.

vital statistics Information derived from registered life events, such as births, deaths, marriages, divorces, and certain diseases.

vital statistics registration system A system for the collection of vital records. In the U.S. vital records are filed with a local vital statistics registrar, forwarded to the state registrar for vital statistics, and then to the Centers for Disease Control and Prevention.

volunteer bias A form of selection bias that can occur because those who volunteer for programs and studies tend to be systematically different from those who do not. Volunteer bias is a form of non-response bias.

W, X

washout period A stage in a crossover design of a randomized controlled trial during which the effects of a previously applied intervention are believed to wear off. In the most basic crossover design, the assignment of the experimental group to the control group and vice versa begins after the washout period has ended. Also see **crossover design**.

weighted kappa A variation of the kappa statistic that can be used with ordinal test results. Weighted kappa provides some credit for agreements that are close but not perfect when measuring interobserver or intraobserver reliability. Also see **kappa**.

Y

years of potential life lost (YPLL) A measure of the impact of premature death on a population. It is calculated by adding together the total years of potential life lost before a specified age (e.g., 65 years). It thus gives more weight to deaths that occur at younger ages in a population. Years of potential life lost can be useful in establishing public health priorities.

yield In the context of screening programs, yield is the number of new cases diagnosed and treated as a result of screening.

YPLL rate For a given population and time period, the YPLL rate is the number of years of potential life lost prior a specified age in relation to all those in the population below the specified age.

Z

zero-time shift A synonym for **lead-time bias**.

z-score A transformed score based on a standardized normal distribution with a mean of zero and a standard deviation of one. For example, a z-score of 2.0 is two standard deviations above the mean, and a z-score of -2.0 is two standard deviations below the mean.

Index

A

Absolute comparisons
  relative comparisons vs., 150, 158,
    162–163, 174
  types of, 158–170
Absolute risk, definition of, 152, 169,
  170, 569
Accuracy of epidemiologic studies. *See*
  also Validity; Precision
  definition of, 196, 226, 458, 569
  major components of, 196–197, 226
  threats to, 198, 226
Accuracy of screening tests, definition
  of, 450. *See also* Overall accuracy
Acquired immune deficiency syndrome
  (AIDS), 2, 18, 24, 36, 107, 186,
  264, 559
Active immunity
  definition of, 46, 52, 569
  passive immunity vs., 47
Active surveillance, 537–538, 547, 569
Active treatment, 385, 388, 399, 569
Actuarial life tables, 90, 95, 126. *See also*
  Life tables
Actuarial method, 92, 569. *See also* Life
  table method; Survival analysis
Additive effects, 295, 354, 359, 569
Additive interaction, 296–297, 569
Additive model, 292, 295–296, 298, 309,
  354, 358, 569
Additivity, 298, 299
Adherence. *See* Compliance
Adjusted odds ratio, definition of, 286,
  569
Adjusted rates
  advantages and disadvantages of,
    135, 136
  calculation of, 141
  definition of, 134, 173, 569
  indirectly standardized rate and, 144

interpretation of, 134–135, 139,
  141–142, 143, 148–149
Adjustment, rate
  comparing methods of, 136–137,
    143, 145, 148–150, 173–174
  definition of, 134–135, 214, 570, 602
  direct method of, 136–142, 143,
    148–150, 173, 579
  indirect method of, 136–137, 142–150,
    173–174, 586
  interpreting findings from, sum-
    mary, 143
  reason for, 135, 148–150
Admission rate bias, 202, 226, 569
Age-adjusted rates. *See* Adjusted rates
Age adjustment. *See* Adjustment, rate
Age distribution, definition of, 133
Age-specific rates. *See* Specific rates
Age standardization, 135, 570. *See also*
  Adjustment, rate
Agent(s)
  infectious, definition of, 36, 37
  types of, 38
Agresti, Alan, 123
AIDS. *See* Acquired immune deficiency
  syndrome (AIDS)
Alpha level
  definition of, 172, 570
  selection of, 174, 224, 227
Alternative hypothesis, definition of,
  171, 570
Altman, Douglas, 405
Ambidirectional cohort studies, 317,
  570. *See also* Mixed cohort studies
Ambispective cohort studies, 317, 570.
  See also Mixed cohort studies
American Cancer Society (ACS), 485
American Heart Association, 487
American Medical Association, 321
American Nurses' Association, 321

615